NCC 国家癌症中心 编
NATIONAL CANCER CENTER

2022
中国肿瘤登记年报

CHINA CANCER REGISTRY ANNUAL REPORT

主 编 赫 捷 魏文强

人民卫生出版社
·北京·

图书在版编目（CIP）数据

2022 中国肿瘤登记年报：汉英对照/国家癌症中心
编. -- 北京：人民卫生出版社，2025.2
ISBN 978-7-117-36276-4

Ⅰ.①2⋯　Ⅱ.①国⋯　Ⅲ.①肿瘤-卫生统计-中国
-2022-年报-汉、英　Ⅳ.①R73-54

中国国家版本馆 CIP 数据核字（2024）第 089359 号

| 人卫智网 | www.ipmph.com | 医学教育、学术、考试、健康，购书智慧智能综合服务平台 |
| 人卫官网 | www.pmph.com | 人卫官方资讯发布平台 |

2022 中国肿瘤登记年报

2022 Zhongguo Zhongliu Dengji Nianbao

编　　写：国家癌症中心
出版发行：人民卫生出版社（中继线 010-59780011）
地　　址：北京市朝阳区潘家园南里 19 号
邮　　编：100021
E - mail：pmph@ pmph.com
购书热线：010-59787592　010-59787584　010-65264830
印　　刷：天津市光明印务有限公司
经　　销：新华书店
开　　本：889×1194　1/16　印张：23
字　　数：665 千字
版　　次：2025 年 2 月第 1 版
印　　次：2025 年 4 月第 1 次印刷
标准书号：ISBN 978-7-117-36276-4
定　　价：188.00 元

打击盗版举报电话：010-59787491　E-mail：WQ @ pmph.com
质量问题联系电话：010-59787234　E-mail：zhiliang @ pmph.com
数字融合服务电话：4001118166　　E-mail：zengzhi @ pmph.com

编 委 会

李宗芬　李诗钰　李建彬　李春艳　李垚俊　李秋月　李秋林　李顺翠　李俊杰　李彦青　李美娜
李美萍　李洁玲　李娅凌　李艳辉　李桂芬　李晓琴　李晓燕　李爱会　李粉妮　李海燕　李悦凤
李彬明　李雪芳　李雪琴　李琼燕　李琰琰　李辉章　李晶晶　李智鹏　李道娟　李慧超　杨　艺
杨　帆　杨　竹　杨　军　杨　玲　杨　俊　杨　亮　杨　涛　杨　娟　杨　爽
杨　琴(重庆市万盛经济技术开发区)　　杨　琴(遵义市汇川区)　　杨　琳　杨　媚
杨　慧(天水市麦积区)　　杨　慧(梅州市梅县区)　　杨小琴　杨永翠　杨宇晨　杨志杰　杨丽萍
杨秀亮　杨体吾　杨茂敏　杨尚波　杨国旗　杨明霞　杨佳娟　杨显路　杨俊杰　杨艳蕾　杨晓静
杨通平　杨雪纷　杨福娣　杨慧君　杨燕琼　杨璐竹　肖　绮　肖　翔　肖艳玲　肖亚洲　肖拥军
肖幸平　吴　丹　吴　刚　吴　会　吴　欢　吴　畅　吴　洁　吴　娅　吴　莹　吴　爽　吴玉福
吴志敏　吴泽宁　吴春晓　吴春陶　吴春燕　吴美秀　吴艳伟　吴晓云　吴晓娟　吴海燕　吴容容
吴逸平　吴锦月　吴新会　邱红　邱林　邱琳　邱玉琼　何飞　何礼　何丽　何柳
何　磊(广元市朝天区)　　何　磊(牟定县)　　何士林　何玉龙　何成丹　何丽明　何秀玲　何保华
何道逢　何新桂　余　敏　余　斌　余小芳　余汉春　余家华　谷朝华　狄　苗　邹　红　邹晓琳
邹跃威　冷江涛　辛　玲　汪有库　汪尚勇　沈　婧　沈飞琼　沈成凤　沈羽翎　沈嘉航　宋冰冰
宋国慧　初玉娜　张　文　张　弘　张　旭　张　军　张　邻　张　青　张　英　张　林　张　明
张　宙　张　荣　张　标　张　思　张　莉　张　莹　张　桃　张　涛　张　敏　张　彩　张　雁
张　婷　张　翼　张乙中　张丁丁　张小玲　张小鹏　张艺杰　张少强　张玉蓉　张世勇　张平稳
张冬梅　张永贞　张永丽　张吉志　张亚莹　张先慧　张乔珍　张红霞　张克燕　张园园　张秀芬
张武武　张坤平　张学强　张建安　张建鲁　张春玉　张思维　张美莲　张艳艳　张振财　张晓芳
张晓林　张晓娜　张晓峰　张晓慧　张倩钰　张徐巾　张海峰　张菲菲　张彩霞　张淑萍　张晶晶
张瑞欣　张韶凯　张慧玲　张赣湘　陆　佩　陆　艳　陆　润　陆小峰　陆玉培　陆素颖　陆家龙
陈　节　陈　冲　陈　英　陈　茹　陈　娜(威远县)　　陈　娜(潼关县)　　陈　娟　陈　萍　陈　琼
陈　霞　陈上清　陈小芳　陈小娜　陈小慧　陈文俊　陈兰芬　陈永刚　陈永群　陈冰霞　陈志虹
陈志艳　陈丽黎　陈妙嫦　陈玥华　陈国荣　陈依琳　陈金武　陈建顺　陈珍莲　陈思红　陈娇娇
陈艳萍　陈晓春　陈海荣　陈海涛　陈雪莲　陈雪筠　陈雯雯　陈紫云　陈紫娟　邵　颖　武　霞
武华倩　拉毛才让　苗佳丽　苟军平　范　颖　范炜钢　范美霞　范莉莉　林　利　林玉成　林海霞
林超兰　欧志秀　欧国琴　欧阳乐　卓　玛　尚明凤　明晓雪　帖映伟　罗　玲　罗　源　罗文云
罗世华　罗丽琼　罗国良　罗春亮　罗艳丽　罗莉菲　和臣慧　和丽娜　和桂芬　季加孚　季佳慧
岳　婷　金红艳　金琦曼　周　丽　周　衍　周　倩　周　浩　周　娟　周　婕　周　琦　周　锐
周小华　周小佳　周川楠　周文武　周永刚　周丽萍　周青霞　周金意　周建容　周建湘　周春林
周艳梅　周素霞　周晓凤　周晓梅　周婷婷　周新玉　周静静　净　昭　郑　玲　郑云枝　郑冬柏
郑永萍　郑欢欢　郑荣寿　郑裕明　单保恩　郎红霞　屈秋琼　孟瑞琳　项莉红　项霞霞　赵　丽
赵　青　赵　莹　赵占峰　赵生明　赵廷明　赵仲刚　赵会联　赵劲良　赵金鸽　赵建华　赵秋萍
赵海荣　赵海洲　赵梦琳　赵朝强　赵雅芳　赵媛丽　赵德坚　郝庆华　郝青青　胡　东　胡　莹
胡　萍　胡　彪　胡艳红　胡素华　胡倩华　南　艳　柯金练　钞利娜　钟　鑫　钟玉美　钟伟文
钟彦丰　钟鲜鲜　段世彬　段乐永　段陈丽　保红莉　侯　亮　俞　亮　俞　敏　施云丽　施长苗
姜　帆　姜　欣　姜金宏　娄培安　洪　波　宫旭志　祝章美　胥璟宸　姚　琳　姚　媛　姚　霜
姚永红　姚信飞　贺　明　贺宇彤　贺军宏　贺绍琼　骆文书　骆秀美　秦　舒　秦大武　秦天燕
秦延锦　秦克波　班琼珍　袁　叶　袁　丽　袁　英　袁　菁　袁晓宇　袁继卫　袁彩红　袁聪玲
耿振强　聂　炜　莫文康　莫淦华　贾文虎　贾丽敏　贾艳芳　贾源瑶　夏　冰　夏　红　夏云磊
夏丽莉　顾　凯　顾晓平　党丽琴　晏　荧　恩荣琳　钱　赟　俸世元　倪　嘉　倪志华　徐　仙
徐　伟　徐　红　徐　芳　徐　珏　徐　玲(沈丘县)　　徐　玲(重庆市璧山区)　　徐　梅　徐　薇
徐玉銮　徐伟晓　徐红斌　徐绍和　徐胜平　徐海霞　徐媛锋　徐新红　徐蔚静　殷　行　殷建湘
凌海杰　高　明　高为民　高生丽　高扬波　高盼盼　高铁柱　高鸿敏　高瑞芳　郭　正　郭　伟
郭　梅　郭　敏(乐安县)　　郭　敏(秀山土家族苗族自治县)　　郭　超　郭天骅　郭凤兰　郭巧红
郭树岚　郭贵周　郭秋献　郭晓雷　郭颖贞　席云峰　唐明月　浦继尹　谈洪芬　陶小红　黄　静
黄一峰　黄小容　黄飞平　黄永杰　黄远田　黄佳玲　黄学敏　黄春广　黄春凤　黄炯媚　黄恢淑

黄海浪　黄锦航　曹　珊　曹　凌　曹良清　曹诗鹏　曹秋菊　曹海洋　曹景军　戚佩玲　龚新洪
龚巍巍　盛根英　常　安　常　蓉　崔玲波　崔海华　符　咏　符地宝　符芳敏　符美艳　庹吉妤
康文慧　康玉霞　章有健　竟广群　淳志明　梁　蒙　梁英凤　梁忠义　梁佳佳　梁树军　梁晓婷
梁赛文　梁翠敏　彭　娜　彭　晔　彭长燕　彭书灵　彭红伟　彭粉茹　董立新　董永年　董亚平
董志鹏　董建梅　敬　琳　蒋　微　蒋东原　蒋素红　蒋蔚林　蒋曙初　韩　霞　韩小玉　韩仁强
韩冰峰　韩贵卫　韩晓康　韩瑞贞　韩嘉仪　覃向清　覃明江　覃荣盼　覃凌峰　覃燕红　智　鑫
程　锋　程　谧　程向东　程志芳　税智群　焦艳莉　鲁婷婷　曾　平　曾　纪　曾红梅　曾映竹
游大勇　游宁静　谢　平　谢威龙　谢美兰　谢海斌　谢淑雯　谢锦荣　婷　婷　靳万春　靳双红
蒙　怡　楚玉梅　雷　林　雷芸华　雷宝琼　鲍月月　鲍克彪　赫　捷　蔡　伟　蔡　林　裴振义
管小琴　管元平　管丽娟　廖　羽　廖　顺　廖　倩　廖　涛　廖冬娟　廖卓航　廖柳艳　廖晓澄
廖凌玲　谭　格　谭万霞　谭家伟　暨丽敏　翟玉庭　熊　君　熊　炜　熊　斌　熊华利　熊润红
熊新征　缪伟刚　樊学琼　黎才刚　黎志芬　颜　玮　颜仕鹏　颜克梅　潘　熙　潘中伟　潘文川
潘希平　穆慧娟　戴　丹　戴　丽　戴　姮　戴曙光　魏　丹　魏九丹　魏文强　魏矿荣　魏翠兰
瞿　媛

Editorial Board

Du Yueqing, Du Lingbin, Du Guoming, Du Xiaofang, Du Tingting, Li Li, Li Feng, Li Ping, Li Gang, Li Yang, Li Hong, Li Lin, Li Ling (Danzhai Xian), Li Ling (Tiandong Xian), Li Li, Li Na, Li Yan, Li Ying, Li Meng, Li Chen, Li Feng, Li Qian, Li Ying, Li Jing, Li Yao, Li Xia, Li Dabing, Li Wanzhong, Li Xiaojian, Li Xiaoqiong, Li Fanka, Li Yunxi, Li Changjian, Li Congmei, Li Wenhua, Li Wenhui, Li Shiyan, Li Shihai, Li Hanfu, Li Yongwei, Li Yafang, Li Yabo, Li Chengyan, Li Weisheng, Li Zhixia, Li Linrong, Li Hangsheng, Li Guoping, Li Guoye, Li Guochun, Li Zhongping, Li Penglin, Li Yuqing, Li Zongfen, Li Shiyu, Li Jianbin, Li Chunyan, Li Yaojun, Li Qiuyue, Li Qiulin, Li Shuncui, Li Junjie, Li Yanqing, Li Meina, Li Meiping, Li Jieling, Li Yaling, Li Yanhui, Li Guifen, Li Xiaoqin, Li Xiaoyan, Li Aihui, Li Fenni, Li Haiyan, Li Yuefeng, Li Binming, Li Xuefang, Li Xueqin, Li Qiongyan, Li Yanyan, Li Huizhang, Li Jingjing, Li Zhipeng, Li Daojuan, Li Huichao, Yang Yi, Yang Fan, Yang Zhu, Yang Jun, Yang Ling, Yang Jun, Yang Liang, Yang Tao, Yang Juan, Yang Shuang, Yang Qin (Wansheng Economic & Technological Development Zone, Chongqing Shi), Yang Qin (Zunyi Shi, Huichuan Qu), Yang Lin, Yang Mei, Yang Hui (Tianshui Shi, Maiji Qu), Yang Hui (Meizhou Shi, Meixian Qu), Yang Xiaoqin, Yang Yongcui, Yang Yuchen, Yang Zhijie, Yang Liping, Yang Xiuliang, Yang Tiwu, Yang Maomin, Yang Shangbo, Yang Guoqi, Yang Mingxia, Yang Jiajuan, Yang Xianlu, Yang Junjie, Yang Yanlei, Yang Xiaojing, Yang Tongping, Yang Xuefen, Yang Fudi, Yang Huijun, Yang Yanqiong, Yang Luzhu, Xiao Qi, Xiao Xiang, Xiao Yanling, Xiao Yazhou, Xiao Yongjun, Xiao Xingping, Wu Dan, Wu Gang, Wu Hui, Wu Huan, Wu Chang, Wu Jie, Wu Ya, Wu Ying, Wu Shuang, Wu Yufu, Wu Zhimin, Wu Zening, Wu Chunxiao, Wu Chuntao, Wu Chunyan, Wu Meixiu, Wu Yanwei, Wu Xiaoyun, Wu Xiaojuan, Wu Haiyan, Wu Rongrong, Wu Yiping, Wu Jinyue, Wu Xinhui, Qiu Hong, Qiu Lin, Qiu Lin, Qiu Yuqiong, He Fei, He Li, He Li, He Liu, He Lei (Chaotian Qu, Guangyuan Shi), He Lei (Mouding Xian), He Shilin, He Yulong, He Chengdan, He Liming, He Xiuling, He Baohua, He Daofeng, He Xingui, Yu Min, Yu Bin, Yu Xiaofang, Yu Hanchun, Yu Jiahua, Gu Chaohua, Di Miao, Zou Hong, Zou Xiaolin, Zou Yuewei, Leng Jiangtao, Xin Ling, Wang Youku, Wang Shangyong, Shen Jing, Shen Feiqiong, Shen Chengfeng, Shen Yuling, Shen Jiahang, Song Bingbing, Song Guohui, Chu Yuna, Zhang Wen, Zhang Hong, Zhang Xu, Zhang Jun, Zhang Lin, Zhang Qing, Zhang Ying, Zhang Lin, Zhang Ming, Zhang Zhou, Zhang Rong, Zhang Biao, Zhang Si, Zhang Li, Zhang Ying, Zhang Tao, Zhang Tao, Zhang Min, Zhang Cai, Zhang Yan, Zhang Ting, Zhang Yi, Zhang Yizhong, Zhang Dingding, Zhang Xiaoling, Zhang Xiaopeng, Zhang Yijie, Zhang Shaoqiang, Zhang Yurong, Zhang Shiyong, Zhang Pingwen, Zhang Dongmei, Zhang Yongzhen, Zhang Yongli, Zhang Jizhi, Zhang Yaying, Zhang Xianhui, Zhang Qiaozhen, Zhang Hongxia, Zhang Keyan, Zhang Yuanyuan, Zhang Xiufen, Zhang Wuwu, Zhang Kunping, Zhang Xueqiang, Zhang Jian'an, Zhang Jianlu, Zhang Chunyu, Zhang Siwei, Zhang Meilian, Zhang Yanyan, Zhang Zhencai, Zhang Xiaofang, Zhang Xiaolin, Zhang Xiaona, Zhang Xiaofeng, Zhang Xiaohui, Zhang Qianyu, Zhang Xujin, Zhang Haifeng, Zhang Feifei, Zhang Caixia, Zhang Shuping, Zhang Jingjing, Zhang Ruixin, Zhang Shaokai, Zhang Huiling, Zhang Ganxiang, Lu Pei, Lu Yan, Lu Run, Lu Xiaofeng, Lu Yupei, Lu Suying, Lu Jialong, Chen Jie, Chen Chong, Chen Ying, Chen Ru, Chen Na (Weiyuan Xian), Chen Na (Tongguan Xian), Chen Juan, Chen Ping, Chen Qiong, Chen Xia, Chen Shangqing, Chen Xiaofang, Chen Xiaona, Chen Xiaohui, Chen Wenjun, Chen Lanfen, Chen Yonggang, Chen Yongqun, Chen Bingxia, Chen Zhihong, Chen Zhiyan, Chen Lili, Chen Miaochang, Chen Yuehua, Chen Guorong, Chen Yilin, Chen Jinwu, Chen Jianshun, Chen Zhenlian, Chen Sihong, Chen Jiaojiao, Chen Yanping, Chen Xiaochun, Chen Hairong, Chen Haitao, Chen Xuelian, Chen Xuejun, Chen Wenwen, Chen Ziyun, Chen Zijuan, Shao Ying, Wu Xia, Wu Huaqian, Lamao Cairang, Miao Jiali, Gou Junping, Fan Ying, Fan Weigang, Fan Meixia, Fan Lili, Lin Li, Lin Yucheng, Lin Haixia, Lin Chaolan, Ou Zhixiu, Ou Guoqin, Ouyang Le, Zhuo Ma, Shang Mingfeng, Ming Xiaoxue, Tie Yingwei, Luo Ling, Luo Yuan, Luo Wenyun, Luo Shihua, Luo Liqiong, Luo Guoliang, Luo Chunliang, Luo Yanli, Luo Lifei, He Chenhui, He Lina, He Guifen, Ji Jiafu, Ji Jiahui, Yue Ting, Jin Hongyan, Jin Qiman, Zhou Li, Zhou Yan, Zhou Qian, Zhou Hao, Zhou Juan, Zhou Jie, Zhou Qi, Zhou Rui, Zhou Xiaohua, Zhou Xiaojia, Zhou Chuannan, Zhou Wenwu, Zhou Yonggang, Zhou Liping, Zhou Qingxia, Zhou Jinyi, Zhou Jianrong, Zhou Jianxiang, Zhou Chunlin, Zhou Yanmei, Zhou Suxia, Zhou Xiaofeng, Zhou Xiaomei, Zhou Tingting, Zhou Xinyu, Zhou Jingjing, Jing Zhao, Zheng Ling, Zheng Yunzhi, Zheng Dongbai, Zheng Yongping, Zheng Huanhuan, Zheng Rongshou, Zheng Yuming, Shan Bao'en, Lang Hongxia, Qu Qiuqiong, Meng Ruilin, Xiang Lihong, Xiang Xiaxia, Zhao Li, Zhao Qing, Zhao Ying, Zhao Zhanfeng, Zhao Shengming, Zhao Tingming, Zhao Zhonggang, Zhao Huilian, Zhao Jinliang, Zhao Jinge, Zhao Jianhua, Zhao Qiuping, Zhao Hairong, Zhao Haizhou, Zhao Menglin, Zhao Chaoqiang, Zhao Yafang, Zhao Yuanli, Zhao Dejian, Hao Qinghua, Hao Qingqing, Hu Dong, Hu Ying, Hu Ping, Hu Biao, Hu Yanhong, Hu Suhua, Hu Qianhua, Nan Yan, Ke Jinlian, Chao Lina, Zhong Xin,

Zhong Yumei, Zhong Weiwen, Zhong Yanfeng, Zhong Xianxian, Duan Shibin, Duan Leyong, Duan Chenli, Bao Hongli, Hou Liang, Yu Liang, Yu Min, Shi Yunli, Shi Changmiao, Jiang Fan, Jiang Xin, Jiang Jinhong, Lou Peian, Hong Bo, Gong Xuzhi, Zhu Zhangmei, Xu Jingchen, Yao Lin, Yao Yuan, Yao Shuang, Yao Yonghong, Yao Xinfei, He Ming, He Yutong, He Junhong, He Shaoqiong, Luo Wenshu, Luo Xiumei, Qin Shu, Qin Dawu, Qin Tianyan, Qin Yanjin, Qin Kebo, Ban Qiongzhen, Yuan Ye, Yuan Li, Yuan Ying, Yuan Jing, Yuan Xiaoyu, Yuan Jiwei, Yuan Caihong, Yuan Congling, Geng Zhenqiang, Nie Wei, Mo Wenkang, Mo Ganhua, Jia Wenhu, Jia Limin, Jia Yanfang, Jia Yuanyao, Xia Bing, Xia Hong, Xia Yunlei, Xia Lili, Gu Kai, Gu Xiaoping, Dang Liqin, Yan Ying, En Ronglin, Qian Yun, Feng Shiyuan, Ni Jia, Ni Zhihua, Xu Xian, Xu Wei, Xu Hong, Xu Fang, Xu Jue, Xu Ling(Shenqiu Xian), Xu Ling(Chongqing Shi, Bishan Qu), Xu Mei, Xu Wei, Xu Yuluan, Xu Weixiao, Xu Hongbin, Xu Shaohe, Xu Shengping, Xu Haixia, Xu Yuanfeng, Xu Xinhong, Xu Weijing, Yin Hang, Yin Jianxiang, Ling Haijie, Gao Ming, Gao Weimin, Gao Shengli, Gao Yangbo, Gao Panpan, Gao Tiezhu, Gao Hongmin, Gao Ruifang, Guo Zheng, Guo Wei, Guo Mei, Guo Min (Le'an Xian), Guo Min(Xiushan Tujiazu Miaozu Zizhixian), Guo Chao, Guo Tianhua, Guo Fenglan, Guo Qiaohong, Guo Shulan, Guo Guizhou, Guo Qiuxian, Guo Xiaolei, Guo Yingzhen, Xi Yunfeng, Tang Mingyue, Pu Jiyin, Tan Hongfen, Tao Xiaohong, Huang Jing, Huang Yifeng, Huang Xiaorong, Huang Feiping, Huang Yongjie, Huang Yuantian, Huang Jialing, Huang Xuemin, Huang Chunguang, Huang Chunfeng, Huang Jiongmei, Huang Huishu, Huang Hailang, Huang Jinhang, Cao Shan, Cao Ling, Cao Liangqing, Cao Shipeng, Cao Qiuju, Cao Haiyang, Cao Jingjun, Qi Peiling, Gong Xinhong, Gong Weiwei, Sheng Genying, Chang An, Chang Rong, Cui Lingbo, Cui Haihua, Fu Yong, Fu Dibao, Fu Fangmin, Fu Meiyan, Tuo Jiyu, Kang Wenhui, Kang Yuxia, Zhang Youjian, Jing Guangqun, Chun Zhiming, Liang Meng, Liang Yingfeng, Liang Zhongyi, Liang Jiajia, Liang Shujun, Liang Xiaoting, Liang Saiwen, Liang Cuimin, Peng Na, Peng Ye, Peng Changyan, Peng Shuling, Peng Hongwei, Peng Fenru, Dong Lixin, Dong Yongnian, Dong Yaping, Dong Zhipeng, Dong Jianmei, Jing Lin, Jiang Wei, Jiang Dongyuan, Jiang Suhong, Jiang Weilin, Jiang Shuchu, Han Xia, Han Xiaoyu, Han Renqiang, Han Bingfeng, Han Guiwei, Han Xiaokang, Han Ruizhen, Han Jiayi, Tan Xiangqing, Tan Mingjiang, Tan Rongpan, Tan Lingfeng, Tan Yanhong, Zhi Xin, Cheng Feng, Cheng Mi, Cheng Xiangdong, Cheng Zhifang, Shui Zhiqun, Jiao Yanli, Lu Tingting, Zeng Ping, Zeng Ji, Zeng Hongmei, Zeng Yingzhu, You Dayong, You Ningjing, Xie Ping, Xie Weilong, Xie Meilan, Xie Haibin, Xie Shuwen, Xie Jinrong, Ting Ting, Jin Wanchun, Jin Shuanghong, Meng Yi, Chu Yumei, Lei Lin, Lei Yunhua, Lei Baoqiong, Bao Yueyue, Bao Kebiao, He Jie, Cai Wei, Cai Lin, Pei Zhenyi, Guan Xiaoqin, Guan Yuanping, Guan Lijuan, Liao Yu, Liao Shun, Liao Qian, Liao Tao, Liao Dongjuan, Liao Zhuohang, Liao Liuyan, Liao Xiaocheng, Liao Lingling, Tan Ge, Tan Wanxia, Tan Jiawei, Ji Limin, Zhai Yuting, Xiong Jun, Xiong Wei, Xiong Bin, Xiong Huali, Xiong Runhong, Xiong Xinzheng, Miao Weigang, Fan Xueqiong, Li Caigang, Li Zhifen, Yan Wei, Yan Shipeng, Yan Kemei, Pan Xi, Pan Zhongwei, Pan Wenchuan, Pan Xiping, Mu Huijuan, Dai Dan, Dai Li, Dai Heng, Dai Shuguang, Wei Dan, Wei Jiudan, Wei Wenqiang, Wei Kuangrong, Wei Cuilan, Qu Yuan

8

前　言

　　恶性肿瘤已成为影响我国居民健康、国家经济和社会发展的重大公共卫生问题。党中央、国务院历来高度重视癌症防治工作，多次将癌症防治纳入国务院《政府工作报告》，并在国家卫生健康相关规划计划中进行重点部署。"十三五"期间，中国政府先后发布《"健康中国2030"规划纲要》《健康中国行动（2019—2030年）》《中国防治慢性病中长期规划（2017—2025年）》《健康中国行动——癌症防治实施方案（2019—2022年）》等一系列政策措施，各地、各部门按照行动要求，积极落实综合防治措施，在体系建设、信息监测、早诊早治、规范诊疗、保障救助、科技攻关、科普宣传等重点领域稳步推进，并取得了显著成果。

　　肿瘤防控，登记先行。恶性肿瘤的发病率、死亡率和生存率数据，是制定卫生政策、评价医疗卫生工作质量和效果的科学依据。不同恶性肿瘤的地理分布和流行趋势不同，将影响全国和地方的癌症防治策略的制定。

　　《2022中国肿瘤登记年报》是自2008年我国首次出版《中国肿瘤登记年报》以来的第16卷。本年报汇总了2019年我国肿瘤登记地区癌症监测数据。国家癌症中心收到来自中国31个省（自治区、直辖市）及新疆生产建设兵团（未包括香港特别行政区、澳门特别行政区和台湾省）的1 073个肿瘤登记处的上报数据。通过对数据审核和质量控制，有919个肿瘤登记处数据入选本年报。此次年报对所有癌症合计及26类癌症的发病与死亡数据进行了详细分析，并分地区、年龄别和性别比较了癌症分布差异。与上卷相同，各省已经开始发布本地区的肿瘤负担数据，为减少篇幅，本年报不再展示各省区县级的肿瘤登记数据。

　　2020年以来，新型冠状病毒感染疫情使全球医疗系统承受巨大压力，世界卫生组织表示，癌症诊疗服务、相关研究及临床试验的参与人数都大幅减少，"诊断延后非常普遍，治疗中断或中止的情况也显著增加"，或将影响到未来数年内因癌症而去世的总人数。新型冠状病毒感染疫情对恶性肿瘤发病与死亡数据的获取及恶性肿瘤患者的生

Foreword

Cancer has become a major public health problem in China, which deeply affects the health of Chinese residents, the national economy and the social development. The CPC Central Committee and the State Council have attached great importance to cancer prevention and control. Cancer prevention and control has been included in the *Government Work Report* for many times and has been prioritized in the national health plans. During the 13th Five-Year Plan period, Chinese government published a series of documents, including the *Outline of the Healthy China 2030 Plan*, the *Healthy China Action (2019-2030)*, the *Medium-to Long-term Plan (2017-2025) on the Prevention and Treatment of Chronic Diseases*, the *Healthy China Action-Implementation Plan for Cancer Prevention and Control (2019-2022)*. Every province and every department comprehensively implemented cancer prevention and control measures according to these plans. Steady progress has been made in key areas such as system construction, surveillance, early diagnosis and treatment, standardized diagnosis and treatment, medical security and medical aid, scientific and technological breakthroughs and popular science propaganda.

Cancer registration is the first step of cancer prevention and control program. Cancer incidence, mortality and survival data provide scientific evidences to develop cancer prevention and control strategies, and to evaluate the effectiveness of the quality of medical and health work. The geographical distribution and epidemiology of cancer will affect the development of the national and local cancer prevention and treatment strategies.

Since the first volume of *China Cancer Registry Annual Report* published in 2008, this book is the 16th Annual Report. In this volume, cancer surveillance data of China cancer registration areas in 2019 was reported. A total of 1 073 cancer registries submitted data to National Cancer Center (NCC) in China, including 31 provinces (autonomous regions and municipalities) and Xinjiang Production and Construction Corps (not including Hongkong Tebiexingzhengqu, Macao Tebiexingzhengqu and Taiwan Sheng). After data quality control, a total of 919 cancer registries were included in the present *China Cancer Registry Annual Report*. In this volume, we summarized and analyzed data of the incidence and mortality for all cancers combined and 26 cancer sites by including

存随访工作均造成持续性影响,数据资料的收集、质量控制和统计分析工作也受到不同程度的影响。

我国的广大肿瘤登记工作者,不忘本职,积极稳妥地及时完成了年报数据收集、审核、上报清理、统计分析、编撰出版工作。《2022 中国肿瘤登记年报》的顺利出版凝结着全国各肿瘤登记处全体工作人员的辛勤付出,也得到了国家卫生健康委员会医疗应急司、国家疾病预防控制局、国家卫生健康委员会宣传司一如既往的指导和大力支持,我们在此表示最衷心的感谢!

编者从登记点选择、数据清理、统计分析、图表呈现、文字描述等方面反复核实,力求做到数字真实、描述准确,竭力避免不必要的失误,然而由于水平和知识有限,加之入选年报的登记点数量剧增,数据体量巨大,工作中难免出现纰漏,敬请国内外同行和广大读者批评指正。

国家癌症中心
2023 年 5 月

overall analysis and analysis by age, sex and area. As in the previous volume, all provinces have begun to release the cancer burden data of their own regions, this national annual report will no longer show the cancer registration data at the county level.

Since 2020, the epidemic of Coronavirus Disease 2019 (COVID-19) has put enormous pressure on the global medical system. The World Health Organization said that the number of participants in cancer diagnosis and treatment services, related research and clinical trials has decreased significantly. "The delay of diagnosis is common, and the interruption or suspension of treatment has also increased significantly", which may affect the total number of deaths due to cancer in the next few years. The epidemic of COVID-19 has a continuous impact on the acquisition of cancer incidence and mortality data and the survival follow-up of patients. The collection, quality control and statistical analysis of data are also affected in some way.

All faculties of cancer registries did not forget their duties and complete the reporting, cleaning, analyzing, and publishing works of the annual report without complaint while actively implementing epidemic prevention and control measures. The successful publication of the *2022 China Cancer Registry Annual Report* embodies the hard work of all staff members in different cancer registries across the country. Department of Medical Emergency Response, National Administration of Disease Prevention and Control, Department of Publicity in National Health Commission of the People's Republic of China have also provided guidance and support in the publication of the *2022 China Cancer Registry Annual Report*. We acknowledge all staff working for the cancer registries and the editorial board who contributed to this publication.

In order to assure the data is real, objective, accurate and without unnecessary mistakes, the authors write carefully and verify repeatedly for choosing the cancer registries, cleaning data, performing statistical analysis, rendering charts, and describing data. However, due to the knowledge limitation and the intensively increased cancer registries, the vast data volume may lead to some mistakes in the work. Colleagues and readers are welcome to criticize and correct.

National Cancer Center
May 2023

目　　录

Contents

第一章　概述

1　中国人群肿瘤登记系统简介

肿瘤登记是癌症防控工作的基础,也是核心的工作内容,为国家和地区的卫生行政部门制定癌症防治策略、开展防治研究、评价防治效果提供科学的数据。建立健全癌症信息监测体系是国家癌症中心最重要的任务之一。

以我国人群为基础的肿瘤登记工作起步于 20 世纪 60 年代初,仅河南林县(林州)和上海等部分地区先后开展。1973—1975 年全国第一次死因回顾性调查后,在肿瘤高发地区相继建立肿瘤登记处。1986 年,随着全国肿瘤防治研究办公室的恢复成立,以及《全国肿瘤防治规划纲要(1986—2000)》的发布,各界对肿瘤防治工作的重视逐步提高,各地又相继建立肿瘤登记处。1990 年,全国肿瘤防治研究办公室在上海市成立"中国肿瘤登记协作组",第一批成员单位共 17 个。为建立既切合我国实际又能与国际接轨的肿瘤发病、死亡及危险因素监测系统,全国肿瘤防治研究办公室在"八五"和"九五"国家科技攻关计划课题"中国恶性肿瘤死亡调查及监测系统的建立"的基础上,开始肿瘤登记试点工作,引起卫生主管部门的重视。2002 年卫生部批准成立全国肿瘤登记中心,挂靠于全国肿瘤防治研究办公室,并发文在全国开展肿瘤登记工作。全国肿瘤登记中心的主要任务是负责经常性系统性地收集、储存、整理、统计和分析癌情资料,进行质量监督,为国家和卫生行政部门制定癌症防治策略、考核评估防治效果、开展防治研究提供依据;建立健全有关登记工作的技术规范和数据库;有计划地开展登记人员的技术培训工作,以及国内外工作及学术交流活动,以提高登记工作的整体水平与质量。2002 年 10 月全国肿瘤登记中心与国际癌症研究机构(International Agency for Research on Cancer,IARC)合作开展的登记工作现状调查报告,全国共有 48 个肿瘤登记处,覆盖人口约 7 527 万。同年 IARC 出版《五大洲癌症发病率》,在第 8 卷中,收录 8 个中国登记处的监测数据。

Chapter 1　Introduction

1　Population-based cancer registration system in China

Cancer registration is the foundation and core of the cancer prevention and control program. It provides scientific evidences for national and local health administrative departments to develop cancer prevention and control strategies, to launch comprehensive researches, and to evaluate the effectiveness of current prevention and control plans. To establish and improve the cancer surveillance system is one of the most important tasks of the National Cancer Center.

Population-based cancer registration initiated in 1960s in China, it was first carried out in Henan Linxian(Linzhou) and Shanghai. After the first national retrospective death cause investigation during 1973－1975, many cancer registries were established in high-risk areas of cancer. In 1986, with the establishment of National Cancer Prevention and Treatment Office(NCPTO) and the publication of the *Outline of National Cancer Prevention and Treatment Program (1986－2000)*, the importance of cancer prevention and control was gradually increasing and numerous of cancer registries were set up. In 1990, NCPTO established "China Cancer Registry Cooperation Group" in Shanghai, including 17 members at that time. To develop a domestically applicable and internationally compatible surveillance system for cancer incidence, mortality, and cancer risk factors, NCPTO started cancer registration pilot study on the basis of previous project "*The Establishment of Malignant Cancer Death Investigation and Monitoring System in China*" during the 8th Five-Year Plan period and 9th Five-Year Plan period, which aroused the attention of health administrative department. In 2002, National Central Cancer Registry(NCCR), which was affiliated with the NCPTO, was approved by the former Ministry of Health and cancer registry was carried out across the country under executive order. The primary missions of NCCR were: to collect continuously and systematically, store, dispose and analysis cancer registry data; to implement quality control and supervision; to provide scientific evidences for cancer prevention and control strategy development and effectiveness evaluation for health administrative departments; to set up operational standards and data base; to provide training, and to carry out exchange activities. In October 2002, NCCR carried out a survey about the current status of cancer registration work in China in cooperation with the International Agency for Research on Cancer(IARC). There were 48 cancer registries in China, with a population coverage of 75 270 000. In the same year, IARC published *Cancer Incidence in Five Continents*, in Volume Ⅷ, 8 cancer registries from China were included.

2003 年,卫生部发布《中国癌症预防与控制规划纲要(2004—2010)》,明确指出加强肿瘤登记工作。全国肿瘤登记中心对《中国恶性肿瘤登记试行规范》进行了重新修订和增补,出版了《中国肿瘤登记工作指导手册》,以此来指导和规范肿瘤登记工作。2006 年,卫生部疾病预防控制局决定将肿瘤登记数据资料每 5 年上报一次改为年报制。当年全国共有 36 个登记处提交了 2003 年恶性肿瘤登记数据。

2008 年,中华人民共和国财政部、卫生部将肿瘤随访登记项目纳入卫生部"医改重大项目"之中,中国的肿瘤登记工作得以迅速发展。到 2020 年,肿瘤随访登记项目每年经费已经达到 5 000 万,支持的登记区县数达 1 000 个以上。2015 年,国家卫生和计划生育委员会、国家中医药管理局联合下发《肿瘤登记管理办法》,从制度上保证了全国肿瘤登记工作的顺利开展。

2018 年国家癌症中心肿瘤登记办公室为建立统一的国家级肿瘤数据库、提高数据的有效利用率,开发"中国肿瘤登记平台",并于 2019 年 7 月正式上线使用。2021 年《中国肿瘤登记数据集标准》(T/CHIA 18—2021)发布,为人群肿瘤登记工作提供一套项目明确、术语规范、定义明确、语义语境无歧义的基本数据集标准,保证肿瘤登记数据质量,便于对肿瘤登记数据实现精准自动化获取,保证信息的有效交换、有效挖掘分析和共享。同时,国家癌症中心积极推进与中国疾病预防控制中心死因监测数据的互联互通,并签订《肿瘤防治战略合作框架协议》与《癌症防控与结局数据共享与应用项目合作协议》。建设完成国家癌症中心随访链接服务平台,后续可自动从死因监测平台抓取死亡数据,减少不必要的人工随访数据采集负担,提高数据质量。

In 2003, the former Ministry of Health published *Cancer Prevention and Control Plan in China(2004-2010)*, which clearly pointed out to strengthen the cancer registration work. NCCR revised and updated the *Regulations on the Work of Cancer Registration(Trial)* into *the Chinese Guideline for Cancer Registration* to guide and standardize the cancer registration work. In 2006, the former Disease Prevention and Control Bureau of the Ministry of Health requested to submit cancer registry data annually instead of by 5 years. 36 cancer registries submitted cancer registry data at 2003.

In 2008, the Ministry of Finance of the People's Republic of China and the former Ministry of Health included the National Cancer Registration and Follow-up Program in the "Major Medical Reform Project", which helped cancer registry to develop rapidly. Till 2020, the National Cancer Registration and Follow-up Program received an annual funding of 50 million yuan, supporting over 1 000 districts/counties to carry out this work. In 2015, the National Health and Family Planning Commission and the National Administration of Traditional Chinese Medicine co-published *Chinese Cancer Registration Management Regulation*, which fundamentally ensured the implementation of cancer registration with the administrative rules and regulations.

In 2018, to establish a standardized national cancer registry data base, as well as to improve the effective utilization rate of cancer registry data, Cancer Registry Office of National Cancer Center developed "National Cancer Registration Platform". This platform was officially put into use in July, 2019. In 2021, the *Standard for Dataset of Cancer Registration in China(T/CHIA 18-2021)* was published, which provided a set of data elements and terminologies with clear definition and unambiguous semantic contexts for PBCR in China. This standard guaranteed the data quality, facilitated the automatic acquisition of cancer registry data, and guaranteed the data exchange, sharing and analysis. What's more, NCC promoted the interconnection of the Cancer Registry Database and National Mortality Database, which was established by the Chinese Center for Disease Control and Prevention. Two institutions signed the *Strategic Cooperation Framework Agreement on Cancer Prevention and Treatment* and the *Cooperation Agreement on Cancer Prevention and Control and Outcome Data Sharing and Application Project*. We completed the construction of National Cancer Data Follow up Linkage Platform. Through this platform, we can automatically capture vital status from the National Mortality Database, which could reduce the unnecessary burden of manual follow-up information collection and promote the data quality.

健康是促进人类全面发展的必然要求,是经济社会发展的基础条件,是民族昌盛和国家富强的重要标志,也是广大人民群众的共同追求。党的十八届五中全会明确提出推进健康中国建设。"十三五"期间,国家发布的系列文件确定了中国癌症防控总体前进方向,并将提高癌症生存率作为癌症防控的重要目标。癌症信息化行动部分也对肿瘤登记工作做了具体部署,明确要求要不断健全肿瘤登记制度,到 2022 年,实现肿瘤登记工作在中国所有县区全覆盖;持续提升肿瘤登记数据质量,完善质量控制标准和评价体系,推进实现多源信息共享应用,提升生存分析与发病死亡趋势预测能力等。

2022 年末,来自 31 个省(自治区、直辖市)及新疆生产建设兵团(未包括香港特别行政区、澳门特别行政区和台湾省)的 2 806 个区县开展肿瘤登记工作,占全国区县总数的 98.6%,肿瘤登记及监测随访网络已经建成,基本实现肿瘤登记县区全覆盖。自 2008 年首次出版《中国肿瘤登记年报》以来,国家癌症中心持续以"年报"形式向社会各界发布我国恶性肿瘤发病与死亡数据,极大地促进了中国肿瘤防控工作。随着肿瘤登记及监测随访网络的建成,以及数据采集体系和工具的不断完善,中国肿瘤登记系统将为我国肿瘤防控工作提供更翔实的数据支持,从而更好地服务"健康中国"战略。

Health is a necessary requirement for all-round development of the individual, a basic condition for economic and social development, an important symbol of national prosperity, and a common pursuit of the people. The Fifth Plenary Session of the 18th CPC Central Committee explicitly called for the need to build a healthy China. During the 13th Five-Year Plan period, the government published a series of documents to point out the direction of cancer prevention and control in China. The improvement of cancer survival rate was set as one of the most important goals of cancer prevention and control work. Specific arrangements were made for cancer registration in Cancer Informalization Action part. In this part, the government requested to continuously improve the cancer registration system, and achieve full coverage of all districts/counties in China in 2022; to continuously improve the quality of cancer registration; to perfect quality control standards and evaluation system; to promote the sharing and application of multi-source data; to promote the ability of survival analysis and prediction analysis.

At the end of 2022, 2 806 districts/counties from 31 provinces(autonomous regions and municipalities) and Xinjiang Production and Construction Corps(not including Hongkong Tebiexingzhengqu, Macao Tebiexingzhengqu and Taiwan Sheng) had carried out cancer registration work, accounting for 98.6% of all districts/counties in the country. We have already established a cancer surveillance system, and basically achieved a full coverage of all districts/counties. Since the first publication of the *China Cancer Registry Annual Report* in 2008, National Cancer Center continued to release data on cancer incidence and mortality to the society in the form of annual report, which greatly improved the cancer prevention and control in China. With the establishment of a mature cancer surveillance system and the perfection of data collection tools, China cancer registration system will provide more detailed and accurate data, so as to better serve the Healthy China Strategy.

2 本年报数据

2.1 数据上报地区及范围

本年报数据收集截止时间为 2022 年 12 月 31 日,数据上报范围为 2019 年 1 月 1 日至 2019 年 12 月 31 日全年新发癌症发病与死亡个案数据(ICD-10 编码范围:C00-C97,D32-D33,D42-D43,D45-D47),以及各肿瘤登记处 2019 年年中人口数据。上报 2019 年肿瘤登记数据的登记处分布在 31 个省(自治区、直辖市)及新疆生产建设兵团(未包括香港特别行政区、澳门特别行政区和台湾省),合计登记处 1 073 个,覆盖人口 691 409 114 人,其中城市登记处 357 个,农村登记处 716 个。

2.2 数据质量控制及最终纳入数据

本年报根据《中国肿瘤登记工作指导手册(2016)》有关数据质量的要求,以及国际癌症研究机构(IARC)/国际癌症登记协会(IACR)肿瘤登记数据的质量控制原则选择登记处,并对各登记处肿瘤登记数据的完整性、可比性和有效性进行评价。具体质量控制指标包括:恶性肿瘤的发病率、死亡率水平及其变化幅度,病理诊断比例(MV%),只有死亡证明书比例(DCO%),死亡/发病比(M/I)等。根据我国各地区实际情况,综合评估该肿瘤登记处数据质量。最终 919 个肿瘤登记处的数据入选,占全部上报数据登记处的 85.6%。

全国 919 个肿瘤登记处 2019 年覆盖人口 628 429 537 人(男性 318 815 999 人,女性 309 613 538 人),占全国 2019 年年末人口数的 44.89%。其中城市地区肿瘤登记处 324 个,覆盖人口 268 481 922 人,占入选年报中国肿瘤登记地区人口数的 42.72%;农村地区肿瘤登记处 595 个,覆盖人口 359 947 615 人,占 57.28%。

2 Data specification in this annual report

2.1 Data collection scope

NCC China required all population-based cancer registries to submit new diagnoses and deaths from cancer in 2019 (ICD-10: C00-C97, D32-D33, D42-D43, D45-D47), as well as the corresponding population data before December 31st, 2022. All those registries who submitted data in 2019 were distributed in 31 provinces (autonomous regions and municipalities) and Xinjiang Production and Construction Corps (not including Hongkong Tebiexingzhengqu, Macao Tebiexingzhengqu and Taiwan Sheng). A total of 1 073 cancer registries submitted data to NCC China, covering a total of 691 409 114 population. Among the 1 073 cancer registries, 357 were urban cancer registries and 716 were rural cancer registries.

2.2 Data quality control and data inclusion

According to the *Chinese Guideline Cancer Registration (2016)* and the standards of International Agency for Research on Cancer/International Association of Cancer Registries (IARC/IACR), we published a national criterion on data quality control to evaluate the completeness, comparability and validity of cancer registry data and select the cancer registries. Specific quality control indicators included the crude incidence rate, the crude mortality rate and their variation between years, morphological verification percent (MV%), death certificate only percent (DCO%), mortality to incidence ratios (M/I). We comprehensively assessed the data quality of cancer registries according to the actual conditions of different regions in our country. A total of 919 cancer registries were included in the present *China Cancer Registry Annual Report*, who made up about 85.6% of all registries.

The 919 cancer registries covered a total of 628 429 537 population (318 815 999 males, 309 613 538 females), accounting for 44.89% of the national population in 2019. Especially, there were 324 urban cancer registries covering 268 481 922 population (42.72%) and 595 rural cancer registries with population coverage of 359 947 615 (57.28%).

2.3 年报内容简介

本年报汇总了 919 个肿瘤登记处 2019 年癌症的发病、死亡及人口数据。详细描述了合计 919 个肿瘤登记处和各肿瘤登记处数据的质量控制指标,并详细报道了合计癌症和 26 种癌症发病和死亡数据指标,包括:发病率、死亡率、中国人口标化率(2000 年中国人口构成)、世界人口标化率(Segi's 世界人口构成)、累积率、分年龄组发病率/死亡率、分性别发病率/死亡率等。部分癌症按亚部位和组织学分型进行了细化描述。分城市农村、东中西部地区、七大行政区比较了各地区癌症发病、死亡差异。

2.3 Content of this annual report

The present annual report summarized data of the cancer incidence, mortality and demography through 919 cancer registration sites in 2019. We reported the quality control indicators, and statistical indicators for all cancer and 26 major cancer sites, including crude incidence rate, crude mortality rate, age-standardized rate(ASR) by 2000 China population, ASR by Segi's world population, cumulative rates, age and sex-specific rates. Moreover, we presented detailed distribution by subsite and morphology for some cancers. We compared cancer incidence and mortality rates by urban and rural areas, three geographic areas(eastern areas, central areas and western areas) and the seven administrative districts(North China, Northeast China, East China, Central China, South China, Southwest China and Northwest China).

第二章 质量控制和统计指标

1 质量控制

质量控制贯穿肿瘤登记工作的全过程。肿瘤登记地区应在各个环节制定工作规范和质量控制程序,并严格执行。质量控制主要包括四个方面:可比性、完整性、有效性和时效性。

1.1 可比性

数据结果真实可比的基本先决条件是采用通用的标准或定义。通常而言,可比性是指发病率间的不同不是因各登记地区之间的数据质量和标准不同而产生。可比性涉及以下几个指标:对"发病"的定义,对原发、复发和转移的诊断标准、分类与编码,死亡医学证明等。

1.2 完整性

完整性是指在登记地区资料库的目标人群中发现所有发病病例的程度。常用的评价指标有死亡/发病比(M/I)、只有死亡证明书比例(DCO%)、病理诊断比例(MV%)、病例的来源数与报告单数、不同时间发病率的稳定性、不同人群发病率的比较、年龄别发病率曲线、儿童癌症评价等。俘获/再俘获方法也用来评价登记报告资料的完整性。

Chapter 2 Quality control and statistical indicators

1 Quality control

The value of cancer registration relies on the data quality. This procedure aims at providing qualified cancer registration data with comparability, completeness, validity, and timeliness.

1.1 Comparability

Comparability is the extent to which coding and classification at a registry, together with the definitions of recording and reporting specific data items, adhere to standardized international guidelines. In the evaluation of the comparability of registration data, the following standards should be identical: the definition of incidence, the identification of primary cancer and cancer recurrence or metastasis of an existing one, the identification for tumor classification and coding, the criteria of death certification.

1.2 Completeness

The completeness of cancer registry data refers to the extent of all the incident cancers occurring in the population included in the cancer registration database. It is an extremely important attribute of a cancer registry's data. The methods which provide indication of the completeness include the following: mortality to incidence ratios (M/I), death certificate only percent (DCO%), morphological verification percent (MV%), reporting avenues, stability of incidence rates over time, comparison of incidence rates in different populations, shape of age-specific curves and incidence rates of childhood cancers, et al. The capture-recapture methods are also used to evaluate the completeness of registration data.

1.3 有效性

有效性是指登记病例中具有给定特征属性（如肿瘤部位、年龄）的病例所占的比例。再摘录与再编码方法是评价有效性的最客观方法，一般由另一个观察者完成对登记地区记录与相关病例文件间的仔细比较。常用的评价指标有病理诊断比例（MV%）、只有死亡证明书比例（DCO%）、其他或未指明部位肿瘤所占比例（O&U%）、年龄不明百分比等。肿瘤登记地区至少进行诸如年龄/出生日期、性别/部位、部位/组织学，以及部位/组织学/年龄、基本变量有无遗漏信息等一致性核对。

1.4 时效性

时效性一般指从发病日期（诊断日期）到数据被利用时（年报、研究报告、论文）的间隔。登记地区应及时报告和获取癌症信息。目前对时效性的要求无统一的国际标准。为平衡与完整性和有效性的关系，国家癌症中心要求各登记地区于诊断年份后的 30 个月内提交数据。

1.3 Validity

Validity is defined as the proportion of cases in a dataset with a given characteristic which truly have the attribute. Re-abstracting and re-coding are the principal methods which permit comparisons with respect to specified subsets of cases. The commonly used evaluation indicators include MV%, DCO%, the percentage of other and unspecified cancer sites (O&U%), and the percentage of unknown age. The cancer registration office shall conduct consistency checks such as age/date of birth, gender/location, location/histology, as well as location/histology/age, and the presence of missing information on basic variables.

1.4 Timeliness

Timeliness relates to the rapidity at which a registry can collect, process and report reliable and complete cancer data. It indicates the time to availability as the interval between date of diagnosis and the date the case was available in the registry for further use. The cancer registries should timely collect and report cancer statistics. While there are no international guidelines for the timeliness of cancer registry data, to balance the relationship between integrity and effectiveness, NCC China requires the cancer registries should report cancer statistics in 30 months.

2 常用质量控制指标

常用质量控制指标有病理诊断比例(MV%)、死亡/发病比(M/I)、只有死亡证明书比例(DCO%),以及信息缺失所占比例,包括其他或未指明部位肿瘤所占比例(O&U%)、诊断依据不明比例(UB%)等。常见恶性肿瘤的逐年发病率和死亡率是否基本稳定等也是评价数据质量的指标。

2.1 病理诊断比例

依靠显微镜下组织学检查做出诊断具有较好的准确性和可靠性,包括脱落细胞学或外周血的血液病检查,是评价有效性和完整性的指标。其绝对指标意义有限,常用的方法是与相似的区域内适当的标准进行比较。

$$病理诊断比例(MV\%)=\frac{有病理诊断的病例}{全部新发病例}\times100\%$$

2.2 死亡/发病比

死亡/发病比为同一时期内死亡病例数与新发病例数之比。死亡数据来源于生命统计,应独立于肿瘤登记数据。M/I 相对过大,提示数据不完整,发病登记存在漏报;M/I 相对过小,提示发病数据中有重复记录可能。同时,还要考虑生命统计数据的完整性和有效性问题。如果死因登记数据质量有保证,那么 M/I 近似等于 1~5 年相对生存率。

$$死亡/发病比(M/I)=\frac{同时期内癌症死亡病例数}{同时期内癌症新发病例数}$$

2 Quality control indicators

Commonly used quality control indicators include morphological verification percent (MV%), mortality to incidence ratios(M/I), and death certificate only percent(DCO%), and proportion of missing information, including proportion of other and unspecified cancer sites(O&U%), proportion of unknown diagnostic basis (UB%), etc. Whether the annual incidence rate and mortality of common cancers are stable or not is also a indicator for evaluating data quality.

2.1 Morphological verification percent

The stated diagnosis of cancer cases based on histological examination under microscope, including exfoliative cytology or hematological examination of peripheral blood, can be more accurate and reliable. MV% is an indicator of the validity and completeness of the diagnostic information. The absolute value of MV% can have little meaning. It is most frequently used to make comparisons with appropriate criteria within similar areas.

$$Morphological\ verification\ percent(MV\%)=\frac{Cases\ with\ histological\ examination\ results}{All\ new\ cases}\times100\%$$

2.2 Mortality to incidence ratios

Mortality to incidence ratios is a comparison of the number of deaths, obtained from a source independent of the registry (usually, the vital statistics system), and the number of new cases of a specific cancer registered, in the same period of time. M/I value greater than expected lead to a suspicion of incompleteness. There might be under-reporting of cancer cases. M/I value smaller than expected lead to a suspicion of duplications of cancer cases. At the same time, the integrity and validity of vital statistical data should also be considered. If the quality of vital statistics system is good, the M/I ratio is approximated by 1-5 years survival probability.

$$Mortality\ to\ incidence\ ratios(M/I)=\frac{Cancer\ deaths\ in\ the\ same\ period\ of\ time}{Cancer\ cases\ in\ the\ same\ period\ of\ time}$$

2.3 只有死亡证明书比例

来自死亡医学证明书(DCN)的病例,指无法追踪到死亡前任何癌症确认信息的病例,称为"只有死亡证明书"(DCO)病例。DCO%是评价有效性的指标之一,也是完整性的指标,与临床或病理诊断的病例记录相比,DCO病例的信息显然准确性差,DCO比例高,提示病例发现流程存在不足。

$$只有死亡证明书比例(DCO\%)= \frac{只有死亡证明书患者}{全部新发病例} \times 100\%$$

2.4 信息缺失所占比例

信息缺失包括年龄不明、性别不明、其他或未指明部位肿瘤所占比例(O&U%)、诊断依据不明比例(UB%)等,是评价有效性的指标。其他或未指明部位肿瘤所占比例(O&U%)的ICD-10编码包括:C26、C39、C48、C75、C76-C80。国家癌症中心要求比例在一个适当的范围内,且比例不能过低。

2.3 Death certificate only percent

Cancer cases notified to registries via death certificates is death certificate notified(DCN)cases. Cancers cases for which no other information other than a death certificate mentioning cancer can be obtained are death certificate only(DCO). DCO% is an indicator of the validity and completeness of the diagnostic information. Compared with cancer cases with clinical or histological diagnosis, the information of DCO cases is less accurate. A high percent of DCO reflects flaws in case tracing procedures.

$$Death\ certificate\ only\ percent(DCO\%)= \frac{DCO\ cases}{All\ new\ cases} \times 100\%$$

2.4 Proportion of missing information

Proportion of missing information is the proportion of cases with unknown age, unknown sex, other and unspecified cancer sites(O&U%) or unknown diagnosis basis(UB%). It is an indicator of the validity of the diagnostic information. The ICD-10 codes for cases with other and unspecified cancer sites are C26, C39, C48, C75, C76-C80. Proportion of missing information should be within an appropriate scope. It shouldn't be too low.

3 统计分类

3.1 癌症分类

参照国际上常用的癌症 ICD-10 分类统计表，根据 ICD-10 前三位"C"类编码，将癌症细分类为 59 部位、25 个大类，其中脑和神经系统包括良性及良恶性未定肿瘤（D32-D33，D42-D43）。真性红细胞增多症（D45）、骨髓增生异常综合征（D46）、淋巴造血和有关组织动态未定肿瘤（D47）归入髓系白血病（C92）。原位癌暂未纳入统计分析（表 2-1、表 2-2）。

3 Classification and coding

3.1 Cancer classification

Taken from the WHO cancer classification publications of ICD-10 version, cancers were classified into 59 types and 25 categories with different anatomic sites. The neoplasms of cerebral and central nervous system including benign and malignant undetermined tumors (D32-D33, D42-D43) are included in the ICD-10 cancer dictionary. For polycythemia vera (D45), myelodysplastic syndrome (D46) and other neoplasms of uncertain or unknown behavior of lymphopoid (D47) are coded as myeloid leukemia (C92). Carcinoma in situ was not included in the analyses (Table 2-1, Table 2-2).

表 2-1　常用癌症分类统计表（细分类）
Table 2-1　Lists for cancer classification by ICD-10 (detailed classification)

部位 Site	ICD-10
唇 Lip	C00
舌 Tongue	C01-C02
口 Mouth	C03-C06
唾液腺 Salivary gland	C07-C08
扁桃体 Tonsil	C09
其他口咽 Other oropharynx	C10
鼻咽 Nasopharynx	C11
下咽 Hypopharynx	C12-C13
咽,部位不明 Pharynx, unspecified	C14
食管 Esophagus	C15
胃 Stomach	C16
小肠 Small intestine	C17
结肠 Colon	C18
直肠 Rectum	C19-C20
肛门 Anus	C21
肝脏 Liver	C22
胆囊及其他 Gallbladder etc.	C23-C24
胰腺 Pancreas	C25
鼻、鼻窦及其他 Nose, sinuses etc.	C30-C31
喉 Larynx	C32
气管、支气管、肺 Trachea, bronchus & lung	C33-C34
其他胸腔器官 Other thoracic organs	C37-C38

部位 Site	ICD-10
骨 Bone	C40-C41
皮肤黑色素瘤 Melanoma of skin	C43
皮肤其他 Other skin	C44
间皮瘤 Mesothelioma	C45
卡波西肉瘤 Kaposi sarcoma	C46
周围神经、其他结缔组织、软组织 Peripheral nerve、Other connective & soft tissue	C47,C49
乳腺 Breast	C50
外阴 Vulva	C51
阴道 Vagina	C52
子宫颈 Cervix uteri	C53
子宫体 Corpus uteri	C54
子宫,部位不明 Uterus,unspecified	C55
卵巢 Ovary	C56
其他女性生殖器官 Other female genital organs	C57
胎盘 Placenta	C58
阴茎 Penis	C60
前列腺 Prostate	C61
睾丸 Testis	C62
其他男性生殖器官 Other male genital organs	C63
肾 Kidney	C64
肾盂 Renal pelvis	C65
输尿管 Ureter	C66
膀胱 Bladder	C67
其他泌尿器官 Other urinary organs	C68
眼 Eye	C69
脑、神经系统 Brain,nervous system	C70-C72,D32-D33,D42-D43
甲状腺 Thyroid	C73
肾上腺 Adrenal gland	C74
其他内分泌腺 Other endocrine	C75
霍奇金淋巴瘤 Hodgkin lymphoma	C81
非霍奇金淋巴瘤 Non-Hodgkin lymphoma	C82-C86,C96
免疫增生性疾病 Immunoproliferative diseases	C88
多发性骨髓瘤 Multiple myeloma	C90
淋巴细胞白血病 Lymphocytic leukemia	C91
髓系白血病 Myeloid leukemia	C92-C94,D45-D47
白血病,未特指 Leukemia,unspecified	C95
其他或未指明部位 Other and unspecified	O&U(C26,C39,C48,C75,C76-C80)
所有部位合计 All sites	C00-C97,D32-D33,D42-D43,D45-D47
所有部位除外 C44 All sites except C44	C00-C97,D32-D33,D42-D43,D45-D47,exc. C44

部位全称 Full title of site	部位缩写 Short title of site	ICD-10
口腔和咽喉（除外鼻咽）Oral cavity & pharynx except nasopharynx	口腔 Oral cavity & pharynx	C00-C10，C12-C14
鼻咽 Nasopharynx	鼻咽 Nasopharynx	C11
食管 Esophagus	食管 Esophagus	C15
胃 Stomach	胃 Stomach	C16
结直肠肛门 Colon，rectum & anus	结直肠 Colorectum	C18-C21
肝脏 Liver	肝 Liver	C22
胆囊及其他 Gallbladder etc.	胆囊 Gallbladder	C23-C24
胰腺 Pancreas	胰腺 Pancreas	C25
喉 Larynx	喉 Larynx	C32
气管、支气管、肺 Trachea，bronchus & lung	肺 Lung	C33-C34
其他胸腔器官 Other thoracic organs	其他胸腔器官 Other thoracic organs	C37-C38
骨 Bone	骨 Bone	C40-C41
皮肤黑色素瘤 Melanoma of skin	皮肤黑色素瘤 Melanoma of skin	C43
乳房 Breast	乳房 Breast	C50
子宫颈 Cervix uteri	子宫颈 Cervix	C53
子宫体及子宫部位不明 Uterus & unspecified	子宫体 Uterus	C54-C55
卵巢 Ovary	卵巢 Ovary	C56
前列腺 Prostate	前列腺 Prostate	C61
睾丸 Testis	睾丸 Testis	C62
肾及泌尿系统不明 Kidney & unspecified urinary organs	肾 Kidney	C64-C66，C68
膀胱 Bladder	膀胱 Bladder	C67
脑、神经系统 Brain，nervous system	脑 Brain	C70-C72，D32-D33，D42-D43
甲状腺 Thyroid	甲状腺 Thyroid	C73
淋巴瘤 Lymphoma	淋巴瘤 Lymphoma	C81-C86，C88，C90，C96
白血病 Leukemia	白血病 Leukemia	C91-C95，D45-D47
其他或未指明部位 Other and unspecified	其他 Other	Other
所有部位合计 All sites	合计 All sites	C00-C97，D32-D33，D42-D43，D45-D47

3.2 自然地区分类

城市、农村地区分类根据《中华人民共和国行政区划代码》(GB/T 2260—2007),将地级以上城市归于城市地区,县及县级市归于农村地区,同时综合考虑地区经济及生活方式等因素。

东、中、西部地区的划分采用国家统计局标准。

东部地区包括:北京市、天津市、河北省、辽宁省、上海市、江苏省、浙江省、福建省、山东省、广东省、海南省、香港特别行政区、澳门特别行政区、台湾省。

中部地区包括:黑龙江省、吉林省、山西省、安徽省、江西省、河南省、湖北省、湖南省。

西部地区包括:内蒙古自治区、广西壮族自治区、重庆市、四川省、贵州省、云南省、西藏自治区、陕西省、甘肃省、青海省、宁夏回族自治区、新疆维吾尔自治区。

七大行政区划分根据民政部区划分类(未包括香港特别行政区、澳门特别行政区和台湾省)。

华北地区:北京市、天津市、河北省、山西省、内蒙古自治区。

东北地区:辽宁省、吉林省、黑龙江省。

华东地区:上海市、江苏省、浙江省、安徽省、福建省、江西省、山东省。

华中地区:河南省、湖北省、湖南省。

华南地区:广东省、广西壮族自治区、海南省。

西南地区:重庆市、四川省、贵州省、云南省、西藏自治区。

西北地区:陕西省、甘肃省、青海省、宁夏回族自治区、新疆维吾尔自治区。

3.2 Natural area classification

According to the *Codes for the administrative divisions of the People's Republic of China* (*GB/T 2260—2007*), prefecture-level cities are classified into urban areas, whereas counties and county-level cities are classified into rural areas. And the socio-economic status of the areas are considered.

The classification of eastern areas, central areas and western areas is based on the standard of National Statistics Bureau.

The eastern areas consists of Beijing Shi, Tianjin Shi, Hebei Sheng, Liaoning Sheng, Shanghai Shi, Jiangsu Sheng, Zhejiang Sheng, Fujian Sheng, Shandong Sheng, Guangdong Sheng, Hainan Sheng, Hongkong Tebiexingzhengqu, Macao Tebiexingzhengqu, Taiwan Sheng.

The central areas consist of Heilongjiang Sheng, Jilin Sheng, Shanxi Sheng, Anhui Sheng, Jiangxi Sheng, Henan Sheng, Hubei Sheng and Hunan Sheng.

The western areas consist of Nei Mongol Zizhiqu, Guangxi Zhuangzu Zizhiqu, Chongqing Shi, Sichuan Sheng, Guizhou Sheng, Yunnan Sheng, Xizang Zizhiqu, Shaanxi Sheng, Gansu Sheng, Qinghai Sheng, Ningxia Huizu Zizhiqu and Xinjiang Uygur Zizhiqu.

According to the standard from Ministry of Civil Affairs of the People's Republic of China, the classification of these seven areas is shown as following(not including Hongkong Tebiexingzhengqu, Macao Tebiexingzhengqu and Taiwan Sheng).

North China: Beijing Shi, Tianjin Shi, Hebei Sheng, Shanxi Sheng, Nei Mongol Zizhiqu.

Northeast China: Liaoning Sheng, Jilin Sheng, Heilongjiang Sheng.

East China: Shanghai Shi, Jiangsu Sheng, Zhejiang Sheng, Anhui Sheng, Fujian Sheng, Jiangxi Sheng, Shandong Sheng.

Central China: Henan Sheng, Hubei Sheng, Hunan Sheng.

South China: Guangdong Sheng, Guangxi Zhuangzu Zizhiqu, Hainan Sheng.

Southwest China: Chongqing Shi, Sichuan Sheng, Guizhou Sheng, Yunnan Sheng, Xizang Zizhiqu.

Northwest China: Shaanxi Sheng, Gansu Sheng, Qinghai Sheng, Ningxia Huizu Zizhiqu, Xinjiang Uygur Zizhiqu.

4 常用统计指标

4.1 年平均人口数

年平均人口数是计算发病（死亡）率指标的分母,精确算法是一年内每一天暴露于发病（死亡）危险的生存人数之和除以年内天数,但实际上很难掌握每一天的生存人数,因而常用年初和年末人口数的算术平均数作为年平均人口数的近似值。公式如下:

$$年平均人口数（人）= \frac{年初（上年末）人口数+年末人口数}{2}$$

年中人口数指 7 月 1 日零时人口数,如果人口数变化均匀,年中人口数等于年平均人口数,可以用年中人口数代替年平均人口数。

4.2 性别、年龄别人口数

性别、年龄别人口数是指按男、女性别和不同年龄分组的人口数,建议用"内插法"推算。规定年龄别划分如下:0 ~ 岁、1 ~ 4 岁、5 ~ 9 岁、10 ~ 14 岁……80 ~ 84 岁、85 岁及以上。

4.3 发病（死亡）率

发病（死亡）率又称为粗发病（死亡）率,是反映人口发病（死亡）情况的基本指标,是指某年该地登记的每 10 万人口癌症新病例（死亡）数,反映人口发病（死亡）水平。

$$发病（死亡）率（1/10 万）= \frac{某时期恶性肿瘤新病例（死亡）数}{某时期年平均人口数} \times 100\,000$$

4 Statistical indicators

4.1 Average annual population

Average annual population is the denominator of the incidence(mortality) rates. The exact method to calculate is the average of persons at risk of incidence(mortality) each day in a specific year. Considering the complexity of the calculation, the arithmetic mean of the population at the beginning and end of the year is commonly used as an approximation of the annual average population. The formula is:

$$\text{Average annual population} = \frac{\text{population at the end of the year} + \text{population in the early of the year}}{2}$$

The mid-year population is the number of populations in 1st July at 0AM. If the population is relatively stable, the mid-year population can be used to represent average annual population.

4.2 Sex-and age-specific population

Sex-specific population is the population by sex. Age-specific population is the population by different age groups. Sex-and age-specific population can be calculated by interpolation. The ages may be grouped into classes of up to five years, for example, 0, 1-4, 5-9, 10-14…80-84, 85+.

4.3 Incidence(mortality) rate

The incidence(mortality) rate, also known as crude incidence(mortality) rate, is a basic indicator reflecting the incidence(mortality) of the population. It refers to the number of new cancer cases(deaths) registered in a certain area for every 100 000 people in a certain year, reflecting the level of incidence(mortality) rate in the population.

$$\text{Incidence(mortality) rate per 100 000} = \frac{\text{new cases(new cancer death) occurring during a given time period}}{\text{average population covered during the same time period}} \times 100\,000$$

4.4 年龄别发病(死亡)率

人口的年龄结构是影响癌症发病(死亡)水平的重要因素,年龄别发病(死亡)率是统计研究的重要指标。

$$某年龄组发病(死亡)率(1/10万) =\frac{某年龄组发病(死亡)人数}{同年龄组人口数} \times 100\,000$$

4.5 年龄调整率(标准化率)

由于粗发病(死亡)率受人口年龄构成的影响较大,因此在对比分析不同地区的发病(死亡)率或同一地区人群不同时期的发病(死亡)水平时,为消除人口年龄结构对发病(死亡)水平的影响,需要计算按年龄标准化的发病(死亡)率,即指按照某一标准人口的年龄结构所计算的发病(死亡)率。本年报使用中国标准人口是2000年第五次全国人口普查的人口构成(简称"中标率"),世界标准人口采用Segi's标准人口构成(简称"世标率")。表2-3为中国人口和世界人口年龄构成,可供计算年龄标准化率时选用。

年龄调整发病(死亡)率的计算(直接法):

(1)计算年龄组发病(死亡)率。

(2)各年龄组发病(死亡)率乘以相应的标准人口年龄构成百分比,得到相应的理论发病(死亡)率。

4.4 Age-specific incidence(mortality)rate

Age is an important factor influencing the cancer incidence and mortality. The age-specific rate is important statistical indicator.

$$\text{Age-specific incidence(mortality)rate per 100\,000} =\frac{\text{cases(cancer death)in a specific age group}}{\text{population in the age group}} \times 100\,000$$

4.5 Age-standardized rate(ASR)

Standardization is necessary when comparing populations with different age structures because age has such a powerful influence on cancer incidence and mortality. ASR is a summary measure of a rate that a population would have if it had a standard age structure.

In this annual cancer report, the population standards we used are the Segi's population and the fifth Chinese national census of 2000. Table 2-3 are the details of the population standards.

Direct method calculating incidence (mortality) rate:

(1)Calculating the rates for subjects in a specific age category in a study population.

(2)Calculating the weighted age-specific rates. The weights applied represent the relative age distribution of the standard population.

表2-3 标准人口构成
Table 2-3 Standard population

年龄组/岁 Age group/ years	2000年中国人口构成 China standard population(2000)	世界人口构成 Segi's population	年龄组/岁 Age group/ years	2000年中国人口构成 China standard population(2000)	世界人口构成 Segi's population
0~	13 793 799	2 400	45~	85 521 045	6 000
1~	55 184 575	9 600	50~	63 304 200	5 000
5~	90 152 587	10 000	55~	46 370 375	4 000
10~	125 396 633	9 000	60~	41 703 848	4 000
15~	103 031 165	9 000	65~	34 780 460	3 000
20~	94 573 174	8 000	70~	25 574 149	2 000
25~	117 602 265	8 000	75~	15 928 330	1 000
30~	127 314 298	6 000	80~	7 989 158	500
35~	109 147 295	6 000	85+	4 001 925	500
40~	81 242 945	6 000	合计	1 242 612 226	100 000

（3）将各年龄组的理论发病（死亡）率相加之和，即年龄标准化发病（死亡）率。

$$年龄标准化发病（死亡）率（1/10 万）= \frac{\sum 标准人口年龄构成×年龄别发病（死亡）率}{\sum 标准人口年龄构成} ×100\ 000$$

4.6 分类构成

各类癌症发病（死亡）构成比可以反映各类癌症对居民健康危害的情况。癌症发病（死亡）分类构成比的计算公式如下。

$$某癌症构成比（\%）= \frac{某癌症发病（死亡）人数}{总发病（死亡）人数} ×100$$

4.7 累积发病（死亡）率

累积发病（死亡）率是指某病在某一年龄阶段内按年龄（岁）的发病（死亡）率进行累积的总指标。累积发病（死亡）率消除了年龄构成不同的影响，故不需要标准化便可以与不同地区的数据直接进行比较。癌症一般是计算 0~74 岁的累积发病（死亡）率。

$$累积发病（死亡）率（\%）= \{\sum [年龄组发病（死亡）率×年龄组距]\}×100$$

4.8 截缩发病（死亡）率

对癌症通常截取 35~64 岁这一易发年龄段计算，其标准人口构成是世界人口。

$$截缩发病（死亡）率（1/10 万）= \frac{\sum 截缩段各年龄组发病（死亡）率×各段标准年龄构成}{\sum 各段标准年龄构成} ×100\ 000$$

因为癌症在 35 岁以前是少发的，而在 65 岁以后其他疾病较多，干扰较大，所以采用 35~64 岁这一阶段的截缩发病（死亡）率比较确切，便于比较。

（3）Adding up each weighted age-specific rate. The summary rates reflect the adjusted rates.

$$ASR\ per\ 100\ 000 = \frac{\sum standard\ population\ in\ corresponding\ age\ group×age\text{-}specific\ rate}{\sum standard\ population} ×100\ 000$$

4.6 Relative frequency

The relative frequency indicates harm of various types of cancer to the health of residents. The formular is：

$$Relative\ frequency\ of\ a\ certain\ type\ of\ cancer（\%）= \frac{number\ of\ cases\ of\ a\ particular\ cancer}{number\ of\ cases\ of\ all\ cancers} ×100$$

4.7 Cumulative incidence（mortality）rate

A cumulative incidence（mortality）rate expresses the probability of the onset of cancer between birth and a specific age. The rate can be compared without age standardization as it is not affected by age structures. This is often expressed for population between 0 and 74 years.

$$Cumulative\ incidence\ （mortality） rate（\%）= [\sum （age\text{-}specific\ incidence\ （mortality）rate×width\ of\ the\ agegroup）]×100$$

4.8 Truncated incidence（mortality）rate

The truncated incidence（mortality）rate is the calculation of rate over the truncated age-range 35-64，using WHO world standard population.

The data are presented as truncated rates mainly because cancer occurred less common before the age of 35，and there are more other diseases and disturbances after the age of 65，using the truncated incidence（mortality）rate between the ages of 35 and 64 is more accurate and easier to compare.

$$Truncated\ incidence\ （mortality） rate\ per\ 100\ 000 = \frac{\sum trancated\ age\text{-}specificincidence（mortality）rate×standard\ proportion\ of\ the\ age\ group}{\sum standard\ population} ×100\ 000$$

5 生存率

生存率是评价癌症治疗是否有效的关键指标。以人群为基础的肿瘤登记工作收集患者的生存资料,计算生存率以反映肿瘤人群的生存状况。某时间生存率是指某一批随访对象中生存期大于等于该时间的研究对象的比例,如5年生存率等。常用的生存率指标有观察生存率、净生存率和相对生存率。生存率实质是累积生存概率。

5.1 观察生存率

观察生存率分析中,以患者死亡为观察终点,包括死于肿瘤和其他原因。肿瘤登记资料常用寿命表法估计观察生存率。寿命表法应用定群寿命表的基本原理计算生存率,可利用截尾数据的不完全信息。

5.2 调整生存率/净生存率

观察生存率反映的是肿瘤患者的整体死亡状况。在很多情况下,人们关注肿瘤患者死于肿瘤的信息。此时,常常需要计算调整生存率/净生存率。净生存率估计的关键是必须依据完整、准确的死因信息。在比较不同年龄、性别、社会经济学状况下癌症患者的生存率时,使用净生存率显得尤为重要,因为肿瘤外其他死因会影响癌症患者的生存状况。

净生存率可通过计算疾病特异性生存率获得,即以患者死于该肿瘤为观察终点。若肿瘤患者死于肿瘤之外的其他原因,将与存活状态同等处理。

5 Survival rate

Survival rate is an overall index for measuring the effectiveness of cancer care. The survival rate calculated based on data from population-based cancer registries will therefore represent the average prognosis in the population. Survival rate can be expressed in terms of the percentage of those cases who were still alive after a specified interval (i. e. 5 years). The measures for survival rate calculation include observed survival rate, net survival rate, and relative survival rate, which are the cumulative probability of survival from diagnosis to the end of each time interval.

5.1 Observed survival rate

In the analysis of the observed survival rate, the endpoint is patient death, including death from cancers and other causes. The life table method is commonly used to estimate the observed survival rate in cancer registration data. The life table method applies the basic principle of fixed group life tables to calculate survival rates, and can utilize incomplete information from truncated data.

5.2 Adjusted survival/net survival rate

The observed survival rate can be interpreted as the probability of survival from cancer and all other causes of deaths combined. In many cases, people pay more attention to information about cancer patients dying from cancers. At this point, it is often necessary to calculate the adjusted survival rate/net survival rate. The key to estimate the net survival rate is to rely on complete and accurate cause of death information. It is a crucial measure for survival rate comparisons among patients with different age, sex and socioeconomic status, because other causes of death other than cancer can affect the survival status of cancer patients.

Net survival rate can be achieved through calculating disease-specific survival rate, which relies on reliable individual cause of death. If the cancer patients die from causes other than cancer, it will be treated as alive.

5.3 相对生存率

当缺乏完整、准确的全死因信息时,净生存率指标往往较难通过疾病特异性生存率获取。此时,净生存率可以通过相对生存率来估计。相对生存率即为特定人群的观察生存率与该人群的期望生存率比值。根据全死因寿命表的死亡率,可以求得一般人群的期望生存率。观察生存率常采用寿命表法,而期望生存率的计算方法有 Ederer Ⅰ、Ederer Ⅱ、Hakulinen 方法等。

$$相对生存率 = \frac{观察生存率}{期望生存率}$$

5.3 Relative survival rate

When death certificate is not publicly available, or certification of the cause of death is not sufficiently reliable, net survival rate is hardly achieved through disease-specific survival rate, which needs the exact cause of death for cancer patients. Relative survival rates are usually expressed as a ratio of the crude survival rate in the group of cancer patients and the corresponding expected survival rate in the general population. The expected survival rate of the general population can be obtained based on the mortality rate of the all-cause life table. Observed survival rate can be achieved by life-table/actual methods, while expected survival rate can be estimated with methods of Ederer Ⅰ, Ederer Ⅱ and Hakulinen, et al.

$$Relative\ survival\ rate = \frac{observed\ survival\ rate}{expected\ survival\ rate}$$

第三章 数据质量评价

1 数据来源

2022 年国家癌症中心收到全国 1 073 个肿瘤登记处提交的 2019 年肿瘤登记资料。登记处分布在 31 个省(自治区、直辖市)及新疆生产建设兵团(未包括香港特别行政区、澳门特别行政区和台湾省),其中地级以上城市 357 个,县和县级市 716 个。四川省上报资料登记处数量最多(121 个),其次为云南省(94 个)、新疆维吾尔自治区(71 个)、广西壮族自治区(56 个)。北京市、天津市、上海市、广州市、石家庄市登记地区覆盖了全部区县,在本年报分城乡按 2 个登记处计(表 3-1)。

Chapter 3 Evaluation of data quality

1 Data sources

A total of 1 073 cancer registries submitted cancer registration data of 2019 to NCC China in 2022. A total of 31provinces(autonomous regions, municipalities) and Xinjiang Production and Construction Corps(not including Hongkong Tebiexingzhengqu, Macao Tebiexingzhengqu and Taiwan Sheng) were covered by these registries, with a total of 357 prefecture-level cities and 716 counties (county-level cities). Sichuan Sheng submitted data from most cancer registries(121), followed by Yunnan Sheng(94), Xinjiang Uygur Zizhiqu (71), and Guangxi Zhuangzu Zizhiqu(56). The data from Beijing Shi, Tianjin Shi, Shanghai Shi, Guangzhou Shi and Shijiazhuang Shi covered all districts and counties. They were classified as urban and rural areas separately in this annual report(Table 3-1).

表 3-1 2019 年全国提交肿瘤登记资料的地区

Table 3-1 The cancer registries which submitted cancer statistics of 2019

省(自治区、直辖市) Province (autonomous region, municipality)	登记处数 No. of cancer registries	登记处名单 List of cancer registries
北京市 Beijing Shi	2	北京市 Beijing Shi、北京市郊区 Rural areas of Beijing Shi
天津市 Tianjin Shi	2	天津市 Tianjin Shi、天津市郊区 Rural areas of Tianjin Shi
河北省 Hebei Sheng	41	石家庄市 Shijiazhuang Shi、石家庄市井陉矿区 Jingxing Kuangqu,Shijiazhuang Shi、石家庄市郊区 Rural areas of Shijiazhuang Shi、井陉县 Jingxing Xian、行唐县 Xingtang Xian、灵寿县 Lingshou Xian、高邑县 Gaoyi Xian、赞皇县 Zanhuang Xian、无极县 Wuji Xian、元氏县 Yuanshi Xian、赵县 Zhao Xian、新乐市 Xinle Shi、迁西县 Qianxi Xian、迁安市 Qian'an Shi、秦皇岛市 Qinhuangdao Shi、邯郸市邯山区 Hanshan Qu,Handan Shi、邯郸市峰峰矿区 Fengfeng Kuangqu,Handan Shi、大名县 Daming Xian、涉县 She Xian、磁县 Ci Xian、武安市 Wu'an Shi、邢台市 Xingtai Shi、临城县 Lincheng Xian、内丘县 Neiqiu Xian、邢台市任泽区 Renze Qu,Xingtai Shi、保定市 Baoding Shi、望都县 Wangdu Xian、安国市 Anguo Shi、张家口市宣化区 Xuanhua Qu,Zhangjiakou Shi、张北县 Zhangbei Xian、承德市双桥区 Shuangqiao Qu, Chengde Shi、丰宁满族自治县 Fengning Manzu Zizhixian、沧州市 Cangzhou Shi、海兴县 Haixing Xian、盐山县 Yanshan Xian、三河市 Sanhe Shi、衡水市桃城区 Taocheng Qu,Hengshui Shi、衡水市冀州区 Jizhou Qu,Hengshui Shi、枣强县 Zaoqiang Xian、景县 Jing Xian、辛集市 Xinji Shi

省(自治区、直辖市) Province (autonomous region, municipality)	登记处数 No. of cancer registries	登记处名单 List of cancer registries
山西省 Shanxi Sheng	29	太原市小店区 Xiaodian Qu,Taiyuan Shi、太原市杏花岭区 Xinghualing Qu,Taiyuan Shi、太原市万柏林区 Wanbailin Qu,Taiyuan Shi、阳泉市 Yangquan Shi、平定县 Pingding Xian、盂县 Yu Xian、襄垣县 Xiangyuan Xian、平顺县 Pingshun Xian、沁源县 Qinyuan Xian、阳城县 Yangcheng Xian、陵川县 Lingchuan Xian、晋中市榆次区 Yuci Qu,Jizhong Shi、晋中市太谷区 Taigu Qu,Jinzhong Shi、昔阳县 Xiyang Xian、寿阳县 Shouyang Xian、稷山县 Jishan Xian、新绛县 Xinjiang Xian、绛县 Jiang Xian、垣曲县 Yuanqu Xian、芮城县 Ruicheng Xian、忻州市忻府区 Xinfu Qu,Xinzhou Shi、定襄县 Dingxiang Xian、原平市 Yuanping Shi、襄汾县 Xiangfen Xian、洪洞县 Hongtong Xian、交城县 Jiaocheng Xian、临县 Lin Xian、孝义市 Xiaoyi Shi、汾阳市 Fenyang Shi
内蒙古自治区 Nei Mongol Zizhiqu	36	武川县 Wuchuan Xian、乌海市 Wuhai Shi、赤峰市红山区 Hongshan Qu,Chifeng Shi、赤峰市元宝山区 Yuanbaoshan Qu,Chifeng Shi、赤峰市松山区 Songshan Qu,Chifeng Shi、巴林左旗 Bairin Zuoqi、敖汉旗 Aohan Qi、通辽市科尔沁区 Horqin Qu,Tongliao Shi、科尔沁左翼中旗 Horqin Zuoyi Zhongqi、科尔沁左翼后旗 Horqin Zuoyi Houqi、开鲁县 Kailu Xian、库伦旗 Hure Qi、奈曼旗 Naiman Qi、扎鲁特旗 Jarud Qi、霍林郭勒市 Holin Gol Shi、呼伦贝尔市海拉尔区 Hailar Qu,Hulun Buir Shi、呼伦贝尔市扎赉诺尔区 Dalai Nur Qu,Hulun Buir Shi、阿荣旗 Arun Qi、莫力达瓦达翰尔族自治旗 Morin Dawa Daurzu Zizhiqi、鄂伦春自治旗 Oroqen Zizhiqi、鄂温克族自治旗 Ewenkizu Zizhiqi、陈巴尔虎旗 Chen Barag Qi、新巴尔虎左旗 Xin Barag Zuoqi、新巴尔虎右旗 Xin Barag Youqi、满洲里市 Manzhouli Shi、牙克石市 Yakeshi Shi、扎兰屯市 Zalantun Shi、根河市 Genhe Shi、巴彦淖尔市临河区 Linhe Qu,Bayannur Shi、五原县 Wuyuan Xian、杭锦后旗 Hanggin Houqi、锡林浩特市 Xilin Hot Shi、苏尼特左旗 Sonid Zuoqi、苏尼特右旗 Sonid Youqi、东乌珠穆沁旗 Dong Ujimqin Qi、太仆寺旗 Taibus Qi
辽宁省 Liaoning Sheng	21	沈阳市 Shenyang Shi、康平县 Kangping Xian、法库县 Faku Xian、新民市 Xinmin Shi、大连市 Dalian Shi、大连市金州区 Jinzhou Qu,Dalian Shi、庄河市 Zhuanghe Shi、鞍山市 Anshan Shi、岫岩满族自治县 Xiuyan Manzu Zizhixian、抚顺市 Fushun Shi、本溪市 Benxi Shi、丹东市 Dandong Shi、东港市 Donggang Shi、锦州市 Jinzhou Shi、营口市 Yingkou Shi、阜新市 Fuxin Shi、彰武县 Zhangwu Xian、辽阳县 Liaoyang Xian、盘锦市 Panjin Shi、盘锦市大洼区 Dawa Qu,Panjin Shi、建平县 Jianping Xian
吉林省 Jilin Sheng	34	长春市朝阳区 Chaoyang Qu,Changchun Shi、德惠市 Dehui Shi、吉林市 Jilin Shi、永吉县 Yongji Xian、蛟河市 Jiaohe Shi、桦甸市 Huadian Shi、舒兰市 Shulan Shi、磐石市 Panshi Shi、四平市铁西区 Tiexi Qu,Siping Shi、四平市铁东区 Tiedong Qu,Siping Shi、梨树县 Lishu Xian、伊通满族自治县 Yitong Manzu Zizhixian、双辽市 Shuangliao Shi、辽源市龙山区 Longshan Qu,Liaoyuan Shi、东辽县 Dongliao Xian、通化市 Tonghua Shi、通化县 Tonghua Xian、梅河口市 Meihekou Shi、集安市 Ji'an Shi、白山市浑江区 Hunjiang Qu,Baishan Shi、抚松县 Fusong Xian、松原市宁江区 Ningjiang Qu,Songyuan Shi、前郭尔罗斯蒙古族自治县 Qian Gorlos Mongolzu Zizhixian、乾安县 Qian'an Xian、通榆县 Tongyu Xian、大安市 Da'an Shi、延吉市 Yanji Shi、图们市 Tumen Shi、敦化市 Dunhua Shi、珲春市 Hunchun Shi、龙井市 Longjing Shi、和龙市 Helong Shi、汪清县 Wangqing Xian、安图县 Antu Xian

省（自治区、直辖市） Province （autonomous region，municipality）	登记处数 No. of cancer registries	登记处名单 List of cancer registries
黑龙江省 Heilongjiang Sheng	11	哈尔滨市道里区 Daoli Qu，Harbin Shi、哈尔滨市南岗区 Nangang Qu，Harbin Shi、哈尔滨市香坊区 Xiangfang Qu，Harbin Shi、尚志市 Shangzhi Shi、五常市 Wuchang Shi、勃利县 Boli Xian、牡丹江市东安区 Dong'an Qu，Mudanjiang Shi、牡丹江市阳明区 Yangming Qu，Mudanjiang Shi、牡丹江市爱民区 Aimin Qu，Mudanjiang Shi、牡丹江市西安区 Xi'an Qu，Mudanjiang Shi、海林市 Hailin Shi
上海市 Shanghai Sheng	2	上海市 Shanghai Shi、上海市郊区 Rural areas of Shanghai Shi
江苏省 Jiangsu Sheng	55	南京市六合区 Luhe Qu，Nanjing Shi、南京市溧水区 Lishui Qu，Nanjing Shi、南京市高淳区 Gaochun Qu，Nanjing Shi、无锡市 Wuxi Shi、江阴市 Jiangyin Shi、宜兴市 Yixing Shi、徐州市 Xuzhou Shi、邳州市 Pizhou Shi、常州市 Changzhou Shi、溧阳市 Liyang Shi、常州市金坛区 Jintan Qu，Changzhou Shi、苏州市 Suzhou Shi、常熟市 Changshu Shi、张家港市 Zhangjiagang Shi、昆山市 Kunshan Shi、太仓市 Taicang Shi、南通市 Nantong Shi、南通市海门区 Haimen Qu，Nantong Shi、如东县 Rudong Xian、启东市 Qidong Shi、如皋市 Rugao Shi、海安市 Hai'an Shi、连云港市 Lianyungang Shi、连云港市赣榆区 Ganyu Qu，Lianyungang Shi、东海县 Donghai Xian、灌云县 Guanyun Xian、灌南县 Guannan Xian、淮安市淮安区 Huai'an Qu，Huai'an Shi、淮安市淮阴区 Huaiyin Qu，Huai'an Shi、淮安市清江浦区 Qingjiangpu Qu，Huai'an Shi、涟水县 Lianshui Xian、淮安市洪泽区 Hongze Qu，Huai'an Shi、盱眙县 Xuyi Xian、金湖县 Jinhu Xian、盐城市亭湖区 Tinghu Qu，Yancheng Shi、盐城市盐都区 Yandu Qu，Yancheng Shi、响水县 Xiangshui Xian、滨海县 Binhai Xian、阜宁县 Funing Xian、射阳县 Sheyang Xian、建湖县 Jianhu Xian、东台市 Dongtai Shi、盐城市大丰区 Dafeng Qu，Yancheng Shi、扬州市广陵区 Guangling Qu，Yangzhou Shi、扬州市邗江区 Hanjiang Qu，Yangzhou Shi、宝应县 Baoying Xian、仪征市 Yizheng Shi、扬州市江都区 Jiangdu Qu，Yangzhou Shi、丹阳市 Danyang Shi、扬中市 Yangzhong Shi、泰兴市 Taixing Shi、宿迁市宿城区 Sucheng Qu，Suqian Shi、沭阳县 Shuyang Xian、泗阳县 Siyang Xian、泗洪县 Sihong Xian
浙江省 Zhejiang Sheng	22	杭州市 Hangzhou Shi、宁波市鄞州区 Yinzhou Qu，Ningbo Shi、慈溪市 Cixi Shi、温州市鹿城区 Lucheng Qu，Wenzhou Shi、乐清市 Yueqing Shi、嘉兴市 Jiaxing Shi、嘉善县 Jiashan Xian、海宁市 Haining Shi、湖州市南浔区 Nanxun Qu，Huzhou Shi、长兴县 Changxing Xian、诸暨市 Zhuji Shi、绍兴市上虞区 Shangyu Qu，Shaoxing Shi、金华市婺城区 Wucheng Qu，Jinhua Shi、永康市 Yongkang Shi、衢州市柯城区 Kecheng Qu，Quzhou Shi、开化县 Kaihua Xian、舟山市定海区 Dinghai Qu，Zhoushan Shi、岱山县 Daishan Xian、仙居县 Xianju Xian、温岭市 Wenling Shi、丽水市莲都区 Liandu Qu，Lishui Shi、龙泉市 Longquan Shi
安徽省 Anhui Sheng	44	合肥市 Hefei Shi、长丰县 Changfeng Xian、肥东县 Feidong Xian、肥西县 Feixi Xian、庐江县 Lujiang Xian、巢湖市 Chaohu Shi、芜湖市 Wuhu Shi、芜湖市繁昌区 Fanchang Qu，Wuhu Shi、南陵县 Nanling Xian、蚌埠市 Bengbu Shi、五河县 Wuhe Xian、淮南市潘集区 Panji Qu，Huainan Shi、凤台县 Fengtai Xian、寿县 Shou Xian、马鞍山市 Ma'anshan Shi、当涂县 Dangtu Xian、濉溪县 Suixi Xian、铜陵市 Tongling Shi、铜陵市义安区 Yi'an Qu，Tongling Shi、安庆市迎江区 Yingjiang Qu，Anqing Shi、安庆市大观区 Daguan Qu，Anqing Shi、安庆市宜秀区 Yixiu Qu，Anqing Shi、怀宁县 Huaining Xian、太湖县 Taihu Xian、望江县 Wangjiang Xian、岳西县 Yuexi Xian、桐城市 Tongcheng Shi、潜山市 Qianshan Shi、定远县 Dingyuan Xian、天长市 Tianchang Shi、阜阳市颍州区 Yingzhou Qu，Fuyang Shi、阜阳市颍东区 Yingdong Qu，Fuyang Shi、阜阳市颍泉区 Yingquan Qu，Fuyang Shi、太和县 Taihe Xian、阜南县 Funan Xian、界首市 Jieshou Shi、宿州市埇桥区 Yongqiao Qu，Suzhou Shi、灵璧县 Lingbi Xian、六安市金安区 Jin'an Qu，Lu'an Shi、金寨县 Jinzhai Xian、蒙城县 Mengcheng Xian、东至县 Dongzhi Xian、泾县 Jing Xian、宁国市 Ningguo Shi

省（自治区、直辖市） Province （autonomous region, municipality）	登记处数 No. of cancer registries	登记处名单 List of cancer registries
福建省 Fujian Sheng	20	罗源县 Luoyuan Xian、永泰县 Yongtai Xian、福清市 Fuqing Shi、福州市长乐区 Changle Qu, Fuzhou Shi、厦门市 Xiamen Shi、厦门市同安区 Tong'an Qu, Xiamen Shi、厦门市翔安区 Xiang'an Qu, Xiamen Shi、莆田市涵江区 Hanjiang Qu, Putian Shi、明溪县 Mingxi Xian、大田县 Datian Xian、建宁县 Jianning Xian、永安市 Yong'an Shi、惠安县 Hui'an Xian、漳州市长泰区 Changtai Qu Zhangzhou Shi、建瓯市 Jian'ou Shi、龙岩市新罗区 Xinluo Qu, Longyan Shi、龙岩市永定区 Yongding Qu, Longyan Shi、上杭县 Shanghang Xian、武平县 Wuping Xian、连城县 Liancheng Xian
江西省 Jiangxi Sheng	40	南昌市东湖区 Donghu Qu, Nanchang Shi、南昌市青山湖区 Qingshanhu Qu, Nanchang Shi、南昌市新建区 Xinjian Qu, Nanchang Shi、萍乡市安源区 Anyuan Qu, Pingxiang Shi、萍乡市湘东区 Xiangdong Qu, Pingxiang Shi、芦溪县 Luxi Xian、九江市浔阳区 Xunyang Qu, Jiujiang Shi、武宁县 Wuning Xian、新余市渝水区 Yushui Qu, Xinyu Shi、鹰潭市余江区 Yujiang Qu, Yingtan Shi、赣州市章贡区 Zhanggong Qu, Ganzhou Shi、赣州市赣县区 Ganxian Qu, Ganzhou Shi、信丰县 Xinfeng Xian、大余县 Dayu Xian、上犹县 Shangyou Xian、崇义县 Chongyi Xian、龙南市 Longnan Shi、于都县 Yudu Xian、峡江县 Xiajiang Xian、新干县 Xingan Xian、安福县 Anfu Xian、万载县 Wanzai Xian、上高县 Shanggao Xian、靖安县 Jing'an Xian、樟树市 Zhangshu Shi、崇仁县 Chongren Xian、乐安县 Le'an Xian、宜黄县 Yihuang Xian、抚州市东乡区 Dongxiang Qu, Fuzhou Shi、上饶市信州区 Xinzhou Qu, Shangrao Shi、上饶市广丰区 Guangfeng Qu, Shangrao Shi、上饶市广信区 Guangxin Qu, Shangrao Shi、铅山县 Yanshan Xian、横峰县 Hengfeng Xian、弋阳县 Yiyang Xian、余干县 Yugan Xian、鄱阳县 Poyang Xian、万年县 Wannian Xian、婺源县 Wuyuan Xian、德兴市 Dexing Shi
山东省 Shandong Sheng	38	济南市 Jinan Shi、济南市章丘区 Zhangqiu Qu, Jinan Shi、济南市莱芜区 Laiwu Qu, Jinan Shi、青岛市 Qingdao Shi、青岛市黄岛区 Huangdao Qu, Qingdao Shi、淄博市临淄区 Linzi Qu, Zibo Shi、沂源县 Yiyuan Xian、滕州市 Tengzhou Shi、东营市东营区 Dongying Qu, Dongying Shi、广饶县 Guangrao Xian、烟台市 Yantai Shi、莱州市 Laizhou Shi、招远市 Zhaoyuan Shi、潍坊市潍城区 Weicheng Qu, Weifang Shi、临朐县 Linqu Xian、青州市 Qingzhou Shi、高密市 Gaomi Shi、济宁市任城区 Rencheng Qu, Jining Shi、汶上县 Wenshang Xian、梁山县 Liangshan Xian、曲阜市 Qufu Shi、邹城市 Zoucheng Shi、宁阳县 Ningyang Xian、肥城市 Feicheng Shi、乳山市 Rushan Shi、日照市东港区 Donggang Qu, Rizhao Shi、莒县 Ju Xian、沂南县 Yinan Xian、沂水县 Yishui Xian、莒南县 Junan Xian、德州市德城区 Decheng Qu, Dezhou Shi、临邑县 Linyi Xian、聊城市东昌府区 Dongchangfu Qu, Liaocheng Shi、高唐县 Gaotang Xian、滨州市滨城区 Bincheng Qu, Binzhou Shi、菏泽市牡丹区 Mudan Qu, Heze Shi、单县 Shan Xian、巨野县 Juye Xian
河南省 Henan Sheng	50	郑州市 Zhengzhou Shi、巩义市 Gongyi Shi、开封市祥符区 Xiangfu Qu, Kaifeng Shi、洛阳市 Luoyang Shi、洛阳市孟津区 Mengjin Qu, Luoyang Shi、新安县 Xin'an Xian、栾川县 Luanchuan Xian、嵩县 Song Xian、汝阳县 Ruyang Xian、宜阳县 Yiyang Xian、洛宁县 Luoning Xian、伊川县 Yichuan Xian、洛阳市偃师区 Yanshi Qu, Luoyang Shi、平顶山市 Pingdingshan Shi、鲁山县 Lushan Xian、郏县 Jia Xian、舞钢市 Wugang Shi、林州市 Linzhou Shi、鹤壁市 Hebi Shi、浚县 Xun Xian、淇县 Qi Xian、辉县市 Huixian Shi、温县 Wen Xian、濮阳市华龙区 Hualong Qu, Puyang Shi、清丰县 Qingfeng Xian、南乐县 Nanle Xian、范县 Fan Xian、濮阳县 Puyang Xian、许昌市魏都区 Weidou Qu, Xuchang Shi、禹州市 Yuzhou Shi、漯河市源汇区 Yuanhui Qu, Luohe Shi、漯河市郾城区 Yancheng Qu, Luohe Shi、漯河市召陵区 Shaoling Qu, Luohe Shi、舞阳县 Wuyang Xian、临颍县 Linying Xian、三门峡市湖滨区 Hubin Qu, Sanmenxia Shi、义马市 Yima Shi、南阳市卧龙区 Wolong Qu, Nanyang Shi、南召县 Nanzhao Xian、方城县 Fangcheng Xian、内乡县 Neixiang Xian、虞城县 Yucheng Xian、信阳市浉河区 Shihe Qu, Xinyang Shi、罗山县 Luoshan Xian、沈丘县 Shenqiu Xian、郸城县 Dancheng Xian、太康县 Taikang Xian、项城市 Xiangcheng Shi、西平县 Xiping Xian、济源市 Jiyuan Shi

省（自治区、直辖市） Province （autonomous region, municipality）	登记处数 No. of cancer registries	登记处名单 List of cancer registries
湖北省 Hubei Sheng	22	武汉市 Wuhan Shi、大冶市 Daye Shi、十堰市郧阳区 Yunyang Qu,Shiyan Shi、丹江口市 Danjiangkou Shi、宜昌市 Yichang Shi、秭归县 Zigui Xian、五峰土家族自治县 Wufeng Tujiazu Zizhixian、宜都市 Yidu Shi、襄阳市 Xiangyang Shi、枣阳市 Zaoyang Shi、宜城市 Yicheng Shi、京山市 Jingshan Shi、钟祥市 Zhongxiang Shi、云梦县 Yunmeng Xian、荆州市 Jingzhou Shi、公安县 Gong'an Xian、洪湖市 Honghu Shi、麻城市 Macheng Shi、嘉鱼县 Jiayu Xian、通城县 Tongcheng Xian、恩施市 Enshi Shi、天门市 Tianmen Shi
湖南省 Hunan Sheng	36	长沙市芙蓉区 Furong Qu,Changsha Shi、长沙市天心区 Tianxin Qu,Changsha Shi、长沙市岳麓 Yuelu Qu,Changsha Shi、长沙市开福区 Kaifu Qu,Changsha Shi、长沙市雨花区 Yuhua Qu,Changsha Shi、长沙市望城区 Wangcheng Qu,Changsha Shi、长沙县 Changsha Xian、宁乡市 Ningxiang Shi、浏阳市 Liuyang Shi、株洲市芦淞区 Lusong Qu,Zhuzhou Shi、株洲市石峰区 Shifeng Qu,Zhuzhou Shi、攸县 You Xian、湘潭市雨湖区 Yuhu Qu,Xiangtan Shi、衡东县 Hengdong Xian、常宁市 Changning Shi、邵东市 Shaodong Shi、新宁县 Xinning Xian、岳阳市岳阳楼区 Yueyanglou Qu,Yueyang Shi、常德市武陵区 Wuling Qu,Changde Shi、安乡县 Anxiang Xian、津市市 Jinshi Shi、张家界市永定区 Yongding Qu,Zhangjiajie Shi、慈利县 Cili Xian、益阳市资阳区 Ziyang Qu,Yiyang Shi、桃江县 Taojiang Xian、临武县 Linwu Xian、资兴市 Zixing Shi、道县 Dao Xian、宁远县 Ningyuan Xian、新田县 Xintian Xian、麻阳苗族自治县 Mayang Miaozu Zizhixian、洪江市 Hongjiang Shi、双峰县 Shuangfeng Xian、冷水江市 Lengshuijiang Shi、涟源市 Lianyuan Shi、泸溪县 Luxi Xian
广东省 Guangdong Sheng	49	广州市 Guangzhou Shi、广州市郊区 Rural areas of Guangzhou Shi、韶关市曲江区 Qujiang Qu,Shaoguan Shi、翁源县 Wengyuan Xian、南雄市 Nanxiong Shi、深圳市 Shenzhen Shi、珠海市 Zhuhai Shi、汕头市澄海区 Chenghai Qu,Shantou Shi、佛山市禅城区 Chancheng Qu,Foshan Shi、佛山市南海区 Nanhai Qu,Foshan Shi、佛山市顺德区 Shunde Qu,Foshan Shi、佛山市三水区 Sanshui Qu,Foshan Shi、佛山市高明区 Gaoming Qu,Foshan Shi、江门市 Jiangmen Shi、湛江市赤坎区 Chikan Qu,Zhanjiang Shi、湛江市霞山区 Xiashan Qu,Zhanjiang Shi、湛江市坡头区 Potou Qu,Zhanjiang Shi、湛江市麻章区 Mazhang Qu,Zhanjiang Shi、遂溪县 Suixi Xian、徐闻县 Xuwen Xian、廉江市 Lianjiang Shi、雷州市 Leizhou Shi、吴川市 Wuchuan Shi、茂名市茂南区 Maonan Qu,Maoming Shi、高州市 Gaozhou Shi、肇庆市端州区 Duanzhou Qu,Zhaoqing Shi、肇庆市鼎湖区 Dinghu Qu,Zhaoqing Shi、肇庆市高要区 Gaoyao Qu,Zhaoqing Shi、肇庆市高新区 Gaoxin Qu,Zhaoqing Shi、广宁县 Guangning Xian、怀集县 Huaiji Xian、封开县 Fengkai Xian、德庆县 Deqing Xian、四会市 Sihui Shi、惠州市惠阳区 Huiyang Qu,Huizhou Shi、梅州市梅江区 Meijiang Qu,Meizhou Shi、梅州市梅县区 Meixian Qu,Meizhou Shi、大埔县 Dabu Xian、汕尾市城区 Chengqu,Shanwei Shi、河源市源城区 Yuancheng Qu,Heyuan Shi、阳江市阳东区 Yangdong Qu,Yangjiang Shi、清远市清城区 Qingcheng Qu,Qingyuan Shi、阳山县 Yangshan Xian、东莞市 Dongguan Shi、中山市 Zhongshan Shi、潮州市潮安区 Chao'an Qu,Chaozhou Shi、揭西县 Jiexi Xian、普宁市 Puning Shi、罗定市 Luoding Shi

省(自治区、直辖市) Province (autonomous region, municipality)	登记处数 No. of cancer registries	登记处名单 List of cancer registries
广西壮族自治区 Guangxi Zhuangzu Zizhiqu	56	南宁市兴宁区 Xingning Qu, Nanning Shi、南宁市青秀区 Qingxiu Qu, Nanning Shi、南宁市江南区 Jiangnan Qu, Nanning Shi、南宁经济技术开发区 Nanning Economic & Technological Development Area、南宁市西乡塘区 Xixiangtang Qu, Nanning Shi、南宁市良庆区 Liangqing Qu, Nanning Shi、南宁市邕宁区 Yongning Qu, Nanning Shi、南宁东盟经济开发区 National Nanning-ASEAN Economic Development Area、南宁市武鸣区 Wuming Qu, Nanning Shi、隆安县 Long'an Xian、马山县 Mashan Xian、上林县 Shanglin Xian、宾阳县 Binyang Xian、横州市 Hengzhou Shi、柳州市 Liuzhou Shi、柳城县 Liucheng Xian、鹿寨县 Luzhai Xian、融安县 Rong'an Xian、桂林市 Guilin Shi、阳朔县 Yangshuo Xian、灵川县 Lingchuan Xian、兴安县 Xing'an Xian、灌阳县 Guanyang Xian、龙胜各族自治县 Longsheng Gezu Zizhixian、资源县 Ziyuan Xian、平乐县 Pingle Xian、荔浦市 Lipu Shi、恭城瑶族自治县 Gongcheng Yaozu Zizhixian、梧州市 Wuzhou Shi、苍梧县 Cangwu Xian、北海市 Beihai Shi、合浦县 Hepu Xian、防城港市港口区 Gangkou Qu, Fangchenggang Shi、钦州市钦南区 Qinnan Qu, Qinzhou Shi、浦北县 Pubei Xian、贵港市港北区 Gangbei Qu, Guigang Shi、贵港市港南区 Gangnan Qu, Guigang Shi、贵港市覃塘区 Qintang Qu, Guigang Shi、平南县 Pingnan Xian、桂平市 Guiping Shi、北流市 Beiliu Shi、百色市右江区 Youjiang Qu, Bose Shi、百色市田阳区 Tianyang Qu, Bose Shi、田东县 Tiandong Xian、凌云县 Lingyun Xian、贺州市八步区 Babu Qu, Hezhou Shi、钟山县 Zhongshan Xian、河池市金城江区 Jinchengjiang Qu, Hechi Shi、罗城仫佬族自治县 Luocheng Mulaozu Zizhixian、来宾市兴宾区 Xingbin Qu, Laibin Shi、合山市 Heshan Shi、崇左市江州区 Jiangzhou Qu, Chongzuo Shi、扶绥县 Fusui Xian、龙州县 Longzhou Xian、大新县 Daxin Xian、天等县 Tiandeng Xian
海南省 Hainan Sheng	9	海口市 Haikou Shi、三亚市 Sanya Shi、儋州市 Danzhou Shi、五指山市 Wuzhishan Shi、琼海市 Qionghai Shi、东方市 Dongfang Shi、定安县 Ding'an Xian、昌江黎族自治县 Changjiang Lizu Zizhixian、陵水黎族自治县 Lingshui Lizu Zizhixian
重庆市 Chongqing Shi	39	重庆市万州区 Wanzhou Qu, Chongqing Shi、重庆市涪陵区 Fuling Qu, Chongqing Shi、重庆市渝中区 Yuzhong Qu, Chongqing Shi、重庆市大渡口区 Dadukou Qu, Chongqing Shi、重庆市江北区 Jiangbei Qu, Chongqing Shi、重庆市沙坪坝区 Shapingba Qu, Chongqing Shi、重庆市九龙坡区 Jiulongpo Qu, Chongqing Shi、重庆市南岸区 Nan'an Qu, Chongqing Shi、重庆市北碚区 Beibei Qu, Chongqing Shi、重庆市綦江区 Qijiang Qu, Chongqing Shi、重庆市大足区 Dazu Qu, Chongqing Shi、重庆市渝北区 Yubei Qu, Chongqing Shi、重庆市巴南区 Banan Qu, Chongqing Shi、重庆市黔江区 Qianjiang Qu, Chongqing Shi、重庆市长寿区 Changshou Qu, Chongqing Shi、重庆市江津区 Jiangjin Qu, Chongqing Shi、重庆市合川区 Hechuan Qu, Chongqing Shi、重庆市永川区 Yongchuan Qu, Chongqing Shi、重庆市南川区 Nanchuan Qu, Chongqing Shi、重庆市万盛经济技术开发区 Wansheng Economic & Technological Development Zone, Chongqing Shi、重庆市潼南区 Tongnan Qu, Chongqing Shi、重庆市铜梁区 Tongliang Qu, Chongqing Shi、重庆市荣昌区 Rongchang Qu, Chongqing Shi、重庆市璧山区 Bishan Qu, Chongqing Shi、重庆市梁平区 Liangping Qu, Chongqing Shi、城口县 Chengkou Xian、丰都县 Fengdu Xian、垫江县 Dianjiang Xian、重庆市武隆区 Wulong Qu, Chongqing Shi、忠县 Zhong Xian、重庆市开州区 Kaizhou Qu, Chongqing Shi、云阳县 Yunyang Xian、奉节县 Fengjie Xian、巫山县 Wushan Xian、巫溪县 Wuxi Xian、石柱土家族自治县 Shizhu Tujiazu Zizhixian、秀山土家族苗族自治县 Xiushan Tujiazu Miaozu Zizhixian、酉阳土家族苗族自治县 Youyang Tujiazu Miaozu Zizhixian、彭水苗族土家族自治县 Pengshui Miaozu Tujiazu Zizhixian

省（自治区、直辖市） Province （autonomous region，municipality）	登记处数 No. of cancer registries	登记处名单 List of cancer registries
四川省 Sichuan Sheng	121	成都市锦江区 Jinjiang Qu，Chengdu Shi、成都市青羊区 Qingyang Qu，Chengdu Shi、成都市金牛区 Jinniu Qu，Chengdu Shi、成都市武侯区 Wuhou Qu，Chengdu Shi、成都市成华区 Chenghua Qu，Chengdu Shi、成都市龙泉驿区 Longquanyi Qu，Chengdu Shi、成都市青白江区 Qingbaijiang Qu，Chengdu Shi、成都市新都区 Xindu Qu，Chengdu Shi、成都市温江区 Wenjiang Qu，Chengdu Shi、金堂县 Jintang Xian、成都市双流区 Shuangliu Qu，Chengdu Shi、成都市天府新区 Tianfu Xinqu，Chengdu Shi、成都市郫都区 Pidu Qu，Chengdu Shi、大邑县 Dayi Xian、蒲江县 Pujiang Xian、成都市新津区 Xinjin Qu，Chengdu Shi、简阳市 Jianyang Shi、都江堰市 Dujiangyan Shi、彭州市 Pengzhou Shi、邛崃市 Qionglai Shi、崇州市 Chongzhou Shi、自贡市自流井区 Ziliujing Qu，Zigong Shi、自贡市贡井区 Gongjing Qu，Zigong Shi、自贡市大安区 Da'an Qu，Zigong Shi、自贡市沿滩区 Yantan Qu，Zigong Shi、荣县 Rong Xian、富顺县 Fushun Xian、攀枝花市东区 Dong Qu，Panzhihua Shi、攀枝花市西区 Xi Qu，Panzhihua Shi、攀枝花市仁和区 Renhe Qu，Panzhihua Shi、米易县 Miyi Xian、泸州市江阳区 Jiangyang Qu，Luzhou Shi、泸州市纳溪区 Naxi Qu，Luzhou Shi、泸州市龙马潭区 Longmatan Qu，Luzhou Shi、泸县 Lu Xian、合江县 Hejiang Xian、叙永县 Xuyong Xian、德阳市旌阳区 Jingyang Qu，Deyang Shi、中江县 Zhongjiang Xian、德阳市罗江区 Luojiang Qu，Deyang Shi、广汉市 Guanghan Shi、什邡市 Shifang Shi、绵竹市 Mianzhu Shi、绵阳市涪城区 Fucheng Qu，Mianyang Shi、绵阳市游仙区 Youxian Qu，Mianyang Shi、绵阳市安州区 Anzhou Qu，Mianyang Shi、三台县 Santai Xian、盐亭县 Yanting Xian、梓潼县 Zitong Xian、北川羌族自治县 Beichuan Qiangzu Zizhixian、平武县 Pingwu Xian、江油市 Jiangyou Shi、广元市利州区 Lizhou Qu，Guangyuan Shi、广元市昭化区 Zhaohua Qu，Guangyuan Shi、广元市朝天区 Chaotian Qu，Guangyuan Shi、旺苍县 Wangcang Xian、青川县 Qingchuan Xian、剑阁县 Jiange Xian、苍溪县 Cangxi Xian、遂宁市船山区 Chuanshan Qu，Suining Shi、遂宁市安居区 Anju Qu，Suining Shi、蓬溪县 Pengxi Xian、射洪市 Shehong Shi、大英县 Daying Xian、内江市市中区 Shizhong Qu，Neijiang Shi、内江市东兴区 Dongxing Qu，Neijiang Shi、威远县 Weiyuan Xian、资中县 Zizhong Xian、隆昌市 Longchang Shi、乐山市市中区 Shizhong Qu，Leshan Shi、乐山市沙湾区 Shawan Qu，Leshan Shi、乐山市五通桥区 Wutongqiao Qu，Leshan Shi、乐山市金口河区 Jinkouhe Qu，Leshan Shi、犍为县 Qianwei Xian、井研县 Jingyan Xian、夹江县 Jiajiang Xian、沐川县 Muchuan Xian、峨眉山市 Emeishan Shi、南充市高坪区 Gaoping Qu，Nanchong Shi、营山县 Yingshan Xian、仪陇县 Yilong Xian、西充县 Xichong Xian、阆中市 Langzhong Shi、眉山市东坡区 Dongpo Qu，Meishan Shi、眉山市彭山区 Pengshan Qu，Meishan Shi、仁寿县 Renshou Xian、洪雅县 Hongya Xian、丹棱县 Danling Xian、青神县 Qingshen Xian、宜宾市翠屏区 Cuiping Qu，Yibin Shi、宜宾市南溪区 Nanxi Qu，Yibin Shi、宜宾市叙州区 Xuzhou Qu，Yibing Shi、江安县 Jiang'an Xian、长宁县 Changning Xian、兴文县 Xingwen Xian、广安市广安区 Guang'an Qu，Guang'an Shi、广安市前锋区 Qianfeng Qu，Guang'an Shi、岳池县 Yuechi Xian、武胜县 Wusheng Xian、邻水县 Linshui Xian、华蓥市 Huaying Shi、达州市达川区 Dachuan Qu，Dazhou Shi、宣汉县 Xuanhan Xian、大竹县 Dazhu Xian、渠县 Qu Xian、雅安市雨城区 Yucheng Qu，Ya'an Shi、雅安市名山区 Mingshan Qu，Ya'an Shi、荥经县 Yingjing Xian、汉源县 Hanyuan Xian、石棉县 Shimian Xian、天全县 Tianquan Xian、芦山县 Lushan Xian、宝兴县 Baoxing Xian、巴中市巴州区 Bazhou Qu，Bazhong Shi、通江县 Tongjiang Xian、南江县 Nanjiang Xian、平昌县 Pingchang Xian、资阳市雁江区 Yanjiang Qu，Ziyang Shi、安岳县 Anyue Xian、乐至县 Lezhi Xian、汶川县 Wenchuan Xian

省（自治区、直辖市） Province （autonomous region, municipality）	登记处数 No. of cancer registries	登记处名单 List of cancer registries
贵州省 Guizhou Sheng	33	开阳县 Kaiyang Xian、息烽县 Xifeng Xian、修文县 Xiuwen Xian、清镇市 Qingzhen Shi、六盘水市钟山区 Zhongshan Qu,Lupanshui Shi、六盘水市六枝特区 Luzhi Tequ,Lupanshui Shi、盘州市 Panzhou Shi、遵义市汇川区 Huichuan Qu,Zunyi Shi、绥阳县 Suiyang Xian、习水县 Xishui Xian、赤水市 Chishui Shi、安顺市西秀区 Xixiu Qu,Anshun Shi、镇宁布依族苗族自治县 Zhenning Buyeizu Miaozu Zizhixian、金沙县 Jinsha Xian、铜仁市碧江区 Bijiang Qu,Tongren Shi、江口县 Jiangkou Xian、玉屏侗族自治县 Yuping Dongzu Zizhixian、印江土家族苗族自治县 YinjiangTujiazu Miaozu Zizhixian、册亨县 Ceheng Xian、黄平县 Huangping Xian、镇远县 Zhenyuan Xian、天柱县 Tianzhu Xian、锦屏县 Jinping Xian、台江县 Taijiang Xian、榕江县 Rongjiang Xian、雷山县 Leishan Xian、麻江县 Majiang Xian、丹寨县 Danzhai Xian、都匀市 Duyun Shi、福泉市 Fuquan Shi、荔波县 Libo Xian、瓮安县 Weng'an Xian、龙里县 Longli Xian
云南省 Yunnan Sheng	94	昆明市五华区 Wuhua Qu,Kunming Shi、昆明市盘龙区 Panlong Qu,Kunming Shi、昆明市官渡区 Guandu Qu,Kunming Shi、昆明市西山区 Xishan Qu,Kunming Shi、昆明市东川区 Dongchuan Qu,Kunming Shi、昆明市呈贡区 Chenggong Qu,Kunming Shi、昆明市晋宁区 Jinning Qu,Kunming Shi、富民县 Fumin Xian、宜良县 Yiliang Xian、石林彝族自治县 Shilin Yizu Zizhixian、嵩明县 Songming Xian、禄劝彝族苗族自治县 Luchuan Yizu Miaozu Zizhixian、寻甸回族彝族自治县 Xundian Huizu Yizu Zizhixian、安宁市 Anning Shi、曲靖市麒麟区 Qilin Qu,Qujing Shi、曲靖市沾益区 Zhanyi Qu,Qujing Shi、曲靖市马龙区 Malong Qu,Qujing Shi、师宗县 Shizong Xian、罗平县 Luoping Xian、富源县 Fuyuan Xian、宣威市 Xuanwei Shi、玉溪市红塔区 Hongta Qu,Yuxi Shi、玉溪市江川区 Jiangchuan Qu,Yuxi Shi、澄江市 Chengjiang Shi、通海县 Tonghai Xian、华宁县 Huaning Xian、易门县 Yimen Xian、峨山彝族自治县 Eshan Yizu Zizhixian、新平彝族傣族自治县 Xinping Yizu Daizu Zizhixian、元江哈尼族彝族傣族自治县 Yuanjiang Hanizu Yizu Daizu Zizhixian、保山市隆阳区 Longyang Qu,Baoshan Shi、施甸县 Shidian Xian、龙陵县 Longling Xian、昌宁县 Changning Xian、腾冲市 Tengchong Shi、绥江县 Suijiang Xian、彝良县 Yiliang Xian、水富市 Shuifu Shi、丽江市古城区 Gucheng Qu,Lijiang Shi、玉龙纳西族自治县 Yulong Naxizu Zizhixian、永胜县 Yongsheng Xian、华坪县 Huaping Xian、宁蒗彝族自治县 Ninglang Yizu Zizhixian、宁洱哈尼族彝族自治县 Ning'er Hanizu Yizu Zizhixian、景东彝族自治县 Jingdong Yizu Zizhixian、景谷傣族彝族自治县 Jinggu Daizu Yizu Zizhixian、镇沅彝族哈尼族拉祜族自治县 Zhengyuan Yizu Hanizu Lahuzu Zizhixian、江城哈尼族彝族自治县 Jiangcheng Hanizu Yizu Zizhixian、澜沧拉祜族自治县 Lancang Lahuzu Zizhixian、临沧市临翔区 Linxiang Qu,Lincang Shi、凤庆县 Fengqing Xian、云县 Yun Xian、永德县 Yongde Xian、镇康县 Zhenkang Xian、双江拉祜族佤族布朗族傣族自治县 Shuangjiang Lahuzu Vazu Blangzu Daizu Zizhixian、沧源佤族自治县 Cangyuan Vazu Zizhixian、楚雄市 Chuxiong Shi、双柏县 Shuangbai Xian、牟定县 Mouding Xian、南华县 Nanhua Xian、姚安县 Yao'an Xian、大姚县 Dayao Xian、永仁县 Yongren Xian、元谋县 Yuanmou Xian、武定县 Wuding Xian、禄丰市 Lufeng Shi、个旧市 Gejiu Shi、开远市 Kaiyuan Shi、蒙自市 Mengzi Shi、屏边苗族自治县 Pingbian Miaozu Zizhixian、建水县 Jianshui Xian、石屏县 Shiping Xian、弥勒市 Mile Shi、泸西县 Luxi Xian、文山市 Wenshan Shi、砚山县 Yanshan Xian、西畴县 Xichou Xian、麻栗坡县 Malipo Xian、马关县 Maguan Xian、丘北县 Qiubei Xian、富宁县 Funing Xian、景洪市 Jinghong Shi、大理市 Dali Shi、祥云县 Xiangyun Xian、宾川县 Bingchuan Xian、弥渡县 Midu Xian、南涧彝族自治县 Nanjian Yizu Zizhixian、永平县 Yongping Xian、洱源县 Eryuan Xian、梁河县 Lianghe Xian、陇川县 Longchuan Xian、泸水市 Lushui Shi、贡山独龙族怒族自治县 Gongshan DerungzuNuzu Zizhixian、香格里拉市 Shangêlila Shi

省(自治区、直辖市) Province (autonomous region, municipality)	登记处数 No. of cancer registries	登记处名单 List of cancer registries
西藏自治区 Xizang Zizhiqu	2	拉萨市城关区 Chengguan Qu, Lhasa Shi、昌都市 Qamdo Shi
陕西省 Shaanxi Sheng	49	西安市新城区 Xincheng Qu, Xi'an Shi、西安市碑林区 Beilin Qu, Xi'an Shi、西安市莲湖区 Lianhu Qu, Xi'an Shi、西安市未央区 Weiyang Qu, Xi'an Shi、西安市雁塔区 Yanta Qu, Xi'an Shi、西安市阎良区 Yanliang Qu, Xi'an Shi、西安市临潼区 Lintong Qu, Xi'an Shi、西安市长安区 Chang'an Qu, Xi'an Shi、西安市高陵区 Gaoling Qu, Xi'an Shi、西安市鄠邑区 Huyi Qu, Xi'an Shi、蓝田县 Lantian Xian、铜川市耀州区 Yaozhou Qu, Tongchuan Shi、宝鸡市渭滨区 Weibin Qu, Baoji Shi、宝鸡市金台区 Jintai Qu, Baoji Shi、宝鸡市陈仓区 Chencang Qu, Baoji Shi、宝鸡市凤翔区 Fengxiang Qu, Baoji Shi、扶风县 Fufeng Xian、眉县 Mei Xian、陇县 Long Xian、千阳县 Qianyang Xian、麟游县 Linyou Xian、太白县 Taibai Xian、泾阳县 Jingyang Xian、武功县 Wugong Xian、渭南市临渭区 Linwei Qu, Weinan Shi、渭南市华州区 Huazhou Qu, Weinan Shi、潼关县 Tongguan Xian、大荔县 Dali Xian、合阳县 Heyang Xian、蒲城县 Pucheng Xian、富平县 Fuping Xian、华阴市 Huayin Shi、延安市宝塔区 Baota Qu, Yan'an Shi、志丹县 Zhidan Xian、富县 Fu Xian、黄龙县 Huanglong Xian、黄陵县 Huangling Xian、汉中市汉台区 Hantai Qu, Hanzhong Shi、城固县 Chenggu Xian、宁强县 Ningqiang Xian、绥德县 Suide Xian、安康市汉滨区 Hanbin Qu, Ankang Shi、汉阴县 Hanyin Xian、宁陕县 Ningshan Xian、紫阳县 Ziyang Xian、旬阳市 Xunyang Shi、商洛市商州区 Shangzhou Qu, Shangluo Shi、丹凤县 Danfeng Xian、镇安县 Zhen'an Xian
甘肃省 Gansu Sheng	23	兰州市城关区 Chengguan Qu, Lanzhou Shi、兰州市七里河区 Qilihe Qu, Lanzhou Shi、兰州市西固区 Xigu Qu, Lanzhou Shi、兰州市安宁区 Anning Qu, Lanzhou Shi、兰州市红古区 Honggu Qu, Lanzhou Shi、白银市白银区 Baiyin Qu, Baiyin Shi、白银市平川区 Pingchuan Qu, Baiyin Shi、靖远县 Jingyuan Xian、会宁县 Huining Xian、景泰县 Jingtai Xian、天水市秦州区 Qinzhou Qu, Tianshui Shi、天水市麦积区 Maiji Qu, Tianshui Shi、武威市凉州区 Liangzhou Qu, Wuwei Shi、民勤县 Minqin Xian、古浪县 Gulang Xian、天祝藏族自治县 Tianzhu Zangzu Zizhixian、张掖市甘州区 Ganzhou Qu, Zhangye Shi、高台县 Gaotai Xian、静宁县 Jingning Xian、敦煌市 Dunhuang Shi、庆城县 Qingcheng Xian、临洮县 Lintao Xian、临潭县 Lintan Xian
青海省 Qinghai Sheng	8	西宁市 Xining Shi、大通回族土族自治县 Datong Huizu Tuzu Zizhixian、西宁市湟中区 Huangzhong Qu, Xining Shi、海东市乐都区 Ledu Qu, Haidong Shi、民和回族土族自治县 Minhe Huizu Tuzu Zizhixian、互助土族自治县 Huzhu Tuzu Zizhixian、循化撒拉族自治县 Xunhua Salarzu Zizhixian、海南藏族自治州 Hainan Zangzu Zizhizhou
宁夏回族自治区 Ningxia Huizu Zizhiqu	11	银川市兴庆区 Xingqing Qu, Yinchuan Shi、银川市西夏区 Xixia Qu, Yinchuan Shi、银川市金凤区 Jinfeng Qu, Yinchuan Shi、贺兰县 Helan Xian、石嘴山市大武口区 Dawukou Qu, Shizuishan Shi、石嘴山市惠农区 Huinong Qu, Shizuishan Shi、平罗县 Pingluo Xian、青铜峡市 Qingtongxia Shi、固原市原州区 Yuanzhou Qu, Guyuan Shi、中卫市沙坡头区 Shapotou Qu, Zhongwei Shi、中宁县 Zhongning Xian

省（自治区、直辖市） Province （autonomous region, municipality）	登记处数 No. of cancer registries	登记处名单 List of cancer registries
新疆维吾尔自治区 Xinjiang Uygur Zizhiqu	71	乌鲁木齐市天山区 Tianshan Qu，Ürümqi Shi、乌鲁木齐市新市区 Xinshi Qu，Ürümqi Shi、乌鲁木齐市水磨沟区 Shuimogou Qu，Ürümqi Shi、乌鲁木齐市达坂城区 Dabancheng Qu，Ürümqi Shi、乌鲁木齐市米东区 Midong Qu，Ürümqi Shi、乌鲁木齐县 Ürümqi Xian、克拉玛依市 Karamay Shi、克拉玛依市乌尔禾区 Orku Qu，Karamay Shi、吐鲁番市高昌区 Gaochang Qu，Turpan Shi、鄯善县 Shanshan Xian、巴里坤哈萨克自治县 Barkol Kazak Zizhixian、伊吾县 Yiwu Xian、昌吉市 Changji Shi、阜康市 Fukang Shi、呼图壁县 Hutubi Xian、玛纳斯县 Manas Xian、奇台县 Qitai Xian、吉木萨尔县 Jimsar Xian、木垒哈萨克自治县 Mori Kazak Zizhixian、博乐市 Bole Shi、阿拉山口市 Alataw Shankou Shi、精河县 Jinghe Xian、温泉县 Wenquan Xian、库尔勒市 Korla Shi、尉犁县 Yuli Xian、焉耆回族自治县 Yanqi Huizu Zizhixian、和静县 Hejing Xian、博湖县 Bohu Xian、阿克苏市 Aksu Shi、温宿县 Wensu Xian、库车市 Kuqa Shi、沙雅县 Xayar Xian、拜城县 Baicheng Xian、阿瓦提县 Awat Xian、柯坪县 Kalpin Xian、阿图什市 Artux Shi、阿克陶县 Akto Xian、阿合奇县 Akqi Xian、疏附县 Shufu Xian、疏勒县 Shule Xian、英吉沙县 Yengisar Xian、泽普县 Zepu Xian、莎车县 Shache Xian、叶城县 Yecheng Xian、麦盖提县 Makit Xian、岳普湖县 Yopurga Xian、伽师县 Jiashi Xian、巴楚县 Bachu Xian、塔什库尔干塔吉克自治县 Taxkorgan Tajik Zizhixian、和田市 Hotan Shi、和田县 Hotan Xian、伊宁市 Yining Shi、伊宁县 Yining Xian、察布查尔锡伯自治县 Qapqal Xibe Zizhixian、霍城县 Huocheng Xian、新源县 Xinyuan Xian、特克斯县 Tekes Xian、尼勒克县 Nilka Xian、塔城市 Tacheng Shi、乌苏市 Usu Shi、沙湾市 Shawan Shi、托里县 Toli Xian、裕民县 Yumin Xian、和布克赛尔蒙古自治县 Hoboksar Mongol Zizhixian、阿勒泰市 Altay Shi、布尔津县 Burqin Xian、富蕴县 Fuyun Xian、福海县 Fuhai Xian、哈巴河县 Habahe Xian、青河县 Qinghe Xian、吉木乃县 Jeminay Xian
新疆生产建设兵团 Xinjiang Production and Construction Corps	3	第二师 Di'ershi、第七师 Diqishi、第八师 Dibashi

2 数据纳入排除标准

国家癌症中心成立肿瘤登记专家委员会和《中国肿瘤登记年报》编委会。在既往《中国肿瘤登记年报》数据入选原则基础上,根据《肿瘤随访登记技术方案》(卫生部疾病预防控制局,2009年)、《中国肿瘤登记工作指导手册(2016)》中的数据质量要求,参照国际癌症研究机构(IARC)/国际癌症登记协会(IACR)对肿瘤登记数据的质量控制规则,经充分研究与讨论,制定了《2022中国肿瘤登记年报》纳入排除标准。

本年报入选标准,注重肿瘤登记数据的真实性、稳定性和均衡性,根据登记地区的特点,综合评估该肿瘤登记处数据质量。重点考核指标要求发病率大于180/10万,死亡率水平基本不低于100/10万,MV%、DCO%、M/I合理。并兼顾地区差异,综合考虑肿瘤登记处各个指标在本地区的合理范围。对于新建立第一次上报数据的登记处,在上述规则的原则上,考虑社会经济发展水平、工作基础、少数民族地区等因素综合评估后择优录取,MV%标准适当放宽。对于曾经被收录的登记处,在行政区划没有变化的情况下,一般粗率变化幅度不能超过±10%。对于曾经上报过数据,但未曾被收录的登记处,变化幅度如果不在上述范围内,根据实际情况进一步核实评估。对于连续5年及以上被纳入年报的登记处数据,若个别指标不符合要求,但为保持连续性适当保留。

2 Data inclusion and exclusion criteria

NCC has established a panel of cancer registry experts and the editorial committee of *China Cancer Registry Annual Report*. According to the principle of selecting the previous annual report data and based on *Technical Protocols of Cancer Registration and Follow Up* by the former Disease Prevention and Control Bureau of the Ministry of Health 2009, *Chinese Guideline for Cancer Registration (2016)* and the quality control rules of cancer registration by the International Agency for Research on Cancer (IARC)/ the International Agency for Cancer Registry (IACR) , the editorial committee has established a comprehensive data inclusion and exclusion criteria of *2022 Chinese Cancer Registry Annual Report* after thorough investigation and discussion.

The data inclusion criteria were focused on the authenticity, stability, and comparability of cancer registry data quality. The quality of data was evaluated based on the characteristics of the corresponding regions. To pass the data inclusion criteria, one registry data should have an incidence of more than 180 per 100 000, while the morality of the data should be greater or equal to 100 per 100 000. The MV%, DCO%, and M/I should be reasonable. Taking regional disparity into account, the proper ranges of quality control indexes of registration data differed by areas. For registries which submitted data for the first time, the quality control index MV% could be flexible. And registries were enrolled with due consideration of their social economic development level, working foundation and ethnic minority conditions. For registries which data have already been included in the report before, changes of crude rates should be less than ±10% if the administrative divisions of the registries remained the same. For registries which have submitted data but have never been included in the report before, over ±10% changes of crude rates should be evaluated according to the actual situation of registries. For registries which have been consecutively included in the report over 5 years, their data were included in this report even if individual indexes were not qualified, in order to guarantee data continuity.

3 肿瘤登记资料评价

3.1 覆盖人口、发病数和死亡数

提交数据的全部肿瘤登记处覆盖人口 691 409 114 人,其中城市地区为 287 694 361 人,占全部覆盖人口的 41.61%,农村地区为 403 714 753 人,占 58.39%。全国登记地区覆盖人口占 2019 年全国年末人口数的 49.03%。2019 年报告癌症新发病例数合计 2 013 495 例,其中城市地区占 46.07%,农村地区占 53.93%。共计报告癌症死亡病例男女合计 1 126 427 例,城市地区占 43.46%,农村地区占 56.54%(表 3-2)。

3.2 数据质量评价

在提交 2019 年资料的 1 073 个登记处中,病理诊断比例(MV%)在 55%~95% 的登记处有 882 个(82.20%),病理诊断比例(MV%)小于 55% 和大于 95% 的分别为 185 个和 6 个,共占 17.80%。只有死亡证明书比例(DCO%)在 0~5% 的登记处有 752 个(70.08%),DCO% 为 0 的登记处有 218 个(20.32%),大于 5% 的登记处有 103 个(9.60%)。死亡/发病比(M/I)为 0.55~0.85 的登记处有 699 个(65.14%),M/I 小于 0.55 和大于 0.85 的登记处分别为 355 个和 19 个,占 34.86%。

2019 年第一次提交数据的登记处有 238 个,占 22.18%。与提交过 2018 年数据的 835 个登记处的癌症发病率相比,变化幅度在 10% 以内的登记处有 585 个,占提交过数据登记处总数的 70.06%。

3 Evaluation of cancer registration data

3.1 Population coverage, new cancer cases and cancer deaths

All cancer registries which submitted cancer data, the population coverage was 691 409 114, with 287 694 361 in urban areas(41.61%) and 403 714 753 in rural areas(58.39%). The covering population accounted for 49.03% of the overall national population of 2019. A total of 2 013 495 new cancer cases were reported in 2019. Among them, 46.07% were from urban areas and 53.93% were from rural areas. There were 1 126 427 new cancer deaths in 2019. The urban cancer deaths accounted for 43.46% of overall cancer deaths and rural cancer deaths accounted for 56.54%(Table 3-2).

3.2 Evaluation of data quality

Among the 1 073 registries which submitted the data of 2019, 882 registries(82.20%) had MV% between 55% and 95%. A total of 185 registries had MV% less than 55%, and 6 had MV% more than 95%, accounting for 17.80% of all registries. There were 752 registries having DCO% between 0 and 5%, accounting for 70.08% of all registries. A total of 218 registries(20.32%) reported no DCO cases, and 103 registries(9.60%) reported more than 5% of DCO cases. Among all registries, there were 699 registries(65.14%) having M/I between 0.55 and 0.85. 355 registries had M/I less than 0.55, 19 registries had M/I more than 0.85, accounting for 34.86%.

There were 238 registries(22.18%) submitted data to NCC for the first time. Compared with 835 cancer incidence rates in 2018(submitted data in 2018), 585 registries reported a change of rate in 2019 less than 10%, accounting for 70.06% of all those registries.

表 3-2　全国肿瘤登记地区覆盖人口、发病数、死亡数及主要质控指标
Table 3-2　The population coverage, new cancer cases, cancer deaths and major
indicators for data quality in cancer registration areas

序号 No.	肿瘤登记处 Cancer registries	人口数 Population	发病数 No. new cases	死亡数 No. deaths	MV%	DCO%	M/I	发病率变化 Change for CR%	接受 Accepted
1	北京市 Beijing Shi	8 543 242	38 726	17 880	82. 24	0. 06	0. 46	10. 05	Y
2	北京市郊区 Rural areas of Beijing Shi	5 322 999	20 540	9 519	79. 17	0. 04	0. 46	11. 34	Y
3	天津市 Tianjin Shi	5 574 694	25 107	12 436	57. 89	0. 22	0. 50	6. 28	Y
4	天津市郊区 Rural areas of Tianjin Shi	5 521 244	17 781	8 423	57. 61	0. 12	0. 47	10. 87	Y
5	石家庄市 Shijiazhuang Shi	2 282 709	6 368	3 407	85. 10	0. 17	0. 54	3. 59	Y
6	石家庄市井陉矿区 Jingxing Kuangqu, Shijiazhuang Shi	88 652	235	172	70. 64	2. 55	0. 73		Y
7	石家庄市郊区 Rural areas of Shijiazhuang Shi	2 439 842	5 548	3 560	80. 89	0. 32	0. 64	−0. 91	Y
8	井陉县 Jingxing Xian	332 299	725	443	83. 31	0. 55	0. 61		Y
9	行唐县 Xingtang Xian	461 762	554	162	63. 90	0. 00	0. 29		
10	灵寿县 Lingshou Xian	340 503	542	151	67. 90	0. 00	0. 28		
11	高邑县 Gaoyi Xian	186 478	433	311	67. 21	0. 69	0. 72		Y
12	赞皇县 Zanhuang Xian	281 343	622	450	69. 45	0. 16	0. 72	−2. 30	Y
13	无极县 Wuji Xian	537 636	758	127	73. 75	0. 00	0. 17		
14	元氏县 Yuanshi Xian	446 568	884	123	69. 12	0. 00	0. 14		
15	赵县 Zhao Xian	621 089	1 257	928	67. 14	0. 16	0. 74		Y
16	新乐市 Xinle Shi	530 349	1 095	669	63. 56	4. 02	0. 61		Y
17	迁西县 Qianxi Xian	418 046	949	638	85. 88	0. 42	0. 67	1. 88	Y
18	迁安市 Qian'an Shi	778 197	1 568	1 242	63. 14	0. 45	0. 79	1. 76	Y
19	秦皇岛市 Qinhuangdao Shi	1 472 212	3 202	2 081	80. 70	3. 40	0. 65	−0. 96	Y
20	邯郸市邯山区 Hanshan Qu, Handan Shi	556 177	1 115	741	75. 07	3. 05	0. 66	7. 28	Y
21	邯郸市峰峰矿区 Fengfeng Kuangqu, Handan Shi	478 001	1 025	705	58. 63	5. 66	0. 69		Y
22	大名县 Daming Xian	797 229	1 635	996	71. 38	0. 37	0. 61	−2. 76	Y
23	涉县 She Xian	434 164	1 423	956	79. 97	0. 35	0. 67	1. 15	Y
24	磁县 Ci Xian	666 412	1 904	1 341	84. 56	0. 68	0. 70	−0. 31	Y
25	武安市 Wu'an Shi	839 491	1 776	1 157	71. 06	1. 91	0. 65	−0. 65	Y
26	邢台市 Xingtai Shi	1 314 797	2 751	2 057	79. 53	0. 51	0. 75	9. 03	Y
27	临城县 Lincheng Xian	212 026	443	287	70. 43	0. 68	0. 65	0. 30	Y
28	内丘县 Neiqiu Xian	259 500	531	360	68. 36	4. 71	0. 68	−3. 92	Y

序号 No.	肿瘤登记处 Cancer registries	人口数 Population	发病数 No. new cases	死亡数 No. deaths	MV%	DCO%	M/I	发病率变化 Change for CR%	接受 Accepted
29	邢台市任泽区 Renze Qu, Xingtai Shi	340 665	756	558	72.35	0.26	0.74	7.62	Y
30	保定市 Baoding Shi	1 186 453	2 397	1 718	69.96	3.00	0.72	−6.94	Y
31	望都县 Wangdu Xian	262 636	586	328	66.89	4.27	0.56	11.27	Y
32	安国市 Anguo Shi	389 003	853	551	67.06	0.70	0.65	−0.65	Y
33	张家口市宣化区 Xuanhua Qu, Zhangjiakou Shi	562 069	1 128	809	66.13	0.18	0.72		Y
34	张北县 Zhangbei Xian	361 410	1 158	748	69.08	0.09	0.65	−5.21	Y
35	承德市双桥区 Shuangqiao Qu, Chengde Shi	327 085	650	395	72.00	0.31	0.61	−1.81	Y
36	丰宁满族自治县 Fengning Manzu Zizhixian	409 460	869	577	69.16	0.81	0.66	5.21	Y
37	沧州市 Cangzhou Shi	543 676	1 092	658	84.25	0.09	0.60	−3.49	Y
38	海兴县 Haixing Xian	220 571	447	261	69.57	1.79	0.58	−3.18	Y
39	盐山县 Yanshan Xian	467 779	923	523	78.66	4.55	0.57	−0.53	Y
40	三河市 Sanhe Shi	721 285	1 186	1 002	44.35	1.01	0.84		
41	衡水市桃城区 Taocheng Qu, Hengshui Shi	507 436	1 089	727	80.72	0.09	0.67		Y
42	衡水市冀州区 Jizhou Qu, Hengshui Shi	345 125	773	548	64.04	4.01	0.71	−3.99	Y
43	枣强县 Zaoqiang Xian	405 000	743	483	64.60	0.67	0.65		Y
44	景县 Jing Xian	546 000	1 054	720	64.61	0.09	0.68		Y
45	辛集市 Xinji Shi	636 701	1 395	834	76.63	0.72	0.60	2.08	Y
46	太原市小店区 Xiaodian Qu, Taiyuan Shi	854 328	938	687	69.94	3.20	0.73	−16.45	
47	太原市杏花岭区 Xinghualing Qu, Taiyuan Shi	673 994	2 305	1 340	61.43	8.42	0.58	5.67	Y
48	太原市万柏林区 Wanbailin Qu, Taiyuan Shi	796 633	267	619	65.17	0.00	2.32		
49	阳泉市 Yangquan Shi	682 092	1 978	1 150	72.35	7.84	0.58	14.72	Y
50	平定县 Pingding Xian	280 632	704	398	59.94	3.84	0.57	13.96	Y
51	盂县 Yu Xian	308 757	541	326	94.45	0.18	0.60	−5.29	Y
52	襄垣县 Xiangyuan Xian	257 873	550	418	62.18	0.18	0.76	−15.87	Y
53	平顺县 Pingshun Xian	151 457	389	320	73.52	0.51	0.82	13.13	Y
54	沁源县 Qinyuan Xian	164 491	256	239	60.55	26.95	0.93	−45.17	
55	阳城县 Yangcheng Xian	382 381	1 126	816	77.09	0.18	0.72	−13.55	Y

序号 No.	肿瘤登记处 Cancer registries	人口数 Population	发病数 No. new cases	死亡数 No. deaths	MV%	DCO%	M/I	发病率变化 Change for CR%	接受 Accepted
56	陵川县 Lingchuan Xian	240 766	149	82	51.68	0.00	0.55	−27.43	
57	晋中市榆次区 Yuci Qu, Jizhong Shi	653 930	1 235	1 006	57.65	0.57	0.81	−31.38	Y
58	晋中市太谷区 Taigu Qu, Jinzhong Shi	293 516	599	416	59.77	0.50	0.69	23.69	Y
59	昔阳县 Xiyang Xian	232 363	164	299	71.34	1.22	1.82	−57.09	
60	寿阳县 Shouyang Xian	214 744	538	413	56.32	5.76	0.77	−18.89	Y
61	稷山县 Jishan Xian	316 114	656	433	61.13	2.44	0.66	28.48	Y
62	新绛县 Xinjiang Xian	346 862	451	287	55.21	1.33	0.64	−5.66	
63	绛县 Jiang Xian	293 096	235	313	34.47	1.28	1.33	−58.72	
64	垣曲县 Yuanqu Xian	236 317	454	320	80.62	0.44	0.70	56.57	Y
65	芮城县 Ruicheng Xian	425 727	212	72	55.19	0.00	0.34	18.22	
66	忻州市忻府区 Xinfu Qu, Xinzhou Shi	552 390	514	171	56.23	0.78	0.33	−19.15	
67	定襄县 Dingxiang Xian	221 395	368	263	58.15	3.80	0.71	267.88	Y
68	原平市 Yuanping Shi	506 954	607	692	78.42	1.65	1.14	−16.33	
69	襄汾县 Xiangfen Xian	425 556	319	179	46.71	0.00	0.56	−5.60	
70	洪洞县 Hongtong Xian	761 104	615	214	43.41	1.95	0.35	−53.46	
71	交城县 Jiaocheng Xian	234 088	434	161	48.62	0.23	0.37	13.66	
72	临县 Lin Xian	660 668	356	172	44.10	0.28	0.48	−45.99	
73	孝义市 Xiaoyi Shi	514 528	529	170	63.71	0.00	0.32	−42.25	
74	汾阳市 Fenyang Shi	434 207	873	551	60.82	5.27	0.63	8.58	Y
75	武川县 Wuchuan Xian	110 123	356	167	82.30	0.84	0.47	121.36	Y
76	乌海市 Wuhai Shi	563 301	1 146	744	63.61	6.20	0.65		Y
77	赤峰市红山区 Hongshan Qu, Chifeng Shi	437 525	979	572	79.06	0.20	0.58	−0.79	Y
78	赤峰市元宝山区 Yuanbaoshan Qu, Chifeng Shi	335 596	1 121	610	53.43	0.18	0.54	−18.96	Y
79	赤峰市松山区 Songshan Qu, Chifeng Shi	572 344	1 458	799	71.06	0.34	0.55	−0.19	Y
80	巴林左旗 Bairin Zuoqi	321 117	834	473	46.04	0.24	0.57		Y
81	敖汉旗 Aohan Qi	532 037	1 278	830	64.79	1.17	0.65	5.54	Y
82	通辽市科尔沁区 Horqin Qu, Tongliao Shi	772 498	2 188	1 150	81.22	0.00	0.53	30.03	Y
83	科尔沁左翼中旗 Horqin Zuoyi Zhongqi	448 526	1 683	749	76.83	0.06	0.45	48.68	Y

序号 No.	肿瘤登记处 Cancer registries	人口数 Population	发病数 No. new cases	死亡数 No. deaths	MV%	DCO%	M/I	发病率变化 Change for CR%	接受 Accepted
84	科尔沁左翼后旗 Horqin Zuoyi Houqi	387 098	822	488	46.35	0.00	0.59	49.86	Y
85	开鲁县 Kailu Xian	383 415	1 221	749	73.63	0.49	0.61	15.84	Y
86	库伦旗 Hure Qi	174 150	430	231	80.47	0.00	0.54	11.92	Y
87	奈曼旗 Naiman Qi	412 397	1 093	626	72.83	0.00	0.57	2.27	Y
88	扎鲁特旗 Jarud Qi	291 907	810	416	67.65	0.12	0.51	26.24	Y
89	霍林郭勒市 Holin Gol Shi	81 213	158	86	76.58	1.90	0.54	25.70	Y
90	呼伦贝尔市海拉尔区 Hailar Qu,Hulun Buir Shi	341 316	1 062	640	71.85	0.56	0.60	3.67	Y
91	呼伦贝尔市扎赉诺尔区 Dalai Nur Qu,Hulun Buir Shi	85 618	207	167	73.43	0.00	0.81	98.95	Y
92	阿荣旗 Arun Qi	272 194	918	575	76.47	0.00	0.63	4.67	Y
93	莫力达瓦达斡尔族自治旗 Morin Dawa Daurzu Zizhiqi	270 892	562	370	56.76	0.00	0.66	6.70	Y
94	鄂伦春自治旗 Oroqen Zizhiqi	205 460	515	228	22.14	0.58	0.44		
95	鄂温克族自治旗 Ewenkizu Zizhiqi	134 877	424	302	75.47	1.89	0.71	-13.69	Y
96	陈巴尔虎旗 Chen Barag Qi	59 328	174	102	74.14	0.57	0.59	91.10	Y
97	新巴尔虎左旗 Xin Barag Zuoqi	40 654	120	79	27.50	4.17	0.66	23.97	
98	新巴尔虎右旗 Xin Barag Youqi	34 178	67	63	7.46	2.99	0.94	180.15	
99	满洲里市 Manzhouli Shi	143 867	378	225	75.66	0.26	0.60	-39.54	Y
100	牙克石市 Yakeshi Shi	331 107	947	606	54.28	0.00	0.64	-6.91	Y
101	扎兰屯市 Zalantun Shi	341 915	859	594	41.21	7.92	0.69	19.43	Y
102	根河市 Genhe Shi	137 343	410	271	86.83	5.12	0.66	-26.02	Y
103	巴彦淖尔市临河区 Linhe Qu,Bayannur Shi	442 858	1024	667	60.74	0.00	0.65	0.49	Y
104	五原县 Wuyuan Xian	258 100	788	295	51.78	0.00	0.37		Y
105	杭锦后旗 Hanggin Houqi	258 401	623	328	55.70	0.00	0.53		Y
106	锡林浩特市 Xilin Hot Shi	261 556	680	408	61.47	6.18	0.60	-16.41	Y
107	苏尼特左旗 Sonid Zuoqi	32 245	99	29	17.17	0.00	0.29		
108	苏尼特右旗 Sonid Youqi	68 104	247	164	52.63	10.53	0.66		Y
109	东乌珠穆沁旗 Dong Ujimqin Qi	68 780	158	112	27.85	1.27	0.71		
110	太仆寺旗 Taibus Qi	120 500	428	318	9.58	3.50	0.74		

序号 No.	肿瘤登记处 Cancer registries	人口数 Population	发病数 No. new cases	死亡数 No. deaths	MV%	DCO%	M/I	发病率变化 Change for CR%	接受 Accepted
111	沈阳市 Shenyang Shi	3 869 807	16 001	9 368	68.00	1.85	0.59		Y
112	康平县 Kangping Xian	341 654	892	610	56.05	1.46	0.68	−17.78	Y
113	法库县 Faku Xian	437 496	1 321	951	62.38	2.12	0.72	−1.83	Y
114	新民市 Xinmin Shi	663 587	1 715	1 092	59.30	11.37	0.64		Y
115	大连市 Dalian Shi	2 413 709	14 253	6 752	83.07	1.02	0.47	6.14	Y
116	大连市金州区 Jinzhou Qu, Dalian Shi	881 675	3 892	1 907	76.00	0.87	0.49		Y
117	庄河市 Zhuanghe Shi	886 935	4 401	2 303	76.03	1.70	0.52	12.46	Y
118	鞍山市 Anshan Shi	1 466 955	7 041	4 570	80.10	0.16	0.65	1.63	Y
119	岫岩满族自治县 Xiuyan Manzu Zizhixian	504 555	1 487	776	62.41	2.29	0.52		Y
120	抚顺市 Fushun Shi	1 301 130	4 913	3 212	65.62	11.22	0.65		Y
121	本溪市 Benxi Shi	882 448	3 322	2 242	63.70	1.75	0.67		Y
122	丹东市 Dandong Shi	773 497	3 164	1 793	74.81	3.00	0.57		Y
123	东港市 Donggang Shi	593 304	2 027	1 500	46.08	0.69	0.74	−10.94	Y
124	锦州市 Jinzhou Shi	954 298	3 321	2 051	68.53	0.42	0.62		Y
125	营口市 Yingkou Shi	553 696	1 644	904	75.18	3.71	0.55		Y
126	阜新市 Fuxin Shi	603 729	2 365	1 781	58.82	0.72	0.75	1.03	Y
127	彰武县 Zhangwu Xian	397 272	1 243	815	46.74	0.00	0.66	13.31	Y
128	辽阳县 Liaoyang Xian	463 104	1 346	1 056	63.00	3.94	0.78	2.36	Y
129	盘锦市 Panjin Shi	633 700	2 393	1 126	80.40	0.92	0.47		Y
130	盘锦市大洼区 Dawa Qu, Panjin Shi	390 684	1 098	766	49.27	0.18	0.70		Y
131	建平县 Jianping Xian	575 605	1 603	1 209	51.28	0.94	0.75	−15.23	Y
132	长春市朝阳区 Chaoyang Qu, Changchun Shi	599 434	2 705	207	88.24	0.04	0.08		
133	德惠市 Dehui Shi	884 504	2 067	1 511	70.63	4.74	0.73	−2.27	Y
134	吉林市 Jilin Shi	1 965 537	6 522	1 540	83.15	0.21	0.24	9.88	
135	永吉县 Yongji Xian	376 941	475	187	61.68	3.79	0.39	23.08	
136	蛟河市 Jiaohe Shi	415 998	682	307	65.69	2.64	0.45	−40.43	
137	桦甸市 Huadian Shi	441 226	1 428	471	34.38	2.73	0.33	72.06	
138	舒兰市 Shulan Shi	585 700	1 249	528	50.76	0.80	0.42	7.69	Y
139	磐石市 Panshi Shi	507 591	912	170	74.12	0.00	0.19	2.77	
140	四平市铁西区 Tiexi Qu, Siping Shi	266 393	766	68	79.24	0.00	0.09		

序号 No.	肿瘤登记处 Cancer registries	人口数 Population	发病数 No. new cases	死亡数 No. deaths	MV%	DCO%	M/I	发病率变化 Change for CR%	接受 Accepted
141	四平市铁东区 Tiedong Qu, Siping Shi	321 077	689	64	80.84	0.00	0.09		
142	梨树县 Lishu Xian	768 096	1 394	135	71.66	0.00	0.10		
143	伊通满族自治县 Yitong Manzu Zizhixian	463 269	966	188	81.47	0.31	0.19		
144	双辽市 Shuangliao Shi	409 876	747	87	79.25	1.74	0.12		
145	辽源市龙山区 Longshan Qu, Liaoyuan Shi	293 386	1 140	608	65.44	1.58	0.53		Y
146	东辽县 Dongliao Xian	352 407	828	435	75.60	1.57	0.53		Y
147	通化市 Tonghua Shi	443 352	1 582	1 190	72.19	1.14	0.75		Y
148	通化县 Tonghua Xian	237 598	898	269	81.29	1.45	0.30	820.59	
149	梅河口市 Meihekou Shi	602 341	1 591	896	49.97	0.25	0.56	-3.64	Y
150	集安市 Ji'an Shi	235 885	600	243	76.33	0.00	0.41	166.87	Y
151	白山市浑江区 Hunjiang Qu, Baishan Shi	338 476	1 201	572	71.61	0.25	0.48		Y
152	抚松县 Fusong Xian	276 875	724	148	64.64	12.02	0.20	94.91	
153	松原市宁江区 Ningjiang Qu, Songyuan Shi	614 616	1 057	337	66.51	0.00	0.32	7.53	
154	前郭尔罗斯蒙古族自治县 Qian Gorlos Mongolzu Zizhixian	573 101	1 944	334	39.61	0.05	0.17	10.83	
155	乾安县 Qian'an Xian	271 046	537	223	63.87	21.97	0.42	76.17	
156	通榆县 Tongyu Xian	343 609	590	35	80.00	0.17	0.06	147.74	
157	大安市 Da'an Shi	415 913	1 237	208	63.38	0.16	0.17	225.26	
158	延吉市 Yanji Shi	556 536	1 422	736	68.21	0.35	0.52	-2.61	Y
159	图们市 Tumen Shi	107 885	303	164	61.06	1.65	0.54	6.22	Y
160	敦化市 Dunhua Shi	452 711	1 829	854	61.73	1.20	0.47	41.75	Y
161	珲春市 Hunchun Shi	227 871	552	309	9.78	2.72	0.56	0.36	
162	龙井市 Longjing Shi	150 387	463	283	52.05	3.46	0.61	5.37	Y
163	和龙市 Helong Shi	185 560	448	222	46.43	0.00	0.50	7.61	Y
164	汪清县 Wangqing Xian	216 309	761	508	69.78	0.79	0.67	-2.75	Y
165	安图县 Antu Xian	221 245	548	160	73.36	0.00	0.29	46.18	
166	哈尔滨市道里区 Daoli Qu, Harbin Shi	787 116	2 357	1 774	73.44	0.38	0.75	-8.62	Y
167	哈尔滨市南岗区 Nangang Qu, Harbin Shi	1 042 302	3 725	1 974	67.38	1.96	0.53	2.53	Y

序号 No.	肿瘤登记处 Cancer registries	人口数 Population	发病数 No. new cases	死亡数 No. deaths	MV%	DCO%	M/I	发病率变化 Change for CR%	接受 Accepted
168	哈尔滨市香坊区 Xiangfang Qu,Harbin Shi	741 246	2 598	1 682	58.78	12.24	0.65	-3.67	Y
169	尚志市 Shangzhi Shi	585 386	1 086	943	80.66	0.00	0.87	-20.21	Y
170	五常市 Wuchang Shi	935 900	2 348	1 448	62.82	4.05	0.62	-4.52	Y
171	勃利县 Boli Xian	287 143	807	607	78.44	1.36	0.75	7.46	Y
172	牡丹江市东安区 Dong'an Qu,Mudanjiang Shi	191 909	658	413	83.89	0.76	0.63	4.84	Y
173	牡丹江市阳明区 Yangming Qu,Mudanjiang Shi	230 304	603	388	84.25	4.48	0.64	11.51	Y
174	牡丹江市爱民区 Aimin Qu,Mudanjiang Shi	263 935	1 038	664	84.97	0.96	0.64	9.05	Y
175	牡丹江市西安区 Xi'an Qu, Mudanjiang Shi	239 197	627	478	87.40	0.80	0.76	-9.52	Y
176	海林市 Hailin Shi	360 308	914	611	70.57	1.20	0.67	-6.30	Y
177	上海市 Shanghai Shi	5 925 555	38 443	16 667	72.68	0.64	0.43	3.81	Y
178	上海市郊区 Rural areas of Shanghai Shi	8 742 006	51 843	24 432	74.97	0.75	0.47	3.49	Y
179	南京市六合区 Luhe Qu, Nanjing Shi	676 338	2 270	1 655	67.62	2.03	0.73		Y
180	南京市溧水区 Lishui Qu, Nanjing Shi	446 177	1 450	959	71.93	0.00	0.66	2.46	Y
181	南京市高淳区 Gaochun Qu,Nanjing Shi	450 061	1 580	897	70.51	1.84	0.57	7.65	Y
182	无锡市 Wuxi Shi	2 663 293	11 736	6 170	78.60	0.25	0.53		Y
183	江阴市 Jiangyin Shi	1 261 946	5 507	2 894	78.79	0.09	0.53	8.61	Y
184	宜兴市 Yixing Shi	1 079 679	4 165	2 794	76.11	0.41	0.67	13.78	Y
185	徐州市 Xuzhou Shi	2 104 430	7 352	3 787	68.35	2.01	0.52		Y
186	邳州市 Pizhou Shi	1 940 176	5 028	3 286	58.67	1.05	0.65	0.44	Y
187	常州市 Changzhou Shi	2 513 749	11 100	5 818	79.85	0.08	0.52		Y
188	溧阳市 Liyang Shi	790 225	2 894	1 625	79.58	0.10	0.56	1.48	Y
189	常州市金坛区 Jintan Qu, Changzhou Shi	546 680	2 547	1 533	79.51	0.00	0.60	4.94	Y
190	苏州市 Suzhou Shi	3 693 332	14 438	7 366	71.64	2.39	0.51	6.83	Y
191	常熟市 Changshu Shi	1 067 423	4 644	2 702	69.66	0.06	0.58	13.33	Y
192	张家港市 Zhangjiagang Shi	929 897	4 786	2 219	66.19	0.46	0.46	6.09	Y
193	昆山市 Kunshan Shi	942 257	4 164	1 764	88.54	0.19	0.42	3.94	Y

序号 No.	肿瘤登记处 Cancer registries	人口数 Population	发病数 No. new cases	死亡数 No. deaths	MV%	DCO%	M/I	发病率变化 Change for CR%	接受 Accepted
194	太仓市 Taicang Shi	497 851	2 063	1 100	71. 35	0. 00	0. 53	−0. 18	Y
195	南通市 Nantong Shi	2 153 429	8 654	5 422	63. 27	1. 03	0. 63		Y
196	海安市 Hai'an Shi	923 774	3 978	2 673	63. 15	0. 15	0. 67	6. 10	Y
197	如东县 Rudong Xian	1 015 610	5 274	2 977	72. 96	0. 00	0. 56	22. 61	Y
198	启东市 Qidong Shi	1 106 936	5 807	3 401	62. 27	0. 03	0. 59	1. 15	Y
199	如皋市 Rugao Shi	1 415 597	6 013	3 853	66. 64	0. 03	0. 64	7. 80	Y
200	南通市海门区 Haimen Qu, Nantong Shi	994 458	4 485	2 865	69. 61	0. 04	0. 64	1. 26	Y
201	连云港市 Lianyungang Shi	1 050 323	3 192	1 782	72. 34	0. 44	0. 56	11. 70	Y
202	连云港市赣榆区 Ganyu Qu, Lianyungang Shi	1 198 854	3 020	1 891	54. 07	0. 93	0. 63	4. 65	Y
203	东海县 Donghai Xian	1 246 152	2 823	1 928	66. 74	2. 52	0. 68	4. 94	Y
204	灌云县 Guanyun Xian	1 031 782	2 411	1 676	63. 33	0. 25	0. 70	1. 64	Y
205	灌南县 Guannan Xian	818 525	1 967	1 251	60. 09	0. 31	0. 64	0. 49	Y
206	淮安市淮安区 Huai'an Qu, Huai'an Shi	1 149 139	3 880	2 742	67. 19	1. 11	0. 71	5. 02	Y
207	淮安市淮阴区 Huaiyin Qu, Huai'an Shi	909 844	2 500	1 726	66. 76	1. 32	0. 69	5. 45	Y
208	淮安市清江浦区 Qingjiang-gpu Qu, Huai'an Shi	574 806	1 293	837	71. 69	1. 93	0. 65	5. 42	Y
209	涟水县 Lianshui Xian	1 124 972	2 854	2 016	73. 34	0. 74	0. 71	5. 99	Y
210	淮安市洪泽区 Hongze Qu, Huai'an Shi	366 331	1 045	809	67. 85	1. 82	0. 77	4. 14	Y
211	盱眙县 Xuyi Xian	795 273	2 179	1 296	60. 90	0. 64	0. 59	7. 52	Y
212	金湖县 Jinhu Xian	338 864	1 277	798	80. 74	0. 94	0. 62	23. 72	Y
213	盐城市亭湖区 Tinghu Qu, Yancheng Shi	692 757	2 398	1 461	65. 39	6. 67	0. 61	3. 36	Y
214	盐城市盐都区 Yandu Qu, Yancheng Shi	709 813	2 971	1 798	73. 85	0. 00	0. 61	4. 47	Y
215	响水县 Xiangshui Xian	621 161	1 570	1 146	67. 20	0. 06	0. 73	−5. 61	Y
216	滨海县 Binhai Xian	1 220 309	3 071	2 217	63. 33	0. 68	0. 72	1. 91	Y
217	阜宁县 Funing Xian	1 114 733	3 498	2 654	74. 36	0. 03	0. 76	3. 65	Y
218	射阳县 Sheyang Xian	947 367	3 577	2 223	68. 94	0. 00	0. 62	6. 23	Y
219	建湖县 Jianhu Xian	776 447	2 738	1 775	56. 57	0. 00	0. 65	5. 77	Y
220	东台市 Dongtai Shi	1 086 830	4 560	2 987	72. 41	0. 02	0. 66	11. 09	Y

序号 No.	肿瘤登记处 Cancer registries	人口数 Population	发病数 No. new cases	死亡数 No. deaths	MV%	DCO%	M/I	发病率变化 Change for CR%	接受 Accepted
221	盐城市大丰区 Dafeng Qu, Yancheng Shi	706 122	3 246	1 951	64.39	0.28	0.60	0.19	Y
222	扬州市广陵区 Guangling Qu, Yangzhou Shi	493 192	1 891	1 320	67.53	0.42	0.70	1.84	Y
223	扬州市邗江区 Hanjiang Qu, Yangzhou Shi	521 528	1 867	1 131	73.86	0.43	0.61		Y
224	宝应县 Baoying Xian	877 104	2 153	1 788	79.05	2.28	0.83	-2.10	Y
225	仪征市 Yizheng Shi	556 327	2 158	1 541	76.69	0.51	0.71	5.21	Y
226	扬州市江都区 Jiangdou Qu, Yangzhou Shi	1 040 479	4 719	3 353	64.67	0.74	0.71		Y
227	丹阳市 Danyang Shi	804 469	3 639	2 682	69.85	0.19	0.74	-0.18	Y
228	扬中市 Yangzhong Shi	282 116	1 123	874	77.47	0.36	0.78	4.35	Y
229	泰兴市 Taixing Shi	1 167 965	4 239	3 175	67.07	0.09	0.75	9.68	Y
230	宿迁市宿城区 Sucheng Qu, Suqian Shi	736 050	2 168	1 301	62.18	0.92	0.60	26.01	Y
231	沭阳县 Shuyang Xian	1 988 771	5 298	2 767	71.52	0.21	0.52		Y
232	泗阳县 Siyang Xian	1 064 397	3 276	2 077	74.51	0.92	0.63	2.98	Y
233	泗洪县 Sihong Xian	1 095 204	2 329	1 472	81.32	0.17	0.63		Y
234	杭州市 Hangzhou Shi	7 784 434	37 678	13 048	87.07	0.62	0.35	10.20	Y
235	宁波市鄞州区 Yinzhou Qu, Ningbo Shi	814 728	4 012	1 479	89.81	0.00	0.37	-1.90	Y
236	慈溪市 Cixi Shi	1 057 654	4 958	2 487	78.54	0.38	0.50	4.57	Y
237	温州市鹿城区 Lucheng Qu, Wenzhou Shi	781 239	3 158	1 449	82.17	1.36	0.46	-4.66	Y
238	乐清市 Yueqing Shi	1 312 832	4 130	2 036	71.67	0.53	0.49		Y
239	嘉兴市 Jiaxing Shi	573 768	2 673	1 093	80.85	1.27	0.41	-3.87	Y
240	嘉善县 Jiashan Xian	402 289	2 350	983	84.30	0.00	0.42	3.31	Y
241	海宁市 Haining Shi	700 533	3 222	1 290	75.11	0.25	0.40	16.17	Y
242	湖州市南浔区 Nanxun Qu, Huzhou Shi	490 855	2 074	1 036	85.49	1.78	0.50		Y
243	长兴县 Changxing Xian	637 509	3 203	1 187	86.26	0.00	0.37	8.17	Y
244	诸暨市 Zhuji Shi	1 084 284	5 762	2 062	79.71	0.00	0.36		Y
245	绍兴市上虞区 Shangyu Qu, Shaoxing Shi	722 407	4 272	1 606	85.23	1.36	0.38	9.23	Y
246	金华市婺城区 Wucheng Qu, Jinhua Shi	655 311	2 989	1 123	86.65	0.00	0.38		Y

序号 No.	肿瘤登记处 Cancer registries	人口数 Population	发病数 No. new cases	死亡数 No. deaths	MV%	DCO%	M/I	发病率变化 Change for CR%	接受 Accepted
247	永康市 Yongkang Shi	619 226	2 460	1 075	83.58	3.46	0.44	−4.51	Y
248	衢州市柯城区 Kecheng Qu, Quzhou Shi	440 289	2 156	684	85.48	0.09	0.32		Y
249	开化县 Kaihua Xian	361 999	1 388	616	77.59	0.07	0.44	20.85	Y
250	舟山市定海区 Dinghai Qu, Zhoushan Shi	398 713	2 044	1 019	74.66	0.78	0.50		Y
251	岱山县 Daishan Xian	177 635	1 410	622	75.96	0.00	0.44	14.00	Y
252	仙居县 Xianju Xian	520 076	2 502	1 119	76.06	0.44	0.45	7.04	Y
253	温岭市 Wenling Shi	1 221 725	5 741	2 411	77.04	0.24	0.42		Y
254	丽水市莲都区 Liandu Qu, Lishui Shi	417 749	2 243	750	79.71	0.00	0.33		Y
255	龙泉市 Longquan Shi	290 311	1 287	526	72.42	0.00	0.41	5.86	Y
256	合肥市 Hefei Shi	2 860 470	8 723	5 037	66.50	2.14	0.58	3.69	Y
257	长丰县 Changfeng Xian	796 085	2 295	1 304	61.53	0.04	0.57	−1.24	Y
258	肥东县 Feidong Xian	1 079 104	3 983	2 295	63.39	0.13	0.58	2.58	Y
259	肥西县 Feixi Xian	842 499	3 795	2 252	60.97	3.00	0.59	0.46	Y
260	庐江县 Lujiang Xian	1 210 086	4 891	3 121	52.10	0.65	0.64	4.37	Y
261	巢湖市 Chaohu Shi	859 758	2 728	1 703	57.88	0.00	0.62	7.17	Y
262	芜湖市 Wuhu Shi	1 499 425	4 886	2 687	69.95	0.39	0.55	5.03	Y
263	芜湖市繁昌区 Fanchang Qu, Wuhu Shi	273 699	975	532	68.00	0.00	0.55	9.83	Y
264	南陵县 Nanling Xian	546 645	1 745	1 053	59.71	0.00	0.60	−0.64	Y
265	蚌埠市 Bengbu Shi	1 164 366	2 512	1 373	72.69	0.08	0.55	2.91	Y
266	五河县 Wuhe Xian	696 517	1 707	1 048	65.85	0.64	0.61	4.38	Y
267	淮南市潘集区 Panji Qu, Huainan Shi	411 997	1 099	508	52.32	0.55	0.46	10.06	Y
268	凤台县 Fengtai Xian	630 654	1 331	803	48.31	0.00	0.60	−7.47	Y
269	马鞍山市 Ma'anshan Shi	636 046	2 245	1 266	82.94	2.18	0.56	5.37	Y
270	当涂县 Dangtu Xian	478 780	1 713	981	77.23	0.93	0.57	5.96	Y
271	濉溪县 Suixi Xian	1 189 278	2 123	1 126	21.06	1.22	0.53		Y
272	铜陵市 Tongling Shi	608 731	1 973	1 334	64.62	4.66	0.68	3.96	Y
273	铜陵市义安区 Yi'an Qu, Tongling Shi	301 289	986	622	66.02	0.00	0.63	−1.18	Y
274	安庆市迎江区 Yingjiang Qu, Anqing Shi	217 847	587	313	82.28	3.07	0.53	5.39	Y

序号 No.	肿瘤登记处 Cancer registries	人口数 Population	发病数 No. new cases	死亡数 No. deaths	MV%	DCO%	M/I	发病率变化 Change for CR%	接受 Accepted
275	安庆市大观区 Daguan Qu, Anqing Shi	259 229	755	448	71.26	0.26	0.59	−7.94	Y
276	安庆市宜秀区 Yixiu Qu, Anqing Shi	171 774	619	319	73.34	3.07	0.52	18.38	Y
277	怀宁县 Huaining Xian	706 265	1 614	905	53.41	6.20	0.56	15.49	Y
278	太湖县 Taihu Xian	578 753	1 326	857	58.67	1.43	0.65	−9.08	Y
279	望江县 Wangjiang Xian	637 437	1 758	1 027	68.83	0.06	0.58	24.42	Y
280	岳西县 Yuexi Xian	413 773	1 053	490	52.99	0.00	0.47	−22.36	Y
281	桐城市 Tongcheng Shi	682 998	2 168	1 301	64.39	2.86	0.60	9.32	Y
282	潜山市 Qianshan Shi	581 151	1 285	771	61.95	3.11	0.60	0.05	Y
283	定远县 Dingyuan Xian	979 833	2 128	1 526	17.48	0.00	0.72		
284	天长市 Tianchang Shi	609 263	1 580	1 245	76.27	1.90	0.79	10.56	Y
285	阜阳市颍州区 Yingzhou Qu, Fuyang Shi	829 823	1 775	992	59.04	1.30	0.56	−4.68	Y
286	阜阳市颍东区 Yingdong Qu, Fuyang Shi	671 345	1 514	1 030	50.13	0.26	0.68	2.00	Y
287	阜阳市颍泉区 Yingquan Qu, Fuyang Shi	746 909	1 742	905	47.36	0.52	0.52		Y
288	太和县 Taihe Xian	1 784 786	4 724	3 085	63.87	0.59	0.65	−8.60	Y
289	阜南县 Funan Xian	1 736 000	3 781	2 567	63.42	1.48	0.68	−6.22	Y
290	界首市 Jieshou Shi	830 932	2 052	928	73.49	1.07	0.45		Y
291	宿州市埇桥区 Yongqiao Qu, Suzhou Shi	1 743 404	4 348	2 870	45.81	2.05	0.66	−0.52	Y
292	灵璧县 Lingbi Xian	1 013 000	2 965	1 405	57.40	0.24	0.47	11.55	Y
293	六安市金安区 Jin'an Qu, Lu'an Shi	849 923	2 010	974	76.62	0.00	0.48	5.79	Y
294	寿县 Shou Xian	1 222 365	3 286	1 991	80.13	3.29	0.61	3.02	Y
295	金寨县 Jinzhai Xian	684 410	1 420	788	66.62	0.56	0.55	−3.00	Y
296	蒙城县 Mengcheng Xian	1 154 104	3 040	1 641	32.53	0.00	0.54	−2.14	Y
297	东至县 Dongzhi Xian	494 243	1 695	1 239	83.54	0.00	0.73	−7.69	Y
298	泾县 Jing Xian	307 001	794	489	81.36	1.26	0.62	−0.40	Y
299	宁国市 Ningguo Shi	383 089	1 069	649	55.47	1.22	0.61	4.53	Y
300	罗源县 Luoyuan Xian	269 457	800	160	76.00	0.00	0.20		
301	永泰县 Yongtai Xian	385 762	1 058	244	73.44	0.00	0.23		
302	福清市 Fuqing Shi	1 387 304	4 769	2 270	79.53	0.86	0.48	19.26	Y

序号 No.	肿瘤登记处 Cancer registries	人口数 Population	发病数 No. new cases	死亡数 No. deaths	MV%	DCO%	M/I	发病率变化 Change for CR%	接受 Accepted
303	福州市长乐区 Changle Qu, Fuzhou Shi	756 979	2 402	1 152	74.77	0.79	0.48	11.95	Y
304	厦门市 Xiamen Shi	1 750 826	6 256	2 608	79.25	0.08	0.42	19.63	Y
305	厦门市同安区 Tong'an Qu, Xiamen Shi	386 955	944	645	76.17	0.11	0.68	−2.06	Y
306	厦门市翔安区 Xiang'an Qu, Xiamen Shi	369 364	1 253	622	75.34	0.00	0.50	24.39	Y
307	莆田市涵江区 Hanjiang Qu, Putian Shi	450 841	1 922	929	84.03	0.00	0.48	32.25	Y
308	明溪县 Mingxi Xian	118 539	330	54	69.70	0.00	0.16		
309	大田县 Datian Xian	415 985	884	136	72.62	0.00	0.15		
310	建宁县 Jianning Xian	155 696	387	56	65.89	0.00	0.14		
311	永安市 Yong'an Shi	330 406	1 061	573	74.55	0.00	0.54	13.25	Y
312	惠安县 Hui'an Xian	820 227	2 636	1 586	73.18	0.42	0.60	19.95	Y
313	漳州市长泰区 Changtai Qu Zhangzhou Shi	212 183	575	358	88.17	0.00	0.62	20.21	Y
314	建瓯市 Jian'ou Shi	552 176	1 669	1 036	65.67	1.32	0.62	24.04	Y
315	龙岩市新罗区 Xinluo Qu, Longyan Shi	543 245	1 988	815	79.18	0.10	0.41	8.87	Y
316	龙岩市永定区 Yongding Qu, Longyan Shi	489 700	1 429	788	79.64	0.35	0.55		Y
317	上杭县 Shanghang Xian	527 966	1 469	492	77.81	0.00	0.33		
318	武平县 Wuping Xian	400 916	1 020	364	76.27	0.00	0.36		
319	连城县 Liancheng Xian	344 542	774	257	83.72	0.00	0.33		
320	南昌市东湖区 Donghu Qu, Nanchang Shi	481 978	1 493	825	72.54	0.47	0.55		Y
321	南昌市青山湖区 Qingshan-hu Qu, Nanchang Shi	441 300	810	489	64.32	2.10	0.60	−29.13	Y
322	南昌市新建区 Xinjian Qu, Nanchang Shi	671 300	1 281	970	65.42	1.17	0.76	−7.30	Y
323	萍乡市安源区 Anyuan Qu, Pingxiang Shi	550 078	1 201	580	74.19	3.66	0.48		Y
324	萍乡市湘东区 Xiangdong Qu, Pingxiang Shi	397 645	766	423	62.79	12.92	0.55		Y
325	芦溪县 Luxi Xian	270 016	630	332	75.24	0.48	0.53	19.78	Y
326	九江市浔阳区 Xunyang Qu, Jiujiang Shi	288 578	707	425	72.84	2.26	0.60	3.51	Y

序号 No.	肿瘤登记处 Cancer registries	人口数 Population	发病数 No. new cases	死亡数 No. deaths	MV%	DCO%	M/I	发病率变化 Change for CR%	接受 Accepted
327	武宁县 Wuning Xian	399 210	733	558	78.04	0.55	0.76	−3.27	Y
328	新余市渝水区 Yushui Qu, Xinyu Shi	902 064	1 999	1 314	63.78	1.75	0.66	1.15	Y
329	鹰潭市余江区 Yujiang Qu, Yingtan Shi	372 074	755	455	60.66	1.19	0.60		Y
330	赣州市章贡区 Zhanggong Qu, Ganzhou Shi	503 446	1 277	688	65.54	0.39	0.54	−2.06	Y
331	赣州市赣县区 Ganxian Qu, Ganzhou Shi	573 512	1 073	607	66.36	1.49	0.57	−12.90	Y
332	信丰县 Xinfeng Xian	687 466	1 437	759	75.85	1.11	0.53	2.03	Y
333	大余县 Dayu Xian	301 048	629	395	61.84	2.07	0.63	9.26	Y
334	上犹县 Shangyou Xian	270 252	626	378	74.76	2.08	0.60	11.13	Y
335	崇义县 Chongyi Xian	193 996	354	239	62.15	1.98	0.68	0.11	Y
336	龙南市 Longnan Shi	319 357	628	429	64.01	0.80	0.68	−11.89	Y
337	于都县 Yudu Xian	872 963	1 937	1 190	69.59	0.15	0.61	3.63	Y
338	峡江县 Xiajiang Xian	190 620	373	201	75.34	0.54	0.54	−0.43	Y
339	新干县 Xingan Xian	215 356	667	324	92.95	0.00	0.49		Y
340	安福县 Anfu Xian	400 731	866	549	66.28	0.58	0.63	6.49	Y
341	万载县 Wanzai Xian	492 294	1 299	744	65.28	1.39	0.57	13.90	Y
342	上高县 Shanggao Xian	340 066	720	453	69.86	2.92	0.63	3.51	Y
343	靖安县 Jing'an Xian	152 762	338	215	67.16	1.18	0.64	14.08	Y
344	樟树市 Zhangshu Shi	570 628	1 336	907	73.50	3.07	0.68	8.10	Y
345	崇仁县 Chongren Xian	302 181	613	372	79.45	3.43	0.61		Y
346	乐安县 Le'an Xian	359 760	652	393	66.41	3.07	0.60	−0.26	Y
347	宜黄县 Yihuang Xian	232 246	420	291	69.29	1.19	0.69	0.09	Y
348	抚州市东乡区 Dongxiang Qu, Fuzhou Shi	454 761	859	507	81.96	0.58	0.59	7.62	Y
349	上饶市信州区 Xinzhou Qu, Shangrao Shi	420 509	1 060	650	65.00	1.23	0.61	−8.06	Y
350	上饶市广丰区 Guangfeng Qu, Shangrao Shi	794 070	1 650	1 139	60.79	0.42	0.69	−0.28	Y
351	上饶市广信区 Guangxin Qu, Shangrao Shi	724 681	1 337	876	63.05	2.54	0.66	2.33	Y
352	铅山县 Yanshan Xian	441 825	867	528	65.74	0.92	0.61	5.60	Y
353	横峰县 Hengfeng Xian	193 367	500	307	65.40	2.80	0.61	9.09	Y
354	弋阳县 Yiyang Xian	365 599	694	439	62.25	5.48	0.63	−3.77	Y

序号 No.	肿瘤登记处 Cancer registries	人口数 Population	发病数 No. new cases	死亡数 No. deaths	MV%	DCO%	M/I	发病率变化 Change for CR%	接受 Accepted
355	余干县 Yugan Xian	919 005	1 703	1 263	60.36	0.47	0.74	2.73	Y
356	鄱阳县 Poyang Xian	1 336 609	2 450	1 499	61.51	0.90	0.61	−1.68	Y
357	万年县 Wannian Xian	371 483	796	564	66.08	1.63	0.71	8.98	Y
358	婺源县 Wuyuan Xian	345 120	753	483	64.67	4.52	0.64	3.16	Y
359	德兴市 Dexing Shi	303 595	551	384	66.61	0.54	0.70	−1.32	Y
360	济南市 Jinan Shi	4 012 375	13 748	7 172	81.15	0.73	0.52	1.05	Y
361	济南市章丘区 Zhangqiu Qu, Jinan Shi	1 042 251	3 808	2 349	68.49	0.92	0.62	−4.06	Y
362	济南市莱芜区 Laiwu Qu, Jinan Shi	994 889	4 047	2 280	66.10	0.37	0.56	6.92	Y
363	青岛市 Qingdao Shi	1 885 077	6 950	3 790	76.55	0.89	0.55	27.53	Y
364	青岛市黄岛区 Huangdao Qu, Qingdao Shi	1 332 967	5 184	2 985	65.37	2.62	0.58	7.82	Y
365	淄博市临淄区 Linzi Qu, Zibo Shi	565 122	2 377	1 279	68.99	2.69	0.54	19.51	Y
366	沂源县 Yiyuan Xian	575 074	2 016	1 191	72.72	0.50	0.59	6.07	Y
367	滕州市 Tengzhou Shi	1 731 615	4 923	2 879	76.48	1.06	0.58	1.44	Y
368	东营市东营区 Dongying Qu, Dongying Shi	675 674	3 000	1 236	81.17	0.07	0.41		Y
369	广饶县 Guangrao Xian	533 893	1 904	1 158	79.94	0.58	0.61	3.49	Y
370	烟台市 Yantai Shi	2 291 507	9 361	4 325	74.97	3.10	0.46	3.24	Y
371	莱州市 Laizhou Shi	839 328	3 544	1 982	68.03	0.34	0.56		Y
372	招远市 Zhaoyuan Shi	560 234	2 527	1 857	66.96	0.28	0.73	11.58	Y
373	潍坊市潍城区 Weicheng Qu, Weifang Shi	359 793	1 495	554	86.69	0.00	0.37	17.73	Y
374	临朐县 Linqu Xian	933 459	3 378	2 005	83.45	0.18	0.59	3.60	Y
375	青州市 Qingzhou Shi	976 067	3 750	2 164	72.19	0.53	0.58	−1.20	Y
376	高密市 Gaomi Shi	902 469	3 118	1 941	72.39	1.38	0.62	0.42	Y
377	济宁市任城区 Rencheng Qu, Jining Shi	1 271 204	3 262	1 456	83.32	5.30	0.45	12.44	Y
378	汶上县 Wenshang Xian	824 545	2 267	1 400	79.40	0.97	0.62	−1.94	Y
379	梁山县 Liangshan Xian	730 683	2 685	1 348	81.08	0.89	0.50	24.02	Y
380	曲阜市 Qufu Shi	649 400	2 148	1 261	72.16	3.21	0.59	25.53	Y
381	邹城市 Zoucheng Shi	1 157 634	3 807	2 122	72.73	3.68	0.56	14.81	Y
382	宁阳县 Ningyang Xian	835 004	2 767	1 675	79.65	2.64	0.61	4.57	Y

序号 No.	肿瘤登记处 Cancer registries	人口数 Population	发病数 No. new cases	死亡数 No. deaths	MV%	DCO%	M/I	发病率变化 Change for CR%	接受 Accepted
383	肥城市 Feicheng Shi	984 673	3 976	2 422	74.20	0.58	0.61	1.40	Y
384	乳山市 Rushan Shi	545 002	2 714	1 407	70.19	6.19	0.52	−1.29	Y
385	日照市东港区 Donggang Qu,Rizhao Shi	1 024 608	2 569	1 328	86.10	0.04	0.52	−15.67	Y
386	莒县 Ju Xian	1 167 328	3 794	2 017	64.23	0.00	0.53	10.75	Y
387	沂南县 Yinan Xian	986 424	2 960	1 730	79.76	0.03	0.58	−9.26	Y
388	沂水县 Yishui Xian	1 168 400	3 494	2 336	64.45	0.83	0.67	14.48	Y
389	莒南县 Junan Xian	859 830	2 636	1 464	64.19	0.30	0.56	9.30	Y
390	德州市德城区 Decheng Qu,Dezhou Shi	412 119	1 633	624	66.32	0.37	0.38	12.40	
391	临邑县 Linyi Xian	554 077	2 592	1 826	83.76	0.04	0.70		Y
392	聊城市东昌府区 Dongchangfu Qu,Liaocheng Shi	1 282 297	3 719	1 523	81.45	2.50	0.41	0.27	Y
393	高唐县 Gaotang Xian	512 634	1 758	996	71.10	6.26	0.57	11.76	Y
394	滨州市滨城区 Bincheng Qu,Binzhou Shi	709 653	2 386	1 216	80.80	0.04	0.51	2.14	Y
395	菏泽市牡丹区 Mudan Qu, Heze Shi	1 388 495	3 561	2 125	40.72	1.40	0.60	−12.70	Y
396	单县 Shan Xian	1 273 899	3 590	1 659	83.65	0.19	0.46	4.70	Y
397	巨野县 Juye Xian	1 090 822	3 292	1 836	44.44	1.73	0.56	9.13	Y
398	郑州市 Zhengzhou Shi	1 445 263	4 697	2 094	80.97	1.55	0.45	18.78	Y
399	开封市祥符区 Xiangfu Qu, Kaifeng Shi	672 701	1 741	858	78.00	0.00	0.49	−0.66	Y
400	洛阳市 Luoyang Shi	1 595 635	4 794	2 654	78.47	0.81	0.55	−6.57	Y
401	洛阳市孟津区 Mengjin Qu, Luoyang Shi	551 261	1 621	958	69.34	1.54	0.59	−1.93	Y
402	新安县 Xin'an Xian	542 133	1 604	974	65.27	0.44	0.61	3.56	Y
403	栾川县 Luanchuan Xian	358 130	969	586	73.48	0.62	0.60	−1.68	Y
404	嵩县 Song Xian	641 860	1 770	1 126	71.69	3.79	0.64	2.20	Y
405	汝阳县 Ruyang Xian	529 426	1 366	764	77.31	0.81	0.56	8.80	Y
406	宜阳县 Yiyang Xian	714 953	1 987	1 238	69.65	0.60	0.62	−0.53	Y
407	洛宁县 Luoning Xian	511 295	1 402	847	72.47	0.50	0.60	1.90	Y
408	伊川县 Yichuan Xian	931 350	2 101	1 446	80.63	3.57	0.69	1.12	Y
409	洛阳市偃师区 Yanshi Qu, Luoyang Shi	634 458	1 731	1 033	76.03	0.64	0.60	−9.15	Y
410	平顶山市 Pingdingshan Shi	917 023	2 734	1 447	81.97	0.77	0.53	0.43	Y

序号 No.	肿瘤登记处 Cancer registries	人口数 Population	发病数 No. new cases	死亡数 No. deaths	MV%	DCO%	M/I	发病率变化 Change for CR%	接受 Accepted
411	鲁山县 Lushan Xian	955 542	2 227	1 297	90.21	0.27	0.58	-6.30	Y
412	郏县 Jia Xian	644 249	1 754	1 090	69.56	2.39	0.62	-1.24	Y
413	舞钢市 Wugang Shi	326 564	998	487	51.20	1.90	0.49		Y
414	林州市 Linzhou Shi	1 130 327	3 957	2 340	83.55	1.11	0.59	5.32	Y
415	鹤壁市 Hebi Shi	656 303	1 789	1 164	67.08	1.40	0.65	-3.65	Y
416	浚县 Xun Xian	681 828	1 683	1 102	70.35	0.12	0.65		Y
417	淇县 Qi Xian	295 700	697	383	63.27	0.14	0.55		Y
418	辉县市 Huixian Shi	904 997	2 302	1 383	76.37	0.26	0.60	-3.12	Y
419	温县 Wen Xian	460 997	1 025	684	90.83	4.20	0.67		Y
420	濮阳市华龙区 Hualong Qu, Puyang Shi	448 818	1 304	713	80.06	0.23	0.55	-22.70	Y
421	清丰县 Qingfeng Xian	755 459	1 898	966	66.75	0.53	0.51		Y
422	南乐县 Nanle Xian	583 142	1 520	735	70.26	0.00	0.48		Y
423	范县 Fan Xian	584 250	1 539	952	76.87	1.95	0.62		Y
424	濮阳县 Puyang Xian	1 135 621	3 698	1 789	77.83	0.08	0.48	9.23	Y
425	许昌市魏都区 Weidou Qu, Xuchang Shi	332 422	1 143	460	85.65	1.49	0.40		Y
426	禹州市 Yuzhou Shi	1 344 570	3 406	2 180	78.54	0.35	0.64	-5.30	Y
427	漯河市源汇区 Yuanhui Qu, Luohe Shi	333 755	893	444	76.15	1.68	0.50		Y
428	漯河市郾城区 Yancheng Qu, Luohe Shi	503 333	1 419	809	70.26	2.75	0.57	7.80	Y
429	漯河市召陵区 Shaoling Qu, Luohe Shi	525 313	1 407	907	73.49	1.14	0.64		Y
430	舞阳县 Wuyang Xian	597 122	1 526	1 013	71.04	5.24	0.66	-2.86	Y
431	临颍县 Linying Xian	727 407	1 969	1 150	75.67	4.27	0.58	33.57	Y
432	三门峡市湖滨区 Hubin Qu, Sanmenxia Shi	289 437	974	555	79.36	1.33	0.57	-1.12	Y
433	义马市 Yima Shi	147 596	370	196	79.46	0.27	0.53		Y
434	南阳市卧龙区 Wolong Qu, Nanyang Shi	939 567	2 566	1 530	70.11	0.31	0.60	1.73	Y
435	南召县 Nanzhao Xian	557 282	1 583	952	77.76	0.32	0.60	-9.52	Y
436	方城县 Fangcheng Xian	1 119 176	2 591	1 641	70.63	5.40	0.63	-7.99	Y
437	内乡县 Neixiang Xian	720 102	2 080	1 328	71.63	1.78	0.64	4.84	Y
438	虞城县 Yucheng Xian	1 143 161	2 796	1 546	66.42	0.00	0.55	-12.76	Y

序号 No.	肿瘤登记处 Cancer registries	人口数 Population	发病数 No. new cases	死亡数 No. deaths	MV%	DCO%	M/I	发病率变化 Change for CR%	接受 Accepted
439	信阳市浉河区 Shihe Qu, Xinyang Shi	660 406	1 632	895	81.62	0.12	0.55	−3.13	Y
440	罗山县 Luoshan Xian	763 366	2 185	1 209	69.34	0.00	0.55	14.81	Y
441	沈丘县 Shenqiu Xian	1 194 472	3 353	2 171	67.13	0.03	0.65	2.31	Y
442	郸城县 Dancheng Xian	1 397 000	3 843	2 474	66.04	2.47	0.64	1.71	Y
443	太康县 Taikang Xian	1 619 114	4 866	2 259	68.50	0.00	0.46	−17.67	
444	项城市 Xiangcheng Shi	1 350 103	4 169	2 115	67.43	0.00	0.51		Y
445	西平县 Xiping Xian	887 846	2 422	1 570	72.50	3.10	0.65	0.68	Y
446	济源市 Jiyuan Shi	728 711	2 074	1 217	73.14	0.24	0.59	−0.44	Y
447	巩义市 Gongyi Shi	852 638	2 093	1 388	57.10	4.87	0.66		Y
448	武汉市 Wuhan Shi	5 256 028	21 017	10 593	87.50	0.10	0.50	4.18	Y
449	大冶市 Daye Shi	842 396	2 310	1 342	85.11	2.81	0.58	4.28	Y
450	十堰市郧阳区 Yunyang Qu, Shiyan Shi	567 928	1 374	1 007	70.01	0.15	0.73	8.79	Y
451	丹江口市 Danjiangkou Shi	446 604	1 151	781	56.39	0.00	0.68	0.32	Y
452	宜昌市 Yichang Shi	1 277 105	4 333	2 280	57.97	5.01	0.53	3.84	Y
453	秭归县 Zigui Xian	368 632	996	727	57.03	10.34	0.73	−11.19	Y
454	五峰土家族自治县 Wufeng Tujiazu Zizhixian	194 069	480	343	62.71	0.42	0.71	−3.87	Y
455	宜都市 Yidu Shi	386 388	1 197	783	57.56	0.50	0.65	−2.90	Y
456	襄阳市 Xiangyang Shi	1 426 167	5 141	2 823	55.71	3.40	0.55	8.89	Y
457	枣阳市 Zaoyang Shi	1 003 795	2 690	1 563	62.94	0.00	0.58	−3.06	Y
458	宜城市 Yicheng Shi	526 797	1 234	829	68.31	5.02	0.67	0.22	Y
459	京山市 Jingshan Shi	623 394	1 418	853	75.18	0.07	0.60	0.54	Y
460	钟祥市 Zhongxiang Shi	1 001 007	2 379	1 487	80.87	0.21	0.63	2.75	Y
461	云梦县 Yunmeng Xian	535 757	1 342	777	62.97	0.00	0.58	−0.18	Y
462	荆州市 Jingzhou Shi	1 248 207	3 962	1 815	73.09	8.40	0.46	15.27	Y
463	公安县 Gong'an Xian	844 500	2 717	1 704	83.55	0.15	0.63	5.11	Y
464	洪湖市 Honghu Shi	809 304	2 207	1 412	71.77	0.00	0.64	2.01	Y
465	麻城市 Macheng Shi	1 153 874	3 200	2 099	74.50	0.38	0.66	4.22	Y
466	嘉鱼县 Jiayu Xian	366 577	827	554	65.30	0.48	0.67	2.59	Y
467	通城县 Tongcheng Xian	416 585	1 033	602	60.50	1.36	0.58	0.20	Y
468	恩施市 Enshi Shi	812 956	2 168	1 169	63.42	0.00	0.54	11.35	Y
469	天门市 Tianmen Shi	1 272 303	3 521	2 341	62.14	0.06	0.66	4.30	Y

序号 No.	肿瘤登记处 Cancer registries	人口数 Population	发病数 No. new cases	死亡数 No. deaths	MV%	DCO%	M/I	发病率变化 Change for CR%	接受 Accepted
470	长沙市芙蓉区 Furong Qu, Changsha Shi	425 835	2 077	922	78.62	3.23	0.44	37.38	Y
471	长沙市天心区 Tianxin Qu, Changsha Shi	501 375	2 345	967	78.08	0.55	0.41	17.89	Y
472	长沙市岳麓区 Yuelu Qu, Changsha Shi	793 603	3 021	1 182	70.41	2.75	0.39	91.58	Y
473	长沙市开福区 Kaifu Qu, Changsha Shi	510 481	2 301	1 280	75.75	2.09	0.56	20.85	Y
474	长沙市雨花区 Yuhua Qu, Changsha Shi	729 635	2 914	1 154	80.78	0.34	0.40	53.95	Y
475	长沙市望城区 Wangcheng Qu, Changsha Shi	639 745	2 481	1 538	78.32	4.03	0.62	45.29	Y
476	长沙县 Changsha Xian	812 354	3 479	1 600	81.37	0.80	0.46	33.84	Y
477	宁乡市 Ningxiang Shi	1 429 941	4 436	1 973	78.81	2.23	0.44		Y
478	浏阳市 Liuyang Shi	1 492 527	4 550	2 474	77.41	0.31	0.54	41.61	Y
479	株洲市芦淞区 Lusong Qu, Zhuzhou Shi	233 215	905	405	76.57	0.22	0.45	26.58	Y
480	株洲市石峰区 Shifeng Qu, Zhuzhou Shi	240 444	977	519	66.53	1.84	0.53	58.49	Y
481	攸县 You Xian	810 033	3 095	1 585	76.45	0.13	0.51	71.86	Y
482	湘潭市雨湖区 Yuhu Qu, Xiangtan Shi	510 096	2 417	963	80.80	0.17	0.40	46.54	Y
483	衡东县 Hengdong Xian	757 199	2 136	1 066	75.28	0.09	0.50	38.38	Y
484	常宁市 Changning Shi	959 900	3 230	1 907	74.58	6.19	0.59	53.37	Y
485	邵东市 Shaodong Shi	1 340 286	3 878	2 269	77.28	0.52	0.59	12.16	Y
486	新宁县 Xinning Xian	649 351	1 359	924	74.76	1.77	0.68	15.75	Y
487	岳阳市岳阳楼区 Yueyanglou Qu, Yueyang Shi	519 217	1 420	788	80.63	0.28	0.55	−3.20	Y
488	常德市武陵区 Wuling Qu, Changde Shi	432 747	1 392	790	74.07	3.38	0.57	15.18	Y
489	安乡县 Anxiang Xian	537 993	2 188	1 110	71.02	5.26	0.51		Y
490	津市市 Jinshi Shi	232 724	911	528	74.20	5.82	0.58	17.14	Y
491	张家界市永定区 Yongding Qu, Zhangjiajie Shi	479 822	1 453	608	81.97	0.41	0.42		Y
492	慈利县 Cili Xian	694 994	2 425	1 281	75.18	0.78	0.53	32.01	Y
493	益阳市资阳区 Ziyang Qu, Yiyang Shi	425 305	1 903	794	77.88	0.84	0.42	88.37	Y

序号 No.	肿瘤登记处 Cancer registries	人口数 Population	发病数 No. new cases	死亡数 No. deaths	MV%	DCO%	M/I	发病率变化 Change for CR%	接受 Accepted
494	桃江县 Taojiang Xian	883 847	2 306	1 374	79.49	1.99	0.60	13.80	Y
495	临武县 Linwu Xian	390 159	1 101	571	78.93	1.36	0.52	35.55	Y
496	资兴市 Zixing Shi	375 947	1 143	591	72.70	7.52	0.52	28.09	Y
497	道县 Dao Xian	800 999	1 594	979	71.20	1.69	0.61	-9.87	Y
498	宁远县 Ningyuan Xian	894 052	2 217	1 273	79.79	0.27	0.57	13.79	Y
499	新田县 Xintian Xian	449 852	1 287	685	69.08	0.16	0.53	6.16	Y
500	麻阳苗族自治县 Mayang Miaozu Zizhixian	397 565	842	586	70.43	2.38	0.70	7.58	Y
501	洪江市 Hongjiang Shi	433 558	1 497	754	71.34	2.61	0.50	74.76	Y
502	双峰县 Shuangfeng Xian	827 390	2 322	1 325	70.50	0.04	0.57		Y
503	冷水江市 Lengshuijiang Shi	366 899	1 059	641	74.32	3.97	0.61	9.51	Y
504	涟源市 Lianyuan Shi	1 146 000	3 006	1 612	79.21	0.17	0.54	30.64	Y
505	泸溪县 Luxi Xian	316 033	1 064	480	73.59	0.09	0.45		Y
506	广州市 Guangzhou Shi	4 589 410	19 614	8 452	77.35	0.47	0.43	8.12	Y
507	广州市郊区 Rural areas of Guangzhou Shi	4 817 626	15 004	6 171	78.35	0.35	0.41	8.59	Y
508	韶关市曲江区 Qujiang Qu, Shaoguan Shi	324 615	1 014	596	71.50	0.00	0.59	-21.78	Y
509	翁源县 Wengyuan Xian	421 756	885	628	55.25	0.00	0.71	-28.99	Y
510	南雄市 Nanxiong Shi	504 520	1 177	745	64.83	4.67	0.63	-1.83	Y
511	深圳市 Shenzhen Shi	4 677 654	12 413	2 472	75.67	0.92	0.20	29.87	Y
512	珠海市 Zhuhai Shi	1 312 887	3 954	1 752	76.43	1.52	0.44	3.34	Y
513	汕头市澄海区 Chenghai Qu, Shantou Shi	789 114	449	1 479	50.33	0.00	3.29		
514	佛山市禅城区 Chancheng Qu, Foshan Shi	700 864	3 062	1 201	75.93	0.98	0.39	13.08	Y
515	佛山市南海区 Nanhai Qu, Foshan Shi	1 608 780	5 123	2 295	78.31	4.98	0.45	6.50	Y
516	佛山市顺德区 Shunde Qu, Foshan Shi	1 528 175	4 860	2 424	59.30	0.04	0.50	-8.13	Y
517	佛山市三水区 Sanshui Qu, Foshan Shi	446 999	1 027	603	71.57	1.95	0.59	3.93	Y
518	佛山市高明区 Gaoming Qu, Foshan Shi	318 367	1 052	547	71.10	0.86	0.52	-23.73	Y
519	江门市 Jiangmen Shi	698 944	2 553	1 352	79.20	1.14	0.53	2.85	Y
520	湛江市赤坎区 Chikan Qu, Zhanjiang Shi	265 297	1 042	347	72.84	0.00	0.33	-21.91	Y

序号 No.	肿瘤登记处 Cancer registries	人口数 Population	发病数 No. new cases	死亡数 No. deaths	MV%	DCO%	M/I	发病率变化 Change for CR%	接受 Accepted
521	湛江市霞山区 Xiashan Qu,Zhanjiang Shi	460 140	2 226	643	67.16	0.00	0.29	−29.24	
522	湛江市坡头区 Potou Qu, Zhanjiang Shi	434 201	994	457	68.61	0.00	0.46		Y
523	湛江市麻章区 Mazhang Qu, Zhanjiang Shi	555 353	1 377	558	70.52	0.00	0.41		Y
524	遂溪县 Suixi Xian	1 108 048	2 603	987	71.69	0.00	0.38		
525	徐闻县 Xuwen Xian	785 512	1 735	509	55.45	0.00	0.29	5081.79	
526	廉江市 Lianjiang Shi	1 845 470	3 462	1 814	70.31	0.00	0.52		Y
527	雷州市 Leizhou Shi	1 860 041	3 593	647	65.43	0.00	0.18		
528	吴川市 Wuchuan Shi	1 227 428	2 486	1 172	58.89	0.00	0.47		Y
529	茂名市茂南区 Maonan Qu, Maoming Shi	1 022 100	2 796	355	99.39	0.00	0.13		
530	高州市 Gaozhou Shi	1 860 442	3 473	1 838	71.15	0.00	0.53		Y
531	肇庆市端州区 Duanzhou Qu,Zhaoqing Shi	425 618	1 352	638	71.45	0.52	0.47	−9.99	Y
532	肇庆市鼎湖区 Dinghu Qu, Zhaoqing Shi	166 980	441	234	59.86	0.45	0.53		Y
533	肇庆市高要区 Gaoyao Qu, Zhaoqing Shi	796 861	1 710	1 109	56.49	0.53	0.65		Y
534	肇庆市高新区 Gaoxin Qu, Zhaoqing Shi	42 662	86	45	54.65	0.00	0.52		Y
535	广宁县 Guangning Xian	585 058	1 130	1 054	55.04	0.00	0.93		Y
536	怀集县 Huaiji Xian	1 116 506	1 586	1 157	41.36	0.69	0.73		
537	封开县 Fengkai Xian	526 654	912	755	40.46	0.00	0.83		Y
538	德庆县 Deqing Xian	412 980	869	624	52.13	1.61	0.72		Y
539	四会市 Sihui Shi	430 673	1 180	730	54.66	0.00	0.62	49.29	Y
540	惠州市惠阳区 Huiyang Qu, Huizhou Shi	416 157	1 018	563	75.64	5.60	0.55	−4.27	Y
541	梅州市梅江区 Meijiang Qu, Meizhou Shi	357 495	1 200	584	72.00	0.33	0.49	2.29	Y
542	梅州市梅县区 Meixian Qu, Meizhou Shi	611 440	1 801	1 068	69.35	3.22	0.59	−3.06	Y
543	大埔县 Dabu Xian	556 308	1 350	919	49.41	10.22	0.68		Y
544	汕尾市城区 Chengqu, Shanwei Shi	499 397	1 657	698	49.97	17.38	0.42		Y
545	河源市源城区 Yuancheng Qu,Heyuan Shi	316 935	752	379	66.89	0.66	0.50	−40.37	Y

序号 No.	肿瘤登记处 Cancer registries	人口数 Population	发病数 No. new cases	死亡数 No. deaths	MV%	DCO%	M/I	发病率变化 Change for CR%	接受 Accepted
546	阳江市阳东区 Yangdong Qu,Yangjiang Shi	518 153	1 189	630	59.71	2.69	0.53		Y
547	清远市清城区 Qingcheng Qu,Qingyuan Shi	768 574	2 424	1 044	45.59	10.40	0.43	261.42	Y
548	阳山县 Yangshan Xian	575 180	1 449	803	53.49	6.07	0.55	3.80	Y
549	东莞市 Dongguan Shi	2 510 586	6 646	2 996	74.16	0.33	0.45	−6.12	Y
550	中山市 Zhongshan Shi	1 823 434	6 320	2 978	79.89	0.00	0.47	7.24	Y
551	潮州市潮安区 Chao'an Qu,Chaozhou Shi	1 072 221	862	1 540	76.91	0.00	1.79	501.00	
552	揭西县 Jiexi Xian	983 602	2 331	1 202	44.32	13.13	0.52	4.53	Y
553	普宁市 Puning Shi	2 483 109	3 524	2 518	44.21	0.00	0.71	−27.41	
554	罗定市 Luoding Shi	1 294 004	2 705	1 606	56.16	4.77	0.59	8.23	Y
555	南宁市兴宁区 Xingning Qu,Nanning Shi	364 748	962	641	53.74	0.10	0.67	0.61	Y
556	南宁市青秀区 Qingxiu Qu,Nanning Shi	766 901	1 713	1 106	88.44	0.00	0.65	−4.36	Y
557	南宁市江南区 Jiangnan Qu,Nanning Shi	385 000	908	591	58.70	0.11	0.65	10.69	Y
558	南宁经济技术开发区 Nanning Economic & Technological Development Area	174 340	327	194	69.72	5.81	0.59	−3.24	Y
559	南宁市西乡塘区 Xixiangtang Qu,Nanning Shi	827 500	2 244	1 323	63.77	1.07	0.59	1.57	Y
560	南宁市良庆区 Liangqing Qu,Nanning Shi	323 193	678	397	72.12	0.29	0.59	0.66	Y
561	南宁市邕宁区 Yongning Qu,Nanning Shi	379 344	679	445	55.82	0.59	0.66	−23.35	Y
562	南宁东盟经济开发区 National Nanning-ASEAN Economic Development Area	39 567	134	64	37.31	0.00	0.48	44.37	Y
563	南宁市武鸣区 Wuming Qu,Nanning Shi	687 435	1 615	938	58.51	0.19	0.58	15.25	Y
564	隆安县 Long'an Xian	424 471	892	607	43.39	5.38	0.68	−6.17	Y
565	马山县 Mashan Xian	574 432	1 189	690	52.23	2.27	0.58	10.54	Y
566	上林县 Shanglin Xian	502 607	1 002	755	53.39	0.20	0.75	5.06	Y
567	宾阳县 Binyang Xian	1 062 183	2 498	1 619	64.49	1.20	0.65	0.13	Y
568	横州市 Hengzhou Shi	1 278 224	2 843	1 810	50.76	2.81	0.64	13.28	Y

序号 No.	肿瘤登记处 Cancer registries	人口数 Population	发病数 No. new cases	死亡数 No. deaths	MV%	DCO%	M/I	发病率变化 Change for CR%	接受 Accepted
569	柳州市 Liuzhou Shi	1 853 333	4 949	3 213	72.26	0.00	0.65	2.23	Y
570	柳城县 Liucheng Xian	373 396	820	539	55.37	0.24	0.66		Y
571	鹿寨县 Luzhai Xian	354 604	737	474	64.86	0.14	0.64	1.33	Y
572	融安县 Rong'an Xian	303 099	556	343	70.14	0.54	0.62		Y
573	桂林市 Guilin Shi	813 396	2 341	1 345	69.84	0.64	0.57	0.47	Y
574	阳朔县 Yangshuo Xian	331 401	668	435	58.68	2.54	0.65		Y
575	灵川县 Lingchuan Xian	395 901	929	595	55.54	1.83	0.64		Y
576	兴安县 Xing'an Xian	392 703	748	462	56.68	2.14	0.62		Y
577	灌阳县 Guanyang Xian	297 200	579	384	51.47	1.38	0.66		Y
578	龙胜各族自治县 Longsheng Gezu Zizhixian	173 701	424	229	47.17	1.89	0.54		Y
579	资源县 Ziyuan Xian	181 500	347	202	57.93	1.73	0.58		Y
580	平乐县 Pingle Xian	465 101	859	683	50.29	1.51	0.80		Y
581	荔浦市 Lipu Shi	385 002	890	594	49.10	2.36	0.67		Y
582	恭城瑶族自治县 Gongcheng Yaozu Zizhixian	305 299	680	454	43.38	1.47	0.67		Y
583	梧州市 Wuzhou Shi	805 838	1 925	1 278	68.42	0.36	0.66	−1.90	Y
584	苍梧县 Cangwu Xian	412 779	819	607	57.51	0.00	0.74	−8.64	Y
585	北海市 Beihai Shi	738 498	2 018	1 267	61.35	3.12	0.63	−9.79	Y
586	合浦县 Hepu Xian	941 504	2 478	1 833	55.08	1.94	0.74	1.85	Y
587	防城港市港口区 Gangkou Qu,Fangchenggang Shi	182 201	359	216	73.54	8.64	0.60		Y
588	钦州市钦南区 Qinnan Qu, Qinzhou Shi	633 271	1 221	753	70.11	0.74	0.62	0.14	Y
589	浦北县 Pubei Xian	956 069	1 698	1 098	53.95	1.88	0.65		Y
590	贵港市港北区 Gangbei Qu, Guigang Shi	736 200	1 525	951	67.28	2.95	0.62	4.23	Y
591	贵港市港南区 Gangnan Qu, Guigang Shi	706 370	1 403	945	64.79	0.14	0.67	3.96	Y
592	贵港市覃塘区 Qintang Qu, Guigang Shi	611 578	1 155	778	66.32	0.00	0.67	0.05	Y
593	平南县 Pingnan Xian	1 549 019	3 727	2 164	67.53	0.21	0.58	−10.74	Y
594	桂平市 Guiping Shi	2 044 083	3 740	2 441	51.87	0.13	0.65	−2.57	Y
595	北流市 Beiliu Shi	1 549 826	2 714	1 922	66.40	0.00	0.71	−4.73	Y
596	百色市右江区 Youjiang Qu, Bose Shi	351 861	934	485	68.09	0.00	0.52	39.70	Y

序号 No.	肿瘤登记处 Cancer registries	人口数 Population	发病数 No. new cases	死亡数 No. deaths	MV%	DCO%	M/I	发病率变化 Change for CR%	接受 Accepted
597	百色市田阳区 Tianyang Qu, Bose Shi	308 785	638	422	53.76	1.57	0.66		Y
598	田东县 Tiandong Xian	434 084	815	624	55.34	0.61	0.77	5.98	Y
599	凌云县 Lingyun Xian	196 899	376	206	75.53	1.60	0.55	10.67	Y
600	贺州市八步区 Babu Qu, Hezhou Shi	658 496	1 775	722	49.46	7.44	0.41		Y
601	钟山县 Zhongshan Xian	464 388	1 007	520	51.84	0.40	0.52		Y
602	河池市金城江区 Jinchengjiang Qu, Hechi Shi	350 700	691	423	70.48	0.29	0.61		Y
603	罗城仫佬族自治县 Luocheng Mulaozu Zizhixian	388 784	920	574	70.98	1.96	0.62	25.21	Y
604	来宾市兴宾区 Xingbin Qu, Laibin Shi	976 399	1 867	1 087	51.42	1.23	0.58	5.65	Y
605	合山市 Heshan Shi	119 101	437	235	67.28	0.23	0.54	22.16	Y
606	崇左市江州区 Jiangzhou Qu, Chongzuo Shi	377 561	690	511	78.55	0.14	0.74	3.52	Y
607	扶绥县 Fusui Xian	461 786	1 211	831	48.55	1.90	0.69	5.58	Y
608	龙州县 Longzhou Xian	270 971	493	359	51.32	4.26	0.73		Y
609	大新县 Daxin Xian	385 495	841	586	77.53	0.24	0.70	13.20	Y
610	天等县 Tiandeng Xian	459 598	892	506	53.03	0.34	0.57		Y
611	海口市 Haikou Shi	1 776 099	4 375	1 173	50.63	2.61	0.27		
612	三亚市 Sanya Shi	615 867	1 584	703	51.64	3.60	0.44	-10.14	Y
613	儋州市 Danzhou Shi	932 356	1 650	273	54.85	1.88	0.17		
614	五指山市 Wuzhishan Shi	106 499	251	115	43.03	0.00	0.46	0.08	Y
615	琼海市 Qionghai Shi	506 098	1 224	903	66.42	0.00	0.74	0.63	Y
616	东方市 Dongfang Shi	437 085	900	255	48.11	2.22	0.28		
617	定安县 Ding'an Xian	297 087	718	333	37.05	1.25	0.46	-27.67	Y
618	昌江黎族自治县 Changjiang Lizu Zizhixian	232 000	529	342	42.16	0.38	0.65	-25.33	Y
619	陵水黎族自治县 Lingshui Lizu Zizhixian	376 192	912	398	41.45	0.22	0.44	0.51	Y
620	重庆市万州区 Wanzhou Qu, Chongqing Shi	1 647 503	5 206	3 846	78.87	0.17	0.74	4.38	Y
621	重庆市涪陵区 Fuling Qu, Chongqing Shi	1 168 002	3 017	1 831	50.91	0.00	0.61	-4.28	Y
622	重庆市渝中区 Yuzhong Qu, Chongqing Shi	660 002	2 238	1 060	71.81	1.61	0.47	1.25	Y

序号 No.	肿瘤登记处 Cancer registries	人口数 Population	发病数 No. new cases	死亡数 No. deaths	MV%	DCO%	M/I	发病率变化 Change for CR%	接受 Accepted
623	重庆市大渡口区 Dadukou Qu,Chongqing Shi	357 005	1 358	596	74.59	0.00	0.44	64.28	Y
624	重庆市江北区 Jiangbei Qu, Chongqing Shi	885 104	2 208	1 394	73.32	0.00	0.63	-9.86	Y
625	重庆市沙坪坝区 Shapingba Qu,Chongqing Shi	1 152 003	3 746	1 925	67.75	1.39	0.51	5.11	Y
626	重庆市九龙坡区 Jiulongpo Qu,Chongqing Shi	968 656	3 186	2 071	63.68	1.07	0.65	37.13	Y
627	重庆市南岸区 Nan'an Qu, Chongqing Shi	909 995	2 684	1 477	42.77	0.26	0.55	-6.34	Y
628	重庆市北碚区 Beibei Qu, Chongqing Shi	811 001	2 600	1 667	49.50	5.92	0.64	-2.99	Y
629	重庆市綦江区 Qijiang Qu, Chongqing Shi	820 971	1 979	1 062	62.35	1.11	0.54	-11.12	Y
630	重庆市大足区 Dazu Qu, Chongqing Shi	788 599	2 972	1 395	62.92	0.03	0.47	19.46	Y
631	重庆市渝北区 Yubei Qu, Chongqing Shi	1 632 301	4 790	2 984	71.88	4.03	0.62	-7.70	Y
632	重庆市巴南区 Banan Qu, Chongqing Shi	1 088 204	3 718	1 702	46.48	3.36	0.46	6.79	Y
633	重庆市黔江区 Qianjiang Qu, Chongqing Shi	483 901	1 340	784	68.36	1.12	0.59	40.22	Y
634	重庆市长寿区 Changshou Qu, Chongqing Shi	854 998	2 770	1 925	70.51	3.86	0.69	-8.40	Y
635	重庆市江津区 Jiangjin Qu, Chongqing Shi	1 387 004	3 837	2 326	63.77	17.88	0.61	0.04	Y
636	重庆市合川区 Hechuan Qu,Chongqing Shi	1 407 201	3 597	1 987	66.69	21.74	0.55	6.64	
637	重庆市永川区 Yongchuan Qu,Chongqing Shi	1 141 997	3 830	2 378	58.62	3.34	0.62	13.38	Y
638	重庆市南川区 Nanchuan Qu,Chongqing Shi	591 096	1 490	771	58.05	9.26	0.52	51.43	Y
639	重庆市万盛经济技术开发区 Wansheng Economic & Technological Development Zone,Chongqing	278 827	694	471	73.63	0.00	0.68	-2.85	Y
640	重庆市潼南区 Tongnan Qu, Chongqing Shi	720 605	2 063	1 174	71.35	2.67	0.57	-14.59	Y
641	重庆市铜梁区 Tongliang Qu,Chongqing Shi	848 316	2 326	1 605	65.78	1.63	0.69	0.61	Y

序号 No.	肿瘤登记处 Cancer registries	人口数 Population	发病数 No. new cases	死亡数 No. deaths	MV%	DCO%	M/I	发病率变化 Change for CR%	接受 Accepted
642	重庆市荣昌区 Rongchang Qu, Chongqing Shi	709 999	1 620	1 085	71.79	2.41	0.67	44.77	Y
643	重庆市璧山区 Bishan Qu, Chongqing Shi	641 485	2 763	1 676	80.09	0.00	0.61	47.83	Y
644	重庆市梁平区 Liangping Qu, Chongqing Shi	654 096	1 444	1 154	60.32	2.15	0.80	19.43	Y
645	城口县 Chengkou Xian	184 405	438	293	77.85	0.00	0.67	5.22	Y
646	丰都县 Fengdu Xian	585 187	1 308	1 062	60.32	0.00	0.81	1.15	Y
647	垫江县 Dianjiang Xian	701 802	1 739	1 228	81.02	0.35	0.71	6.22	Y
648	重庆市武隆区 Wulong Qu, Chongqing Shi	348 207	1 196	824	62.96	7.11	0.69	−12.10	Y
649	忠县 Zhong Xian	738 767	2 392	1 462	70.94	0.67	0.61	6.42	Y
650	重庆市开州区 Kaizhou Qu, Chongqing Shi	1 181 104	4 433	2 876	65.91	0.02	0.65	4.45	Y
651	云阳县 Yunyang Xian	931 399	2 969	2 258	79.08	0.07	0.76	3.47	Y
652	奉节县 Fengjie Xian	733 303	2 289	1 399	69.55	3.36	0.61	−11.73	Y
653	巫山县 Wushan Xian	446 803	1 394	917	61.41	1.00	0.66	3.16	Y
654	巫溪县 Wuxi Xian	383 203	825	590	75.27	0.00	0.72	−6.00	Y
655	石柱土家族自治县 Shizhu Tujiazu Zizhixian	377 995	947	614	51.32	0.00	0.65	1.93	Y
656	秀山土家族苗族自治县 Xiushan Tujiazu Miaozu Zizhixian	485 695	1 122	845	59.36	7.66	0.75	49.54	Y
657	酉阳土家族苗族自治县 Youyang Tujiazu Miaozu Zizhixian	547 101	1 443	893	50.66	0.35	0.62	38.99	Y
658	彭水苗族土家族自治县 Pengshui Miaozu Tujiazu Zizhixian	488 497	1 477	902	55.38	0.34	0.61	0.88	Y
659	成都市锦江区 Jinjiang Qu, Chengdu Shi	607 835	1 857	1 299	69.90	2.05	0.70	45.33	Y
660	成都市青羊区 Qingyang Qu, Chengdu Shi	714 160	2 492	1 505	76.32	0.04	0.60	−2.55	Y
661	成都市金牛区 Jinniu Qu, Chengdu Shi	763 608	2 468	1 652	66.41	0.08	0.67	−2.10	Y
662	成都市武侯区 Wuhou Qu, Chengdu Shi	658 014	1 781	1 071	78.83	1.24	0.60	6.78	Y
663	成都市成华区 Chenghua Qu, Chengdu Shi	783 176	2 348	1 427	69.51	2.94	0.61	−2.28	Y

序号 No.	肿瘤登记处 Cancer registries	人口数 Population	发病数 No. new cases	死亡数 No. deaths	MV%	DCO%	M/I	发病率变化 Change for CR%	接受 Accepted
664	成都市龙泉驿区 Longquanyi Qu,Chengdu Shi	749 912	2 180	1 446	68.99	1.42	0.66	-0.94	Y
665	成都市青白江区 Qingbaijiang Qu,Chengdu Shi	422 495	1 737	1 114	70.24	0.29	0.64	-0.69	Y
666	成都市新都区 Xindu Qu, Chengdu Shi	799 448	2 521	1 520	70.88	0.40	0.60	9.28	Y
667	成都市温江区 Wenjiang Qu,Chengdu Shi	512 032	1 666	686	84.09	10.62	0.41	-6.89	Y
668	金堂县 Jintang Xian	903 134	3 388	2 037	76.06	0.03	0.60	14.93	Y
669	成都市双流区 Shuangliu Qu,Chengdu Shi	611 066	1 824	1 133	78.73	0.00	0.62	3.73	Y
670	成都市天府新区 Tianfu Xinqu,Chengdu Shi	690 361	1 727	1 062	83.44	5.21	0.61	26.52	Y
671	成都市郫都区 Pidu Qu, Chengdu Shi	643 892	1 553	1 048	69.29	1.42	0.67	1.42	Y
672	大邑县 Dayi Xian	510 017	1 447	1 070	62.27	2.00	0.74	37.02	Y
673	蒲江县 Pujiang Xian	268 193	879	540	81.46	2.50	0.61	39.53	Y
674	成都市新津区 Xinjin Qu, Chengdu Shi	318 817	1 128	684	67.64	0.80	0.61	-0.06	Y
675	简阳市 Jianyang Shi	934 346	3 052	1 864	47.90	0.39	0.61	48.76	Y
676	都江堰市 Dujiangyan Shi	622 380	2 416	1 451	71.73	2.11	0.60	59.70	Y
677	彭州市 Pengzhou Shi	796 682	2 939	1 800	71.28	0.68	0.61	4.49	Y
678	邛崃市 Qionglai Shi	652 459	1 912	1 239	66.58	0.00	0.65	-26.31	Y
679	崇州市 Chongzhou Shi	660 339	2 116	1 273	73.68	6.00	0.60	3.17	Y
680	自贡市自流井区 Ziliujing Qu,Zigong Shi	403 317	1 586	1 077	76.86	0.13	0.68	-9.69	Y
681	自贡市贡井区 Gongjing Qu,Zigong Shi	282 165	1 232	767	62.99	0.81	0.62	-2.93	Y
682	自贡市大安区 Da'an Qu, Zigong Shi	428 742	1 140	843	68.68	0.18	0.74	6.05	Y
683	自贡市沿滩区 Yantan Qu, Zigong Shi	356 845	850	594	56.12	1.41	0.70	7.40	Y
684	荣县 Rong Xian	664 045	1 703	1 417	45.63	4.11	0.83	1.39	Y
685	富顺县 Fushun Xian	1 065 825	2 645	2 065	64.31	0.04	0.78	0.74	Y
686	攀枝花市东区 Dong Qu, Panzhihua Shi	287 086	1 069	639	83.82	4.30	0.60	23.00	Y
687	攀枝花市西区 Xi Qu,Panzhihua Shi	127 227	487	299	76.59	0.21	0.61	5.34	Y

序号 No.	肿瘤登记处 Cancer registries	人口数 Population	发病数 No. new cases	死亡数 No. deaths	MV%	DCO%	M/I	发病率变化 Change for CR%	接受 Accepted
688	攀枝花市仁和区 Renhe Qu,Panzhihua Shi	235 155	595	356	83.03	0.84	0.60	11.62	Y
689	米易县 Miyi Xian	225 181	552	298	74.64	1.09	0.54	18.86	Y
690	泸州市江阳区 Jiangyang Qu,Luzhou Shi	686 329	2 264	1 593	67.84	0.35	0.70	15.76	Y
691	泸州市纳溪区 Naxi Qu, Luzhou Shi	464 673	1 178	767	68.76	2.72	0.65	17.71	Y
692	泸州市龙马潭区 Longmatan Qu,Luzhou Shi	372 966	1 395	978	76.42	0.50	0.70	0.44	Y
693	泸县 Lu Xian	1 067 160	3 529	2 690	47.24	0.23	0.76	-1.26	Y
694	合江县 Hejiang Xian	895 273	2 883	1 980	72.18	0.97	0.69	1.01	Y
695	叙永县 Xuyong Xian	722 986	1 373	1 077	50.40	1.53	0.78	6.23	Y
696	德阳市旌阳区 Jingyang Qu,Deyang Shi	700 375	2 837	1 838	69.72	0.78	0.65	14.30	Y
697	中江县 Zhongjiang Xian	1 378 571	3 619	2 332	65.21	3.32	0.64	12.77	Y
698	德阳市罗江区 Luojiang Qu,Deyang Shi	244 673	880	540	73.18	0.68	0.61	8.21	Y
699	广汉市 Guanghan Shi	602 144	2 040	1 409	70.34	0.69	0.69	0.25	Y
700	什邡市 Shifang Shi	426 860	1 523	996	71.24	0.20	0.65	13.53	Y
701	绵竹市 Mianzhu Shi	497 723	1 759	1 290	60.20	1.48	0.73	-3.33	Y
702	绵阳市涪城区 Fucheng Qu,Mianyang Shi	756 807	1 924	1 204	69.80	7.59	0.63	2.00	Y
703	绵阳市游仙区 YouxianQu, Mianyang Shi	488 063	1 624	1 080	78.51	0.18	0.67	25.72	Y
704	绵阳市安州区 Anzhou Qu, Mianyang Shi	441 538	1 164	847	52.32	0.52	0.73	14.37	Y
705	三台县 Santai Xian	1 401 840	4 012	2 764	68.12	0.15	0.69	29.96	Y
706	盐亭县 Yanting Xian	589 285	2 259	1 681	70.69	0.09	0.74	-0.63	Y
707	梓潼县 Zitong Xian	368 628	989	685	48.43	4.45	0.69	11.07	Y
708	北川羌族自治县 Beichuan Qiangzu Zizhixian	232 717	544	361	46.88	0.18	0.66	8.96	Y
709	平武县 Pingwu Xian	165 000	283	218	59.01	13.78	0.77	69.05	Y
710	江油市 Jiangyou Shi	858 251	2 358	1 703	73.24	0.04	0.72	-4.61	Y
711	广元市利州区 Lizhou Qu, Guangyuan Shi	491 711	1 409	910	75.59	1.06	0.65	10.23	Y
712	广元市昭化区 Zhaohua Qu,Guangyuan Shi	231 340	506	349	56.92	0.79	0.69	-15.53	Y

序号 No.	肿瘤登记处 Cancer registries	人口数 Population	发病数 No. new cases	死亡数 No. deaths	MV%	DCO%	M/I	发病率变化 Change for CR%	接受 Accepted
713	广元市朝天区 Chaotian Qu,Guangyuan Shi	201 390	452	297	81.42	0.00	0.66	6.87	Y
714	旺苍县 Wangcang Xian	442 737	905	702	67.07	1.77	0.78	−2.20	Y
715	青川县 Qingchuan Xian	226 524	543	347	65.75	3.13	0.64	4.86	Y
716	剑阁县 Jiange Xian	647 940	2 151	1 324	69.08	0.46	0.62	3.35	Y
717	苍溪县 Cangxi Xian	754 024	1 571	1 115	60.34	0.51	0.71	−2.35	Y
718	遂宁市船山区 Chuanshan Qu,Suining Shi	694 804	1 993	1 292	83.19	0.15	0.65	−7.71	Y
719	遂宁市安居区 Anju Qu, Suining Shi	767 307	1 801	1 292	68.74	0.39	0.72	0.12	Y
720	蓬溪县 Pengxi Xian	680 490	2 057	1 340	76.62	0.05	0.65	4.11	Y
721	射洪市 Shehong Shi	949 179	2 651	1 727	66.16	0.57	0.65	−0.72	Y
722	大英县 Daying Xian	531 358	1 374	927	71.47	0.07	0.67	10.78	Y
723	内江市市中区 Shizhong Qu,Neijiang Shi	505 555	1 761	1 116	72.23	1.76	0.63	2.45	Y
724	内江市东兴区 Dongxing Qu,Neijiang Shi	882 428	2 536	1 684	67.55	0.91	0.66	18.63	Y
725	威远县 Weiyuan Xian	701 330	1 911	1 219	70.80	0.52	0.64	32.59	Y
726	资中县 Zizhong Xian	1 228 608	4 303	2 747	72.81	0.02	0.64	14.02	Y
727	隆昌市 Longchang Shi	760 504	2 155	1 395	72.67	0.79	0.65	13.06	Y
728	乐山市市中区 Shizhong Qu,Leshan Shi	643 738	2 069	1 137	54.52	0.29	0.55	63.58	Y
729	乐山市沙湾区 Shawan Qu, Leshan Shi	169 165	445	291	71.69	0.45	0.65	−8.98	Y
730	乐山市五通桥区 Wutongqiao Qu,Leshan Shi	294 096	754	509	78.12	1.33	0.68	−1.35	Accepted
731	乐山市金口河区 Jinkouhe Qu,Leshan Shi	48 649	102	66	78.43	4.90	0.65	160.81	Y
732	犍为县 Qianwei Xian	552 082	1 150	709	73.22	3.91	0.62	2.04	Y
733	井研县 Jingyan Xian	390 534	1 133	818	66.46	0.00	0.72	18.48	Y
734	夹江县 Jiajiang Xian	343 281	825	552	72.61	0.12	0.67	5.91	Y
735	沐川县 Muchuan Xian	249 121	516	309	52.33	2.91	0.60	45.78	Y
736	峨眉山市 Emeishan Shi	427 140	963	711	64.38	1.14	0.74	−6.63	Y
737	南充市高坪区 Gaoping Qu,Nanchong Shi	595 184	1 480	1 040	83.04	0.34	0.70	16.37	Y
738	营山县 Yingshan Xian	897 114	2 885	1 612	61.56	0.14	0.56	77.35	Y

序号 No.	肿瘤登记处 Cancer registries	人口数 Population	发病数 No. new cases	死亡数 No. deaths	MV%	DCO%	M/I	发病率变化 Change for CR%	接受 Accepted
739	仪陇县 Yilong Xian	1 068 036	2 374	1 804	66.13	0.34	0.76	-9.76	Y
740	西充县 Xichong Xian	593 306	1 751	1 077	61.11	0.17	0.62	44.93	Y
741	阆中市 Langzhong Shi	831 088	2 580	1 906	67.87	0.70	0.74	-4.29	Y
742	眉山市东坡区 Dongpo Qu, Meishan Shi	874 018	2 183	1 615	73.39	0.82	0.74	-0.43	Y
743	眉山市彭山区 Pengshan Qu, Meishan Shi	326 067	910	511	56.81	0.22	0.56	0.76	Y
744	仁寿县 Renshou Xian	1 524 807	4 317	3 058	50.87	1.78	0.71	3.20	Y
745	洪雅县 Hongya Xian	342 697	656	458	78.20	0.00	0.70	38.75	Y
746	丹棱县 Danling Xian	162 645	386	228	55.18	5.96	0.59	-9.64	Y
747	青神县 Qingshen Xian	192 185	492	347	76.63	0.41	0.71	14.81	Y
748	宜宾市翠屏区 Cuiping Qu, Yibin Shi	854 075	2 058	1 462	66.23	0.39	0.71	-12.52	Y
749	宜宾市南溪区 Nanxi Qu, Yibin Shi	432 688	890	646	50.34	1.35	0.73	-0.45	Y
750	宜宾市叙州区 Xuzhou Qu, Yibing Shi	1 004 613	2 237	1 399	61.69	1.39	0.63	12.47	Y
751	江安县 Jiang'an Xian	586 129	1 344	839	53.42	0.15	0.62	11.69	Y
752	长宁县 Changning Xian	461 332	1 060	702	72.74	0.28	0.66	-4.45	Y
753	兴文县 Xingwen Xian	484 100	1 028	716	58.17	2.53	0.70	33.19	Y
754	广安市广安区 Guang'an Qu, Guang'an Shi	894 988	2 666	1 825	69.58	3.49	0.68	3.18	Y
755	广安市前锋区 Qianfeng Qu, Guang'an Shi	367 683	974	619	62.83	0.51	0.64	13.13	Y
756	岳池县 Yuechi Xian	1 156 813	3 031	2 037	70.27	0.63	0.67	22.73	Y
757	武胜县 Wusheng Xian	818 164	2 142	1 496	50.23	2.15	0.70	26.64	Y
758	邻水县 Linshui Xian	1 012 770	2 415	1 545	56.89	2.69	0.64	7.27	Y
759	华蓥市 Huaying Shi	354 865	975	590	64.00	0.31	0.61	21.86	Y
760	达州市达川区 Dachuan Qu, Dazhou Shi	1 164 084	3 010	2 023	69.00	0.23	0.67	48.63	Y
761	宣汉县 Xuanhan Xian	1 278 273	2 785	2 153	74.36	0.86	0.77	-9.22	Y
762	大竹县 Dazhu Xian	1 082 257	2 493	1 723	72.28	0.40	0.69	0.28	Y
763	渠县 Qu Xian	1 321 868	2 782	2 112	66.75	2.19	0.76	5.68	Y
764	雅安市雨城区 Yucheng Qu, Ya'an Shi	340 493	976	634	70.80	4.71	0.65	6.36	Y

序号 No.	肿瘤登记处 Cancer registries	人口数 Population	发病数 No. new cases	死亡数 No. deaths	MV%	DCO%	M/I	发病率变化 Change for CR%	接受 Accepted
765	雅安市名山区 Mingshan Qu,Ya'an Shi	278 261	684	409	70.47	1.90	0.60	2.47	Y
766	荥经县 Yingjing Xian	146 012	407	245	81.57	1.23	0.60	3.68	Y
767	汉源县 Hanyuan Xian	319 009	814	481	68.92	0.86	0.59	5.32	Y
768	石棉县 Shimian Xian	120 831	317	218	68.14	1.58	0.69	1.14	Y
769	天全县 Tianquan Xian	150 398	448	272	67.63	0.45	0.61	6.45	Y
770	芦山县 Lushan Xian	118 639	360	215	76.94	0.56	0.60	2.93	Y
771	宝兴县 Baoxing Xian	58 226	179	115	68.16	2.23	0.64	22.83	Y
772	巴中市巴州区 Bazhou Qu, Bazhong Shi	772 504	1 898	1 166	49.32	0.53	0.61	−4.85	Y
773	通江县 Tongjiang Xian	741 668	1 472	872	63.59	0.20	0.59	6.30	Y
774	南江县 Nanjiang Xian	652 842	1 380	850	73.91	0.00	0.62	7.58	Y
775	平昌县 Pingchang Xian	943 108	1 756	1 325	62.87	1.03	0.75	33.94	Y
776	资阳市雁江区 Yanjiang Qu,Ziyang Shi	1 072 433	3 194	2 148	59.92	0.06	0.67	−0.28	Y
777	安岳县 Anyue Xian	1 565 136	2 901	2 033	63.87	0.59	0.70	22.28	Y
778	乐至县 Lezhi Xian	798 948	2 352	1 618	73.21	0.89	0.69	0.64	Y
779	汶川县 Wenchuan Xian	91 682	177	150	75.71	0.56	0.85	55.30	Y
780	开阳县 Kaiyang Xian	383 403	808	684	68.81	4.21	0.85	−8.23	Y
781	息烽县 Xifeng Xian	243 308	626	407	80.19	6.87	0.65	12.62	Y
782	修文县 Xiuwen Xian	280 900	533	319	86.12	1.13	0.60	1.19	Y
783	清镇市 Qingzhen Shi	496 300	782	545	74.94	2.30	0.70	−16.95	
784	六盘水市钟山区 Zhongshan Qu,Lupanshui Shi	609 796	822	602	80.29	2.92	0.73	−44.51	
785	六盘水市六枝特区 Luzhi Tequ,Lupanshui Shi	505 504	1 242	785	60.55	0.89	0.63	−7.38	Y
786	盘州市 Panzhou Shi	1 065 105	3 432	2 018	69.03	0.50	0.59		Y
787	遵义市汇川区 Huichuan Qu,Zunyi Shi	574 601	1 341	922	76.44	2.09	0.69	−9.17	Y
788	绥阳县 Suiyang Xian	384 703	551	409	61.89	9.80	0.74		
789	习水县 Xishui Xian	524 497	1 248	898	68.27	4.97	0.72	74.19	Y
790	赤水市 Chishui Shi	245 498	917	560	60.85	3.60	0.61	8.09	Y
791	安顺市西秀区 Xixiu Qu, Anshun Shi	621 300	1 486	824	80.82	1.55	0.55	0.53	Y
792	镇宁布依族苗族自治县 Zhenning Buyeizu Miaozu Zizhixian	271 300	762	577	69.42	0.39	0.76	6.44	Y

序号 No.	肿瘤登记处 Cancer registries	人口数 Population	发病数 No. new cases	死亡数 No. deaths	MV%	DCO%	M/I	发病率变化 Change for CR%	接受 Accepted
793	金沙县 Jinsha Xian	573 400	965	715	67.05	4.04	0.74		Y
794	铜仁市碧江区 Bijiang Qu，Tongren Shi	336 095	900	594	77.67	0.56	0.66	9.64	Y
795	江口县 Jiangkou Xian	176 011	378	268	66.40	2.38	0.71		Y
796	玉屏侗族自治县 Yuping Dongzu Zizhixian	137 203	325	161	89.85	0.31	0.50	−23.03	Y
797	印江土家族苗族自治县 YinjiangTujiazu Miaozu Zizhixian	277 893	526	364	69.01	4.37	0.69		Y
798	册亨县 Ceheng Xian	186 898	523	310	82.22	0.76	0.59	35.72	Y
799	黄平县 Huangping Xian	266 816	535	311	69.53	1.87	0.58	0.32	Y
800	镇远县 Zhenyuan Xian	206 808	396	241	72.22	2.27	0.61		Y
801	天柱县 Tianzhu Xian	264 725	664	341	66.11	3.61	0.51		Y
802	锦屏县 Jinping Xian	156 212	343	142	70.26	2.92	0.41		Y
803	台江县 Taijiang Xian	112 804	172	111	58.14	8.72	0.65		
804	榕江县 Rongjiang Xian	290 307	447	275	54.59	6.94	0.62	33.72	
805	雷山县 Leishan Xian	118 700	345	202	66.96	2.32	0.59	80.57	Y
806	麻江县 Majiang Xian	124 167	201	138	65.67	1.00	0.69	15.69	Y
807	丹寨县 Danzhai Xian	124 405	333	192	67.87	2.40	0.58	5.27	Y
808	都匀市 Duyun Shi	468 904	1 335	591	76.25	0.97	0.44	18.09	Y
809	福泉市 Fuquan Shi	296 907	572	371	68.88	1.40	0.65	−1.85	Y
810	荔波县 Libo Xian	132 424	266	171	71.80	1.50	0.64	49.21	Y
811	瓮安县 Wengan Xian	394 274	933	554	66.99	6.00	0.59	199.06	Y
812	龙里县 Longli Xian	162 102	456	231	65.79	3.51	0.51	−2.66	Y
813	昆明市五华区 Wuhua Qu，Kunming Shi	614 611	1 517	1 021	56.03	0.00	0.67	−9.42	Y
814	昆明市盘龙区 Panlong Qu，Kunming Shi	585 244	1 467	960	55.15	9.88	0.65	−8.94	Y
815	昆明市官渡区 Guandu Qu，Kunming Shi	542 592	1 360	762	62.06	0.22	0.56	7.86	Y
816	昆明市西山区 Xishan Qu，Kunming Shi	565 572	1 489	1 064	76.23	0.34	0.71	−0.66	Y
817	昆明市东川区 Dongchuan Qu，Kunming Shi	305 159	629	366	61.05	1.43	0.58		Y
818	昆明市呈贡区 Chenggong Qu，Kunming Shi	133 427	237	117	85.65	0.00	0.49	−15.41	Y

序号 No.	肿瘤登记处 Cancer registries	人口数 Population	发病数 No. new cases	死亡数 No. deaths	MV%	DCO%	M/I	发病率变化 Change for CR%	接受 Accepted
819	昆明市晋宁区 Jinning Qu, Kunming Shi	287 991	667	426	75. 11	0. 00	0. 64	5. 22	Y
820	富民县 Fumin Xian	153 708	284	144	1. 76	0. 00	0. 51	4. 07	
821	宜良县 Yiliang Xian	435 471	705	473	34. 33	0. 00	0. 67	−57. 06	Y
822	石林彝族自治县 Shilin Yi-zu Zizhixian	254 882	411	241	64. 72	0. 00	0. 59	26. 93	Y
823	嵩明县 Songming Xian	311 518	661	377	53. 56	0. 15	0. 57	19. 82	Y
824	禄劝彝族苗族自治县 Lu-chuan Yizu Miaozu Zizhix-ian	489 858	924	539	52. 27	0. 00	0. 58	8. 58	Y
825	寻甸回族彝族自治县 Xun-dian Huizu Yizu Zizhixian	574 965	926	550	80. 45	0. 11	0. 59		Y
826	安宁市 Anning Shi	282 703	701	413	53. 64	0. 00	0. 59	−1. 89	Y
827	曲靖市麒麟区 Qilin Qu, Qujing Shi	768 449	1 541	939	52. 50	2. 86	0. 61	−3. 08	Y
828	曲靖市沾益区 Zhanyi Qu, Qujing Shi	440 116	875	663	65. 37	0. 00	0. 76	6. 86	Y
829	曲靖市马龙区 Malong Qu, Qujing Shi	213 429	397	260	60. 20	3. 53	0. 65	3. 85	Y
830	师宗县 Shizong Xian	438 920	1 138	740	33. 48	12. 83	0. 65	23. 52	Y
831	罗平县 Luoping Xian	655 206	1 375	790	52. 22	3. 56	0. 57	142. 55	Y
832	富源县 Fuyuan Xian	838 515	2 269	1 096	62. 71	0. 40	0. 48	1. 46	Y
833	宣威市 Xuanwei Shi	1 547 961	3 544	2 624	54. 15	8. 94	0. 74	−0. 02	Y
834	玉溪市红塔区 Hongta Qu, Yuxi Shi	460 203	1 008	572	70. 24	2. 28	0. 57	2. 59	Y
835	玉溪市江川区 Jiangchuan Qu, Yuxi Shi	286 300	549	298	73. 22	1. 46	0. 54	−4. 19	Y
836	澄江市 Chengjiang Shi	148 195	327	169	71. 87	0. 00	0. 52	0. 79	Y
837	通海县 Tonghai Xian	292 080	664	375	54. 97	0. 00	0. 56	3. 10	Y
838	华宁县 Huaning Xian	213 635	460	215	51. 30	0. 00	0. 47	18. 63	Y
839	易门县 Yimen Xian	165 433	409	254	65. 04	0. 00	0. 62	−4. 98	Y
840	峨山彝族自治县 Eshan Yi-zu Zizhixian	155 946	401	254	59. 60	1. 25	0. 63	−9. 55	Y
841	新平彝族傣族自治县 Xin-ping Yizu Daizu Zizhixian	280 461	560	310	61. 25	0. 00	0. 55	8. 07	Y
842	元江哈尼族彝族傣族自治县 Yuanjiang Hanizu Yizu Daizu Zizhixian	211 685	398	220	67. 09	0. 00	0. 55	−15. 47	Y

序号 No.	肿瘤登记处 Cancer registries	人口数 Population	发病数 No. new cases	死亡数 No. deaths	MV%	DCO%	M/I	发病率变化 Change for CR%	接受 Accepted
843	保山市隆阳区 Longyang Qu,Baoshan Shi	947 125	1 802	1 118	62.93	2.55	0.62	5.53	Y
844	施甸县 Shidian Xian	348 159	638	356	60.34	0.31	0.56	4.35	Y
845	龙陵县 Longling Xian	305 971	555	304	73.15	0.72	0.55	2.05	Y
846	昌宁县 Changning Xian	355 427	649	378	71.65	0.31	0.58	1.10	Y
847	腾冲市 Tengchong Shi	673 310	1 220	718	71.80	2.30	0.59	−9.81	Y
848	绥江县 Suijiang Xian	171 188	398	185	42.96	0.00	0.46	19.95	Y
849	彝良县 Yiliang Xian	563 562	921	548	19.65	0.00	0.60		Y
850	水富市 Shuifu Shi	109 885	272	131	50.74	0.37	0.48	31.09	Y
851	丽江市古城区 Gucheng Qu,Lijiang Shi	160 307	364	222	77.47	3.30	0.61	3.53	Y
852	玉龙纳西族自治县 Yulong Naxizu Zizhixian	221 975	443	272	74.27	2.93	0.61	8.55	Y
853	永胜县 Yongsheng Xian	403 035	706	422	76.06	2.41	0.60		Y
854	华坪县 Huaping Xian	162 105	300	183	73.00	4.33	0.61	1.86	Y
855	宁蒗彝族自治县 Ninglang Yizu Zizhixian	271 468	503	378	65.01	3.78	0.75	0.09	Y
856	宁洱哈尼族彝族自治县 Ning'er Hanizu Yizu Zizhixian	191 111	464	259	75.86	0.00	0.56		Y
857	景东彝族自治县 Jingdong Yizu Zizhixian	364 836	862	526	82.60	11.83	0.61	−5.23	Y
858	景谷傣族彝族自治县 Jinggu Daizu Yizu Zizhixian	301 044	553	371	78.84	0.00	0.67	5.50	Y
859	镇沅彝族哈尼族拉祜族自治县 Zhengyuan Yizu Hanizu Lahuzu Zizhixian	213 812	396	161	72.73	0.25	0.41		Y
860	江城哈尼族彝族自治县 Jiangcheng Hanizu Yizu Zizhixian	117 922	201	125	58.21	4.48	0.62	−6.89	Y
861	澜沧拉祜族自治县 Lancang Lahuzu Zizhixian	490 230	924	504	69.91	0.43	0.55		Y
862	临沧市临翔区 Linxiang Qu,Lincang Shi	330 417	629	407	76.31	0.00	0.65	−1.23	Y
863	凤庆县 Fengqing Xian	443 851	973	561	60.95	4.73	0.58	7.58	Y
864	云县 Yun Xian	442 544	808	444	45.17	3.47	0.55		Y
865	永德县 Yongde Xian	364 441	650	362	78.31	1.08	0.56		Y
866	镇康县 Zhenkang Xian	185 285	332	188	65.36	0.00	0.57	−2.85	Y

序号 No.	肿瘤登记处 Cancer registries	人口数 Population	发病数 No. new cases	死亡数 No. deaths	MV%	DCO%	M/I	发病率变化 Change for CR%	接受 Accepted
867	双江拉祜族佤族布朗族傣族自治县 Shuangjiang Lahuzu Vazu Blangzu Daizu Zizhixian	177 852	329	177	53.50	0.00	0.54		Y
868	沧源佤族自治县 Cangyuan Vazu Zizhixian	171 832	328	195	65.85	10.67	0.59	8.88	Y
869	楚雄市 Chuxiong Shi	540 596	1 293	736	73.16	1.86	0.57	23.98	Y
870	双柏县 Shuangbai Xian	161 099	286	183	87.76	1.75	0.64	3.06	Y
871	牟定县 Mouding Xian	212 785	416	239	75.96	0.00	0.57	−1.79	Y
872	南华县 Nanhua Xian	242 916	447	285	78.97	0.00	0.64		Y
873	姚安县 Yao'an Xian	205 502	431	216	74.94	0.00	0.50	9.24	Y
874	大姚县 Dayao Xian	280 075	579	313	60.10	0.00	0.54	4.19	Y
875	永仁县 Yongren Xian	111 604	163	114	20.86	0.00	0.70	−31.06	Y
876	元谋县 Yuanmou Xian	221 389	429	238	76.92	0.00	0.55	10.14	Y
877	武定县 Wuding Xian	280 136	498	315	52.81	3.61	0.63	20.14	Y
878	禄丰市 Lufeng Shi	432 271	915	499	62.62	0.22	0.55	10.76	Y
879	个旧市 Gejiu Shi	379 243	1 000	540	55.50	0.00	0.54	7.89	Y
880	开远市 Kaiyuan Shi	286 788	641	418	51.33	7.96	0.65	−3.23	Y
881	蒙自市 Mengzi Shi	435 986	974	479	79.06	0.00	0.49	12.74	Y
882	屏边苗族自治县 Pingbian Miaozu Zizhixian	160 841	326	197	65.64	0.00	0.60	−4.65	Y
883	建水县 Jianshui Xian	549 020	1 047	643	69.53	0.86	0.61	12.32	Y
884	石屏县 Shiping Xian	318 545	691	415	59.77	0.00	0.60	−4.10	Y
885	弥勒市 Mile Shi	547 800	956	563	67.78	0.00	0.59	−2.59	Y
886	泸西县 Luxi Xian	448 758	888	543	72.18	0.00	0.61	0.50	Y
887	文山市 Wenshan Shi	503 477	877	538	60.89	0.00	0.61		Y
888	砚山县 Yanshan Xian	481 011	833	514	71.31	1.08	0.62	44.12	Y
889	西畴县 Xichou Xian	264 303	424	291	75.24	0.47	0.69	−8.48	Y
890	麻栗坡县 Malipo Xian	288 498	515	310	75.53	0.00	0.60		Y
891	马关县 Maguan Xian	381 401	772	448	70.60	0.00	0.58		Y
892	丘北县 Qiubei Xian	495 926	930	527	62.15	1.61	0.57	7.11	Y
893	富宁县 Funing Xian	423 900	710	508	64.51	0.42	0.72	12.33	Y
894	景洪市 Jinghong Shi	544 123	1 346	681	84.55	0.00	0.51	3.07	Y
895	大理市 Dali Shi	645 350	1 327	662	28.33	0.00	0.50	72.40	Y
896	祥云县 Xiangyun Xian	473 092	885	505	63.84	0.00	0.57	−19.27	Y

序号 No.	肿瘤登记处 Cancer registries	人口数 Population	发病数 No. new cases	死亡数 No. deaths	MV%	DCO%	M/I	发病率变化 Change for CR%	接受 Accepted
897	宾川县 Bingchuan Xian	363 204	684	368	22.51	0.73	0.54	77.57	
898	弥渡县 Midu Xian	324 815	584	331	69.35	1.37	0.57	11.11	Y
899	南涧彝族自治县 Nanjian Yizu Zizhixian	220 782	396	226	52.53	0.25	0.57	28.28	Y
900	永平县 Yongping Xian	186 306	361	202	39.34	0.55	0.56		Y
901	洱源县 Eryuan Xian	280 140	525	292	32.57	21.52	0.56		
902	梁河县 Lianghe Xian	161 300	306	170	14.71	9.15	0.56		
903	陇川县 Longchuan Xian	196 201	369	201	13.01	31.17	0.54		
904	泸水市 Lushui Shi	191 287	377	209	63.40	5.04	0.55		Y
905	贡山独龙族怒族自治县 Gongshan Derungzu Nuzu Zizhixian	38 802	71	54	21.13	0.00	0.76		
906	香格里拉市 Shangêlila Shi	150 743	269	162	44.24	0.00	0.60	-0.12	Y
907	拉萨市城关区 Chengguan Qu,Lhasa Shi	345 803	119	87	21.01	47.06	0.73	-36.06	Y
908	昌都市 Qamdo Shi	122 626	9	0	11.11	0.00	0.00	-81.69	Y
909	西安市新城区 Xincheng Qu,Xi'an Shi	537 316	1 575	1 021	79.30	6.86	0.65		Y
910	西安市碑林区 Beilin Qu,Xi'an Shi	677 942	1 626	1 093	82.35	0.98	0.67	13.29	Y
911	西安市莲湖区 Lianhu Qu,Xi'an Shi	761 267	1 862	1 328	66.43	6.34	0.71	-12.36	Y
912	西安市未央区 Weiyang Qu,Xi'an Shi	653 101	1 348	805	83.61	0.07	0.60	-39.69	Y
913	西安市雁塔区 Yanta Qu,Xi'an Shi	814 201	1 858	1 128	68.68	4.57	0.61	12.32	Y
914	西安市阎良区 Yanliang Qu,Xi'an Shi	294 882	726	223	69.28	0.00	0.31		Y
915	西安市临潼区 Lintong Qu,Xi'an Shi	696 906	1 353	1 125	84.18	0.15	0.83		Y
916	西安市长安区 Chang'an Qu,Xi'an Shi	723 080	1 466	1 074	71.69	0.00	0.73		Y
917	西安市高陵区 Gaoling Qu,Xi'an Shi	362 596	781	542	74.01	0.00	0.69	-0.14	Y
918	西安市鄠邑区 Huyi Qu,Xi'an Shi	453 325	1 085	698	79.91	4.70	0.64	25.31	Y
919	蓝田县 Lantian Xian	450 001	887	663	76.10	0.00	0.75		Y

序号 No.	肿瘤登记处 Cancer registries	人口数 Population	发病数 No. new cases	死亡数 No. deaths	MV%	DCO%	M/I	发病率变化 Change for CR%	接受 Accepted
920	铜川市耀州区 Yaozhou Qu,Tongchuan Shi	349 606	641	413	64.12	3.12	0.64	25.88	Y
921	宝鸡市渭滨区 Weibin Qu, Baoji Shi	368 642	748	645	78.07	0.13	0.86	48.85	Y
922	宝鸡市金台区 Jintai Qu, Baoji Shi	384 448	699	546	65.95	1.00	0.78	8.32	Y
923	宝鸡市陈仓区 Chencang Qu,Baoji Shi	438 682	837	587	65.95	0.48	0.70	2.37	Y
924	宝鸡市凤翔区 Fengxiang Qu,Baoji Shi	492 100	913	603	77.11	0.33	0.66	−8.74	Y
925	扶风县 Fufeng Xian	423 700	745	490	60.94	0.54	0.66	57.95	Y
926	眉县 Mei Xian	305 000	550	495	63.27	1.45	0.90	0.55	Y
927	陇县 Long Xian	271 377	536	374	75.56	0.19	0.70	−5.93	Y
928	千阳县 Qianyang Xian	125 900	271	229	79.70	0.00	0.85	0.18	Y
929	麟游县 Linyou Xian	92 292	174	125	74.14	2.87	0.72	−9.09	Y
930	太白县 Taibai Xian	51 791	94	64	75.53	4.26	0.68	−6.56	Y
931	泾阳县 Jingyang Xian	316 600	833	591	69.03	1.08	0.71	14.90	Y
932	武功县 Wugong Xian	417 391	768	564	64.71	1.17	0.73	−9.16	Y
933	渭南市临渭区 Linwei Qu, Weinan Shi	753 899	1 681	1 297	61.33	3.51	0.77	−1.58	Y
934	渭南市华州区 Huazhou Qu,Weinan Shi	328 001	637	464	65.93	2.04	0.73	−5.38	Y
935	潼关县 Tongguan Xian	154 200	290	220	59.31	0.34	0.76	42.64	Y
936	大荔县 Dali Xian	704 400	1 405	1 042	66.69	0.28	0.74	−11.13	Y
937	合阳县 Heyang Xian	444 098	803	480	64.01	0.12	0.60	5.25	Y
938	蒲城县 Pucheng Xian	743 604	1 343	1 055	72.30	1.94	0.79	−8.91	Y
939	富平县 Fuping Xian	753 701	1 503	1 270	57.75	9.25	0.84	−1.25	Y
940	华阴市 Huayin Shi	251 803	462	347	73.38	0.22	0.75	−4.30	Y
941	延安市宝塔区 Baota Qu, Yan'an Shi	475 003	1 089	676	76.12	1.10	0.62	21.28	Y
942	志丹县 Zhidan Xian	143 460	252	176	64.29	0.00	0.70		Y
943	富县 Fu Xian	159 298	293	204	71.33	0.68	0.70	−25.15	Y
944	黄龙县 Huanglong Xian	45 740	101	77	72.28	0.99	0.76	52.09	Y
945	黄陵县 Huangling Xian	119 670	227	142	83.26	0.00	0.63	−6.22	Y
946	汉中市汉台区 Hantai Qu, Hanzhong Shi	540 198	1 117	765	66.88	0.98	0.68	−5.87	Y

序号 No.	肿瘤登记处 Cancer registries	人口数 Population	发病数 No. new cases	死亡数 No. deaths	MV%	DCO%	M/I	发病率变化 Change for CR%	接受 Accepted
947	城固县 Chenggu Xian	559 515	1 019	659	67.71	0.29	0.65	−5.66	Y
948	宁强县 Ningqiang Xian	324 318	690	483	73.19	0.00	0.70	−9.63	Y
949	绥德县 Suide Xian	353 341	470	407	37.23	0.85	0.87	3.89	
950	安康市汉滨区 Hanbin Qu, Ankang Shi	959 848	2 066	1 251	74.10	0.05	0.61	17.14	Y
951	汉阴县 Hanyin Xian	249 703	492	345	75.00	0.20	0.70	6.42	Y
952	宁陕县 Ningshan Xian	70 321	166	107	73.49	5.42	0.64	8.59	Y
953	紫阳县 Ziyang Xian	286 700	670	484	77.46	0.60	0.72	−12.83	Y
954	旬阳市 Xunyang Shi	434 681	1 017	702	78.76	1.18	0.69	−0.29	Y
955	商洛市商州区 Shangzhou Qu, Shangluo Shi	557 332	1 603	1 013	79.79	0.00	0.63	13.50	Y
956	丹凤县 Danfeng Xian	313 058	540	477	45.19	0.00	0.88		Y
957	镇安县 Zhen'an Xian	253 786	515	379	77.09	0.00	0.74	−8.02	Y
958	兰州市城关区 Chengguan Qu, Lanzhou Shi	956 821	3 580	1 812	69.05	0.00	0.51	−7.54	Y
959	兰州市七里河区 Qilihe Qu, Lanzhou Shi	583 443	1 606	677	52.37	2.93	0.42	48.23	Y
960	兰州市西固区 Xigu Qu, Lanzhou Shi	320 551	966	501	65.22	1.04	0.52	65.27	Y
961	兰州市安宁区 Anning Qu, Lanzhou Shi	219 471	608	246	58.22	1.48	0.40	280.71	Y
962	兰州市红古区 Honggu Qu, Lanzhou Shi	141 780	276	175	46.38	0.00	0.63	80.99	Y
963	白银市白银区 Baiyin Qu, Baiyin Shi	317 968	770	471	62.08	1.56	0.61	1.56	Y
964	白银市平川区 Pingchuan Qu, Baiyin Shi	212 371	592	240	45.10	8.61	0.41	−6.46	Y
965	靖远县 Jingyuan Xian	468 163	1 000	496	50.60	0.90	0.50	4.82	Y
966	会宁县 Huining Xian	543 900	1 585	667	72.62	6.94	0.42	29.76	Y
967	景泰县 Jingtai Xian	238 941	636	386	66.51	2.04	0.61	5.42	Y
968	天水市秦州区 Qinzhou Qu, Tianshui Shi	665 999	1 355	672	64.50	7.38	0.50	536.56	Y
969	天水市麦积区 Maiji Qu, Tianshui Shi	552 928	680	668	61.47	0.00	0.98	696.30	Y
970	武威市凉州区 Liangzhou Qu, Wuwei Shi	1 087 856	2 959	1 446	78.98	0.07	0.49	−3.06	Y
971	民勤县 Minqin Xian	241 541	803	396	68.24	2.37	0.49	10.62	Y

序号 No.	肿瘤登记处 Cancer registries	人口数 Population	发病数 No. new cases	死亡数 No. deaths	MV%	DCO%	M/I	发病率变化 Change for CR%	接受 Accepted
972	古浪县 Gulang Xian	264 100	923	466	60. 02	0. 22	0. 50	51. 85	Y
973	天祝藏族自治县 Tianzhu Zangzu Zizhixian	204 401	404	226	52. 48	2. 72	0. 56	−13. 66	Y
974	张掖市甘州区 Ganzhou Qu,Zhangye Shi	518 502	1 519	860	63. 92	1. 84	0. 57	21. 93	Y
975	高台县 Gaotai Xian	146 709	412	228	70. 87	5. 34	0. 55	2. 51	Y
976	静宁县 Jingning Xian	481 972	1 325	666	73. 13	3. 85	0. 50	−9. 90	Y
977	敦煌市 Dunhuang Shi	144 080	314	176	55. 73	0. 32	0. 56	−9. 37	Y
978	庆城县 Qingcheng Xian	273 676	617	315	79. 25	1. 94	0. 51	−1. 56	Y
979	临洮县 Lintao Xian	544 414	1 110	547	46. 76	0. 00	0. 49	26. 19	Y
980	临潭县 Lintan Xian	142 468	379	171	70. 45	2. 11	0. 45	18. 63	Y
981	西宁市 Xining Shi	1 014 473	3 294	1 618	81. 72	1. 24	0. 49	3. 32	Y
982	大通回族土族自治县 Datong Huizu Tuzu Zizhixian	468 334	882	577	55. 90	0. 00	0. 65	1. 77	Y
983	西宁市湟中区 Huangzhong Qu,Xining Shi	482 027	820	735	75. 24	0. 00	0. 90	−37. 30	Y
984	海东市乐都区 Ledu Qu, Haidong Shi	287 526	584	380	59. 42	0. 00	0. 65	4. 10	Y
985	民和回族土族自治县 Minhe Huizu Tuzu Zizhixian	438 067	689	463	68. 51	0. 29	0. 67	−0. 90	Y
986	互助土族自治县 Huzhu Tuzu Zizhixian	401 605	964	625	75. 73	0. 00	0. 65	44. 76	Y
987	循化撒拉族自治县 Xunhua Salarzu Zizhixian	165 082	183	181	66. 12	0. 55	0. 99	−39. 53	
988	海南藏族自治州 Hainan Zangzu Zizhizhou	471 520	849	595	55. 12	0. 59	0. 70	−18. 02	Y
989	银川市兴庆区 Xingqing Qu,Yinchuan Shi	592 381	1 723	528	77. 60	0. 46	0. 31	56. 00	Y
990	银川市西夏区 Xixia Qu, Yinchuan Shi	246 958	714	308	65. 27	4. 34	0. 43	−23. 55	Y
991	银川市金凤区 Jinfeng Qu, Yinchuan Shi	327 200	1 002	456	69. 96	0. 40	0. 46	6. 63	Y
992	贺兰县 Helan Xian	249 152	748	390	67. 38	0. 27	0. 52	22. 55	Y
993	石嘴山市大武口区 Dawukou Qu,Shizuishan Shi	262 498	855	507	79. 06	0. 35	0. 59	−3. 40	Y
994	石嘴山市惠农区 Huinong Qu,Shizuishan Shi	179 925	473	380	69. 77	1. 06	0. 80	−17. 52	Y

序号 No.	肿瘤登记处 Cancer registries	人口数 Population	发病数 No. new cases	死亡数 No. deaths	MV%	DCO%	M/I	发病率变化 Change for CR%	接受 Accepted
995	平罗县 Pingluo Xian	310 989	660	441	69.85	0.45	0.67	-3.17	Y
996	青铜峡市 Qingtongxia Shi	297 836	849	492	78.33	0.35	0.58	11.29	Y
997	固原市原州区 Yuanzhou Qu, Guyuan Shi	431 032	731	496	74.15	1.23	0.68	-17.29	Y
998	中卫市沙坡头区 Shapotou Qu, Zhongwei Shi	406 181	908	665	77.86	0.88	0.73	-18.42	Y
999	中宁县 Zhongning Xian	351 612	650	382	73.38	4.92	0.59	1.76	Y
1000	乌鲁木齐市天山区 Tianshan Qu, Ürümqi Shi	478 382	2 040	917	69.61	12.50	0.45	31.89	Y
1001	乌鲁木齐市新市区 Xinshi Qu, Ürümqi Shi	816 822	1 563	115	87.01	0.45	0.07	-37.48	
1002	乌鲁木齐市水磨沟区 Shuimogou Qu, Ürümqi Shi	437 360	271	45	76.75	2.58	0.17	-13.54	
1003	乌鲁木齐市达坂城区 Dabancheng Qu, Ürümqi Shi	45 726	11	1	81.82	0.00	0.09		
1004	乌鲁木齐市米东区 Midong Qu, Ürümqi Shi	281 567	665	343	66.47	10.68	0.52	39.82	Y
1005	乌鲁木齐县 Ürümqi Xian	94 504	22	0	72.73	0.00	0.00		
1006	克拉玛依市 Karamay Shi	309 930	888	552	70.05	1.91	0.62	-37.79	Y
1007	克拉玛依市乌尔禾区 Orku Qu, Karamay Shi	2 353	7	2	85.71	0.00	0.29		
1008	吐鲁番市高昌区 Gaochang Qu, Turpan Shi	314 273	11	3	36.36	9.09	0.27		
1009	鄯善县 Shanshan Xian	267 171	7	1	71.43	0.00	0.14		
1010	巴里坤哈萨克自治县 Barkol Kazak Zizhixian	87 351	17	0	47.06	5.88	0.00		
1011	伊吾县 Yiwu Xian	28 236	2	0	50.00	0.00	0.00		
1012	昌吉市 Changji Shi	487 556	124	16	66.94	16.94	0.13		
1013	阜康市 Fukang Shi	122 706	171	139	35.09	1.17	0.81	118.54	
1014	呼图壁县 Hutubi Xian	248 009	50	2	74.00	6.00	0.04		
1015	玛纳斯县 Manas Xian	282 851	94	43	75.53	1.06	0.46		
1016	奇台县 Qitai Xian	246 854	116	87	8.62	64.66	0.75		
1017	吉木萨尔县 Jimsar Xian	132 447	14	5	21.43	7.14	0.36		
1018	木垒哈萨克自治县 Mori Kazak Zizhixian	67 045	44	4	52.27	40.91	0.09		
1019	博乐市 Bole Shi	260 296	6	3	33.33	16.67	0.50		

序号 No.	肿瘤登记处 Cancer registries	人口数 Population	发病数 No. new cases	死亡数 No. deaths	MV%	DCO%	M/I	发病率变化 Change for CR%	接受 Accepted
1020	阿拉山口市 Alataw Shank-ou Shi	8 764	1	0	0.00	0.00	0.00		
1021	精河县 Jinghe Xian	136 489	1	0	100.00	0.00	0.00		
1022	温泉县 Wenquan Xian	72 971	1	0	100.00	0.00	0.00		
1023	库尔勒市 Korla Shi	458 067	200	52	87.00	0.50	0.26	−35.41	
1024	尉犁县 Yuli Xian	119 593	4	0	50.00	0.00	0.00		
1025	焉耆回族自治县 Yanqi Huizu Zizhixian	158 874	96	3	53.13	0.00	0.03		
1026	和静县 Hejing Xian	200 147	70	8	64.29	1.43	0.11		
1027	博湖县 Bohu Xian	58 926	1	1	0.00	100.00	1.00		
1028	阿克苏市 Aksu Shi	580 194	555	60	26.49	4.32	0.11	309.09	
1029	温宿县 Wensu Xian	235 539	168	1	36.90	0.00	0.01		
1030	库车市 Kuqa Shi	505 612	112	17	9.82	0.89	0.15		
1031	沙雅县 Xayar Xian	264 138	216	9	27.31	2.78	0.04		
1032	拜城县 Baicheng Xian	240 344	175	5	28.57	1.14	0.03	464.62	
1033	阿瓦提县 Awat Xian	260 528	122	2	45.90	0.00	0.02		
1034	柯坪县 Kalpin Xian	48 177	40	0	2.50	0.00	0.00		
1035	阿图什市 Artux Shi	282 437	7	0	57.14	0.00	0.00		
1036	阿克陶县 Akto Xian	237 057	2	0	100.00	0.00	0.00		
1037	阿合奇县 Akqi Xian	46 121	12	0	16.67	0.00	0.00		
1038	疏附县 Shufu Xian	335 005	19	0	89.47	0.00	0.00		
1039	疏勒县 Shule Xian	336 952	10	4	50.00	20.00	0.40		
1040	英吉沙县 Yengisar Xian	293 542	48	3	27.08	2.08	0.06		
1041	泽普县 Zepu Xian	221 883	21	0	76.19	0.00	0.00		
1042	莎车县 Shache Xian	829 949	31	1	70.97	3.23	0.03		
1043	叶城县 Yecheng Xian	493 222	6	2	66.67	0.00	0.33		
1044	麦盖提县 Makit Xian	281 692	84	3	44.05	1.19	0.04		
1045	岳普湖县 Yopurga Xian	162 274	20	2	50.00	5.00	0.10		
1046	伽师县 Jiashi Xian	424 615	19	0	89.47	0.00	0.00		
1047	巴楚县 Bachu Xian	361 703	8	2	87.50	12.50	0.25		
1048	塔什库尔干塔吉克自治县 Taxkorgan Tajik Zizhixian	40 608	1	0	0.00	0.00	0.00		
1049	和田市 Hotan Shi	393 794	231	54	51.95	0.43	0.23	−20.64	
1050	和田县 Hotan Xian	353 214	28	57	17.86	0.00	2.04	−78.73	

序号 No.	肿瘤登记处 Cancer registries	人口数 Population	发病数 No. new cases	死亡数 No. deaths	MV%	DCO%	M/I	发病率变化 Change for CR%	接受 Accepted
1051	伊宁市 Yining Shi	626 913	153	2	24.84	7.19	0.01		
1052	伊宁县 Yining Xian	453 474	7	0	57.14	0.00	0.00		
1053	察布查尔锡伯自治县 Qapqal Xibe Zizhixian	194 407	10	0	50.00	40.00	0.00		
1054	霍城县 Huocheng Xian	333 871	44	3	50.00	4.55	0.07	176.96	
1055	新源县 Xinyuan Xian	292 611	434	228	82.95	0.23	0.53	−23.95	Y
1056	特克斯县 Tekes Xian	169 011	2	1	100.00	0.00	0.50		
1057	尼勒克县 Nilka Xian	191 979	14	0	42.86	57.14	0.00		
1058	塔城市 Tacheng Shi	184 986	5	1	60.00	20.00	0.20		
1059	乌苏市 Usu Shi	345 652	6	4	33.33	33.33	0.67		
1060	沙湾市 Shawan Shi	427 939	8	3	62.50	12.50	0.38		
1061	托里县 Toli Xian	106 680	3	0	66.67	33.33	0.00		
1062	裕民县 Yumin Xian	59 875	3	0	33.33	0.00	0.00		
1063	和布克赛尔蒙古自治县 Hoboksar Mongol Zizhixian	70 253	9	2	33.33	11.11	0.22		
1064	阿勒泰市 Altay Shi	217 106	14	3	50.00	7.14	0.21		
1065	布尔津县 Burqin Xian	77 719	39	3	46.15	2.56	0.08		
1066	富蕴县 Fuyun Xian	102 306	5	2	40.00	40.00	0.40		
1067	福海县 Fuhai Xian	95 379	2	0	50.00	0.00	0.00		
1068	哈巴河县 Habahe Xian	96 562	2	0	50.00	0.00	0.00		
1069	青河县 Qinghe Xian	69 145	1	0	100.00	0.00	0.00		
1070	吉木乃县 Jeminay Xian	40 949	2	0	50.00	50.00	0.00		
1071	第二师 Di'ershi	214 820	382	288	58.12	4.71	0.75	19.25	Y
1072	第七师 Diqishi	125 854	383	268	85.64	0.00	0.70	4.64	Y
1073	第八师 Dibashi	691 049	1 295	714	69.50	3.71	0.55	−38.61	Y

4 本年报收录登记地区的选取与数据质量评价

4.1 年报收录登记地区的选取

国家癌症中心审核了 1 073 个登记地区提交的 2019 年登记资料,经质量控制,919 个肿瘤登记地区的数据被本年报收录,覆盖了 31 个省(自治区、直辖市)及新疆生产建设兵团(未包括香港特别行政区、澳门特别行政区和台湾省)。该数据作为全国肿瘤登记地区样本数据,用于分析中国癌症的发病与死亡情况。

4.2 全国登记地区数据质量评价指标

919 个肿瘤登记地区合计病理诊断比例为 70.61%,只有死亡证明书比例为 1.34%,死亡/发病比为 0.57;全国城市登记地区合计病理诊断比例为 72.67%,只有死亡证明书比例为 1.50%,死亡/发病比为 0.53;全国农村登记地区合计病理诊断比例为 68.81%,只有死亡证明书比例为 1.20%,死亡/发病比为 0.60(表 3-3)。

4 Coverage and data quality of cancer registries in this annual report

4.1 Coverage of cancer registries in this annual report

NCC reviewed cancer registration data of 2019 from 1073 cancer registries, 919 cancer registries' data were included in this annual report after quality control, covering all 31 provinces (autonomous regions and municipalities) and Xinjiang Production and Construction Corps in China(data of Hongkong Tebiexingzhengqu, Macao Tebiexingzhengqu and Taiwan Sheng is not included). The qualified data were included in the final database for further analysis.

4.2 Evaluation of data quality

Among the 919 cancer registries, the MV%, DCO%, M/I was 70.61%, 1.34% and 0.57, respectively. In urban cancer registries, the MV%, DCO% and M/I was 72.67%, 1.50% and 0.53, respectively. In rural cancer registries, the MV%, DCO% and M/I was 68.81%, 1.20% and 0.60, respectively(Table 3-3).

部位 Site	ICD-10 编码范围	全国合计 All			城市 Urban			农村 Rural		
		MV%	DCO%	M/I	MV%	DCO%	M/I	MV%	DCO%	M/I
口腔和咽喉（除外鼻咽癌）Oral Cavity & pharynx but nasopharynx	C00-C10，C12-C14	76.99	1.00	0.48	78.71	1.17	0.49	75.46	0.85	0.48
鼻咽癌 Nasopharynx	C11	75.07	1.09	0.51	74.79	1.23	0.50	75.28	0.98	0.52
食管 Esophagus	C15	74.04	1.41	0.81	73.17	1.89	0.82	74.50	1.15	0.80
胃 Stomach	C16	74.98	1.51	0.74	75.01	1.76	0.72	74.96	1.33	0.75
结直肠肛门 Colon, rectum & anus	C18-C21	80.22	0.94	0.47	80.83	1.07	0.47	79.59	0.80	0.48
肝脏 Liver	C22	42.26	2.48	0.88	42.05	2.95	0.87	42.40	2.16	0.89
胆囊及其他 Gallbladder etc.	C23-C24	52.32	1.64	0.73	52.86	1.96	0.74	51.82	1.34	0.72
胰腺 Pancreas	C25	43.60	2.28	0.90	43.82	2.73	0.93	43.40	1.86	0.88
喉 Larynx	C32	74.55	1.62	0.58	77.04	1.53	0.54	72.15	1.70	0.63
气管，支气管，肺 Trachea, bronchus & lung	C33-C34	63.45	1.79	0.72	66.34	2.00	0.69	60.98	1.62	0.75
其他胸腔器官 Other thoracic organs	C37-C38	60.08	1.41	0.49	62.94	1.75	0.50	57.34	1.08	0.47
骨 Bone	C40-C41	46.22	2.45	0.73	48.52	2.60	0.70	44.78	2.36	0.74
皮肤黑色素瘤 Melanoma of skin	C43	94.39	0.18	0.55	93.24	0.26	0.59	95.41	0.11	0.51
乳房 Breast	C50	86.35	0.36	0.22	87.22	0.43	0.21	85.41	0.30	0.23
子宫颈 Cervix uteri	C53	83.99	0.58	0.31	85.05	0.71	0.30	83.27	0.49	0.31
子宫体及子宫部位不明 Uterus & unspecified	C54-C55	82.75	0.60	0.25	85.15	0.57	0.23	80.64	0.63	0.27
卵巢 Ovary	C56	75.63	0.73	0.46	76.23	0.98	0.48	75.08	0.50	0.43
前列腺 Prostate	C61	73.88	0.74	0.39	75.25	0.79	0.38	72.23	0.69	0.40
睾丸 Testis	C62	76.07	0.34	0.24	78.68	0.30	0.21	73.86	0.38	0.27
肾及泌尿系统不明 Kidney & unspecified urinary organs	C64-C66，C68	73.81	0.83	0.36	76.15	0.96	0.36	70.81	0.67	0.36
膀胱 Bladder	C67	74.60	0.88	0.42	77.27	0.99	0.41	71.89	0.77	0.43
脑，神经系统 Brain & central nervous system	C70-C72	52.87	1.95	0.52	56.89	1.93	0.48	49.60	1.97	0.55
甲状腺 Thyroid gland	C73	91.50	0.06	0.04	93.23	0.05	0.03	89.20	0.09	0.04
淋巴瘤 Lymphoma	C81-C85，C88，C90，C96	94.18	0.50	0.53	94.02	0.55	0.52	94.35	0.44	0.55
白血病 Leukemia	C91-C95	92.71	0.87	0.60	91.73	0.95	0.59	93.54	0.80	0.61
不明及其他癌症 Other and unspecified	O&U	62.05	2.09	0.50	63.30	2.77	0.51	60.93	1.47	0.49
所有部位合计 All sites	C00-C97，D32-D33，D42-D43，D45-D47	70.61	1.34	0.57	72.67	1.50	0.53	68.81	1.20	0.60

第四章　中国肿瘤登记地区癌症发病与死亡

本年报收录的 919 个肿瘤登记处数据作为全国肿瘤登记地区数据,以反映目前我国癌症的发病与死亡情况,为我国的癌症防治与研究提供了基础数据。

1　中国肿瘤登记地区覆盖人口

纳入年报的中国肿瘤登记地区覆盖人口628 429 537 人(男性 318 815 999 人,女性 309 613 538人),占 2019 年中国总人口(1 410 008 000)的44.89%。其中城市人口 268 481 922 人(男性134 446 031 人,女性 134 035 891 人),占全国登记地区人口的 42.72%;农村人口 359 947 615 人(男性 184 369 968,女性 175 577 647 人),占全国登记地区人口的 57.28%(表 4-1a,图 4-1)。

东部登记地区覆盖人口 253 675 446 人(男性127 474 807 人,女性 126 200 639 人),占全国登记地区人口的 40.37%;中部登记地区覆盖人口150 352 686 人(男性 76 544 468 人,女性 73 808 218人),占全国登记地区人口的 23.93%;西部登记地区覆盖人口 224 401 405 人(男性 114 796 724 人,女性 109 604 681 人),占全国登记地区人口的35.71%(表 4-1b,图 4-1)。

Chapter 4　Cancer incidence and mortality in the registration areas of China

In this annual report, 919 cancer registry data included are used as data for national cancer registration regions in China. This annual report represented the current status of cancer incidence and mortality rates in China and provided the basic data for cancer prevention and control.

1　Population coverage in cancer registration areas of China

The population covered by cancer registration areas included in thethis annual report was 628 429 537 (318 815 999 males and 309 613 538 females), accounting for 44.89% of the total population (1 410 008 000) in 2019. There were 268 481 922 people in urban areas (134 446 031 males and 134 035 891 females) and 359 947 615 people in the rural areas (184 369 968 males and 175 577 647 females), accounting for 42.72% and 57.28% of the covered population in all cancer registration areas, respectively (Table 4-1a, Figure 4-1).

The population covered by cancer registration in eastern areas was 253 675 446 (127 474 807 males and 126 200 639 females), which accounted for 40.37% of the covered population in all cancer registration areas. The population covered by the cancer registration in central areas was 150 352 686 (76 544 468 males and 73 808 218 females), which accounted for 23.93% of the population in all cancer registration areas. The population covered by the cancer registration in western areas was 224 401 405 (114 796 724 males and 109 604 681 females), which accounted for 35.71% of the population in all cancer registration areas (Table 4-1b, Figure 4-1).

表 4-1a 中国肿瘤登记地区覆盖人口
Table 4-1a Population in all cancer registration areas of China

年龄组/岁 Age group/years	全国 All areas			城市地区 Urban areas			农村地区 Rural areas		
	合计 All	男性 Male	女性 Female	合计 All	男性 Male	女性 Female	合计 All	男性 Male	女性 Female
合计 All	628 429 537	318 815 999	309 613 538	268 481 922	134 446 031	134 035 891	359 947 615	184 369 968	175 577 647
0~	6 265 574	3 285 886	2 979 688	2 747 869	1 435 954	1 311 915	3 517 705	1 849 932	1 667 773
1~	28 744 448	15 109 022	13 635 426	12 260 904	6 416 276	5 844 628	16 483 544	8 692 746	7 790 798
5~	35 357 889	18 756 858	16 601 031	14 369 046	7 573 770	6 795 276	20 988 843	11 183 088	9 805 755
10~	33 568 704	17 860 859	15 707 845	12 791 934	6 743 294	6 048 640	20 776 770	11 117 565	9 659 205
15~	32 324 417	17 141 257	15 183 160	12 464 064	6 539 366	5 924 698	19 860 353	10 601 891	9 258 462
20~	37 052 892	19 240 619	17 812 273	15 153 952	7 775 979	7 377 973	21 898 940	11 464 640	10 434 300
25~	44 895 919	22 999 457	21 896 462	19 137 793	9 625 426	9 512 367	25 758 126	13 374 031	12 384 095
30~	49 719 987	24 967 620	24 752 367	22 150 994	10 834 305	11 316 689	27 568 993	14 133 315	13 435 678
35~	45 768 481	23 068 128	22 700 353	21 116 636	10 390 762	10 725 874	24 651 845	12 677 366	11 974 479
40~	46 065 225	23 321 055	22 744 170	20 246 267	10 073 251	10 173 016	25 818 958	13 247 804	12 571 154
45~	54 120 641	27 381 029	26 739 612	22 883 578	11 471 016	11 412 562	31 237 063	15 910 013	15 327 050
50~	51 281 016	25 886 354	25 394 662	21 095 434	10 605 057	10 490 377	30 185 582	15 281 297	14 904 285
55~	41 813 257	21 020 376	20 792 881	18 533 364	9 292 708	9 240 656	23 279 893	11 727 668	11 552 225
60~	37 356 497	18 765 405	18 591 092	16 719 671	8 314 717	8 404 954	20 636 826	10 450 688	10 186 138
65~	31 790 219	15 654 908	16 135 311	13 810 335	6 727 548	7 082 787	17 979 884	8 927 360	9 052 524
70~	21 350 389	10 443 171	10 907 218	9 168 563	4 437 632	4 730 931	12 181 826	6 005 539	6 176 287
75~	14 305 073	6 776 392	7 528 681	6 172 062	2 885 388	3 286 674	8 133 011	3 891 004	4 242 007
80~	9 696 055	4 340 497	5 355 558	4 389 974	1 961 260	2 428 714	5 306 081	2 379 237	2 926 844
85+	6 952 854	2 797 106	4 155 748	3 269 482	1 342 322	1 927 160	3 683 372	1 454 784	2 228 588

表 4-1b 中国肿瘤登记地区东、中、西部地区覆盖人口

Table4-1b Population in eastern, central and western areas in cancer registration areas of China

年龄组/ 岁 Age group/ years	东部地区 Eastern areas			中部地区 Central areas			西部地区 Western areas		
	合计 All	男性 Male	女性 Female	合计 All	男性 Male	女性 Female	合计 All	男性 Male	女性 Female
合计 All	253 675 446	127 474 807	126 200 639	150 352 686	76 544 468	73 808 218	224 401 405	114 796 724	109 604 681
0~	2 504 672	1 316 341	1 188 331	1 506 088	794 501	711 587	2 254 814	1 175 044	1 079 770
1~	11 708 506	6 165 884	5 542 622	7 140 789	3 788 636	3 352 153	9 895 153	5 154 502	4 740 651
5~	14 001 739	7 435 484	6 566 255	9 067 905	4 862 665	4 205 240	12 288 245	6 458 709	5 829 536
10~	12 135 293	6 461 617	5 673 676	8 787 879	4 725 561	4 062 318	12 645 532	6 673 681	5 971 851
15~	10 766 351	5 721 491	5 044 860	8 423 832	4 515 791	3 908 041	13 134 234	6 903 975	6 230 259
20~	13 196 712	6 875 067	6 321 645	9 108 971	4 750 978	4 357 993	14 747 209	7 614 574	7 132 635
25~	17 704 657	9 045 218	8 659 439	10 966 580	5 560 267	5 406 313	16 224 682	8 393 972	7 830 710
30~	21 002 556	10 415 276	10 587 280	11 958 921	5 976 103	5 982 818	16 758 510	8 576 241	8 182 269
35~	19 146 595	9 502 903	9 643 692	11 108 825	5 601 833	5 506 992	15 513 061	7 963 392	7 549 669
40~	17 543 534	8 732 782	8 810 752	11 071 391	5 613 392	5 457 999	17 450 300	8 974 881	8 475 419
45~	20 314 721	10 112 211	10 202 510	12 819 249	6 485 736	6 333 513	20 986 671	10 783 082	10 203 589
50~	20 606 746	10 305 615	10 301 131	12 224 197	6 148 010	6 076 187	18 450 073	9 432 729	9 017 344
55~	18 453 892	9 232 077	9 221 815	9 631 693	4 838 712	4 792 981	13 727 672	6 949 587	6 778 085
60~	17 063 198	8 503 740	8 559 458	8 130 990	4 091 777	4 039 213	12 162 309	6 169 888	5 992 421
65~	14 105 610	6 914 377	7 191 233	6 981 351	3 451 497	3 529 854	10 703 258	5 289 034	5 414 224
70~	9 222 139	4 475 213	4 746 926	4 776 602	2 340 000	2 436 602	7 351 648	3 627 958	3 723 690
75~	6 107 203	2 868 650	3 238 553	3 191 021	1 511 479	1 679 542	5 006 849	2 396 263	2 610 586
80~	4 504 636	1 986 850	2 517 786	2 082 440	929 087	1 153 353	3 108 979	1 424 560	1 684 419
85+	3 586 686	1 404 011	2 182 675	1 373 962	558 443	815 519	1 992 206	834 652	1 157 554

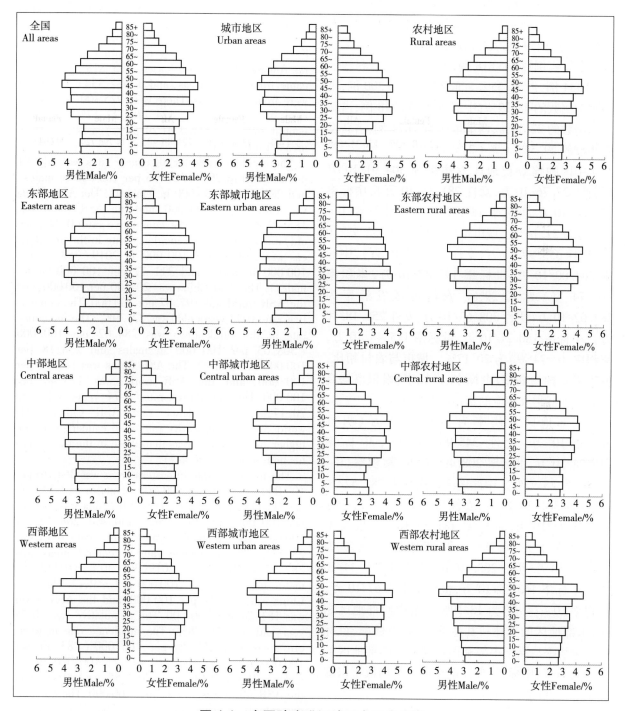

图 4-1　中国肿瘤登记地区人口金字塔

Figure 4-1　Population pyramid in cancer registration areas of China

2 中国肿瘤登记地区全部癌症发病与死亡

2.1 中国肿瘤登记地区全部癌症发病情况

中国肿瘤登记地区新发病例数 1 916 152 例（男性 1 044 959 例，女性 871 193 例），其中城市地区的新发病例数 893 818 例，占 46.65%，农村地区 1 022 334 例，占 53.35%。东部地区 925 300 例，占新发病例数的 48.29%；中部地区 424 778 例，占新发病例数的 22.17%；西部地区 566 074 例，占新发病例数的 29.54%（表 4-2）。

中国肿瘤登记地区发病率为 304.91/10 万（男性 327.76/10 万，女性 281.38/10 万），中标率 190.66/10 万，世标率 185.32/10 万，累积率（0～74 岁）为 21.14%。城市地区发病率为 332.92/10 万（男性 353.99/10 万，女性 311.77/10 万），中标率 204.00/10 万，世标率 197.87/10 万，累积率（0～74 岁）为 22.39%。农村地区发病率为 284.02/10 万（男性 308.63/10 万，女性 258.18/10 万），中标率 180.21/10 万，世标率 175.48/10 万，累积率（0～74 岁）为 20.17%。城市与农村相比，城市男女的发病率、中标率、世标率、累积率均高于农村地区男女相应的指标（表 4-2）。

东部地区发病率为 364.76/10 万（男性 383.43/10 万，女性 345.90/10 万），中标率 215.78/10 万，世标率 208.49/10 万，累积率（0～74 岁）为 23.72%。中部地区发病率为 282.52/10 万（男性 301.30/10 万，女性 263.05/10 万），中标率 185.94/10 万，世标率 181.54/10 万，累积率（0～74 岁）为 20.78%。西部地区发病率为 252.26/10 万（男性 283.60/10 万，女性 219.44/10 万），中标率 163.55/10 万，世标率 159.67/10 万，累积率（0～74 岁）为 18.19%。东中西部地区相比，东部地区的男性和女性发病率、中标率、世标率和累积率均高于中部和西部地区。西部地区的女性发病率、中标率、世标率和累积率均低于东部和中部地区（表 4-2）。

2 Incidence and mortality for all cancer sites in the registration areas of China

2.1 Incidence for all cancer sites in the registration areas of China

There were 1 916 152 new cases(1 044 959 males and 871 193 females) in cancer registration areas of China. Among all the new cases, 893 818 (46.65%) came from urban areas, and 1 022 334 (53.35%) were from rural areas. There were 925 300(48.29%) cases in eastern areas, 424 778 (22.17%) cases in central areas, and 566 074(29.54%)cases in western areas(Table 4-2).

The incidence rate for all cancer sites was 304.91 per 100 000 in 2019(327.76 per 100 000 in males, and 281.38 per 100 000 in females). The ASR China was 190.66 per 100 000, and the ASR world was 185.32 per 100 000. The cumulative rate(0-74 years old) was 21.14%. The incidence rate in the urban areas was 332.92 per 100 000 in 2019(353.99 per 100 000 in males and 311.77 per 100 000 in females). The ASR China was 204.00 per 100 000, and the ASR world was 197.87 per 100 000. The cumulative rate(0-74 years old) was 22.39%. The incidence rate in the rural areas was 284.02 per 100 000 (308.63 per 100 000 in males and 258.18 per 100 000 in females). The ASR China was 180.21 per 100 000, and the ASR world was 175.48 per 100 000. The cumulative rate (0-74 years old) was 20.17%. The incidence rate, ASR China, ASR world, and the cumulative rate of all cancer sites were higher in the urban areas than those in the rural areas for both sexes(Table 4-2).

The incidence rate in eastern areas was 364.76 per 100 000(383.43 per 100 000 in males and 345.90 per 100 000 in females). The ASR China was 215.78 per 100 000, and the ASR world was 208.49 per 100 000. The cumulative rate (0-74 years old) was 23.72%. The incidence rate in central areas was 282.52 per 100 000 in 2019(301.30 per 100 000 in males and 263.05 per 100 000 in females). The ASR China was 185.94 per 100 000, and the ASR world was 181.54 per 100 000. The cumulative rate(0-74 years old) was 20.78%. The incidence rate in western areas was 252.26 per 100 000 (283.60 per 100 000 in males and 219.44 per 100 000 in females). The ASR China was 163.55 per 100 000, and the ASR world was 159.67 per 100 000. The cumulative rate(0-74 years old) was 18.20%. The incidence rate, ASR China, ASR world, and the cumulative rate of both males and females in eastern areas were higher than those in central and western areas. The incidence rate, ASR China, ASR world, and cumulative rate for females in western areas were lower than those in eastern and central areas(Table 4-2).

表 4-2 中国肿瘤登记地区全部癌症发病情况

Table 4-2 Incidence for all cancer sites in the registration areas of China

地区 Area	性别 Sex	病例数 No. cases	发病率 Incidence rate/ 100 000⁻¹	中标率 ASR China/ 100 000⁻¹	世标率 ASR world/ 100 000⁻¹	累积率 Cum. rate 0~74/%
全国 All areas	合计 Both	1 916 152	304. 91	190. 66	185. 32	21. 14
	男性 Male	1 044 959	327. 76	203. 52	201. 24	23. 65
	女性 Female	871 193	281. 38	180. 15	171. 73	18. 76
城市地区 Urban areas	合计 Both	893 818	332. 92	204. 00	197. 87	22. 39
	男性 Male	475 932	353. 99	213. 59	211. 10	24. 62
	女性 Female	417 886	311. 77	196. 73	187. 06	20. 33
农村地区 Rural areas	合计 Both	1 022 334	284. 02	180. 21	175. 48	20. 17
	男性 Male	569 027	308. 63	195. 70	193. 52	22. 90
	女性 Female	453 307	258. 18	166. 95	159. 57	17. 52
东部地区 Eastern areas	合计 Both	925 300	364. 76	215. 78	208. 49	23. 72
	男性 Male	488 775	383. 43	221. 62	218. 36	25. 68
	女性 Female	436 525	345. 90	212. 38	201. 15	21. 91
中部地区 Central areas	合计 Both	424 778	282. 52	185. 94	181. 54	20. 78
	男性 Male	230 625	301. 30	199. 07	197. 43	23. 28
	女性 Female	194 153	263. 05	175. 06	167. 86	18. 38
西部地区 Western areas	合计 Both	566 074	252. 26	163. 55	159. 67	18. 20
	男性 Male	325 559	283. 60	184. 31	182. 59	21. 36
	女性 Female	240 515	219. 44	144. 53	138. 43	15. 10

2. 2 中国肿瘤登记地区全部癌症年龄别发病率

中国肿瘤登记地区全部癌症的年龄别发病率在 0~34 岁时处于较低水平,35~39 岁年龄组发病率快速上升,为 105.79/10 万,80~84 岁年龄组发病率处于最高水平,为 1 416.08/10 万,85 岁及以上年龄组的发病率有所下降,为 1 332.04/10 万。城市和农村地区的癌症年龄别发病率变化模式基本相同。除 10~19 岁年龄组农村发病率略高于城市以外,城市发病率均高于农村。城市男性癌症发病率在 5~9 岁、15~19 岁年龄组低于农村,其他年龄组高于农村;城市女性除 10~19 岁年龄组外,各年龄组癌症发病率均高于农村(表 4-3a,图 4-2)。

东部、中部和西部地区的年龄别发病率均在 80~84 岁年龄组达到最高,85 岁及以上年龄组有所下降。除少数几个年龄组外,东部地区男女性年龄组发病率均高于中部和西部地区。三个区域的城市癌症发病率均高于农村,分城乡、分性别的年龄别发病率曲线基本类似(表 4-3b,图 4-2)。

2. 2 Age-specific incidence rates for all cancer sites in the registration areas of China

The incidence rate for all cancer sites was relatively low in the age group of 0-34 years, and dramatically increased from age group 35-39 years old(105. 79 per 100 100), and reached the peak at the age of 80-84 years old(1 416. 08 per 100 000) and then decreased slightly after 85 years old(1 332. 04 per 100 000). The overall trends of the age-specific incidence in urban areas were similar as that in rural areas. The incidence rate in urban areas was higher than that in rural areas except the age group of 10-19. The incidence rates for males in urban areas were lower than those in rural areas in the age group of 5-9 and 15-19, and higher in other age groups, and the incidence rates for females were higher in urban areas that those in rural areas except the age group of 10-19(Table 4-3a, Figure 4-2).

The age-specific incidence rates in eastern, central and western areas reached peak at the age group of 80-84 years old, and declined after 85 years old. Overall, the age-specific incidence rates in eastern areas were higher than those in central and western areas for both sexes except for a few age groups. The incidence rates in urban areas were higher than those in rural areas in the all three geographic areas and the age-specific incidence curves by urban and rural areas and by sex are basically similar(Table 4-3b, Figure 4-2).

表 4-3a　中国肿瘤登记地区癌症年龄别发病率

Table 4-3a　Age-specific incidence rates for all cancer sites in the registration areas of China

单位：100 000^{-1}

年龄组/ 岁 Age group/ years	全国 All areas			城市地区 Urban areas			农村地区 Rural areas		
	合计 All	男性 Male	女性 Female	合计 All	男性 Male	女性 Female	合计 All	男性 Male	女性 Female
合计 All	304.91	327.76	281.38	332.92	353.99	311.77	284.02	308.63	258.18
0~	12.93	13.48	12.32	13.39	14.00	12.73	12.57	13.08	11.99
1~	12.03	12.95	11.02	12.74	13.82	11.55	11.50	12.30	10.62
5~	8.33	9.03	7.54	8.34	8.97	7.64	8.32	9.07	7.47
10~	9.26	9.76	8.68	9.04	9.80	8.18	9.39	9.73	9.00
15~	13.53	13.44	13.63	13.38	13.32	13.45	13.62	13.51	13.75
20~	20.55	15.90	25.58	21.99	16.71	27.55	19.56	15.35	24.18
25~	43.02	30.77	55.88	49.26	35.52	63.17	38.37	27.34	50.28
30~	70.59	49.36	92.00	82.29	56.48	106.99	61.20	43.91	79.38
35~	105.79	72.00	140.13	119.06	78.92	157.95	94.43	66.33	124.18
40~	160.59	114.15	208.21	172.52	117.15	227.35	151.24	111.88	192.72
45~	249.54	191.89	308.56	268.35	198.37	338.68	235.76	187.22	286.13
50~	360.20	328.37	392.65	380.75	337.85	424.12	345.83	321.79	370.49
55~	480.13	502.83	457.18	522.20	538.56	505.74	446.63	474.51	418.33
60~	688.36	814.43	561.11	734.99	859.62	611.70	650.59	778.48	519.37
65~	900.04	1 134.14	672.90	942.11	1 176.03	719.93	867.72	1 102.58	636.11
70~	1 106.13	1 430.02	796.02	1 141.71	1 462.29	841.00	1 079.35	1 406.17	761.57
75~	1 308.37	1 718.70	939.04	1 375.54	1 790.37	1 011.36	1 257.39	1 665.56	883.00
80~	1 416.08	1 868.43	1 049.47	1 537.69	2 001.67	1 163.00	1 315.47	1 758.59	955.26
85+	1 332.04	1 809.19	1 010.89	1 474.91	1 993.78	1 113.50	1 205.23	1 638.87	922.15

表 4-3b 中国不同肿瘤登记地区癌症年龄别发病率
Table 4-3b Age-specific incidence rates for all cancer sites in different registration areas of China

单位: 100 000⁻¹

年龄组/岁 Age group/years	东部地区 Eastern areas			中部地区 Central areas			西部地区 Western areas		
	合计 All	男性 Male	女性 Female	合计 All	男性 Male	女性 Female	合计 All	男性 Male	女性 Female
合计 All	364.76	383.43	345.90	282.52	301.30	263.05	252.26	283.60	219.44
0~	15.85	17.17	14.39	12.68	12.96	12.37	9.85	9.70	10.00
1~	13.21	14.37	11.93	12.62	13.59	11.51	10.21	10.77	9.60
5~	8.26	8.96	7.46	9.37	9.91	8.75	7.63	8.44	6.74
10~	9.67	10.11	9.17	10.21	10.77	9.55	8.20	8.71	7.64
15~	15.89	15.63	16.19	12.58	12.40	12.79	12.20	12.30	12.09
20~	25.82	19.46	32.74	18.15	13.91	22.76	17.32	13.92	20.95
25~	56.12	39.31	73.68	40.10	28.61	51.92	30.68	22.98	38.94
30~	88.70	59.45	117.47	62.07	42.60	81.52	53.98	41.82	66.72
35~	136.80	88.72	184.17	88.70	58.82	119.08	79.77	61.32	99.24
40~	195.19	128.42	261.36	147.08	102.24	193.20	134.38	107.72	162.61
45~	290.25	207.07	372.69	242.75	182.82	304.13	214.27	183.12	247.19
50~	391.36	335.50	447.25	355.21	314.00	396.89	328.70	329.94	327.40
55~	539.35	546.27	532.42	469.34	486.93	451.58	408.09	456.19	358.77
60~	763.97	878.99	649.70	670.58	793.08	546.49	594.18	739.62	444.43
65~	976.76	1 206.53	755.84	913.52	1 149.10	683.17	790.13	1 029.75	556.05
70~	1 232.67	1 576.51	908.52	1 103.13	1 436.54	782.93	949.34	1 245.11	661.17
75~	1 420.73	1 851.53	1 039.14	1 310.18	1 737.11	925.97	1 170.16	1 548.08	823.26
80~	1 541.43	2 036.89	1 150.46	1 441.91	1 907.14	1 067.15	1 217.15	1 608.22	886.42
85+	1 387.05	1 884.96	1 066.76	1 360.66	1 826.33	1 041.79	1 213.28	1 670.28	883.76

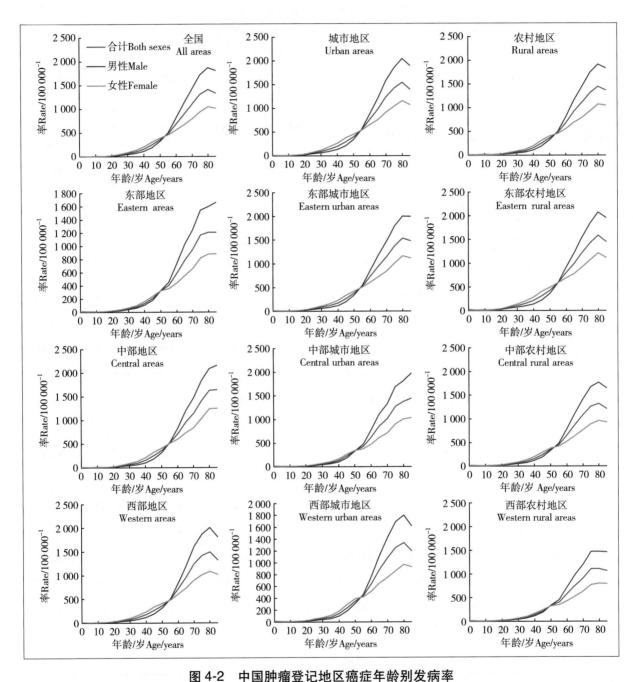

图 4-2　中国肿瘤登记地区癌症年龄别发病率

Figure 4-2　Age-specific incidence rates for all cancer sites in the registration areas of China

2.3 中国肿瘤登记地区全部癌症死亡情况

中国肿瘤登记地区报告癌症死亡 1 087 549 例（男性 698 492 例，女性 389 057 例），其中城市地区 477 415 例，占全国癌症死亡的 43.90%，农村地区 610 134 例，占全国癌症死亡的 56.10%。东部地区 483 539 例，占全国癌症死亡的 44.46%；中部地区 245 436 例，占全国癌症死亡的 22.57%；西部地区 358 574 例，占全国癌症死亡的 32.97%（表 4-4）。

中国肿瘤登记地区癌症死亡率为 173.06/10万（男性 219.09/10 万，女性 125.66/10 万），中标率 97.19/10 万，世标率 96.51/10 万，累积率（0~74 岁）为 10.79%。城市地区癌症死亡率为 177.82/10 万（男性 225.72/10 万，女性 129.78/10 万），中标率 95.88/10 万，世标率 95.42/10 万，累积率（0~74 岁）为 10.47%。农村地区癌症死亡率为 169.51/10 万（男性 214.26/10 万，女性 122.52/10 万），中标率 98.10/10 万，世标率 97.21/10 万，累积率（0~74 岁）为 11.03%。城市与农村相比，城市地区男性和女性癌症死亡率均高于农村，而城市男性和女性的中标率、世标率和累积率均低于农村（表 4-4）。

东部、中部和西部地区癌症死亡率分别为 190.61/10 万（男性 239.52/10 万，女性 141.21/10 万）、163.24/10 万（男性 204.75/10 万，女性 120.19/10 万）和 159.79/10 万（男性 205.96/10 万，女性 111.43/10 万）。东部地区的中标率为 95.98/10 万、中部地区 98.86/10 万、西部地区 97.01/10 万。东部地区的世标率为 95.27/10 万、中部地区 98.13/10 万、西部地区 96.33/10 万。东部、中部和西部地区累积率（0~74 岁）分别为 10.54%、11.09% 和 10.89%。东部地区男女性的癌症死亡率均高于中部和西部，男女合计的中标率、世标率和累积率均低于中部和西部地区（表 4-4）。

2.3 Mortality for all cancer sites in the registration areas of China

There were 1 087 549 cancer deaths (698 492 males and 389 057 females) in the registration areas of China. Among those, 477 415 (43.90%) came from urban areas, and 610 134 (56.10%) came from rural areas. There were 483 539 (44.46%) death cases in eastern areas, 245 436 (22.57%) in central areas and 358 574 (32.97%) in western areas (Table 4-4).

The mortality rate of all cancer sites was 173.06 per 100 000 (219.09 per 100 000 in males and 125.66 per 100 000 in females). The ASR China was 97.19 per 100 000, and the ASR world was 96.51 per 100 000. The cumulative rate (0-74 years old) was 10.79%. The mortality rate for all cancer sites in urban areas was 177.82 per 100 000 (225.72 per 100 000 in males and 129.78 per 100 000 in females). The ASR China was 95.88 per 100 000, and the ASR world was 95.42 per 100 000. The cumulative rate (0-74 years old) was 10.47%. The mortality rate for all cancer sites in rural areas was 169.51 per 100 000 in 2019 (214.26 per 100 000 in males and 122.52 per 100 000 in females). The ASR China was 98.10 per 100 000, and the ASR world was 97.21 per 100 000. The cumulative rate (0-74 years old) was 11.03%. The mortality rates for all cancer sites in urban areas were higher than those in rural areas for both sexes. The ASR China, ASR world and cumulative rates of all cancer sites were lower in urban areas than those in rural areas for both sexes (Table 4-4).

The mortality rates for all cancer sites in eastern, central and western areas were 190.61 per 100 000 (239.52 per 100 000 in males and 141.21 per 100 000 in females), 163.24 per 100 000 (204.75 per 100 000 in males and 120.19 per 100 000 in females), and 159.79 per 100 000 (205.96 per 100 000 in males and 111.43 per 100 000 in females), respectively. The ASR China were 95.98 per 100 000 in eastern areas, 98.86 per 100 000 in central areas, and 97.01 per 100 000 in western areas, respectively. The ASRworld were 95.27 per 100 000 in eastern areas, 98.13 per 100 000 in central areas, and 96.33 per 100 000 in western areas. The cumulative rates (0-74 years old) in eastern, central and western areas were 10.54%, 11.09% and 10.89%, respectively. The mortality rate for all cancer sites in eastern areas was higher than that in central and western areas for both sexes. The ASR China, ASR world and cumulative rates were the lowest in eastern areas for both sexes combined (Table 4-4).

表 4-4　中国肿瘤登记地区全部癌症死亡情况

Table 4-4　Mortality for all cancer sites in the registration areas of China

地区 Area	性别 Sex	死亡数 No. deaths	粗率 Crude rate/ 100 000⁻¹	中标率 ASR China/ 100 000⁻¹	世标率 ASR world/ 100 000⁻¹	累积率 Cum. rate 0~74/%
全国 All areas	合计 Both	1 087 549	173. 06	97. 19	96. 51	10. 79
	男性 Male	698 492	219. 09	129. 10	128. 62	14. 52
	女性 Female	389 057	125. 66	67. 13	66. 33	7. 13
城市地区 Urban areas	合计 Both	477 415	177. 82	95. 88	95. 42	10. 47
	男性 Male	303 467	225. 72	127. 26	127. 26	14. 16
	女性 Female	173 948	129. 78	66. 85	66. 02	6. 91
农村地区 Rural areas	合计 Both	610 134	169. 51	98. 10	97. 21	11. 03
	男性 Male	395 025	214. 26	130. 31	129. 43	14. 79
	女性 Female	215 109	122. 52	67. 30	66. 51	7. 30
东部地区 Eastern areas	合计 Both	483 539	190. 61	95. 98	95. 27	10. 54
	男性 Male	305 326	239. 52	127. 12	126. 74	14. 17
	女性 Female	178 213	141. 21	67. 33	66. 41	7. 04
中部地区 Central areas	合计 Both	245 436	163. 24	98. 86	98. 13	11. 09
	男性 Male	156 727	204. 75	130. 17	129. 46	14. 74
	女性 Female	88 709	120. 19	69. 42	68. 73	7. 50
西部地区 Western areas	合计 Both	358 574	159. 79	97. 01	96. 33	10. 89
	男性 Male	236 439	205. 96	130. 02	129. 55	14. 80
	女性 Female	122 135	111. 43	64. 91	64. 12	6. 99

2. 4　中国肿瘤登记地区全部癌症年龄别死亡率

中国肿瘤登记地区癌症年龄别死亡率在 25~29 岁组为 7. 53/10 万(男性 8. 44/10 万,女性 6. 58/10 万),在 40~44 岁年龄组时达到 42. 12/10 万,在这以后死亡率随年龄增长而明显升高,85 岁以上年龄组达最高,为 1 503. 21/10 万。城乡年龄别死亡率的变化模式基本相似,城市地区和农村地区的癌症死亡率均在 85 岁及以上年龄组达到最高,分别为 1 649. 89 /10 万和 1 373. 01/10 万。城市多数年龄组的死亡率低于农村(表 4-5a,图 4-3)。

东部、中部和西部地区的年龄别癌症死亡率曲线与全国的基本一致。东部、中部和西部地区男性和女性年龄别死亡率均在 85 岁以后达到高峰,分别为 1 615. 34/10 万、1 503. 10/10 万和 1 301. 42/10 万。在 0~64 岁的各个组别中,西部多数年龄组的死亡率高于东部和中部,65~74 岁年龄组以中部最高,而 80~84 岁年龄组以东部地区最高。三个区域的城市癌症死亡率均高于农村,城市与农村的年龄别死亡率曲线基本相似(表 4-5b,图 4-3)。

2. 4　Age-specific mortality rates for all cancer sites in the registration areas of China

The age-specific mortality rate for all cancer sites was 7. 53 per 100 000 (8. 44 per 100 000 in males and 6. 58 per 100 000 in females) in the 25-29 age group and 42. 12 per 100 000 in the 40-44 age group. The mortality rate increased significantly after the age group of 40-44 years old and reached the peak in the over 85 years old, with a mortality rate of 1 503. 21/ 100 000. The trends of age-specific mortality in urban and rural areas were similar, the mortality rate in urban areas and rural areas reaches the highest in the age group of 85 years and above, with a mortality rate of 1 649. 89 per 100 000 and 1 373. 01 per 100 000, respectively. Most age groups had lower mortality rates in urban areas than in rural areas(Table 4-5a, Figure 4-3).

The trends of age-specific mortality rates in different areas(eastern areas, central areas, and western areas) were similar to those of the overall country. The age-specific mortality rates for both sexes in eastern, central and western areas reached peak after 85 years old, with mortality rates of 1 615. 34 per 100 000, 1 503. 10 per 100 000 and 1 301. 42 per 100 000, respectively. Most age groups in the age range of 0-64 had the highest mortality rate in western areas. The mortality rate was the highest in central areas in the 65-74 age group, and it was the highest in eastern areas in 80-84 age groups. The trends of the age-specific mortality rates were similar in urban and rural areas, although the rates in urban areas were generally higher than those in rural areas in all three geographic areas(Table 4-5b, Figure 4-3).

表 4-5a 中国肿瘤登记地区癌症年龄别死亡率

Table 4-5a Age-specific mortality rates for all cancer sites in the registration areas of China

单位:100 000⁻¹

年龄组/岁 Age group/years	全国 All areas			城市地区 Urban areas			农村地区 Rural areas		
	合计 All	男性 Male	女性 Female	合计 All	男性 Male	女性 Female	合计 All	男性 Male	女性 Female
合计 All	173.06	219.09	125.66	177.82	225.72	129.78	169.51	214.26	122.52
0~	6.11	6.39	5.81	4.11	3.90	4.34	7.68	8.32	6.96
1~	3.59	3.77	3.39	3.55	3.72	3.35	3.62	3.81	3.41
5~	2.80	3.08	2.48	2.63	2.83	2.41	2.92	3.25	2.53
10~	3.21	3.44	2.94	3.10	3.38	2.78	3.28	3.48	3.04
15~	5.03	5.92	4.04	5.60	6.87	4.20	4.68	5.33	3.93
20~	4.66	5.33	3.94	4.10	4.60	3.58	5.05	5.83	4.20
25~	7.53	8.44	6.58	6.57	7.10	6.04	8.25	9.41	6.99
30~	13.33	15.30	11.34	12.08	13.08	11.12	14.33	17.00	11.53
35~	21.91	24.93	18.85	20.02	21.78	18.31	23.54	27.52	19.32
40~	42.12	49.34	34.72	38.47	43.46	33.53	44.98	53.81	35.68
45~	78.97	94.94	62.61	74.53	87.10	61.90	82.22	100.59	63.14
50~	139.55	176.15	102.25	132.97	167.47	98.09	144.15	182.17	105.17
55~	206.73	274.47	138.25	206.86	275.05	138.28	206.63	274.00	138.23
60~	351.64	483.42	218.63	344.89	480.55	210.70	357.11	485.71	225.17
65~	526.80	729.41	330.21	515.39	720.86	320.23	535.56	735.86	338.03
70~	749.50	1 025.90	484.86	722.52	994.72	467.20	769.81	1 048.95	498.39
75~	1 037.78	1 408.01	704.55	1 045.15	1 410.21	724.65	1 032.19	1 406.37	688.97
80~	1 327.42	1 776.80	963.20	1 408.76	1 856.71	1 047.02	1 260.12	1 710.93	893.66
85+	1 503.21	2 059.20	1 128.99	1 649.89	2 247.75	1 233.47	1 373.01	1 885.23	1 038.64

表 4-5b 中国不同肿瘤登记地区癌症年龄别死亡率

Table 4-5b Age-specific mortality rates for all cancer sites in different registration areas of China

单位:100 000^{-1}

年龄组/岁 Age group/ years	东部地区 Eastern areas			中部地区 Central areas			西部地区 Western areas		
	合计 All	男性 Male	女性 Female	合计 All	男性 Male	女性 Female	合计 All	男性 Male	女性 Female
合计 Total	190.61	239.52	141.21	163.24	204.75	120.19	159.79	205.96	111.43
0~	3.87	3.57	4.21	3.65	3.15	4.22	10.24	11.74	8.61
1~	2.87	3.23	2.47	3.02	2.75	3.34	4.85	5.18	4.49
5~	2.36	2.73	1.95	3.22	3.29	3.14	2.99	3.33	2.61
10~	2.93	2.99	2.87	3.43	3.85	2.93	3.32	3.60	3.01
15~	4.76	5.47	3.96	5.00	6.11	3.71	5.28	6.16	4.30
20~	4.24	4.67	3.78	4.30	4.84	3.72	5.26	6.24	4.22
25~	6.42	7.04	5.77	8.21	9.28	7.10	8.29	9.39	7.11
30~	11.05	11.78	10.32	13.11	14.78	11.45	16.34	19.93	12.58
35~	20.27	21.97	18.59	19.92	21.81	18.00	25.37	30.67	19.79
40~	37.78	41.99	33.61	39.38	44.11	34.52	48.22	59.76	36.00
45~	71.80	84.20	59.50	76.86	88.56	64.88	87.19	108.85	64.31
50~	124.44	155.76	93.12	138.46	167.52	109.07	157.14	204.04	108.08
55~	200.54	266.01	135.01	210.30	271.95	148.05	212.55	287.46	135.75
60~	341.40	468.66	214.96	353.92	478.86	227.35	364.49	506.78	217.99
65~	512.35	707.63	324.59	550.27	752.54	352.48	530.53	742.80	323.17
70~	764.63	1 048.96	496.57	788.09	1 078.21	509.48	705.46	963.74	453.82
75~	1 076.30	1 454.76	741.07	1 072.92	1 471.21	714.48	968.39	1 312.17	652.84
80~	1 452.64	1 941.41	1 066.93	1 342.56	1 836.64	944.55	1 135.84	1 508.18	820.94
85+	1 615.34	2 227.69	1 221.44	1 503.10	2 032.79	1 140.38	1 301.42	1 793.44	946.65

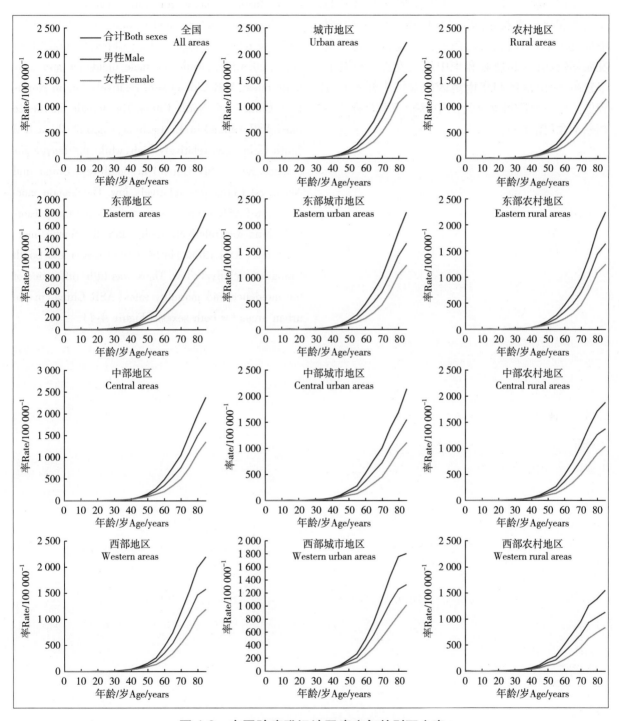

图 4-3　中国肿瘤登记地区癌症年龄别死亡率

Figure 4-3　Age-specific mortality rates for all cancer sites in the registration areas of China

2.5 中国不同肿瘤登记地区全部癌症标化发病与死亡情况

总体而言,七大行政区中标发病率与死亡率相差不大。华东、华中和华南地区男性中标发病率和死亡率相对较高,西北和华北地区男性中标发病率和死亡率较低;华东、华中和华北地区女性中标发病率相对较高,西南和西北地区女性中标发病率较低;东北地区和华中地区女性中标死亡率较高,西南地区和华南地区的女性中标死亡率较低。城市地区男女合计的中标发病率与死亡率相差不大(图4-4)。

2.5 Age-standardized incidence and mortality for all cancer sites in different registration areas of China

In general, the incidence and mortality rates (ASR China) in the seven administrative districts were similar. The male incidence and mortality rates (ASR China) were relatively high in East China, Central China and South China, while the male incidence and mortality rates (ASR China) were relatively low in Northwest China and North China. The female incidence rate (ASR China) in East China, Central China and North China was relatively high, while the female incidence rate (ASR China) in Southwest China and Northwest China was relatively low. The female mortality rate (ASR China) in Northeast China and Central China was relatively high, while the female mortality rate (ASR China) in Southwest China and South China was relatively low. There was little difference of the incidence and mortality rates (ASR China) in the urban areas for both sexes. (Figure 4-4).

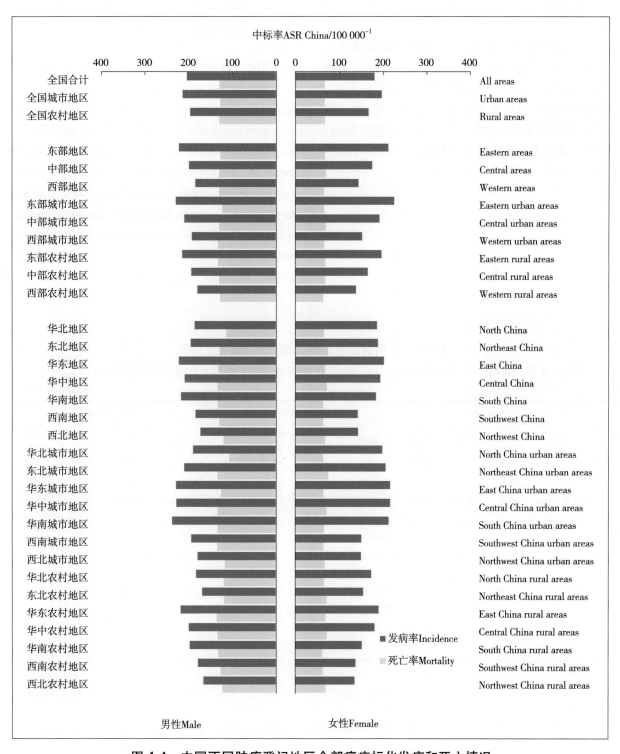

中标率ASR China/100 000^{-1}

全国合计		All areas
全国城市地区		Urban areas
全国农村地区		Rural areas
东部地区		Eastern areas
中部地区		Central areas
西部地区		Western areas
东部城市地区		Eastern urban areas
中部城市地区		Central urban areas
西部城市地区		Western urban areas
东部农村地区		Eastern rural areas
中部农村地区		Central rural areas
西部农村地区		Western rural areas
华北地区		North China
东北地区		Northeast China
华东地区		East China
华中地区		Central China
华南地区		South China
西南地区		Southwest China
西北地区		Northwest China
华北城市地区		North China urban areas
东北城市地区		Northeast China urban areas
华东城市地区		East China urban areas
华中城市地区		Central China urban areas
华南城市地区		South China urban areas
西南城市地区		Southwest China urban areas
西北城市地区		Northwest China urban areas
华北农村地区		North China rural areas
东北农村地区		Northeast China rural areas
华东农村地区		East China rural areas
华中农村地区		Central China rural areas
华南农村地区		South China rural areas
西南农村地区		Southwest China rural areas
西北农村地区		Northwest China rural areas

■ 发病率Incidence
■ 死亡率Mortality

男性Male　　　　女性Female

图 4-4　中国不同肿瘤登记地区全部癌症标化发病和死亡情况
Figure 4-4　Age-standardized incidence and mortality for all cancer sites in different registration areas of China

3 中国肿瘤登记地区前 10 位癌症发病与死亡

3.1 中国肿瘤登记地区前 10 位癌症发病情况

中国肿瘤登记地区癌症发病第 1 位的是肺癌,其次为女性乳腺癌、结直肠癌、肝癌和胃癌。男性发病第 1 位癌症为肺癌,其次为肝癌、结直肠癌、胃癌和食管癌;女性发病第 1 位癌症为肺癌,其次为乳腺癌、甲状腺癌、结直肠癌和子宫颈癌(表 4-6,图 4-5a,图 4-5b)。

3 Top ten leading causes of new cancer cases and deaths in the registration areas of China

3.1 Top ten leading causes of new cancer cases in the registration areas of China

Lung cancer was the most common cancer in cancer registration areas of China, followed by female breast cancer, colorectum cancer, liver cancer and stomach cancer. The top five cancers in males were lung cancer, liver cancer, colorectal cancer, stomach cancer, and esophageal cancer. The most common cancer in females was lung cancer, followed by breast cancer, thyroid cancer, colorectal cancer and cervix cancer (Table 4-6, Figure 4-5a, Figure 4-5b).

表 4-6 中国肿瘤登记地区前 10 位癌症发病率

Table 4-6 Incidence rates of top ten leading cancer sites in the registration areas of China

单位:100 000^{-1}

顺位 Rank	合计 All				男性 Male				女性 Female			
	部位 Site	粗率 Crude rate	世标率 ASR world	中标率 ASR China	部位 Site	粗率 Crude rate	世标率 ASR world	中标率 ASR China	部位 Site	粗率 Crude rate	世标率 ASR world	中标率 ASR China
1	肺 Lung	67.22	38.45	38.58	肺 Lung	84.99	50.28	50.14	肺 Lung	48.93	27.28	27.67
2	乳腺 Breast	43.10	28.08	30.11	肝 Liver	39.64	24.86	25.37	乳腺 Breast	43.10	28.08	30.11
3	结直肠 Colorectum	31.23	17.97	18.19	结直肠 Colorectum	36.33	21.81	21.96	甲状腺 Thyroid	28.98	21.33	24.77
4	肝 Liver	26.99	16.20	16.50	胃 Stomach	35.57	21.02	21.02	结直肠 Colorectum	25.99	14.30	14.58
5	胃 Stomach	25.89	14.68	14.79	食管 Esophagus	24.62	14.43	14.28	子宫颈 Cervix	18.16	11.80	12.74
6	甲状腺 Thyroid	18.96	14.09	16.46	前列腺 Prostate	13.62	7.41	7.53	胃 Stomach	15.91	8.62	8.85
7	子宫颈 Cervix	18.16	11.80	12.74	膀胱 Bladder	9.41	5.45	5.48	肝 Liver	13.96	7.64	7.73
8	食管 Esophagus	16.72	9.25	9.20	甲状腺 Thyroid	9.23	6.99	8.31	子宫体 Uterus	10.83	6.84	7.08
9	前列腺 Prostate	13.62	7.41	7.53	胰腺 Pancreas	8.01	4.72	4.72	脑 Brain	9.22	6.09	6.18
10	子宫体 Uterus	10.83	6.84	7.08	淋巴瘤 Lymphoma	7.63	4.99	5.09	食管 Esophagus	8.58	4.27	4.31

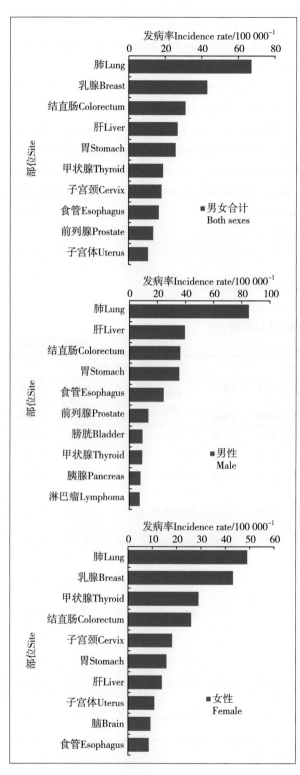

图 4-5a 中国肿瘤登记地区前 10 位癌症发病率
Figure 4-5a Incidence rates of top ten leading cancer sites in the registration areas of China

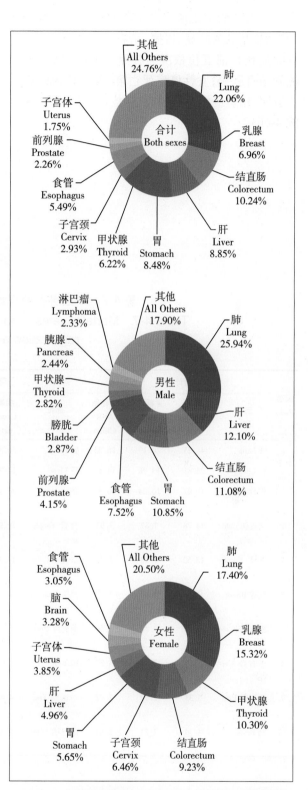

图 4-5b 中国肿瘤登记地区前 10 位癌症发病构成
Figure 4-5b Distribution of top ten leading causes of new cancer cases in the registration areas of China

3.2 中国肿瘤登记地区前 10 位癌症死亡情况

中国肿瘤登记地区男女合计癌症死亡第 1 位为肺癌,其次为肝癌、胃癌、结直肠癌和食管癌;男性癌症死亡前五位依次为肺癌、肝癌、胃癌、食管癌和结直肠癌;女性癌症死亡第 1 位为肺癌,其次为肝癌、结直肠癌、胃癌和乳腺癌(表 4-7,图 4-6a,图 4-6b)。

3.2 Top ten leading causes of cancer deaths in the registration areas of China

For both sexes combined, lung cancer was the leading cause of cancer deaths, followed by liver cancer, stomach cancer, colorectal cancer and esophageal cancer. For males, the five leading causes of cancer deaths were lung cancer, liver cancer, stomach cancer, esophageal cancer and colorectal cancer. For females, the five leading causes of cancer deaths were lung cancer, liver cancer, colorectal cancer, stomach cancer and breast cancer(Table 4-7, Figure 4-6a, Figure 4-6b).

表 4-7 中国肿瘤登记地区前 10 位癌症死亡率
Table 4-7 Mortality rates of top ten leading cancer sites in the registration areas of China

单位:100 000^{-1}

顺位 Rank	合计 All				男性 Male				女性 Female			
	部位 Site	粗率 Crude rate	世标率 ASR world	中标率 ASR China	部位 Site	粗率 Crude rate	世标率 ASR world	中标率 ASR China	部位 Site	粗率 Crude rate	世标率 ASR world	中标率 ASR China
1	肺 Lung	48.25	26.19	26.23	肺 Lung	66.80	38.43	38.39	肺 Lung	29.15	14.65	14.77
2	肝 Liver	23.81	13.96	14.20	肝 Liver	34.77	21.47	21.88	肝 Liver	12.52	6.58	6.65
3	胃 Stomach	19.07	10.24	10.36	胃 Stomach	26.11	14.88	14.98	结直肠 Colorectum	12.14	5.99	6.07
4	结直肠 Colorectum	14.78	7.87	7.93	食管 Esophagus	19.96	11.40	11.37	胃 Stomach	11.82	5.92	6.04
5	食管 Esophagus	13.50	7.18	7.18	结直肠 Colorectum	17.34	9.91	9.93	乳腺 Breast	9.24	5.42	5.57
6	乳腺 Breast	9.24	5.42	5.57	胰腺 Pancreas	7.27	4.22	4.22	食管 Esophagus	6.84	3.16	3.20
7	胰腺 Pancreas	6.43	3.50	3.50	前列腺 Prostate	5.33	2.77	2.72	胰腺 Pancreas	5.57	2.80	2.81
8	子宫颈 Cervix	5.55	3.27	3.39	脑 Brain	4.66	3.16	3.18	子宫颈 Cervix	5.55	3.27	3.39
9	前列腺 Prostate	5.33	2.77	2.72	白血病 Leukemia	4.40	3.06	3.08	脑 Brain	3.93	2.45	2.45
10	脑 Brain	4.30	2.81	2.81	淋巴瘤 Lymphoma	4.31	2.61	2.65	卵巢 Ovary	3.57	2.09	2.12

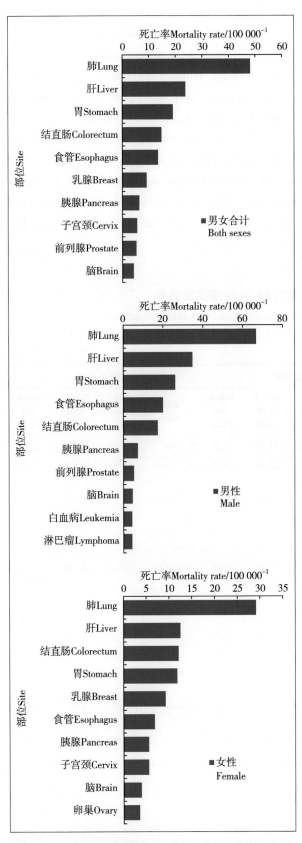

图 4-6a 中国肿瘤登记地区前 10 位癌症死亡率
Figure 4-6a Mortality rates of top ten leading cancer sites in the registration areas of China

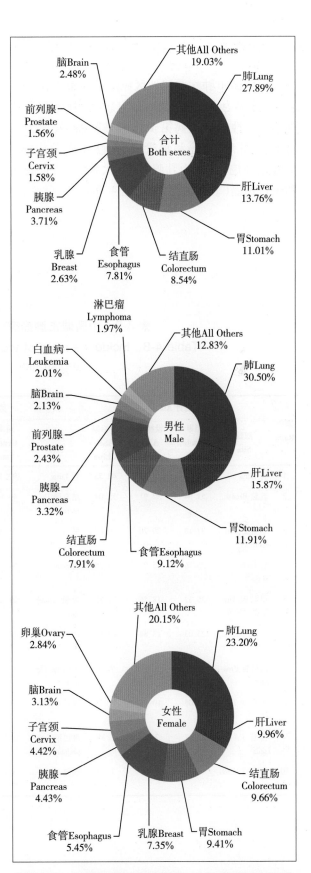

图 4-6b 中国肿瘤登记地区前 10 位癌症死亡构成
Figure 4-6b Distribution of top ten leading causes of cancer deaths in the registration areas of China

3.3 中国城市肿瘤登记地区前 10 位癌症发病情况

中国城市肿瘤登记地区癌症发病第 1 位的是肺癌,其次为女性乳腺癌、结直肠癌、肝癌和甲状腺癌。男性癌症发病第 1 位的是肺癌,其次为结直肠癌、肝癌、胃癌和食管癌;女性癌症发病第 1 位的是肺癌,其次为乳腺癌、甲状腺癌、结直肠癌和子宫颈癌(表 4-8,图 4-7a,图 4-7b)。

3.3 Top ten leading causes of new cancer cases in urban registration areas of China

Lung cancer was the most common cancer in urban areas of China, followed by female breast cancer, colorectal cancer, liver cancer and thyroid cancer. In males, lung cancer was the most common cancer, followed by colorectal cancer, liver cancer, stomach cancer and esophageal cancer. In females, lung cancer was the most common cancer, followed by breast cancer, thyroid cancer, colorectal cancer and cervix cancer (Table 4-8, Figure 4-7a, Figure 4-7b).

表 4-8 中国城市肿瘤登记地区前 10 位癌症发病率

Table 4-8 Incidence rates of top ten leading cancer sites in urban registration areas of China

单位:100 000^{-1}

顺位 Rank	合计 All				男性 Male				女性 Female			
	部位 Site	粗率 Crude rate	世标率 ASR world	中标率 ASR China	部位 Site	粗率 Crude rate	世标率 ASR world	中标率 ASR China	部位 Site	粗率 Crude rate	世标率 ASR world	中标率 ASR China
1	肺 Lung	72.36	40.39	40.53	肺 Lung	90.35	51.82	51.60	肺 Lung	54.31	29.79	30.28
2	乳腺 Breast	51.94	32.91	35.04	结直肠 Colorectum	43.89	25.43	25.49	乳腺 Breast	51.94	32.91	35.04
3	结直肠 Colorectum	37.18	20.70	20.87	肝 Liver	38.35	23.39	23.74	甲状腺 Thyroid	37.55	27.25	31.83
4	肝 Liver	25.76	15.06	15.26	胃 Stomach	34.56	19.81	19.79	结直肠 Colorectum	30.44	16.24	16.53
5	甲状腺 Thyroid	25.32	18.56	21.85	食管 Esophagus	21.22	12.13	11.96	子宫颈 Cervix	17.05	10.94	11.78
6	胃 Stomach	25.03	13.84	13.95	前列腺 Prostate	17.62	9.24	9.37	胃 Stomach	15.46	8.24	8.48
7	前列腺 Prostate	17.62	9.24	9.37	甲状腺 Thyroid	13.13	9.81	11.77	肝 Liver	13.13	6.97	7.03
8	子宫颈 Cervix	17.05	10.94	11.78	膀胱 Bladder	11.19	6.24	6.26	子宫体 Uterus	11.70	7.28	7.50
9	食管 Esophagus	13.67	7.42	7.35	淋巴瘤 Lymphoma	9.08	5.75	5.88	脑 Brain	9.78	6.32	6.41
10	子宫体 Uterus	11.70	7.28	7.50	胰腺 Pancreas	9.04	5.15	5.13	卵巢 Ovary	8.63	5.63	5.93

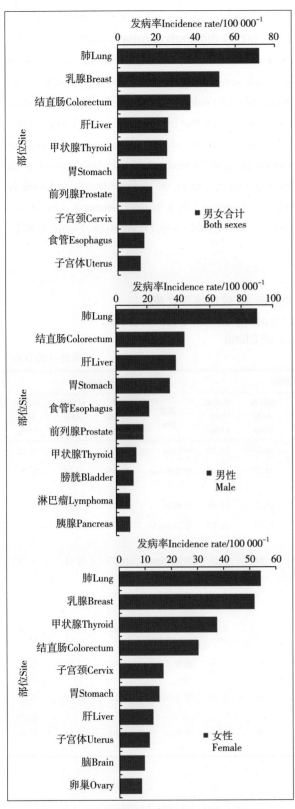

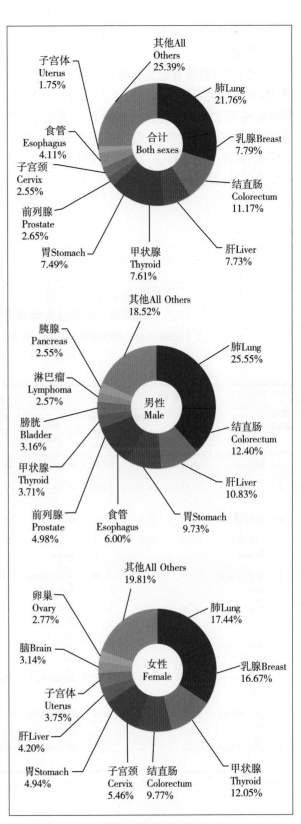

图 4-7a　中国城市肿瘤登记地区前 10 位
癌症发病率

Figure 4-7a　Incidence rates of top ten leading cancer sites in urban registration areas of China

图 4-7b　中国城市肿瘤登记地区前 10 位
癌症发病构成

Figure 4-7b　Distribution of top ten leading causes of new cancer cases in urban registration areas of China

3.4 中国城市肿瘤登记地区前10位癌症死亡情况

中国城市肿瘤登记地区合计癌症死亡第1位的为肺癌,其次为肝癌、胃癌、结直肠癌和食管癌。男性癌症死亡第1位的为肺癌,其次为肝癌、胃癌、结直肠癌和食管癌;女性癌症死亡率第1位的为肺癌,其次为结直肠癌、肝癌、胃癌和乳腺癌(表4-9,图4-8a,图4-8b)。

3.4 Top ten leading causes of cancer deaths in urban registration areas of China

Lung cancer was the leading cause of cancer deaths in urban areas of China, followed by cancers of the liver, stomach, colorectum and esophagus. In males, lung cancer was the leading cause of cancer deaths, followed by cancers of the liver, stomach, colorectum and esophageal. In females, lung cancer ranked as the leading cancer cause of cancer deaths, followed by colorectal cancer, liver cancer, stomach cancer and breast cancer(Table 4-9, Figure 4-8a, Figure 4-8b).

表 4-9 中国城市肿瘤登记地区前 10 位癌症死亡率

Table 4-9 Mortality rates of top ten leading cancer sites in urban registration areas of China

单位:100 000⁻¹

顺位 Rank	合计 All				男性 Male				女性 Female			
	部位 Site	粗率 Crude rate	世标率 ASR world	中标率 ASR China	部位 Site	粗率 Crude rate	世标率 ASR world	中标率 ASR China	部位 Site	粗率 Crude rate	世标率 ASR world	中标率 ASR China
1	肺 Lung	49.58	25.87	25.89	肺 Lung	69.34	38.37	38.25	肺 Lung	29.75	14.28	14.43
2	肝 Liver	22.45	12.72	12.90	肝 Liver	33.07	19.75	20.04	结直肠 Colo-rectum	14.19	6.70	6.77
3	胃 Stomach	17.91	9.30	9.40	胃 Stomach	24.66	13.52	13.59	肝 Liver	11.79	5.94	6.00
4	结直肠 Colo-rectum	17.31	8.80	8.83	结直肠 Colo-rectum	20.43	11.12	11.07	胃 Stomach	11.14	5.43	5.56
5	食管 Esoph-agus	11.18	5.81	5.79	食管 Esoph-agus	17.35	9.64	9.56	乳腺 Breast	10.70	6.05	6.19
6	乳腺 Breast	10.70	6.05	6.19	胰腺 Pancre-as	8.41	4.71	4.69	胰腺 Pancre-as	6.51	3.15	3.18
7	胰腺 Pancre-as	7.46	3.91	3.91	前列腺 Pros-tate	6.76	3.29	3.22	子宫颈 Cer-vix	5.09	2.97	3.09
8	前列腺 Pros-tate	6.76	3.29	3.22	淋巴瘤 Lym-phoma	5.05	2.92	2.96	食管 Esoph-agus	4.98	2.22	2.26
9	子宫颈 Cer-vix	5.09	2.97	3.09	白血病 Leu-kemia	4.68	3.08	3.10	卵巢 Ovary	4.18	2.39	2.42
10	淋巴瘤 Lym-phoma	4.20	2.32	2.36	脑 Brain	4.52	2.99	2.99	脑 Brain	3.80	2.32	2.31

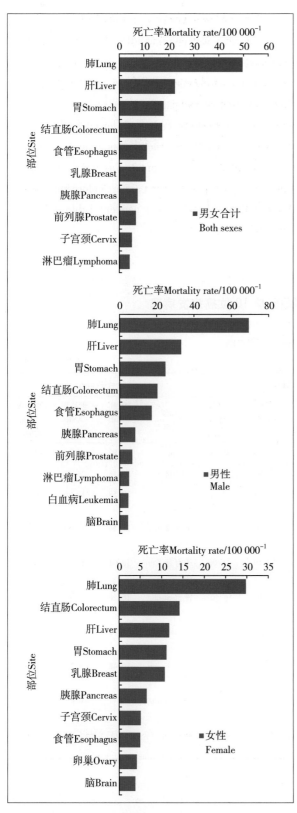

图 4-8a　中国城市肿瘤登记地区前 10 位
癌症死亡率

Figure 4-8a　Mortality rates of top ten leading cancer sites in urban registration areas of China

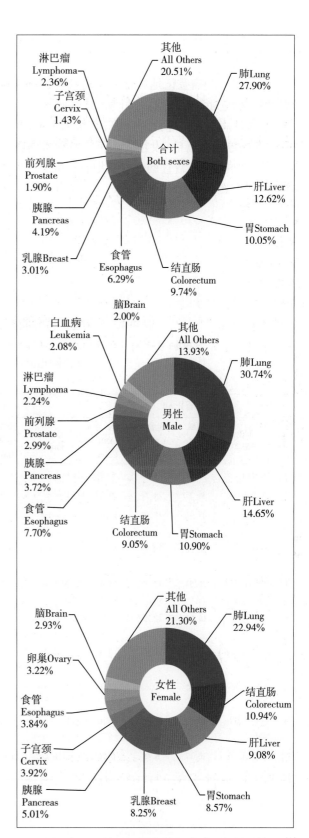

图 4-8b　中国城市肿瘤登记地区前 10 位
癌症死亡构成

Figure 4-8b　Distribution of top ten leading causes of cancer deaths in urban registration areas of China

3.5 中国农村肿瘤登记地区前 10 位癌症发病情况

中国农村肿瘤登记地区合计发病第 1 位癌症为肺癌,其次为女性乳腺癌、肝癌、结直肠癌和胃癌。男性发病第 1 位癌症为肺癌,其次为肝癌、胃癌、结直肠癌和食管癌;女性发病第 1 位癌症为肺癌,其次为乳腺癌、结直肠癌、甲状腺癌和子宫颈癌(表 4-10,图 4-9a,图 4-9b)。

3.5 Top ten leading causes of new cancer cases in rural registration areas of China

Lung cancer was the most common cancer in rural areas of China, followed by cancers of female breast, liver, colorectum and stomach. In males, lung cancer was the most common cancer, followed by liver cancer, stomach cancer, colorectal cancer and esophageal cancer. In females, lung cancer was the most common cancer, followed by breast cancer, colorectal cancer, thyroid cancer and cervical cancer (Table 4-10, Figure 4-9a, Figure 4-9b).

表 4-10 中国农村肿瘤登记地区前 10 位癌症发病率

Table 4-10 Incidence rates of top ten leading cancer sites in rural registration areas of China

单位:100 000^{-1}

顺位 Rank	合计 All				男性 Male				女性 Female			
	部位 Site	粗率 Crude rate	世标率 ASR world	中标率 ASR China	部位 Site	粗率 Crude rate	世标率 ASR world	中标率 ASR China	部位 Site	粗率 Crude rate	世标率 ASR world	中标率 ASR China
1	肺 Lung	63.39	36.92	37.05	肺 Lung	81.08	49.05	48.99	肺 Lung	44.82	25.30	25.61
2	乳腺 Breast	36.35	24.28	26.23	肝 Liver	40.58	25.96	26.60	乳腺 Breast	36.35	24.28	26.23
3	肝 Liver	27.91	17.08	17.46	胃 Stomach	36.31	21.93	21.95	结直肠 Colo-rectum	22.58	12.76	13.04
4	结直肠 Colo-rectum	26.80	15.83	16.10	结直肠 Colo-rectum	30.82	19.00	19.24	甲状腺 Thy-roid	22.44	16.63	19.11
5	胃 Stomach	26.53	15.33	15.43	食管 Esoph-agus	27.10	16.19	16.06	子宫颈 Cer-vix	19.01	12.48	13.48
6	子宫颈 Cer-vix	19.01	12.48	13.48	前列腺 Pros-tate	10.70	5.99	6.10	胃 Stomach	16.26	8.93	9.13
7	食管 Esoph-agus	19.00	10.69	10.64	膀胱 Bladder	8.11	4.84	4.88	肝 Liver	14.60	8.17	8.27
8	甲状腺 Thy-roid	14.22	10.63	12.26	胰腺 Pancre-as	7.26	4.39	4.41	食管 Esoph-agus	10.48	5.33	5.37
9	前列腺 Pros-tate	10.70	5.99	6.10	脑 Brain	7.22	5.27	5.36	子宫体 Ute-rus	10.17	6.49	6.76
10	子宫体 Ute-rus	10.17	6.49	6.76	白血病 Leu-kemia	6.64	5.34	5.22	脑 Brain	8.78	5.90	6.00

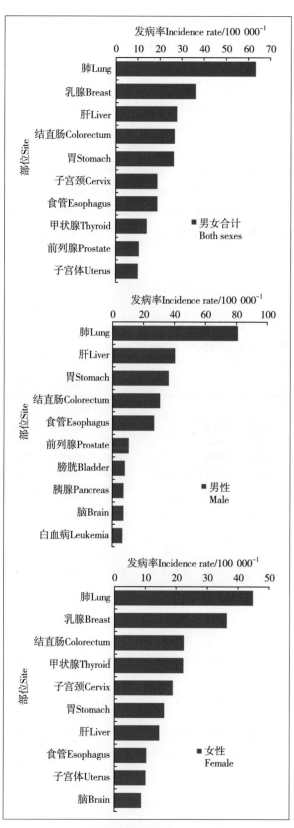

图 4-9a 中国农村肿瘤登记地区前 10 位
癌症发病率

Figure 4-9a Incidence rates of top ten leading cancer sites in rural registration areas of
China

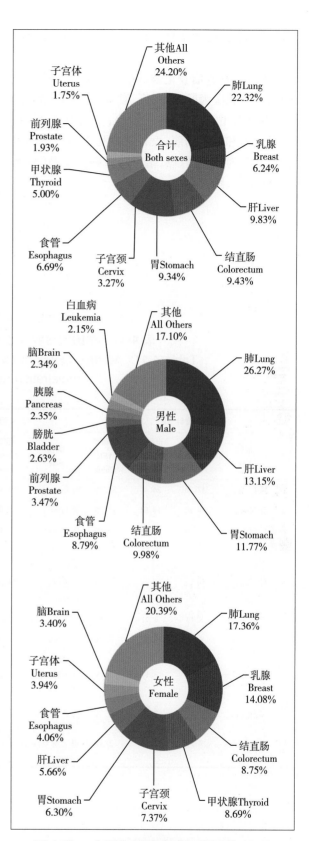

图 4-9b 中国农村肿瘤登记地区前 10 位
癌症发病构成

Figure 4-9b Distribution of top ten leading causes of new cancer cases in rural registration areas of China

3.6 中国农村肿瘤登记地区前 10 位癌症死亡情况

中国农村肿瘤登记地区合计癌症死亡第 1 位的是肺癌,其次为肝癌、胃癌、食管癌和结直肠癌。男性癌症死亡第 1 位的是肺癌,其次为肝癌、胃癌、食管癌和结直肠癌;女性癌症死亡第 1 位的是肺癌,其次为肝癌、胃癌、结直肠癌和食管癌(表 4-11,图 4-10a,图 4-10b)。

3.6 Top ten leading causes of cancer deaths in rural registration areas of China

Lung cancer was the leading cause of cancer deaths in rural areas of China, followed by cancers of liver, stomach, esophagus and colorectum. In males, lung cancer was the leading cause of cancer deaths, followed by liver cancer, stomach cancer, esophageal cancer and colorectal cancer. In females, lung cancer ranked as the leading cause of cancer deaths, followed by liver cancer, stomach cancer, colorectal cancer and esophageal cancer (Table 4-11, Figure 4-10a, Figure 4-10b).

表 4-11 中国农村肿瘤登记地区前 10 位癌症死亡率

Table 4-11 Mortality rates of top ten leading cancer sites in rural registration areas of China

单位:100 000^{-1}

顺位 Rank	合计 All				男性 Male				女性 Female			
	部位 Site	粗率 Crude rate	世标率 ASR world	中标率 ASR China	部位 Site	粗率 Crude rate	世标率 ASR world	中标率 ASR China	部位 Site	粗率 Crude rate	世标率 ASR world	中标率 ASR China
1	肺 Lung	47.26	26.40	26.48	肺 Lung	64.95	38.41	38.45	肺 Lung	28.68	14.93	15.03
2	肝 Liver	24.82	14.91	15.20	肝 Liver	36.02	22.76	23.26	肝 Liver	13.07	7.09	7.15
3	胃 Stomach	19.94	10.98	11.10	胃 Stomach	27.17	15.91	16.04	胃 Stomach	12.34	6.30	6.42
4	食管 Esophagus	15.23	8.25	8.26	食管 Esophagus	21.87	12.77	12.75	结直肠 Colorectum	10.58	5.42	5.50
5	结直肠 Colorectum	12.89	7.12	7.21	结直肠 Colorectum	15.09	8.93	9.01	食管 Esophagus	8.26	3.91	3.95
6	乳腺 Breast	8.13	4.91	5.07	胰腺 Pancreas	6.44	3.84	3.85	乳腺 Breast	8.13	4.91	5.07
7	子宫颈 Cervix	5.91	3.51	3.63	脑 Brain	4.76	3.29	3.33	子宫颈 Cervix	5.91	3.51	3.63
8	胰腺 Pancreas	5.66	3.17	3.18	前列腺 Prostate	4.29	2.34	2.31	胰腺 Pancreas	4.85	2.51	2.52
9	脑 Brain	4.40	2.93	2.95	白血病 Leukemia	4.20	3.03	3.07	脑 Brain	4.03	2.56	2.56
10	前列腺 Prostate	4.29	2.34	2.31	淋巴瘤 Lymphoma	3.77	2.37	2.40	白血病 Leukemia	3.12	2.17	2.17

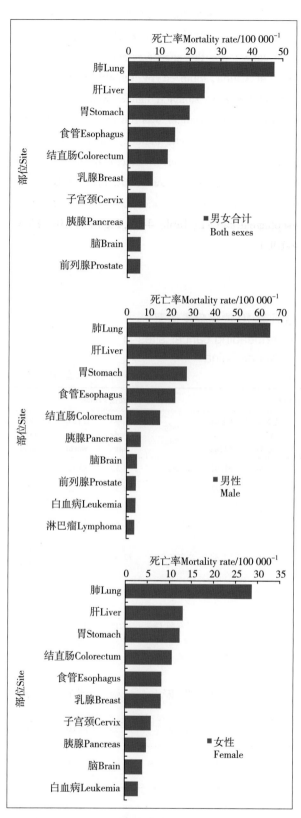

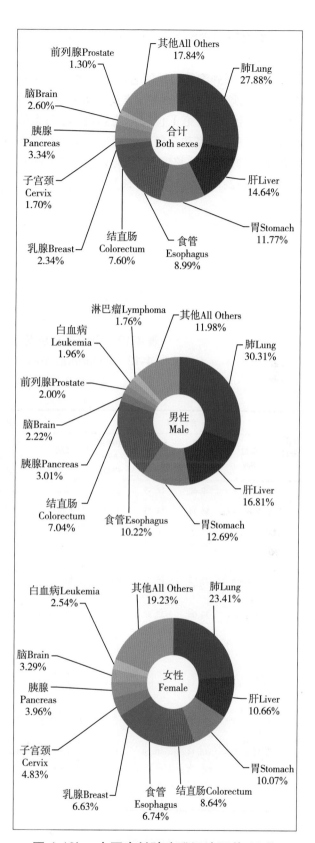

图 4-10a　中国农村肿瘤登记地区前 10 位
癌症死亡率

Figure 4-10a　Mortality rates of top ten leading cancer sites in rural registration areas of China

图 4-10b　中国农村肿瘤登记地区前 10 位
癌症死亡构成

Figure 4-10b　Distribution of top ten leading causes of cancer deaths in rural registration areas of China

3.7 中国东部肿瘤登记地区前 10 位癌症发病情况

中国东部肿瘤登记地区合计发病第 1 位癌症为肺癌,其次为女性乳腺癌、结直肠癌、胃癌和甲状腺癌。男性发病第 1 位癌症为肺癌,其次为结直肠癌、胃癌、肝癌和食管癌;女性发病第 1 位癌症为肺癌,其次为乳腺癌、甲状腺癌、结直肠癌和胃癌(表 4-12,图 4-11a,图 4-11b)。

3.7 Top ten leading causes of new cancer cases in eastern registration areas of China

Lung cancer was the most common cancer in eastern areas of China, followed by female breast cancer, colorectal cancer, stomach cancer and thyroid cancer. In males, lung cancer was the most common cancer, followed by colorectal cancer, stomach cancer, liver cancer and esophageal cancer. In females, lung cancer was the most common cancer, followed by breast cancer, thyroid cancer, colorectal cancer and stomach cancer (Table 4-12, Figure 4-11a, Figure 4-11b).

表 4-12 中国东部肿瘤登记地区前 10 位癌症发病率

Table 4-12 Incidence rates of top ten leading cancer sites in eastern registration areas of China

单位:100 000^{-1}

顺位 Rank	合计 All				男性 Male				女性 Female			
	部位 Site	粗率 Crude rate	世标率 ASR world	中标率 ASR China	部位 Site	粗率 Crude rate	世标率 ASR world	中标率 ASR China	部位 Site	粗率 Crude rate	世标率 ASR world	中标率 ASR China
1	肺 Lung	79.47	42.15	42.49	肺 Lung	95.26	51.64	51.62	肺 Lung	63.53	33.45	34.15
2	乳腺 Breast	56.34	35.25	37.75	结直肠 Colo-rectum	46.30	25.60	25.72	乳腺 Breast	56.34	35.25	37.75
3	结直肠 Colo-rectum	39.20	20.75	20.98	胃 Stomach	43.06	23.26	23.30	甲状腺 Thy-roid	44.91	32.94	38.36
4	胃 Stomach	31.02	16.11	16.28	肝 Liver	37.57	22.03	22.34	结直肠 Colo-rectum	32.03	16.17	16.51
5	甲状腺 Thy-roid	30.06	22.28	26.14	食管 Esoph-agus	25.08	13.42	13.27	胃 Stomach	18.86	9.41	9.70
6	肝 Liver	25.43	14.16	14.33	前列腺 Pros-tate	19.48	9.65	9.81	子宫颈 Cer-vix	16.14	10.20	11.05
7	前列腺 Pros-tate	19.48	9.65	9.81	甲状腺 Thy-roid	15.36	11.64	13.91	肝 Liver	13.16	6.52	6.56
8	食管 Esoph-agus	17.05	8.54	8.50	膀胱 Bladder	12.17	6.45	6.49	子宫体 Ute-rus	12.69	7.68	7.92
9	子宫颈 Cer-vix	16.14	10.20	11.05	胰腺 Pancreas	10.32	5.53	5.53	脑 Brain	11.29	7.00	7.13
10	子宫体 Ute-rus	12.69	7.68	7.92	淋巴瘤 Lym-phoma	10.00	6.06	6.21	食管 Esoph-agus	8.93	3.91	3.97

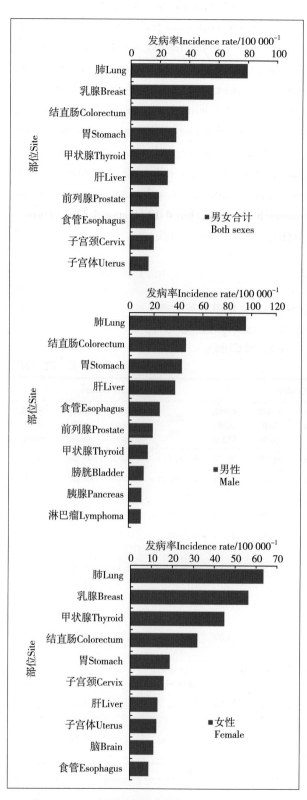

图 4-11a　中国东部肿瘤登记地区前 10 位癌症发病率

Figure 4-11a　Incidence rates of top ten leading cancer sites in eastern registration areas of China

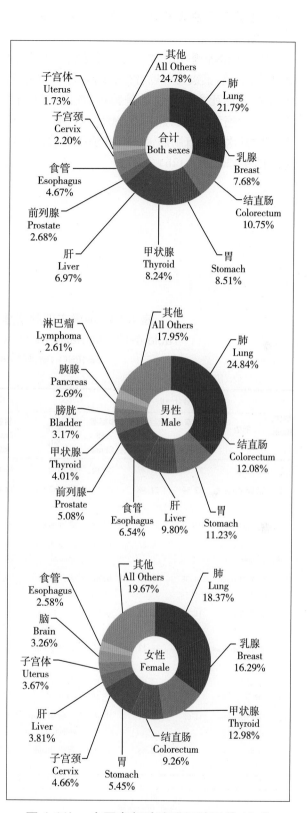

图 4-11b　中国东部肿瘤登记地区前 10 位癌症发病构成

Figure 4-11b　Distribution of top ten leading causes of new cancer cases in eastern registration areas of China

3.8 中国东部肿瘤登记地区前10位癌症死亡情况

中国东部肿瘤登记地区男女合计癌症死亡第1位的为肺癌,其次为肝癌、胃癌、结直肠癌和食管癌;男性癌症死亡第1位的是肺癌,其次是肝癌、胃癌、食管癌和结直肠癌;女性癌症死亡第1位的是肺癌,其次为结直肠癌、胃癌、肝癌和乳腺癌(表4-13,图4-12a,图4-12b)。

3.8 Top ten leading causes of cancer deaths in eastern registration areas of China

Lung cancer was the leading cause of cancer deaths in eastern areas of China, followed by liver cancer, stomach cancer, colorectal cancer and esophageal cancer. In males, lung cancer was the leading cause of cancer deaths, followed by liver cancer, stomach cancer, esophageal cancer and colorectal cancer. In females, lung cancer was still the leading cause of cancer deaths, followed by colorectal cancer, stomach cancer, liver cancer and breast cancer (Table 4-13, Figure 4-12a, Figure 4-12b).

表4-13　中国东部肿瘤登记地区前10位癌症死亡率

Table 4-13　Mortality rates of top ten leading cancer sites in eastern registration areas of China

单位:100 000^{-1}

顺位 Rank	合计 All				男性 Male				女性 Female			
	部位 Site	粗率 Crude rate	世标率 ASR world	中标率 ASR China	部位 Site	粗率 Crude rate	世标率 ASR world	中标率 ASR China	部位 Site	粗率 Crude rate	世标率 ASR world	中标率 ASR China
1	肺 Lung	52.13	25.27	25.40	肺 Lung	71.05	36.70	36.78	肺 Lung	33.02	14.74	14.91
2	肝 Liver	22.34	11.98	12.12	肝 Liver	32.69	18.65	18.88	结直肠 Colorectum	14.47	6.25	6.32
3	胃 Stomach	22.08	10.62	10.79	胃 Stomach	30.40	15.56	15.72	胃 Stomach	13.67	6.11	6.29
4	结直肠 Colorectum	17.51	8.27	8.30	食管 Esophagus	20.65	10.63	10.62	肝 Liver	11.87	5.55	5.60
5	食管 Esophagus	14.08	6.67	6.70	结直肠 Colorectum	20.53	10.50	10.48	乳腺 Breast	11.24	6.00	6.15
6	乳腺 Breast	11.24	6.00	6.15	胰腺 Pancreas	9.46	4.98	4.97	食管 Esophagus	7.45	2.98	3.04
7	胰腺 Pancreas	8.46	4.12	4.14	前列腺 Prostate	6.81	3.08	3.00	胰腺 Pancreas	7.44	3.32	3.34
8	前列腺 Prostate	6.81	3.08	3.00	淋巴瘤 Lymphoma	5.49	3.01	3.06	子宫颈 Cervix	4.61	2.55	2.65
9	淋巴瘤 Lymphoma	4.62	2.41	2.46	白血病 Leukemia	5.45	3.38	3.42	脑 Brain	4.21	2.39	2.40
10	子宫颈 Cervix	4.61	2.55	2.65	膀胱 Bladder	4.85	2.27	2.22	卵巢 Ovary	4.17	2.26	2.29

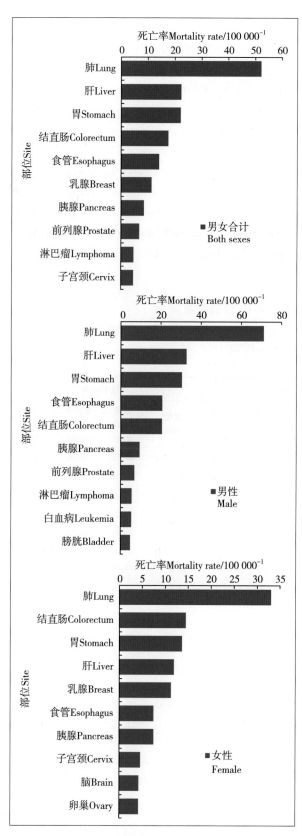

图 4-12a　中国东部肿瘤登记地区前 10 位癌症死亡率

Figure 4-12a　Mortality rates of top ten leading cancer sites in eastern registration areas of China

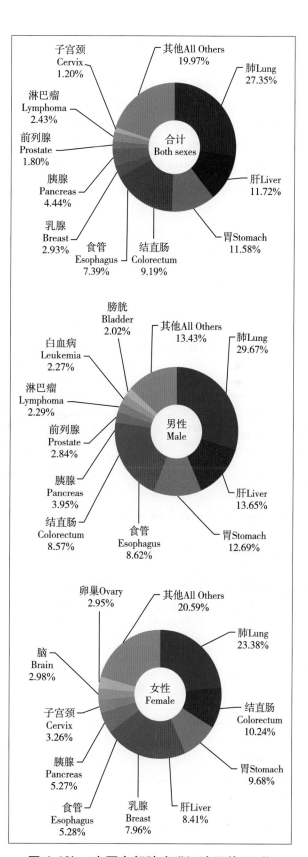

图 4-12b　中国东部肿瘤登记地区前 10 位癌症死亡构成

Figure 4-12b　Distribution of top ten leading causes of cancer deaths in eastern registration areas of China

3.9 中国中部肿瘤登记地区前 10 位癌症发病情况

中国中部肿瘤登记地区男女合计发病第 1 位癌症为肺癌,其次为女性乳腺癌、胃癌、肝癌和结直肠癌。男性发病第 1 位癌症为肺癌,其次为肝癌、胃癌、结直肠癌和食管癌;女性发病第 1 位症为乳腺癌,其次为肺癌、甲状腺癌、结直肠癌和子宫颈癌(表 4-14,图 4-13a、图 4-13b)。

3.9 Top ten leading causes of new cancer cases in central registration areas of China

Lung cancer was the most common cancer in central areas of China, followed by female breast cancer, stomach cancer, liver cancer and colorectal cancer. In males, lung cancer was the most common cancer, followed by liver cancer, stomach cancer, colorectal cancer and esophageal cancer. In females, breast cancer was the most common cancer, followed by lung cancer, thyroid cancer, colorectal cancer and cervical cancer (Table 4-14, Figure 4-13a, Figure 4-13b).

表 4-14　中国中部肿瘤登记地区前 10 位癌症发病率

Table 4-14　Incidence rates of top ten leading cancer sites in central registration areas of China

单位:100 000⁻¹

顺位 Rank	合计 All				男性 Male				女性 Female			
	部位 Site	粗率 Crude rate	世标率 ASR world	中标率 ASR China	部位 Site	粗率 Crude rate	世标率 ASR world	中标率 ASR China	部位 Site	粗率 Crude rate	世标率 ASR world	中标率 ASR China
1	肺 Lung	61.21	37.20	37.19	肺 Lung	82.31	52.17	52.06	乳腺 Breast	41.55	28.06	30.11
2	乳腺 Breast	41.55	28.06	30.11	肝 Liver	37.20	24.55	24.94	肺 Lung	39.34	22.95	23.06
3	胃 Stomach	26.82	16.36	16.44	胃 Stomach	36.62	23.32	23.28	甲状腺 Thyroid	24.44	17.86	20.43
4	肝 Liver	26.19	16.53	16.78	结直肠 Colorectum	29.47	19.03	19.22	结直肠 Colorectum	22.29	13.18	13.45
5	结直肠 Colorectum	25.94	16.05	16.28	食管 Esophagus	23.55	14.83	14.73	子宫颈 Cervix	21.75	14.45	15.49
6	子宫颈 Cervix	21.75	14.45	15.49	前列腺 Prostate	9.58	5.68	5.78	胃 Stomach	16.67	9.71	9.91
7	食管 Esophagus	17.14	10.21	10.17	膀胱 Bladder	7.89	4.96	4.97	肝 Liver	14.77	8.64	8.72
8	甲状腺 Thyroid	15.56	11.55	13.27	脑 Brain	7.40	5.59	5.63	食管 Esophagus	10.50	5.77	5.79
9	子宫体 Uterus	10.49	6.85	7.09	甲状腺 Thyroid	7.00	5.34	6.23	子宫体 Uterus	10.49	6.85	7.09
10	前列腺 Prostate	9.58	5.68	5.78	淋巴瘤 Lymphoma	6.82	4.78	4.83	脑 Brain	8.56	5.93	5.99

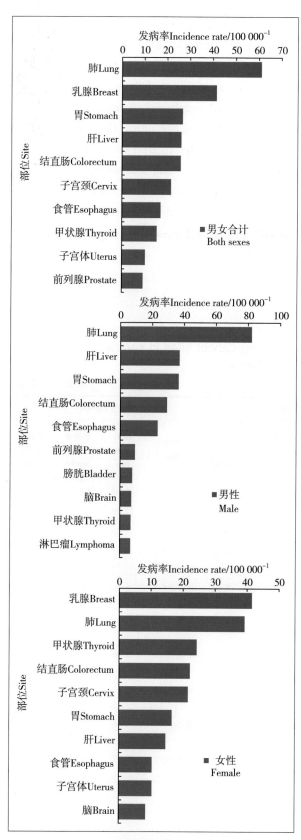

图 4-13a 中国中部肿瘤登记地区前 10 位癌症发病率

Figure 4-13a Incidence rates of top ten leading cancer sites in central registration areas of China

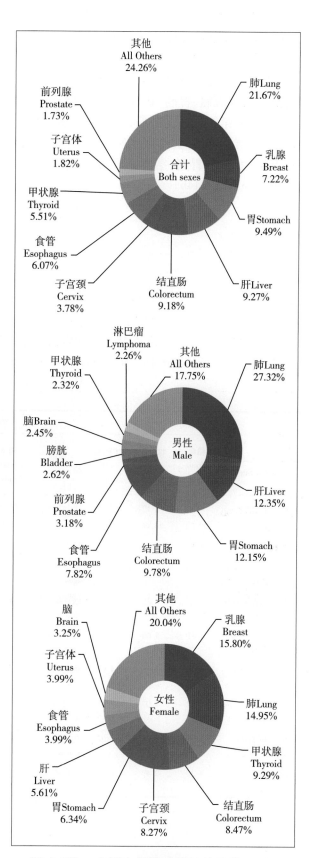

图 4-13b 中国中部肿瘤登记地区前 10 位癌症发病构成

Figure 4-13b Distribution of top ten leading causes of new cancer cases in central registration areas of China

3.10 中国中部肿瘤登记地区前10位癌症死亡情况

中国中部肿瘤登记地区癌症死亡第1位的是肺癌,其次为肝癌、胃癌、食管癌和结直肠癌。男性癌症死亡第1位的是肺癌,其次是肝癌、胃癌、食管癌和结直肠癌;女性癌症死亡第1位的是肺癌,其次为肝癌、胃癌、结直肠癌和乳腺癌(表4-15,图4-14a,图4-14b)。

3.10 Top ten leading causes of cancer deaths in central registration areas of China

Lung cancer was the leading cause of cancer deaths in central areas of China, followed by liver cancer, stomach cancer, esophageal cancer and colorectal cancer. In males, lung cancer was the leading cause of cancer deaths, followed by liver cancer, stomach cancer, esophageal cancer and colorectal cancer. In females, lung cancer was still the leading cause of cancer deaths, followed by liver cancer, stomach cancer, colorectal cancer and breast cancer(Table 4-15, Figure 4-14a, Figure 4-14b).

表 4-15　中国中部肿瘤登记地区前 10 位癌症死亡率

Table 4-15　Mortality rates of top ten leading cancer sites in central registration areas of China

单位:100 000^{-1}

顺位 Rank	合计 All				男性 Male				女性 Female			
	部位 Site	粗率 Crude rate	世标率 ASR world	中标率 ASR China	部位 Site	粗率 Crude rate	世标率 ASR world	中标率 ASR China	部位 Site	粗率 Crude rate	世标率 ASR world	中标率 ASR China
1	肺 Lung	46.03	27.04	27.08	肺 Lung	65.28	40.59	40.61	肺 Lung	26.08	14.28	14.34
2	肝 Liver	22.72	14.06	14.27	肝 Liver	32.11	20.89	21.26	肝 Liver	12.98	7.37	7.43
3	胃 Stomach	19.67	11.47	11.58	胃 Stomach	26.88	16.62	16.74	胃 Stomach	12.20	6.65	6.76
4	食管 Esophagus	13.14	7.52	7.53	食管 Esophagus	18.28	11.25	11.23	结直肠 Colorectum	10.35	5.65	5.72
5	结直肠 Colorectum	12.41	7.25	7.33	结直肠 Colorectum	14.39	8.96	9.04	乳腺 Breast	9.11	5.66	5.83
6	乳腺 Breast	9.11	5.66	5.83	胰腺 Pancreas	5.90	3.70	3.71	食管 Esophagus	7.81	4.00	4.03
7	子宫颈 Cervix	6.46	3.96	4.07	脑 Brain	4.71	3.35	3.37	子宫颈 Cervix	6.46	3.96	4.07
8	胰腺 Pancreas	5.17	3.07	3.08	前列腺 Prostate	4.30	2.49	2.47	胰腺 Pancreas	4.42	2.46	2.47
9	脑 Brain	4.39	3.02	3.02	白血病 Leukemia	3.93	2.91	2.97	脑 Brain	4.06	2.70	2.67
10	前列腺 Prostate	4.30	2.49	2.47	淋巴瘤 Lymphoma	3.85	2.52	2.56	卵巢 Ovary	3.39	2.10	2.13

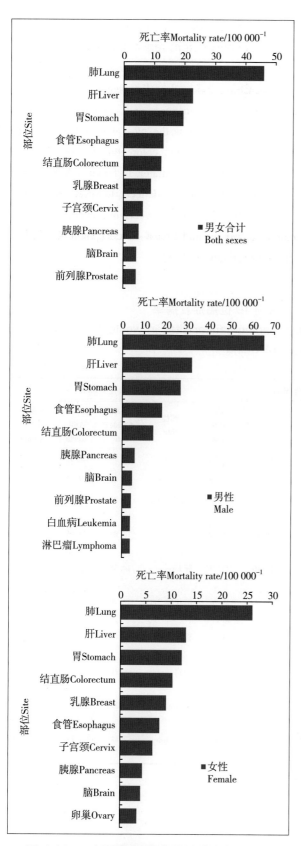

图 4-14a 中国中部肿瘤登记地区前 10 位
癌症死亡率

Figure 4-14a Mortality rates of top ten leading cancer sites in central registration areas of China

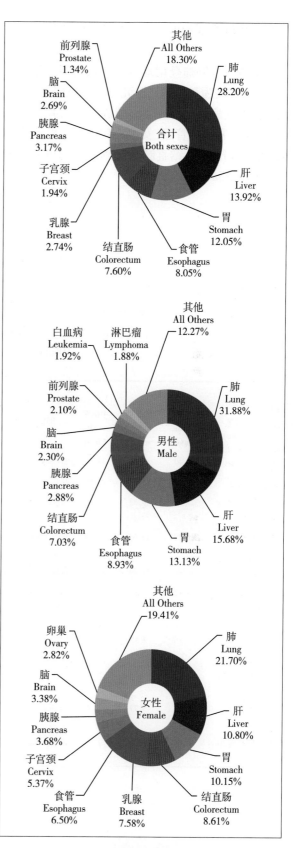

图 4-14b 中国中部肿瘤登记地区前 10 位
癌症死亡构成

Figure 4-14b Distribution of top ten leading causes of cancer deaths in central registration areas of China

3.11 中国西部肿瘤登记地区前 10 位癌症发病情况

中国西部肿瘤登记地区合计发病第 1 位癌症为肺癌,其次为肝癌、女性乳腺癌、结直肠癌、胃癌。男性发病第 1 位癌症为肺癌,其次为肝癌、结直肠癌、胃癌和食管癌;女性发病第 1 位癌症为肺癌,其次为乳腺癌、结直肠癌、子宫颈癌和肝癌(表 4-16,图 4-15a,图 4-15b)。

3.11 Top ten leading causes of new cancer cases in western registration areas of China

Lung cancer was the most common cancer in western areas of China, followed by liver cancer, female breast cancer, colorectal cancer and stomach cancer. In males, lung cancer was the most common cancer, followed by liver cancer, colorectal cancer, stomach cancer and esophageal cancer. In females, lung cancer was the most common cancer, followed by breast cancer, colorectal cancer, cervical cancer and liver cancer(Table 4-16, Figure 4-15a, Figure 4-15b).

表 4-16 中国西部肿瘤登记地区前 10 位癌症发病率

Table 4-16 Incidence rates of top ten leading cancer sites in western registration areas of China

单位:100 000^{-1}

顺位 Rank	合计 All				男性 Male				女性 Female			
	部位 Site	粗率 Crude rate	世标率 ASR world	中标率 ASR China	部位 Site	粗率 Crude rate	世标率 ASR world	中标率 ASR China	部位 Site	粗率 Crude rate	世标率 ASR world	中标率 ASR China
1	肺 Lung	57.40	34.71	34.70	肺 Lung	75.37	47.29	47.00	肺 Lung	38.58	22.45	22.72
2	肝 Liver	29.29	18.50	18.99	肝 Liver	43.56	28.47	29.28	乳腺 Breast	28.90	19.33	20.87
3	乳腺 Breast	28.90	19.33	20.87	结直肠 Colo-rectum	29.83	18.81	19.01	结直肠 Colo-rectum	21.52	12.57	12.82
4	结直肠 Colo-rectum	25.77	15.64	15.87	胃 Stomach	26.57	16.67	16.65	子宫颈 Cer-vix	18.08	11.99	12.94
5	胃 Stomach	19.45	11.73	11.80	食管 Esoph-agus	24.82	15.46	15.28	肝 Liver	14.35	8.41	8.55
6	子宫颈 Cer-vix	18.08	11.99	12.94	前列腺 Pros-tate	9.80	5.63	5.74	甲状腺 Thy-roid	13.70	10.22	11.91
7	食管 Esoph-agus	16.07	9.55	9.46	膀胱 Bladder	7.37	4.50	4.54	胃 Stomach	12.00	6.90	7.05
8	前列腺 Pros-tate	9.80	5.63	5.74	胰腺 Pancreas	6.55	4.11	4.11	子宫体 Ute-rus	8.91	5.77	6.03
9	子宫体 Ute-rus	8.91	5.77	6.03	脑 Brain	6.24	4.60	4.67	脑 Brain	7.27	5.04	5.13
10	甲状腺 Thy-roid	8.69	6.50	7.58	鼻咽 Naso-pharynx	5.56	3.83	4.09	卵巢 Ovary	7.11	4.88	5.17

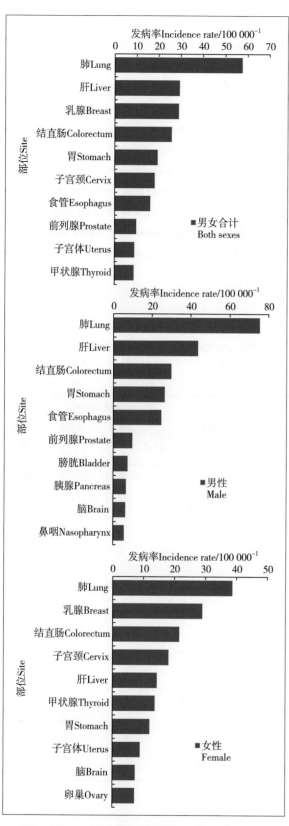

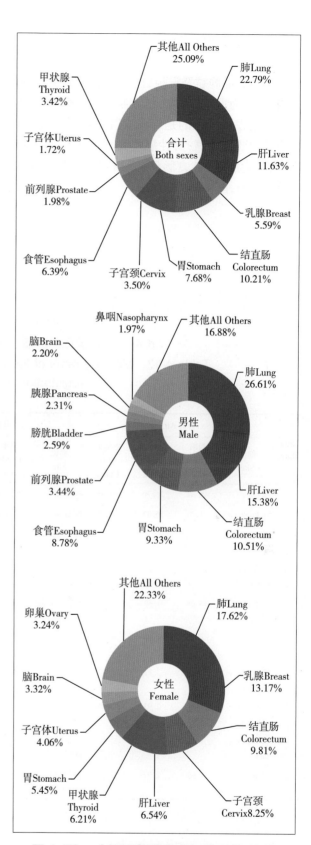

图 4-15a　中国西部肿瘤登记地区前 10 位癌症发病率

Figure 4-15a　Incidence rates of top ten leading cancer sites in western registration areas of China

图 4-15b　中国西部肿瘤登记地区前 10 位癌症发病构成

Figure 4-15b　Distribution of top ten leading causes of new cancer cases in western registration areas of China

3.12 中国西部肿瘤登记地区前 10 位癌症死亡情况

中国西部肿瘤登记地区癌症死亡第 1 位的为肺癌,其次为肝癌、胃癌、结直肠癌和食管癌。男性癌症死亡第 1 位的是肺癌,其次是肝癌、胃癌、食管癌和结直肠癌;女性癌症死亡第 1 位的是肺癌,其次为肝癌、结直肠癌、胃癌和乳腺癌(表 4-17,图 4-16a,图 4-16b)。

3.12 Top ten leading causes of cancer deaths in western registration areas of China

Lung cancer was the leading cause of cancer deaths in western areas of China, followed by liver cancer, stomach cancer, colorectal cancer and esophageal cancer. In males, lung cancer ranked as the leading cause of cancer deaths, followed by liver cancer, stomach cancer, esophageal cancer and colorectal cancer. In females, lung cancer was also the leading cause of cancer deaths, followed by liver cancer, colorectal cancer, stomach cancer and breast cancer (Table 4-17, Figure 4-16a, Figure 4-16b).

表 4-17 中国西部肿瘤登记地区前 10 位癌症死亡率

Table 4-17 Mortality rates of top ten leading cancer sites in western registration areas of China

单位:100 000^{-1}

顺位 Rank	合计 All				男性 Male				女性 Female			
	部位 Site	粗率 Crude rate	世标率 ASR world	中标率 ASR China	部位 Site	粗率 Crude rate	世标率 ASR world	中标率 ASR China	部位 Site	粗率 Crude rate	世标率 ASR world	中标率 ASR China
1	肺 Lung	45.34	26.70	26.63	肺 Lung	63.10	39.05	38.80	肺 Lung	26.75	14.71	14.81
2	肝 Liver	26.20	16.33	16.69	肝 Liver	38.86	25.21	25.83	肝 Liver	12.94	7.37	7.45
3	胃 Stomach	15.27	8.91	8.96	胃 Stomach	20.84	12.80	12.83	结直肠 Colorectum	10.68	5.80	5.89
4	结直肠 Colorectum	13.28	7.67	7.76	食管 Esophagus	20.33	12.48	12.39	胃 Stomach	9.44	5.16	5.22
5	食管 Esophagus	13.08	7.59	7.55	结直肠 Colorectum	15.77	9.63	9.71	乳腺 Breast	7.03	4.44	4.60
6	乳腺 Breast	7.03	4.44	4.60	胰腺 Pancreas	5.76	3.57	3.57	子宫颈 Cervix	6.04	3.73	3.87
7	子宫颈 Cervix	6.04	3.73	3.87	脑 Brain	4.43	3.17	3.19	食管 Esophagus	5.48	2.83	2.85
8	胰腺 Pancreas	4.99	2.93	2.94	前列腺 Prostate	4.38	2.49	2.47	胰腺 Pancreas	4.18	2.29	2.32
9	前列腺 Prostate	4.38	2.49	2.47	白血病 Leukemia	3.55	2.69	2.70	脑 Brain	3.52	2.35	2.35
10	脑 Brain	3.98	2.77	2.77	淋巴瘤 Lymphoma	3.30	2.15	2.16	卵巢 Ovary	2.99	1.86	1.89

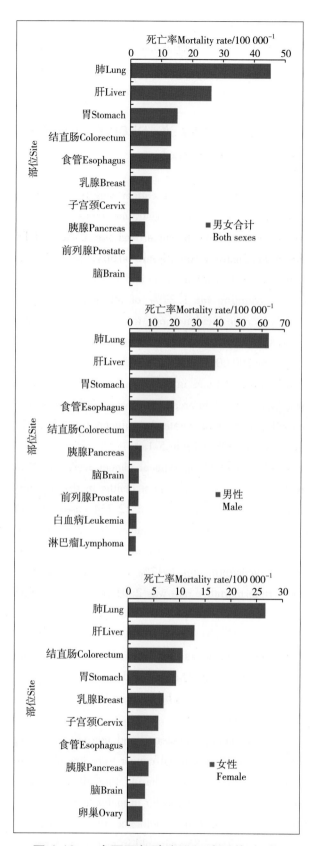

图 4-16a　中国西部肿瘤登记地区前 10 位癌症死亡率

Figure 4-16a　Mortality rates of top ten leading cancer sites in western registration areas of China

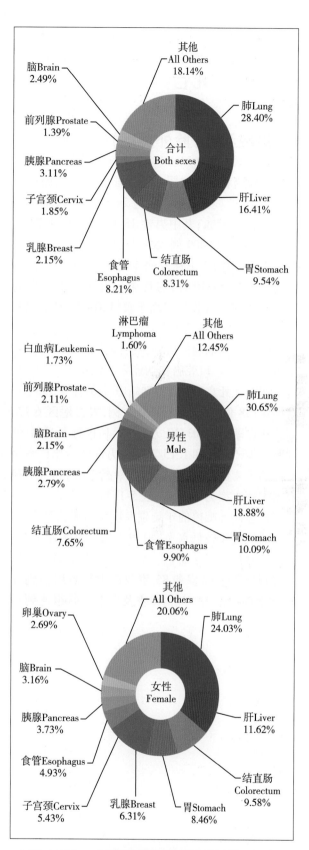

图 4-16b　中国西部肿瘤登记地区前 10 位癌症死亡构成

Figure 4-16b　Distribution of top ten leading causes of cancer deaths in western registration areas of China

第五章 各部位癌症的发病与死亡

1 口腔和咽(除外鼻咽)

口腔癌和咽癌位居中国肿瘤登记地区癌症发病谱第 19 位。新发病例数为 26 338 例,占全部癌症发病的 1.37%;其中男性 18 413 例,女性 7 925 例,城市地区 12 409 例,农村地区 13 929 例。发病率为 4.19/10 万,中标发病率为 2.63/10 万,世标发病率为 2.58/10 万;男性中标发病率为女性的 2.3 倍,城市中标发病率高于农村,0~74 岁累积发病率为 0.30%(表 5-1a)。

口腔癌和咽癌位居中国肿瘤登记地区癌症死亡谱第 17 位。口腔癌和咽癌死亡病例 12 754 例,占全部癌症死亡数的 1.17%;其中男性 9 596 例,女性 3 158 例,城市地区 6 028 例,农村地区 6 726 例。死亡率为 2.03/10 万,中标和世标死亡率分别为 1.16/10 万和 1.15/10 万;男性中标死亡率为女性的 3.4 倍,城市中标死亡率高于农村。0~74 岁累积死亡率为 0.13%(表 5-1b)。

口腔癌和咽癌的年龄别发病率和死亡率在 40 岁以前均处于较低水平,40 岁之后开始快速上升,男性上升速度快于女性。男性和女性年龄别发病率分别在 75~79 岁和 85 岁及以上年龄组达到高峰,年龄别死亡率均在 85 岁及以上年龄组达到高峰(图 5-1a)。

1 Oral cavity & pharynx (except nasopharynx)

Oral cavity and pharyngeal cancer were the 19th most common cancer in the registration areas of China. There were 26 338 new cases diagnosed as oral cavity and pharyngeal cancer (18 413 males and 7 925 females, 12 409 in urban areas and 13 929 in rural areas), accounting for 1.37% of all new cancer cases. The crude incidence rate was 4.19 per 100 000, with ASR China 2.63 per 100 000 and ASR world 2.58 per 100 000, respectively. The incidence of ASR China was 2.3 times in males as that in females, and was higher in urban areas than that in rural areas. The cumulative incidence rate for subjects aged 0 to 74 years was 0.30% (Table 5-1a).

Oral cavity and pharyngeal cancer were the 17th most common cause of cancer deaths in the registration areas of China. A total of 12 754 cases died of oral cavity and pharyngeal cancer (9 596 males and 3 158 females, 6 028 in urban areas and 6 726 in rural areas), accounting for 1.17% of all cancer deaths. The crude mortality rate was 2.03 per 100 000, with ASR China of 1.16 per 100 000 and ASR world of 1.15 per 100 000. The mortality of ASR China was 3.4 times in males as that in females, and was higher in urban areas than that in rural areas. The cumulative mortality rate for subjects aged 0 to 74 years was 0.13% (Table 5-1b).

The age-specific incidence and mortality rates for oral cavity and pharyngeal cancer were low before 40 years old, but increased sharply thereafter. The age-specific rates increased faster in males than that in females. The age-specific incidence rates reached its peak at 75-79 and 85 years old in males and females, respectively. The age-specific mortality rates peaked at the age group of 85 years old for both sexes (Figure 5-1a).

城市地区口腔癌和咽癌的发病率和死亡率均略高于农村地区。男性中标发病率中部地区最高,西部地区70~84岁年龄组出现明显的高峰,中标死亡率西部地区最高。女性中标发病率和死亡率西部地区最高。在七大行政区中,口腔癌和咽癌的中标发病率男性在华中地区最高,女性在华南地区最高,中标死亡率男性和女性均在华南地区最高(表5-1a,表5-1b,图5-1b)。

全部口腔癌和咽癌新发病例中,口腔是最常见的发病部位,占27.94%;其次是舌、唾液腺和下咽,分别占全部口腔癌和咽癌的21.26%、15.17%和12.45%(图5-1c)。

The incidence and mortality rates of oral cavity and pharyngeal cancer were slightly higher in urban areas than that in rural areas. For males, the incidence rate (ASR China) was the highest in central areas and showed an obvious peak at the age group of 70-84 years in western areas, and the mortality rate (ASR China) was the highest in western areas. For females, the incidence and mortality rates (ASR China) were the highest in western areas. Among the seven administrative districts, the incidence rates (ASR China) were the highest in Central China for males and in South China for females, and the mortality rates (ASR China) were the highest in South China for both sexes (Table 5-1a, Table 5-1b, Figure 5-1b).

Mouth was the most common subsite of the oral cavity and pharyngeal cancer, accounting for 27.94% of the total cases, followed by tongue, salivary gland, and hypopharynx, with proportions of 21.26%, 15.17%, and 12.45%, respectively (Figure 5-1c).

表 5-1a　中国肿瘤登记地区口腔癌和咽癌发病情况

地区 Area	性别 Sex	发病数 No. cases	粗率 Crude rate/ 100 000⁻¹	构成比 Freq./%	中标率 ASR China/ 100 000⁻¹	世标率 ASR world/ 100 000⁻¹	累积率 Cum. rate 0~74/%	顺位 Rank
合计 All	合计 Both	26 338	4.19	1.37	2.63	2.58	0.30	19
	男性 Male	18 413	5.78	1.76	3.68	3.64	0.43	14
	女性 Female	7 925	2.56	0.91	1.60	1.54	0.17	17
城市地区 Urban areas	合计 Both	12 409	4.62	1.39	2.81	2.76	0.32	19
	男性 Male	8 720	6.49	1.83	4.02	3.97	0.47	14
	女性 Female	3 689	2.75	0.88	1.65	1.59	0.18	18
农村地区 Rural areas	合计 Both	13 929	3.87	1.36	2.48	2.43	0.28	19
	男性 Male	9 693	5.26	1.70	3.42	3.38	0.40	13
	女性 Female	4 236	2.41	0.93	1.55	1.49	0.16	17
东部地区 Eastern areas	合计 Both	11 420	4.50	1.23	2.62	2.58	0.30	19
	男性 Male	7 886	6.19	1.61	3.65	3.63	0.44	14
	女性 Female	3 534	2.80	0.81	1.62	1.57	0.17	18
中部地区 Central areas	合计 Both	6 122	4.07	1.44	2.74	2.67	0.30	18
	男性 Male	4 433	5.79	1.92	4.00	3.92	0.45	13
	女性 Female	1 689	2.29	0.87	1.49	1.44	0.16	17
西部地区 Western areas	合计 Both	8 796	3.92	1.55	2.55	2.50	0.29	18
	男性 Male	6 094	5.31	1.87	3.49	3.45	0.41	13
	女性 Female	2 702	2.47	1.12	1.63	1.56	0.17	18

表 5-1b　中国肿瘤登记地区口腔癌和咽癌死亡情况

地区 Area	性别 Sex	死亡数 No. deaths	粗率 Crude rate/ 100 000⁻¹	构成比 Freq./%	中标率 ASR China/ 100 000⁻¹	世标率 ASR world/ 100 000⁻¹	累积率 Cum. rate 0~74/%	顺位 Rank
合计 All	合计 Both	12 754	2.03	1.17	1.16	1.15	0.13	17
	男性 Male	9 596	3.01	1.37	1.80	1.81	0.21	12
	女性 Female	3 158	1.02	0.81	0.53	0.52	0.06	17
城市 Urban areas	合计 Both	6 028	2.25	1.26	1.24	1.24	0.14	18
	男性 Male	4 529	3.37	1.49	1.95	1.96	0.23	12
	女性 Female	1 499	1.12	0.86	0.55	0.54	0.05	17
农村 Rural areas	合计 Both	6 726	1.87	1.10	1.09	1.09	0.13	18
	男性 Male	5 067	2.75	1.28	1.69	1.69	0.20	13
	女性 Female	1 659	0.94	0.77	0.51	0.50	0.06	18
东部地区 Eastern areas	合计 Both	5 305	2.09	1.10	1.08	1.09	0.13	18
	男性 Male	3 910	3.07	1.28	1.67	1.69	0.20	14
	女性 Female	1 395	1.11	0.78	0.51	0.51	0.05	17
中部地区 Central areas	合计 Both	2 743	1.82	1.12	1.13	1.12	0.13	17
	男性 Male	2 102	2.75	1.34	1.79	1.78	0.21	12
	女性 Female	641	0.87	0.72	0.49	0.48	0.05	19
西部地区 Western areas	合计 Both	4 706	2.10	1.31	1.27	1.26	0.14	18
	男性 Male	3 584	3.12	1.52	1.97	1.96	0.23	12
	女性 Female	1 122	1.02	0.92	0.58	0.57	0.06	17

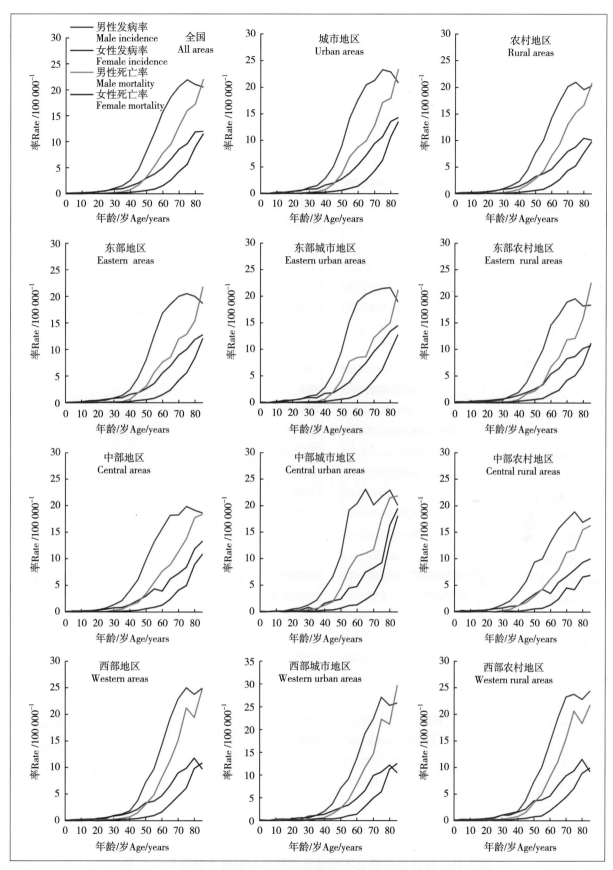

图 5-1a　中国肿瘤登记地区口腔癌和咽癌年龄别发病率和死亡率
Figure 5-1a　Age-specific incidence and mortality rates of oral cavity and pharyngeal cancer in the registration areas of China

x

中标率ASR China/100 000⁻¹

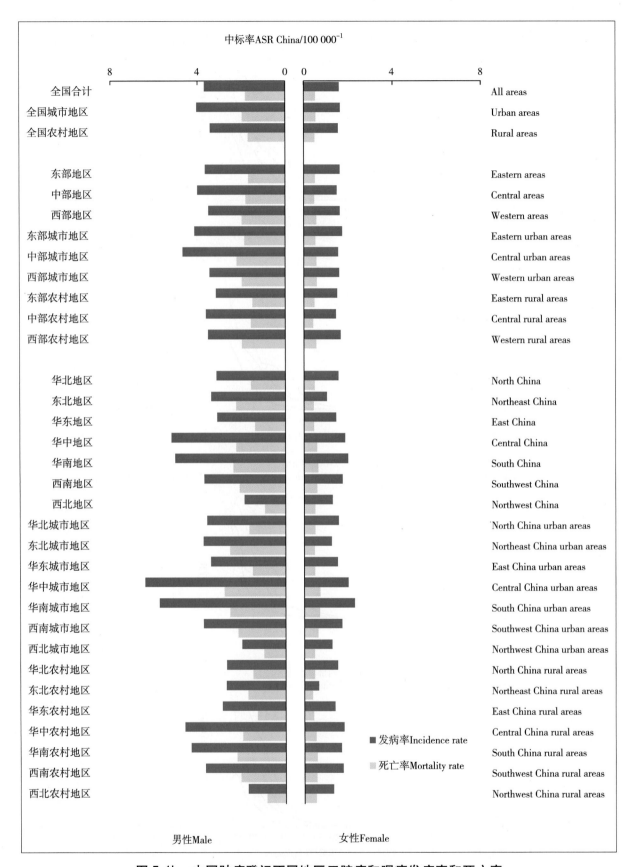

图 5-1b　中国肿瘤登记不同地区口腔癌和咽癌发病率和死亡率
Figure 5-1b　Incidence and mortality rates of oral cavity and pharyngeal cancer in
different registration areas of China

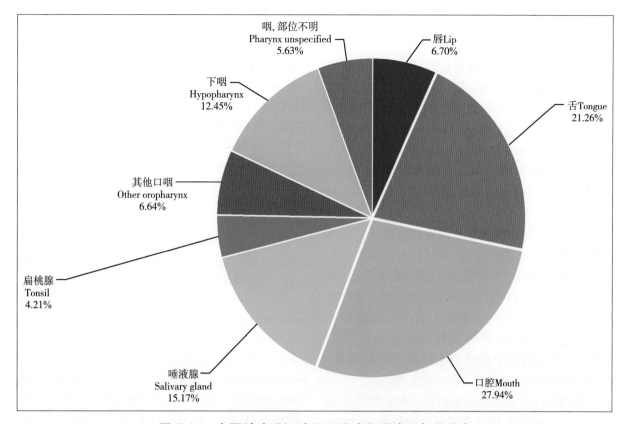

图 5-1c　中国肿瘤登记地区口腔癌和咽癌亚部位分布

Figure 5-1c　Subsite distribution of oral cavity and pharyngeal cancer in the registration areas of China

2 鼻咽

鼻咽癌位居中国肿瘤登记地区癌症发病谱第20位。新发病例 23 651 例，占全部癌症发病的1.23%。其中男性 16 823 例，女性 6 828 例；城市地区 10 041 例，农村地区 13 610 例。发病率为 3.76/10 万，中标发病率为 2.71/10 万，世标发病率为 2.52/10 万；男性中标发病率为女性的 2.40 倍，城市地区中标发病率与农村地区接近。0~74 岁累积发病率为 0.27%（表 5-2a）。

鼻咽癌位居中国肿瘤登记地区癌症死亡谱第18位。鼻咽癌死亡病例 12 138 例，占全部癌症死亡人数的 1.12%。其中男性 9 055 例，女性 3 083 例；城市地区 5 048 例，农村地区 7 090 例。死亡率为 1.93/10 万，中标死亡率为 1.21/10 万，世标死亡率为 1.18/10 万；男性中标死亡率为女性的 3.07 倍，城市地区中标死亡率略低于农村地区。0~74 岁累积死亡率为 0.14%（表 5-2b）。

鼻咽癌的年龄别发病率和死亡率男性明显高于女性。发病率在 20 岁之前处于较低水平，20 岁以后开始快速上升，男性和女性均在 60~64 岁组出现最高峰，随后下降。鼻咽癌的年龄别死亡率男性和女性 30 岁之前均处于较低水平，随后快速上升，男性和女性均在 80~84 岁组达到最高峰（图5-2a）。

城市地区鼻咽癌中标发病率和死亡率与农村地区接近。中标发病率和死亡率均是西部地区最高，东部和中部地区相似。在七大行政区中，华南地区中标发病率和死亡率均最高，华北地区最低（表 5-2a，表 5-2b，图 5-2b）。

2　Nasopharynx

Nasopharyngeal cancer was the 20th most common cancer in the registration areas of China. There were 23 651 new cases of nasopharyngeal cancer (16 823 males and 6 828 females, 10 041 in urban areas and 13 610 in rural areas), accounting for 1.23% of all new cancer cases. The crude incidence rate was 3.76 per 100 000, with ASR China 2.71 per 100 000 and ASR world 2.52 per 100 000, respectively. The incidence of ASR China in males was 2.40 times as that in females, while the rate in urban areas was close to that in rural areas. The cumulative incidence rate for subjects aged 0-74 years was 0.27% (Table 5-2a).

Nasopharyngeal cancer was the 18th most common cause of cancer deaths. A total of 12 138 cases died of nasopharyngeal cancer (9 055 males and 3 083 females, 5 048 in urban areas and 7 090 in rural areas), accounting for 1.12% of all cancer deaths. The crude mortality rate was 1.93 per 100 000, with ASR China 1.21 per 100 000 and ASR world 1.18 per 100 000, respectively. The ASR China in males was 3.07 times as that in females, while the rate in urban areas was slightly lower than that in rural areas. The cumulative mortality rate for subjects aged 0-74 years was 0.14% (Table 5-2b).

The age-specific incidence and mortality rates of nasopharyngeal cancer were higher in males than that in females. For both sexes, the age-specific incidence rates were low before 20 years old but increased sharply thereafter. Then the incidence rates reached the peak at the age group of 60-64 years for both sexes, and decreased thereafter. For both sexes, the age-specific mortality rates were low before 30 years old and increased fast thereafter, with a peak age group of 80-84 years (Figure 5-2a).

The incidence and mortality rates (ASR China) of nasopharyngeal cancer in urban areas were closed to that in rural areas. The incidence and mortality rates (ASR China) were the highest in western areas, and were similar in the eastern areas and central areas. Among the seven administrative districts, the incidence and mortality rates (ASR China) were the highest in South China and the lowest in North China (Table 5-2a, Table 5-2b, Figure 5-2b).

表 5-2a　中国肿瘤登记地区鼻咽癌发病情况

Table 5-2a　Incidence of nasopharyngeal cancer in the registration areas of China

地区 Area	性别 Sex	发病数 No. cases	粗率 Crude rate/ 100 000^{-1}	构成比 Freq./%	中标率 ASR China/ 100 000^{-1}	世标率 ASR world/ 100 000^{-1}	累积率 Cum. rate 0~74/%	顺位 Rank
合计 All	合计 Both	23 651	3.76	1.23	2.71	2.52	0.27	20
	男性 Male	16 823	5.28	1.61	3.82	3.57	0.39	15
	女性 Female	6 828	2.21	0.78	1.59	1.46	0.15	19
城市地区 Urban areas	合计 Both	10 041	3.74	1.12	2.66	2.47	0.26	20
	男性 Male	7 148	5.32	1.50	3.79	3.53	0.38	15
	女性 Female	2 893	2.16	0.69	1.56	1.43	0.15	19
农村地区 Rural areas	合计 Both	13 610	3.78	1.33	2.74	2.55	0.28	20
	男性 Male	9 675	5.25	1.70	3.84	3.60	0.39	14
	女性 Female	3 935	2.24	0.87	1.61	1.49	0.16	18
东部地区 Eastern areas	合计 Both	9 670	3.81	1.05	2.72	2.50	0.26	20
	男性 Male	7 010	5.50	1.43	3.93	3.63	0.39	15
	女性 Female	2 660	2.11	0.61	1.53	1.38	0.14	19
中部地区 Central areas	合计 Both	4 887	3.25	1.15	2.32	2.21	0.24	20
	男性 Male	3 431	4.48	1.49	3.25	3.11	0.35	15
	女性 Female	1 456	1.97	0.75	1.40	1.32	0.14	19
西部地区 Western areas	合计 Both	9 094	4.05	1.61	2.96	2.76	0.30	17
	男性 Male	6 382	5.56	1.96	4.09	3.83	0.41	10
	女性 Female	2 712	2.47	1.13	1.80	1.67	0.18	17

表 5-2b　中国肿瘤登记地区鼻咽癌死亡情况

Table 5-2b　Mortality of nasopharyngeal cancer in the registration areas of China

地区 Area	性别 Sex	死亡数 No. deaths	粗率 Crude rate/ 100 000^{-1}	构成比 Freq./%	中标率 ASR China/ 100 000^{-1}	世标率 ASR world/ 100 000^{-1}	累积率 Cum. rate 0~74/%	顺位 Rank
合计 All	合计 Both	12 138	1.93	1.12	1.21	1.18	0.14	18
	男性 Male	9 055	2.84	1.30	1.84	1.79	0.21	14
	女性 Female	3 083	1.00	0.79	0.60	0.58	0.07	18
城市地区 Urban areas	合计 Both	5 048	1.88	1.06	1.15	1.12	0.13	19
	男性 Male	3 779	2.81	1.25	1.76	1.72	0.20	15
	女性 Female	1 269	0.95	0.73	0.56	0.54	0.06	18
农村地区 Rural areas	合计 Both	7 090	1.97	1.16	1.26	1.23	0.14	17
	男性 Male	5 276	2.86	1.34	1.90	1.84	0.21	12
	女性 Female	1 814	1.03	0.84	0.62	0.61	0.07	17
东部地区 Eastern areas	合计 Both	5 117	2.02	1.06	1.19	1.15	0.14	19
	男性 Male	3 845	3.02	1.26	1.83	1.78	0.21	15
	女性 Female	1 272	1.01	0.71	0.57	0.55	0.06	18
中部地区 Central areas	合计 Both	2 263	1.51	0.92	0.98	0.97	0.11	19
	男性 Male	1 657	2.16	1.06	1.46	1.44	0.17	14
	女性 Female	606	0.82	0.68	0.51	0.50	0.06	20
西部地区 Western areas	合计 Both	4 758	2.12	1.33	1.40	1.36	0.15	17
	男性 Male	3 553	3.10	1.50	2.10	2.03	0.23	13
	女性 Female	1 205	1.10	0.99	0.69	0.67	0.07	15

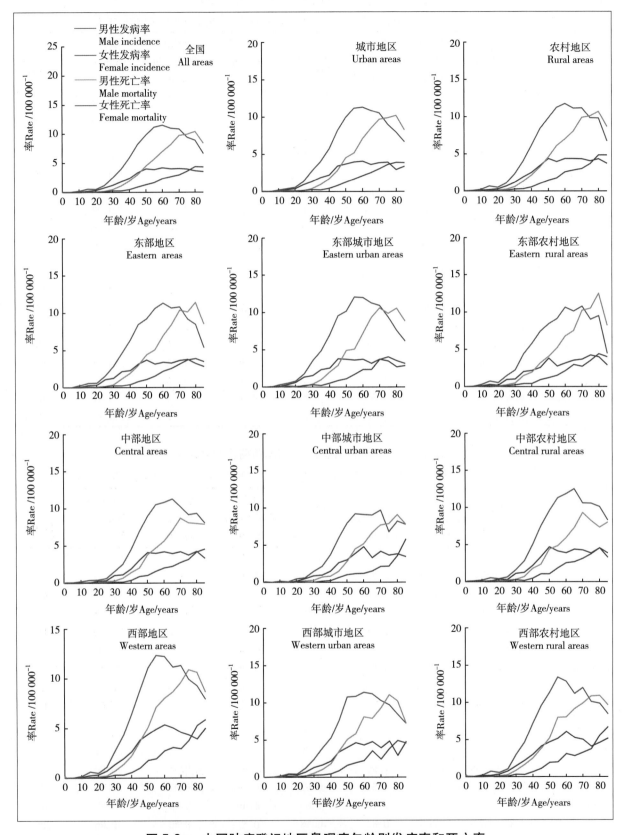

图 5-2a　中国肿瘤登记地区鼻咽癌年龄别发病率和死亡率

Figure 5-2a　Age-specific incidence and mortality rates of nasopharyngeal cancer
in the registration areas of China

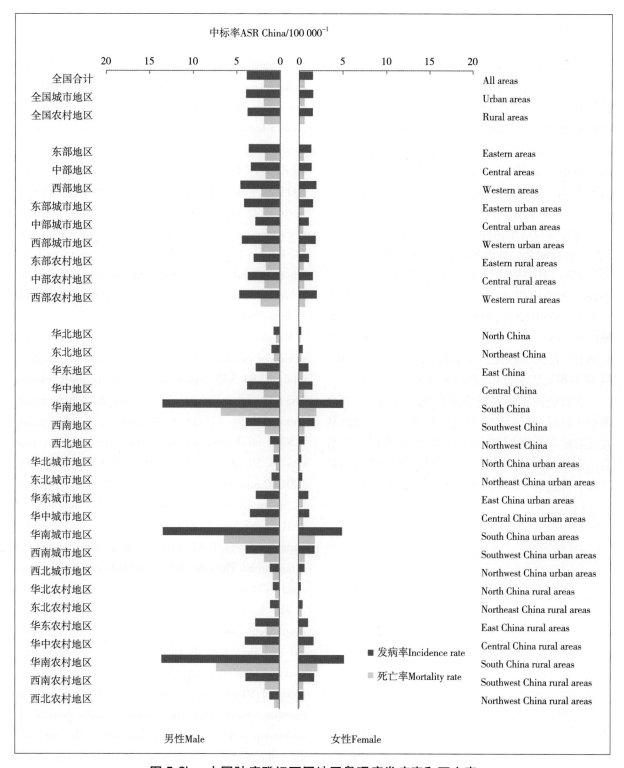

中标率ASR China/100 000^{-1}

全国合计	All areas
全国城市地区	Urban areas
全国农村地区	Rural areas
东部地区	Eastern areas
中部地区	Central areas
西部地区	Western areas
东部城市地区	Eastern urban areas
中部城市地区	Central urban areas
西部城市地区	Western urban areas
东部农村地区	Eastern rural areas
中部农村地区	Central rural areas
西部农村地区	Western rural areas
华北地区	North China
东北地区	Northeast China
华东地区	East China
华中地区	Central China
华南地区	South China
西南地区	Southwest China
西北地区	Northwest China
华北城市地区	North China urban areas
东北城市地区	Northeast China urban areas
华东城市地区	East China urban areas
华中城市地区	Central China urban areas
华南城市地区	South China urban areas
西南城市地区	Southwest China urban areas
西北城市地区	Northwest China urban areas
华北农村地区	North China rural areas
东北农村地区	Northeast China rural areas
华东农村地区	East China rural areas
华中农村地区	Central China rural areas
华南农村地区	South China rural areas
西南农村地区	Southwest China rural areas
西北农村地区	Northwest China rural areas

发病率Incidence rate
死亡率Mortality rate

男性Male　　　女性Female

图 5-2b　中国肿瘤登记不同地区鼻咽癌发病率和死亡率

Figure 5-2b　Incidence and mortality rates of nasopharyngeal cancer in different registration areas of China

3 食管

食管癌位居中国肿瘤登记地区癌症发病谱第8位。新发病例数为 105 070 例，占全部癌症发病的 5.48%；其中男性 78 494 例，女性 26 576 例，城市地区 36 693 例，农村地区 68 377 例。食管癌发病率为 16.72/10 万，中标发病率为 9.20/10 万，世标发病率为 9.25/10 万；男性中标发病率为女性的 3.31 倍，农村中标发病率为城市的 1.45 倍。0~74 岁累积发病率为 1.16%（表 5-3a）。

食管癌位居中国肿瘤登记地区癌症死亡谱第5位。食管癌死亡病例 84 828 例，占全部癌症死亡的 7.80%；其中男性 63 651 例，女性 21 177 例，城市地区 30 006 例，农村地区 54 822 例。食管癌死亡率为 13.50/10 万，中标死亡率 7.18/10 万，世标死亡率 7.18/10 万；男性中标死亡率为女性的 3.56 倍，农村中标死亡率为城市的 1.42 倍。0~74 岁累积死亡率为 0.84%（表 5-3b）。

食管癌的年龄别发病率和死亡率在 40 岁之前处于较低水平，自 40 岁之后快速上升。男性和女性发病率分别于 80~84 岁和 85 岁及以上年龄组达到高峰，死亡率均在 85 岁及以上年龄组达到高峰。男性各年龄别发病率和死亡率均明显高于女性（图 5-3a）。

3 Esophagus

Esophageal cancer was the 8th most common cancer in the registration areas of China. There were 105 070 new cases of esophageal cancer (78 494 males and 26 576 females, 36 693 in urban areas and 68 377 in rural areas), accounting for 5.48% of new cases of all cancers. The crude incidence rate was 16.72 per 100 000, with ASR China 9.20 per 100 000 and ASR world 9.25 per 100 000, respectively. Subgroup analyses showed that the incidence of ASR China was 3.31 times in males as that in females, and was 1.45 times in rural areas as that in urban areas. The cumulative incidence rate for subjects aged 0-74 years was 1.16% (Table 5-3a).

Esophageal cancer was the 5th most common cause of cancer deaths in the registration areas of China. A total of 84 828 cases died of esophageal cancer (63 651 males and 21 177 females, 30 006 in urban areas and 54 822 in rural areas), accounting for 7.80% of all cancer deaths. The crude mortality rate was 13.50 per 100 000, with ASR China 7.18 per 100 000 and ASR world 7.18 per 100 000, respectively. Subgroup analyses showed that the mortality of ASR China was 3.56 times in males as that in females, and was 1.42 times in rural areas as that in urban areas. The cumulative mortality rate for subjects aged 0-74 years was 0.84% (Table 5-3b).

The age-specific incidence and mortality rates of esophageal cancer were relatively low before 40 years old and increased dramatically since then. The age-specific incidence rates were the highest in the age group of 80-84 yearsand 85 years old for males and females, respectively. The mortality rates peaked in age group of 85 years old for both sexes. The age-specific incidence and mortality rates were generally higher in males than those in females (Figure 5-3a).

农村地区食管癌的发病率和死亡率均高于城市地区。男性中标发病率和死亡率西部地区最高，东部地区最低。女性中标发病率和死亡率在中部地区最高，西部地区最低。七大行政区中，男性中标发病率和死亡率在西南地区最高，中标发病率在东北地区最低，中标死亡率在华南地区最低；女性中标发病率和死亡率在华中地区最高，东北地区最低（表5-3a，表5-3b，图5-3b）。

食管癌病例中有明确亚部位信息的占31.54%，其中50.42%的病例发生在食管中段，其次是食管上段占21.71%，食管下段占19.28%，交搭跨越占8.59%（图5-3c）。

全部食管癌病例中有明确组织学类型的病例占66.03%，其中鳞状细胞癌是最主要的病理类型，占84.65%；其次是腺癌，占10.57%；腺鳞癌占1.18%（图5-3d）。

The incidence and mortality rates of esophageal cancer were higher in rural areas than those in urban areas. The incidence and mortality rates(ASR China) in males were the highest in western areas and the lowest in eastern areas. The incidence and mortality rates(ASR China) in females were the highest in central areas, and the lowest in western areas. Among the seven administrative districts, the incidence and mortality rates(ASR China) in males were the highest in Southwest China, and the lowest in Northeast China and South China, respectively. The incidence and mortality rates(ASR China) in females were the highest in Central China and the lowest in Northeast China(Table 5-3a, Table 5-3b, Figure 5-3b).

There were 31.54% of the esophageal cancer cases having specific subsite information. Esophageal cancer occurred the most frequently in the middle third of the esophagus(50.42%), followed by upper third(21.71%), lower third(19.28%) and overlapping esophagus(8.59%)(Figure 5-3c).

About 66.03% of the esophageal cancer cases had morphological verification. Among those, esophageal squamous cell carcinoma was the most common type, accounting for 84.65% of all cases, followed by adenocarcinoma(10.57%) and adenosquamous carcinoma(1.18%)(Figure 5-3d).

表 5-3a　中国肿瘤登记地区食管癌发病情况

表 5-3a　中国肿瘤登记地区食管癌发病情况

Table 5-3a　Incidence of esophageal cancer in the registration areas of China

地区 Area	性别 Sex	发病数 No. cases	粗率 Crude rate/ 100 000^{-1}	构成比 Freq. /%	中标率 ASR China/ 100 000^{-1}	世标率 ASR world/ 100 000^{-1}	累积率 Cum. rate 0~74/%	顺位 Rank
合计 All	合计 Both	105 070	16.72	5.48	9.20	9.25	1.16	8
	男性 Male	78 494	24.62	7.51	14.28	14.43	1.84	5
	女性 Female	26 576	8.58	3.05	4.31	4.27	0.50	10
城市地区 Urban areas	合计 Both	36 693	13.67	4.11	7.35	7.42	0.93	9
	男性 Male	28 526	21.22	5.99	11.96	12.13	1.54	5
	女性 Female	8 167	6.09	1.95	2.97	2.93	0.34	13
农村地区 Rural areas	合计 Both	68 377	19.00	6.69	10.64	10.69	1.34	7
	男性 Male	49 968	27.10	8.78	16.06	16.19	2.06	5
	女性 Female	18 409	10.48	4.06	5.37	5.33	0.63	8
东部地区 Eastern areas	合计 Both	43 242	17.05	4.67	8.50	8.54	1.07	8
	男性 Male	31 974	25.08	6.54	13.27	13.42	1.70	5
	女性 Female	11 268	8.93	2.58	3.97	3.91	0.45	10
中部地区 Central areas	合计 Both	25 777	17.14	6.07	10.17	10.21	1.27	7
	男性 Male	18 026	23.55	7.82	14.73	14.83	1.87	5
	女性 Female	7 751	10.50	3.99	5.79	5.77	0.68	8
西部地区 Western areas	合计 Both	36 051	16.07	6.37	9.46	9.55	1.21	7
	男性 Male	28 494	24.82	8.75	15.28	15.46	1.98	5
	女性 Female	7 557	6.89	3.14	3.76	3.74	0.45	11

表 5-3b　中国肿瘤登记地区食管癌死亡情况

Table 5-3b　Mortality of esophageal cancer in the registration areas of China

地区 Area	性别 Sex	死亡数 No. deaths	粗率 Crude rate/ 100 000^{-1}	构成比 Freq. /%	中标率 ASR China/ 100 000^{-1}	世标率 ASR world/ 100 000^{-1}	累积率 Cum. rate 0~74/%	顺位 Rank
合计 All	合计 Both	84 828	13.50	7.80	7.18	7.18	0.84	5
	男性 Male	63 651	19.96	9.11	11.37	11.40	1.36	4
	女性 Female	21 177	6.84	5.44	3.20	3.16	0.32	6
城市地区 Urban areas	合计 Both	30 006	11.18	6.29	5.79	5.81	0.68	5
	男性 Male	23 326	17.35	7.69	9.56	9.64	1.16	5
	女性 Female	6 680	4.98	3.84	2.26	2.22	0.22	8
农村地区 Rural areas	合计 Both	54 822	15.23	8.99	8.26	8.25	0.96	4
	男性 Male	40 325	21.87	10.21	12.75	12.77	1.52	4
	女性 Female	14 497	8.26	6.74	3.95	3.91	0.40	5
东部地区 Eastern areas	合计 Both	35 726	14.08	7.39	6.70	6.67	0.76	5
	男性 Male	26 325	20.65	8.62	10.62	10.63	1.25	4
	女性 Female	9 401	7.45	5.28	3.04	2.98	0.29	6
中部地区 Central areas	合计 Both	19 756	13.14	8.05	7.53	7.52	0.86	4
	男性 Male	13 989	18.28	8.93	11.23	11.25	1.32	4
	女性 Female	5 767	7.81	6.50	4.03	4.00	0.42	6
西部地区 Western areas	合计 Both	29 346	13.08	8.18	7.55	7.59	0.92	5
	男性 Male	23 337	20.33	9.87	12.39	12.48	1.54	4
	女性 Female	6 009	5.48	4.92	2.85	2.83	0.30	7

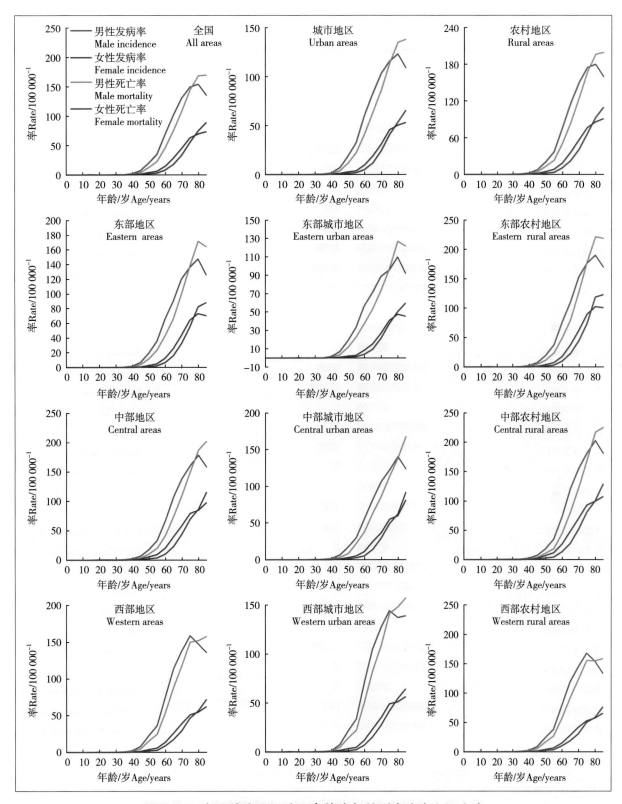

图 5-3a　中国肿瘤登记地区食管癌年龄别发病率和死亡率

Figure 5-3a　Age-specific incidence and mortality rates of esophageal cancer
in the registration areas of China

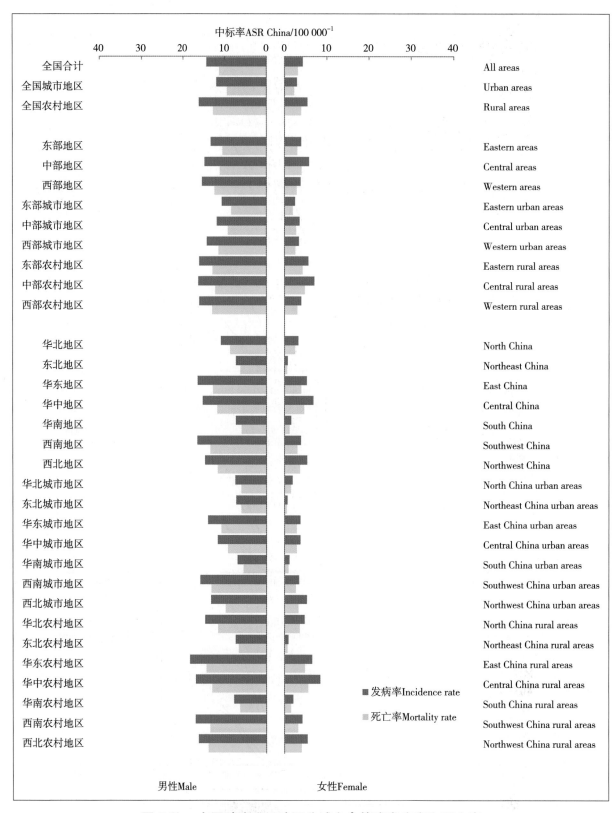

中标率ASR China/100 000^{-1}

全国合计		All areas
全国城市地区		Urban areas
全国农村地区		Rural areas
东部地区		Eastern areas
中部地区		Central areas
西部地区		Western areas
东部城市地区		Eastern urban areas
中部城市地区		Central urban areas
西部城市地区		Western urban areas
东部农村地区		Eastern rural areas
中部农村地区		Central rural areas
西部农村地区		Western rural areas
华北地区		North China
东北地区		Northeast China
华东地区		East China
华中地区		Central China
华南地区		South China
西南地区		Southwest China
西北地区		Northwest China
华北城市地区		North China urban areas
东北城市地区		Northeast China urban areas
华东城市地区		East China urban areas
华中城市地区		Central China urban areas
华南城市地区		South China urban areas
西南城市地区		Southwest China urban areas
西北城市地区		Northwest China urban areas
华北农村地区		North China rural areas
东北农村地区		Northeast China rural areas
华东农村地区		East China rural areas
华中农村地区		Central China rural areas
华南农村地区		South China rural areas
西南农村地区		Southwest China rural areas
西北农村地区		Northwest China rural areas

发病率Incidence rate

死亡率Mortality rate

男性Male　　　　女性Female

图 5-3b　中国肿瘤登记地区分城乡食管癌发病率和死亡率

Figure 5-3b　Incidence and mortality rates of esophageal cancer in different registration areas of China

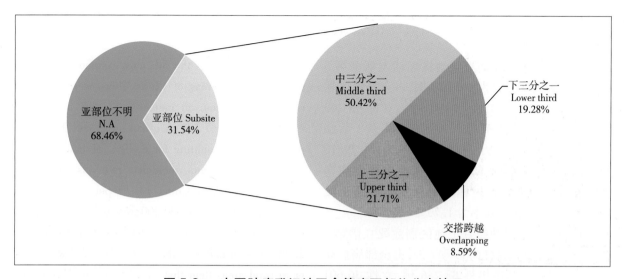

图 5-3c   中国肿瘤登记地区食管癌亚部位分布情况
Figure 5-3c   Subsite distribution of esophageal cancer in the registration areas of China

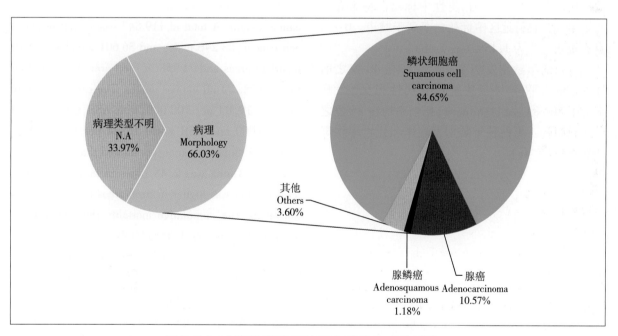

图 5-3d   中国肿瘤登记地区食管癌病理分型情况
Figure 5-3d   Morphological distribution of esophageal cancer in the
registration areas of China

4 胃

胃癌位居中国肿瘤登记地区癌症发病谱第 5 位。胃癌新发病例数为 162 680 例,占全部癌症发病的 8.49%。其中男性 113 418 例,女性 49 262 例;城市地区 67 192 例,农村地区 95 488 例。胃癌发病率为 25.89/10 万,中标发病率为 14.79/10 万,世标发病率为 14.68/10 万,男性中标发病率为女性的 2.38 倍,农村地区中标发病率高于城市。0~74 岁累积发病率为 1.79%(表 5-4a)。

胃癌位居中国肿瘤登记地区癌症死亡谱第 3 位。胃癌死亡病例数为 119 847 例,占全部癌症死亡的 11.02%。其中男性 83 246 例,女性 36 601 例;城市地区 48 089 例,农村地区 71 758 例。胃癌死亡率为 19.07/10 万,中标死亡率 10.36/10 万,世标死亡率 10.24/10 万,男性中标死亡率为女性的 2.48 倍,农村地区中标死亡率高于城市。0~74 岁累积死亡率为 1.15%(表 5-4b)。

胃癌的年龄别发病率和死亡率在 40 岁之前处于较低水平,40 岁后快速上升,男性和女性发病率均于 80~84 岁组达到高峰,死亡率均在 85 岁之后达到高峰。男性各年龄别发病率和死亡率均高于女性(图 5-4a)。

4　Stomach

Stomach cancer was the 5th most common cancer in the registration areas of China. There were 162 680 new cases of stomach cancer (113 418 males and 49 262 females, 67 192 in urban areas and 95 488 in rural areas), accounting for 8.49% of new cases of all cancers. The crude incidence rate was 25.89 per 100 000, with ASR China 14.79 per 100 000 and ASR world 14.68 per 100 000, respectively. Subgroup analyses showed that the incidence of ASR China was 2.38 times in males as that in females, and was higher in rural areas than that in urban areas. The cumulative incidence rate for subjects aged 0-74 years was 1.79% (Table 5-4a).

Stomach cancer was the 3rd most common cause of cancer deaths. A total of 119 847 cases died of stomach cancer (83 246 males and 36 601 females, 48 089 in urban areas and 71 758 in rural areas), accounting for 11.02% of all cancer deaths. The crude mortality rate was 19.07 per 100 000, with ASR China 10.36 per 100 000 and ASR world 10.24 per 100 000, respectively. Subgroup analyses showed that the mortality of ASR China was 2.48 times in males as that in females, and was higher in rural areas than that in urban areas. The cumulative mortality rate for subjects aged 0-74 years was 1.15% (Table 5-4b).

The age-specific incidence and mortality rates of stomach cancer were relatively low before 40 years old and increased rapidly since then. For both sexes, the incidence ratesand mortality rates peaked at the age group of 80-84 years and 85 years old, respectively. Age-specific incidence and mortality rates in males were generally higher than those in females across all age groups (Figure 5-4a).

农村地区胃癌的发病率和死亡率均高于城市地区。中标发病率和死亡率在中部地区和东部地区均较高,西部地区较低。七大行政区中,中标发病率男性在西北地区最高,女性在华东地区最高,男性和女性均在华南地区最低;男性和女性中标死亡率均在西北地区最高,华南地区最低(表5-4a,表5-4b,图5-4b)。

全部胃癌病例中有明确亚部位信息的病例占41.29%。其中贲门病例最多,占36.05%,其次是幽门窦(22.52%)、胃体(17.99%)、胃底(8.12%)、胃小弯(6.90%)、交搭跨越(5.68%)、幽门(1.37%)和胃大弯(1.37%)(图5-4c)。

全部胃癌病例中有明确组织学类型的病例占67.05%。其中腺癌是最主要的病理类型,占90.39%,其次是其他类型(5.26%)、鳞状细胞癌(3.52%)、类癌(0.63%)和腺鳞癌(0.20%)(图5-4d)。

The incidence and mortality rates of stomach cancer were higher in rural areas than those in urban areas. The incidence and mortality rates (ASR China) were high in centraland eastern areas, and low in western areas. Among the seven administrative districts, the incidence rates(ASR China) were the highest in Northwest China for males and in East China for females, and the lowest in South China for both sexes. The mortality rates(ASR China) were the highest in Northwest China and the lowest in South China for both sexes(Table 5-4a, Table 5-4b, Figure 5-4b).

About 41. 29% of the stomach cancer cases had complete information on subsite. Among those, cardia was the most common subsite and accounted for 36. 05% of the total cases, followed by pyloric antrum (22. 52%), body(17. 99%), fundus(8. 12%), lesser curvature(6. 90%), overlapping (5. 68%), pylorus(1. 37%) and greater curvature(1. 37%) (Figure 5-4c).

About 67. 05% of the stomach cancer cases had morphological verification. Among those, adenocarcinoma was the most common histological type, accounting for 90. 39% of all cases, followed by other type(5. 26%), squamous cell carcinoma(3. 52%), carcinoid (0. 63%) and adenosquamous carcinoma (0. 20%) (Figure 5-4d).

表 5-4a　中国肿瘤登记地区胃癌发病情况

Table 5-4a　Incidence of stomach cancer in the registration areas of China

地区 Area	性别 Sex	发病数 No. cases	粗率 Crude rate/ 100 000⁻¹	构成比 Freq./%	中标率 ASR China/ 100 000⁻¹	世标率 ASR world/ 100 000⁻¹	累积率 Cum. rate 0~74/%	顺位 Rank
合计 All	合计 Both	162 680	25.89	8.49	14.79	14.68	1.79	5
	男性 Male	113 418	35.57	10.85	21.02	21.02	2.62	4
	女性 Female	49 262	15.91	5.65	8.85	8.62	0.99	6
城市地区 Urban areas	合计 Both	67 192	25.03	7.52	13.95	13.84	1.68	6
	男性 Male	46 471	34.56	9.76	19.79	19.81	2.46	4
	女性 Female	20 721	15.46	4.96	8.48	8.24	0.94	6
农村地区 Rural areas	合计 Both	95 488	26.53	9.34	15.43	15.33	1.88	5
	男性 Male	66 947	36.31	11.77	21.95	21.93	2.74	3
	女性 Female	28 541	16.26	6.30	9.13	8.93	1.03	6
东部地区 Eastern areas	合计 Both	78 701	31.02	8.51	16.28	16.11	1.99	4
	男性 Male	54 894	43.06	11.23	23.30	23.26	2.91	3
	女性 Female	23 807	18.86	5.45	9.70	9.41	1.09	5
中部地区 Central areas	合计 Both	40 330	26.82	9.49	16.44	16.36	2.01	3
	男性 Male	28 027	36.62	12.15	23.28	23.32	2.92	3
	女性 Female	12 303	16.67	6.34	9.91	9.71	1.11	6
西部地区 Western areas	合计 Both	43 649	19.45	7.71	11.80	11.73	1.41	5
	男性 Male	30 497	26.57	9.37	16.65	16.67	2.04	4
	女性 Female	13 152	12.00	5.47	7.05	6.90	0.77	7

表 5-4b　中国肿瘤登记地区胃癌死亡情况

Table 5-4b　Mortality of stomach cancer in the registration areas of China

地区 Area	性别 Sex	死亡数 No. deaths	粗率 Crude rate/ 100 000⁻¹	构成比 Freq./%	中标率 ASR China/ 100 000⁻¹	世标率 ASR world/ 100 000⁻¹	累积率 Cum. rate 0~74/%	顺位 Rank
合计 All	合计 Both	119 847	19.07	11.02	10.36	10.24	1.15	3
	男性 Male	83 246	26.11	11.92	14.98	14.88	1.71	3
	女性 Female	36 601	11.82	9.41	6.04	5.92	0.61	4
城市地区 Urban areas	合计 Both	48 089	17.91	10.07	9.40	9.30	1.03	3
	男性 Male	33 157	24.66	10.93	13.59	13.52	1.52	3
	女性 Female	14 932	11.14	8.58	5.56	5.43	0.55	4
农村地区 Rural areas	合计 Both	71 758	19.94	11.76	11.10	10.98	1.25	3
	男性 Male	50 089	27.17	12.68	16.04	15.91	1.85	3
	女性 Female	21 669	12.34	10.07	6.42	6.30	0.66	3
东部地区 Eastern areas	合计 Both	56 002	22.08	11.58	10.79	10.62	1.18	3
	男性 Male	38 749	30.40	12.69	15.72	15.56	1.76	3
	女性 Female	17 253	13.67	9.68	6.29	6.11	0.63	3
中部地区 Central areas	合计 Both	29 578	19.67	12.05	11.58	11.47	1.31	3
	男性 Male	20 573	26.88	13.13	16.74	16.62	1.93	3
	女性 Female	9 005	12.20	10.15	6.76	6.65	0.70	3
西部地区 Western areas	合计 Both	34 267	15.27	9.56	8.96	8.91	1.02	3
	男性 Male	23 924	20.84	10.12	12.83	12.80	1.50	3
	女性 Female	10 343	9.44	8.47	5.22	5.16	0.55	4

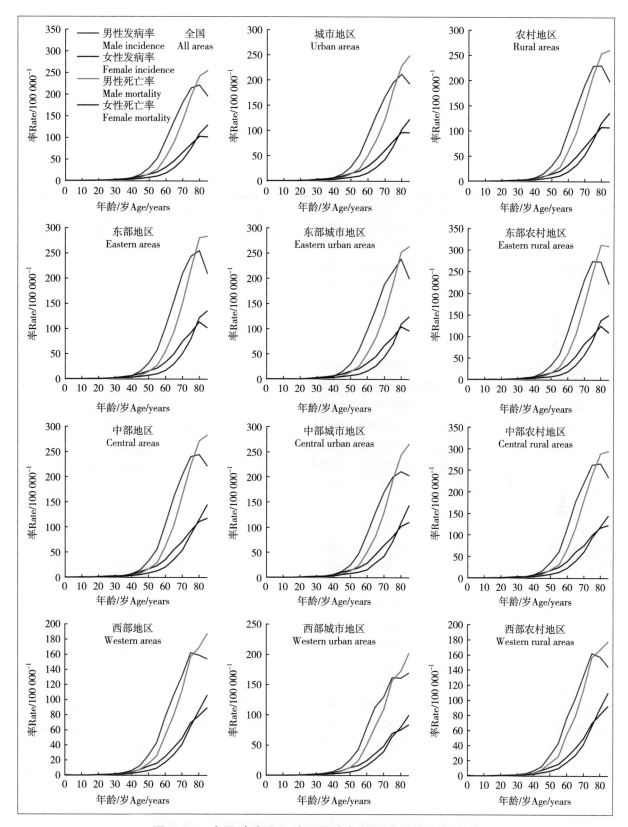

图 5-4a　中国肿瘤登记地区胃癌年龄别发病率和死亡率

Figure 5-4a　Age-specific incidence and mortality rates of stomach cancer in the registration areas of China

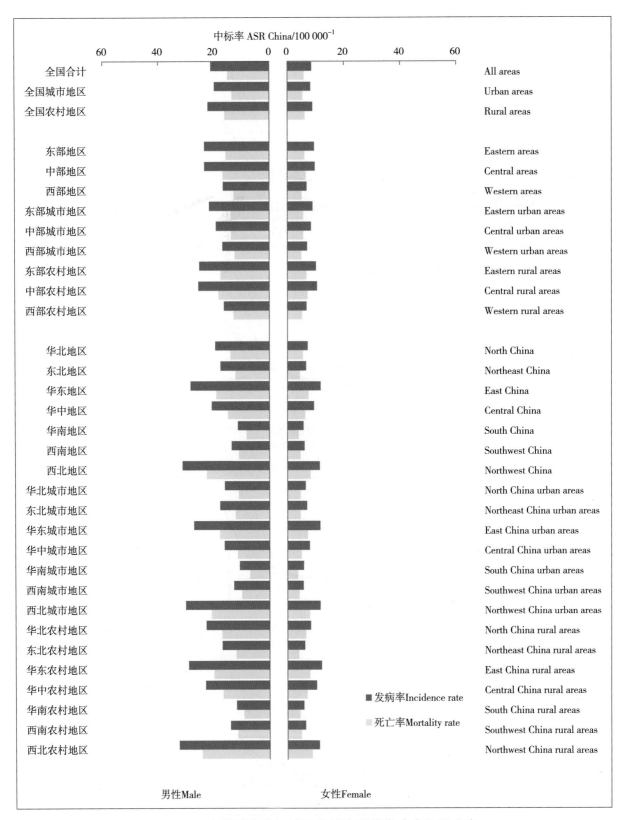

图 5-4b 中国肿瘤登记地区分城乡胃癌发病率和死亡率

Figure 5-4b Incidence and mortality rates of stomach cancer in different registration areas of China

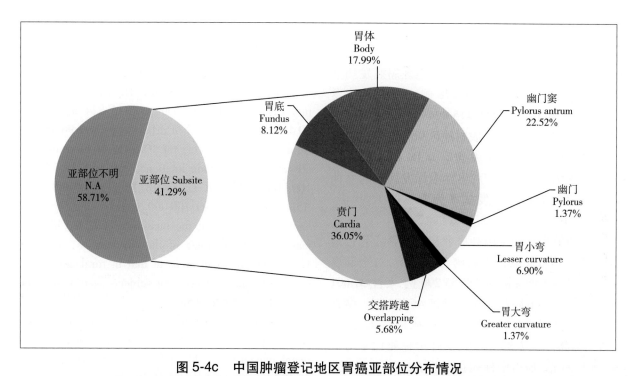

图 5-4c　中国肿瘤登记地区胃癌亚部位分布情况

Figure 5-4c　Subsite distribution of stomach cancer in the registration areas of China

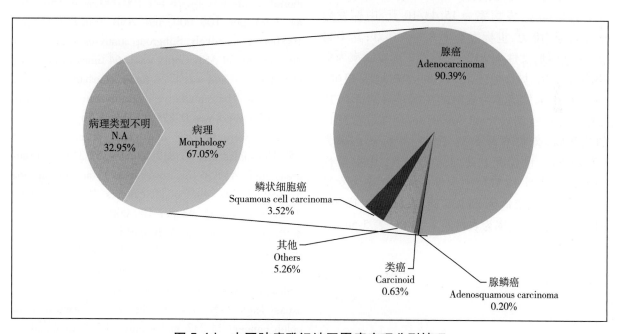

图 5-4d　中国肿瘤登记地区胃癌病理分型情况

Figure 5-4d　Morphological distribution of stomach cancer in the
registration areas of China

5 结直肠

结直肠癌位居中国肿瘤登记地区癌症发病谱第 3 位。新发病例数为 196 278 例，占全部癌症发病的 10.24%；其中男性 115 824 例，女性 80 454 例，城市地区 99 809 例，农村地区 96 469 例。发病率为 31.23/10 万，中标发病率为 18.19/10 万，世标发病率为 17.97/10 万；男性中标发病率为女性的 1.51 倍，城市中标发病率为农村的 1.30 倍。0~74 岁累积发病率为 2.14%（表 5-5a）。

结直肠癌位居中国肿瘤登记地区癌症死亡谱第 4 位。结直肠癌死亡病例 92 891 例，占全部癌症死亡的 8.54%；其中男性 55 290 例，女性 37 601 例，城市地区 46 487 例，农村地区 46 404 例。结直肠癌死亡率为 14.78/10 万，中标死亡率 7.93/10 万，世标死亡率 7.87/10 万；男性中标死亡率为女性的 1.64 倍，城市中标死亡率为农村的 1.22 倍。0~74 岁累积死亡率为 0.82%（表 5-5b）。

结肠癌新发病例数为 96 967 例，占全部癌症发病的 5.06%，发病率为 15.43/10 万，中标发病率为 8.98/10 万，世标发病率 8.84/10 万；其中男性 55 155 例，女性 41 812 例，男性中标发病率为女性的 1.39 倍；城市地区 53 311 例，农村地区 43 656 例，城市中标发病率为农村的 1.51 倍（表 5-5c）。结肠癌死亡病例数为 42 809 例，占全部癌症死亡的 3.94%，死亡率为 6.81/10 万，中标死亡率为 3.63/10 万，世标死亡率 3.61/10 万；其中男性 24 232 例，女性 18 577 例，男性中标死亡率为女性的 1.46 倍；城市地区 23 936 例，农村地区 18 873 例，城市中标死亡率为农村的 1.53 倍（表 5-5d）。

5 Colorectum

Colorectal cancer was the 3rd most common cancer in the registration areas of China. There were 196 278 new cases of colorectal cancer (115 824 males and 80 454 females, 99 809 in urban areas and 96 469 in rural areas), accounting for 10.24% of new cases of all cancers. The crude incidence rate was 31.23 per 100 000, with ASR China 18.19 per 100 000 and ASR world 17.97 per 100 000, respectively. Subgroup analyses showed that the incidence of ASR China in males was 1.51 times of that in females, and was 1.30 times in urban areas of that in rural areas. The cumulative incidence rate for subjects aged 0-74 years was 2.14% (Table 5-5a).

Colorectal cancer was the 4th most common cause of cancer deaths. A total of 92 891 cases died of colorectal cancer (55 290 males and 37 601 females, 46 487 in urban areas and 46 404 in rural areas), accounting for 8.54% of all cancer deaths. The crude mortality rate was 14.78 per 100 000, with ASR China 7.93 per 100 000 and ASR world 7.87 per 100 000, respectively. Subgroup analyses showed that the mortality of ASR China was 1.64 times in males as of in females, and was 1.22 times in urban areas of in rural areas. The cumulative mortality rate for subjects aged 0-74 years was 0.82% (Table 5-5b).

There were 96 967 new cases of colon cancer (55 155 males and 41 812 females, 53 311 in urban areas and 43 656 in rural areas), accounting for 5.06% of new cases of all cancers. The crude incidence rate was 15.43 per 100 000, with ASR China 8.98 per 100 000 and ASR world 8.84 per 100 000, respectively. Subgroup analyses showed that the incidence of ASR China was 1.39 times in males of in females, and was 1.51 times in urban areas of in rural areas (Table 5-5c). A total of 42 809 cases died of colon cancer (24 232 males and 18 577 in females, 23 936 in urban areas and 18 873 in rural areas), accounting for 3.94% of all cancer deaths. The crude mortality rate was 6.81 per 100 000, with ASR China 3.63 per 100 000 and ASR world 3.61 per 100 000, respectively. Subgroup analyses showed that the mortality of ASR China was 1.46 times in males of in females, and was 1.53 times in urban areas of in rural areas (Table 5-5d).

直肠癌新发病例数为 97 038 例,占全部癌症发病的 5.06%,发病率为 15.44/10 万,中标发病率为 9.00/10 万,世标发病率 8.92/10 万;其中男性 59 391 例,女性 37 647 例,男性中标发病率为女性的 1.64 倍;城市地区 45 625 例,农村地区 51 413 例,城市中标发病率为农村的 1.13 倍(表 5-5e)。直肠癌死亡病例数为 48 477 例,占全部癌症死亡的 4.46%,死亡率为 7.71/10 万,中标死亡率为 4.16/10 万,世标死亡率 4.13/10 万;其中男性 30 126 例,女性 18 351 例,男性中标死亡率为女性的 1.82 倍;城市地区 21 944 例,农村地区 26 533 例,城市中标死亡率和农村接近(表 5-5f)。

结直肠癌年龄别发病率和死亡率在男性和女性中均随年龄呈上升趋势,40～44 岁组开始上升明显,发病率在 80～84 岁组达高峰,死亡率在 85 岁及以上组达到高峰,男性各年龄别发病率和死亡率均明显高于女性(图 5-5a)。

城市地区结直肠癌的发病率和死亡率均高于农村地区,中标发病率和死亡率东部地区高于西部和中部地区(表 5-5a,表 5-5b,图 5-5a)。七大行政区中,男性和女性中标发病率均在东北地区最高,西北地区最低。男性和女性中标死亡率分别在华南地区和东北地区最高,西北地区最低(图 5-5b)。

在全部结肠癌病例中,有明确亚部位的病例占 60.65%,其中乙状结肠发生癌症的比例最高,占 42.66%,其次是升结肠、横结肠和降结肠,分别占 23.38%、8.53% 和 8.15%(图 5-5c)。

There were 97 038 new cases of rectal cancer (59 391 males and 37 647 females, 45 625 in urban areas and 51 413 in rural areas), accounting for 5.06% of new cases of all cancers. The crude incidence rate was 15.44 per 100 000, with ASR China 9.00 per 100 000 and ASR world 8.92 per 100 000, respectively. Subgroup analyses showed that the incidence of ASR China was 1.64 times in males of in females, and was 1.13 times in urban areas of in rural areas(Table 5-5e). A total of 48 477 cases died of rectal cancer (30 126 males and 18 351 females, 21 944 in urban areas and 26 533 in rural areas), accounting for 4.46% of all cancer deaths. The crude mortality rate was 7.71 per 100 000, with ASR China 4.16 per 100 000 and ASR world 4.13 per 100 000, respectively. Subgroup analyses showed that the mortality of ASR China was 1.82 times in males of that in females, and that was similar in urban and rural areas(Table 5-5f).

The age-specific incidence and mortality rates of colorectal cancer increased with age in both sexes, especially after the age group of 40-44 years, and reached the peak at the age group of 80-84 years for the incidence rates and at the age group of 85 years old for the mortality rates in both sexes. Age-specific incidence and mortality rates in males were generally higher than those in females across all age groups (Figure 5-5a).

The incidence and mortality rates of colorectal cancer were higher in urban areas than those in rural areas. The incidence and mortality rates(ASR China) were higher in eastern than in western and central areas(Table 5-5a, Table 5-5b, Figure 5-5a). Among the seven administrative districts, the incidence rates (ASR China) were the highest in Northeast for males and females, and the lowest in Northwest China for both sexes. The mortality rates(ASR China) were the highest in South China and Northeast China for males and females, respectively, and the lowest in Northwest China for both sexes(Figure 5-5b).

Approximately 60.65% of the colon cancer cases had complete information onsubsite. Among those, sigmoid colon was the most common subsite(42.66%), followed by ascending colon (23.38%), transverse colon(8.53%) and descending colon(8.15%)(Figure 5-5c).

表 5-5a　中国肿瘤登记地区结直肠癌发病情况

Table 5-5a　Incidence of colorectal cancer in the registration areas of China

地区 Area	性别 Sex	发病数 No. cases	粗率 Crude rate/ 100 000^{-1}	构成比 Freq./%	中标率 ASR China/ 100 000^{-1}	世标率 ASR world/ 100 000^{-1}	累积率 Cum. rate 0~74/%	顺位 Rank
合计 All	合计 Both	196 278	31.23	10.24	18.19	17.97	2.14	3
	男性 Male	115 824	36.33	11.08	21.96	21.81	2.62	3
	女性 Female	80 454	25.99	9.23	14.58	14.30	1.67	4
城市地区 Urban areas	合计 Both	99 809	37.18	11.17	20.87	20.70	2.46	3
	男性 Male	59 005	43.89	12.40	25.49	25.43	3.05	2
	女性 Female	40 804	30.44	9.76	16.53	16.24	1.88	4
农村地区 Rural areas	合计 Both	96 469	26.80	9.44	16.10	15.83	1.90	4
	男性 Male	56 819	30.82	9.99	19.24	19.00	2.29	4
	女性 Female	39 650	22.58	8.75	13.04	12.76	1.50	3
东部地区 Eastern areas	合计 Both	99 439	39.20	10.75	20.98	20.75	2.49	3
	男性 Male	59 021	46.30	12.08	25.72	25.60	3.10	2
	女性 Female	40 418	32.03	9.26	16.51	16.17	1.89	4
中部地区 Central areas	合计 Both	39 008	25.94	9.18	16.28	16.05	1.91	5
	男性 Male	22 559	29.47	9.78	19.22	19.03	2.28	4
	女性 Female	16 449	22.29	8.47	13.45	13.18	1.54	4
西部地区 Western areas	合计 Both	57 831	25.77	10.22	15.87	15.64	1.85	4
	男性 Male	34 244	29.83	10.52	19.01	18.81	2.23	3
	女性 Female	23 587	21.52	9.81	12.82	12.57	1.47	3

表 5-5b　中国肿瘤登记地区结直肠癌死亡情况

Table 5-5b　Mortality of colorectal cancer in the registration areas of China

地区 Area	性别 Sex	死亡数 No. deaths	粗率 Crude rate/ 100 000^{-1}	构成比 Freq./%	中标率 ASR China/ 100 000^{-1}	世标率 ASR world/ 100 000^{-1}	累积率 Cum. Rate 0~74/%	顺位 Rank
合计 All	合计 Both	92 891	14.78	8.54	7.93	7.87	0.82	4
	男性 Male	55 290	17.34	7.92	9.93	9.91	1.05	5
	女性 Female	37 601	12.14	9.66	6.07	5.99	0.60	3
城市地区 Urban areas	合计 Both	46 487	17.31	9.74	8.83	8.80	0.90	4
	男性 Male	27 468	20.43	9.05	11.07	11.12	1.16	4
	女性 Female	19 019	14.19	10.93	6.77	6.70	0.65	2
农村地区 Rural areas	合计 Both	46 404	12.89	7.61	7.21	7.12	0.76	5
	男性 Male	27 822	15.09	7.04	9.01	8.93	0.96	5
	女性 Female	18 582	10.58	8.64	5.50	5.42	0.57	4
东部地区 Eastern areas	合计 Both	44 423	17.51	9.19	8.30	8.27	0.84	4
	男性 Male	26 167	20.53	8.57	10.48	10.50	1.09	5
	女性 Female	18 256	14.47	10.24	6.32	6.25	0.61	2
中部地区 Central areas	合计 Both	18 657	12.41	7.60	7.33	7.25	0.77	5
	男性 Male	11 017	14.39	7.03	9.04	8.96	0.96	5
	女性 Female	7 640	10.35	8.61	5.72	5.65	0.59	4
西部地区 Western areas	合计 Both	29 811	13.28	8.31	7.76	7.67	0.83	4
	男性 Male	18 106	15.77	7.66	9.71	9.63	1.05	5
	女性 Female	11 705	10.68	9.58	5.89	5.80	0.61	3

表 5-5c 中国肿瘤登记地区结肠癌发病情况
Table 5-5c Incidence of colon cancer in the registration areas of China

地区 Area	性别 Sex	发病数 No. cases	粗率 Crude rate/ 100 000^{-1}	构成比 Freq./%	中标率 ASR China/ 100 000^{-1}	世标率 ASR world/ 100 000^{-1}	累积率 Cum. rate 0~74/%
合计 All	合计 Both	96 967	15.43	5.06	8.98	8.84	1.04
	男性 Male	55 155	17.30	5.28	10.48	10.38	1.23
	女性 Female	41 812	13.50	4.80	7.54	7.38	0.85
城市地区 Urban areas	合计 Both	53 311	19.86	5.96	11.08	10.96	1.28
	男性 Male	30 283	22.52	6.36	13.03	12.98	1.53
	女性 Female	23 028	17.18	5.51	9.24	9.07	1.04
农村地区 Rural areas	合计 Both	43 656	12.13	4.27	7.34	7.18	0.85
	男性 Male	24 872	13.49	4.37	8.51	8.36	1.00
	女性 Female	18 784	10.70	4.14	6.20	6.04	0.71
东部地区 Eastern areas	合计 Both	53 935	21.26	5.83	11.33	11.16	1.32
	男性 Male	30 839	24.19	6.31	13.41	13.30	1.59
	女性 Female	23 096	18.30	5.29	9.37	9.14	1.06
中部地区 Central areas	合计 Both	18 797	12.50	4.43	7.85	7.71	0.90
	男性 Male	10 585	13.83	4.59	9.06	8.94	1.05
	女性 Female	8 212	11.13	4.23	6.69	6.53	0.76
西部地区 Western areas	合计 Both	24 235	10.80	4.28	6.70	6.58	0.76
	男性 Male	13 731	11.96	4.22	7.69	7.58	0.88
	女性 Female	10 504	9.58	4.37	5.73	5.61	0.65

表 5-5d 中国肿瘤登记地区结肠癌死亡情况
Table 5-5d Mortality of colon cancer in the registration areas of China

地区 Area	性别 Sex	死亡数 No. deaths	粗率 Crude rate/ 100 000^{-1}	构成比 Freq./%	中标率 ASR China/ 100 000^{-1}	世标率 ASR world/ 100 000^{-1}	累积率 Cum. rate 0~74/%
合计 All	合计 Both	42 809	6.81	3.94	3.63	3.61	0.37
	男性 Male	24 232	7.60	3.47	4.34	4.33	0.44
	女性 Female	18 577	6.00	4.77	2.97	2.94	0.29
城市地区 Urban areas	合计 Both	23 936	8.92	5.01	4.50	4.49	0.45
	男性 Male	13 502	10.04	4.45	5.41	5.43	0.55
	女性 Female	10 434	7.78	6.00	3.67	3.64	0.35
农村地区 Rural areas	合计 Both	18 873	5.24	3.09	2.94	2.90	0.30
	男性 Male	10 730	5.82	2.72	3.49	3.46	0.36
	女性 Female	8 143	4.64	3.79	2.41	2.37	0.25
东部地区 Eastern areas	合计 Both	23 592	9.30	4.88	4.38	4.36	0.43
	男性 Male	13 253	10.40	4.34	5.30	5.30	0.54
	女性 Female	10 339	8.19	5.80	3.55	3.51	0.33
中部地区 Central areas	合计 Both	8 609	5.73	3.51	3.39	3.35	0.36
	男性 Male	4 866	6.36	3.10	4.01	3.98	0.42
	女性 Female	3 743	5.07	4.22	2.81	2.77	0.29
西部地区 Western areas	合计 Both	10 608	4.73	2.96	2.76	2.73	0.29
	男性 Male	6 113	5.33	2.59	3.28	3.26	0.34
	女性 Female	4 495	4.10	3.68	2.27	2.23	0.24

表 5-5e　中国肿瘤登记地区直肠癌发病情况

Table 5-5e　Incidence of rectal cancer in the registration areas of China

地区 Area	性别 Sex	发病数 No. cases	粗率 Crude rate/ 100 000⁻¹	构成比 Freq./%	中标率 ASR China/ 100 000⁻¹	世标率 ASR world/ 100 000⁻¹	累积率 Cum. Rate 0~74/%
合计 All	合计 Both	97 038	15.44	5.06	9.00	8.92	1.08
	男性 Male	59 391	18.63	5.68	11.24	11.19	1.36
	女性 Female	37 647	12.16	4.32	6.85	6.74	0.80
城市地区 Urban areas	合计 Both	45 625	16.99	5.10	9.61	9.56	1.16
	男性 Male	28 234	21.00	5.93	12.24	12.25	1.49
	女性 Female	17 391	12.97	4.16	7.12	7.02	0.83
农村地区 Rural areas	合计 Both	51 413	14.28	5.03	8.53	8.42	1.02
	男性 Male	31 157	16.90	5.48	10.47	10.37	1.26
	女性 Female	20 256	11.54	4.47	6.64	6.52	0.78
东部地区 Eastern areas	合计 Both	44 711	17.63	4.83	9.49	9.42	1.15
	男性 Male	27 745	21.77	5.68	12.12	12.11	1.49
	女性 Female	16 966	13.44	3.89	6.99	6.88	0.82
中部地区 Central areas	合计 Both	19 705	13.11	4.64	8.21	8.13	0.98
	男性 Male	11 701	15.29	5.07	9.92	9.86	1.20
	女性 Female	8 004	10.84	4.12	6.56	6.46	0.77
西部地区 Western areas	合计 Both	32 622	14.54	5.76	8.91	8.80	1.05
	男性 Male	19 945	17.37	6.13	11.02	10.92	1.32
	女性 Female	12 677	11.57	5.27	6.86	6.75	0.79

表 5-5f　中国肿瘤登记地区直肠癌死亡情况

Table 5-5f　Mortality of rectal cancer in the registration areas of China

地区 Area	性别 Sex	死亡数 No. deaths	粗率 Crude rate/ 100 000⁻¹	构成比 Freq./%	中标率 ASR China/ 100 000⁻¹	世标率 ASR world/ 100 000⁻¹	累积率 Cum. rate 0~74/%
合计 All	合计 Both	48 477	7.71	4.46	4.16	4.13	0.44
	男性 Male	30 126	9.45	4.31	5.42	5.40	0.58
	女性 Female	18 351	5.93	4.72	2.98	2.94	0.30
城市地区 Urban areas	合计 Both	21 944	8.17	4.60	4.21	4.20	0.44
	男性 Male	13 621	10.13	4.49	5.52	5.55	0.60
	女性 Female	8 323	6.21	4.78	3.00	2.96	0.30
农村地区 Rural areas	合计 Both	26 533	7.37	4.35	4.12	4.07	0.44
	男性 Male	16 505	8.95	4.18	5.33	5.28	0.58
	女性 Female	10 028	5.71	4.66	2.97	2.93	0.31
东部地区 Eastern areas	合计 Both	20 324	8.01	4.20	3.82	3.82	0.40
	男性 Male	12 625	9.90	4.13	5.06	5.09	0.54
	女性 Female	7 699	6.10	4.32	2.69	2.67	0.27
中部地区 Central areas	合计 Both	9 687	6.44	3.95	3.79	3.76	0.40
	男性 Male	5 953	7.78	3.80	4.87	4.82	0.52
	女性 Female	3 734	5.06	4.21	2.79	2.76	0.29
西部地区 Western areas	合计 Both	18 466	8.23	5.15	4.81	4.75	0.52
	男性 Male	11 548	10.06	4.88	6.20	6.14	0.68
	女性 Female	6 918	6.31	5.66	3.47	3.42	0.36

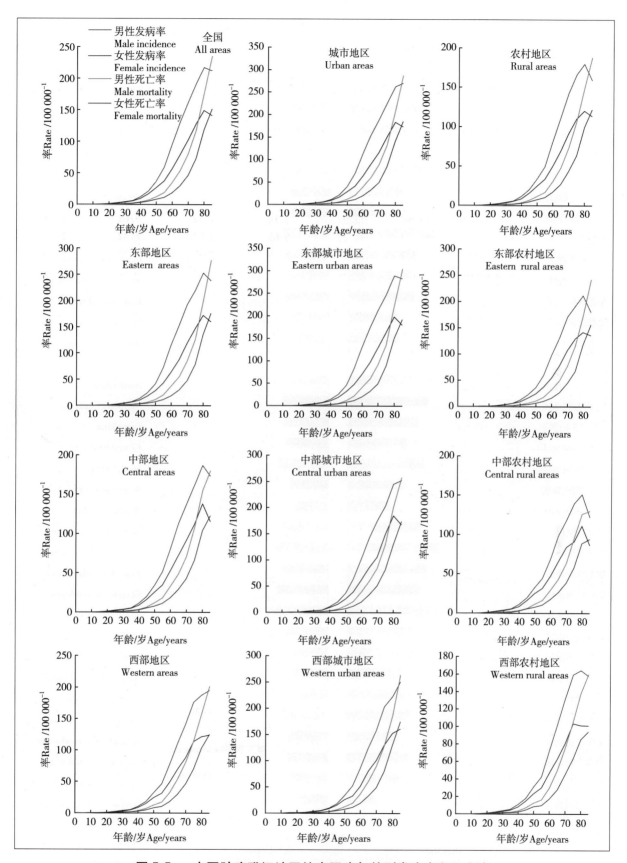

图 5-5a　中国肿瘤登记地区结直肠癌年龄别发病率和死亡率

Figure 5-5a　Age-specific incidence and mortality rates of colorectal cancer in the registration areas of China

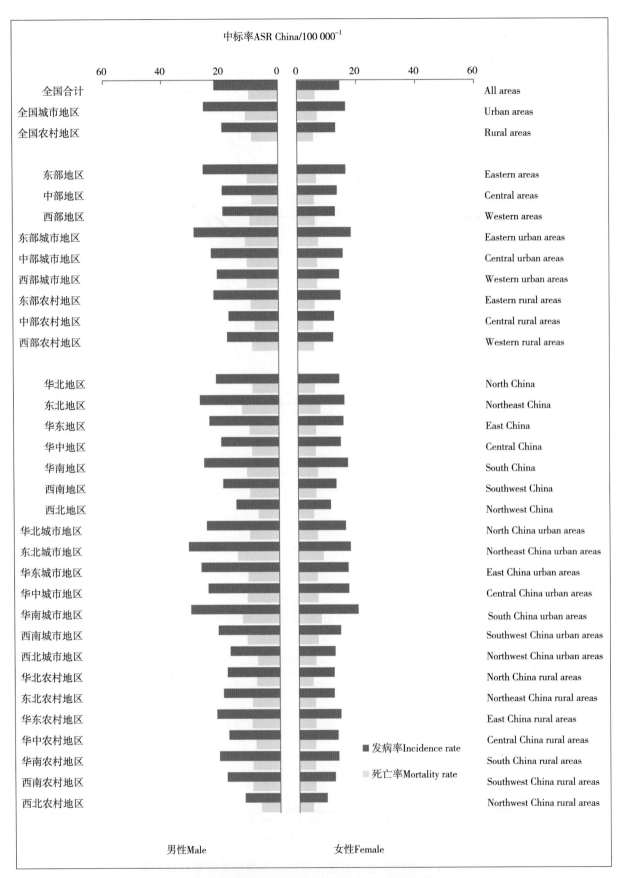

中标率ASR China/100 000^{-1}

	全国合计	All areas
全国城市地区	Urban areas
全国农村地区	Rural areas
东部地区	Eastern areas
中部地区	Central areas
西部地区	Western areas
东部城市地区	Eastern urban areas
中部城市地区	Central urban areas
西部城市地区	Western urban areas
东部农村地区	Eastern rural areas
中部农村地区	Central rural areas
西部农村地区	Western rural areas
华北地区	North China
东北地区	Northeast China
华东地区	East China
华中地区	Central China
华南地区	South China
西南地区	Southwest China
西北地区	Northwest China
华北城市地区	North China urban areas
东北城市地区	Northeast China urban areas
华东城市地区	East China urban areas
华中城市地区	Central China urban areas
华南城市地区	South China urban areas
西南城市地区	Southwest China urban areas
西北城市地区	Northwest China urban areas
华北农村地区	North China rural areas
东北农村地区	Northeast China rural areas
华东农村地区	East China rural areas
华中农村地区	Central China rural areas
华南农村地区	South China rural areas
西南农村地区	Southwest China rural areas
西北农村地区	Northwest China rural areas

发病率Incidence rate
死亡率Mortality rate

男性Male   女性Female

图 5-5b 中国肿瘤登记地区分城乡结直肠癌发病率和死亡率
Figure 5-5b Incidence and mortality rates of colorectal cancer in different registration areas of China

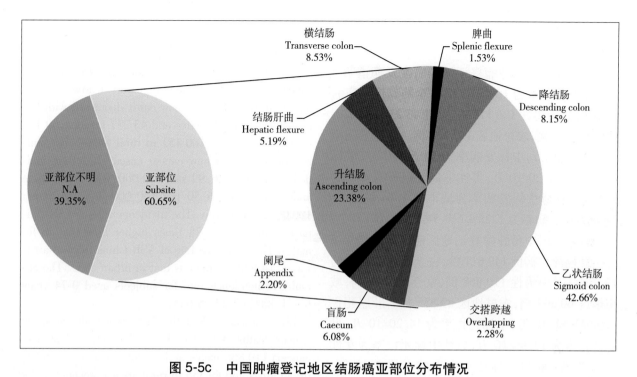

图 5-5c 中国肿瘤登记地区结肠癌亚部位分布情况

Figure 5-5c Subsite distribution of colon cancer in the registration areas of China

6 肝

　　肝癌位居中国肿瘤登记地区癌症发病谱第 4 位。新发病例数为 169 609 例,占全部癌症发病的 8.85%;其中男性 126 372 例,女性 43 237 例,城市地区 69 156 例,农村地区 100 453 例。肝癌发病率为 26.99/10 万,中标发病率为 16.50/10 万,世标发病率为 16.20/10 万;男性中标发病率为女性的 3.28 倍,农村中标发病率为城市的 1.14 倍。0~74 岁累积发病率为 1.88%(表 5-6a)。

　　肝癌位居中国肿瘤登记地区癌症死亡谱第 2 位。肝癌死亡病例 149 617 例,占全部癌症死亡的 13.76%;其中男性 110 868 例,女性 38 749 例,城市地区 60 262 例,农村地区 89 355 例。肝癌死亡率为 23.81/10 万,中标死亡率为 14.20/10 万,世标死亡率为 13.96/10 万;男性中标死亡率为女性的 3.29 倍,农村中标死亡率为城市的 1.18 倍。0~74 岁累积死亡率为 1.60%(表 5-6b)。

　　肝癌年龄别发病率、年龄别死亡率呈现性别差异。男性年龄别发病率和死亡率在 0~34 岁处于较低水平,35~39 岁组后显著上升;女性在 0~54 岁处于较低水平,55~59 岁组后上升。各年龄组男性发病率和死亡率一般高于女性(图 5-6a)。

　　农村地区肝癌发病率和死亡率均略高于城市地区。西部地区中标发病率最高。七大行政区中,男性肝癌的中标发病率和死亡率最高的地区均为华南地区,华北地区最低;女性中标发病率和死亡率最高的是西北地区,华北地区最低(表 5-6a,表 5-6b,图 5-6b)。

6　Liver

The incidence of liver cancer rankedthe 4th among all cancer types in the cancer registration areas of China. There were 169 609 new cases diagnosed with liver cancer(126 372 males and 43 237 females, 69 156 in urban areas and 100 453 in rural areas), accounting for 8.85% of new cancer cases. The crude incidence rate was 26.99 per 100 000, with ASR China and ASR world 16.50 per 100 000 and 16.20 per 100 000, respectively. The incidence rate of ASR China in males was 3.28 times higher than that in females. The incidence rate of ASR China in rural areas was 1.14 folds as high as that in urban areas. The cumulative incidence rate for subjects aged 0-74 years was 1.88% (Table 5-6a).

Liver cancer ranked the 2nd among all causes of cancer deaths. A total of 149 617 cases died of liver cancer(110 868 males and 38 749 females, 60 262 in urban areas and 89 355 in rural areas), accounting for 13.76% of all cancer deaths. The crude mortality rate was 23.81 per 100 000. The ASR China was 14.20 per 100 000 and ASR world was 13.96 per 100 000. The mortality rate of ASR China in males was 3.29 times higher than that in females. The mortality rate of ASR China in rural areas was 1.18 times as high as that in urban areas. The cumulative mortality rate for subjects aged 0-74 years was 1.60% (Table 5-6b).

The age-specific incidence and mortality rates showed differences between males and females. The incidence and mortality rates for males were relatively low inthe age group of 0-34 years, but increased sharply thereafter. For females, the age-specific rates were relatively low in the age group of 0-54 years and increased thereafter. Age-specific incidence and mortality rates in males were generally higher than those in females(Figure 5-6a).

The incidence and mortality rates of liver cancer in rural areas were higher than those in urban areas. Western areas had the highest incidence rate(ASR China). Among the seven administrative districts, for males, South China had the highest incidence and mortality rates(ASR China), while North China had the lowest rates. For females, the highest incidence and mortality rates (ASR China) were in Northwest China and the lowest incidence and mortality rates (ASR China) were in North China(Table 5-6a, Table 5-6b, Figure 5-6b).

表 5-6a 中国肿瘤登记地区肝癌发病情况
Table 5-6a Incidence of liver cancer in registration areas of China

地区 Area	性别 Sex	发病数 No. cases	粗率 Crude rate/ 100 000⁻¹	构成比 Freq./%	中标率 ASR China/ 100 000⁻¹	世标率 ASR world/ 100 000⁻¹	累积率 Cum. rate 0~74/%	顺位 Rank
合计 All	合计 Both	169 609	26.99	8.85	16.50	16.20	1.88	4
	男性 Male	126 372	39.64	12.09	25.37	24.86	2.88	2
	女性 Female	43 237	13.96	4.96	7.73	7.64	0.88	7
城市地区 Urban areas	合计 Both	69 156	25.76	7.74	15.26	15.06	1.74	4
	男性 Male	51 559	38.35	10.83	23.74	23.39	2.71	3
	女性 Female	17 597	13.13	4.21	7.03	6.97	0.79	7
农村地区 Rural areas	合计 Both	100 453	27.91	9.83	17.46	17.08	1.99	3
	男性 Male	74 813	40.58	13.15	26.60	25.96	3.01	2
	女性 Female	25 640	14.60	5.66	8.27	8.17	0.95	7
东部地区 Eastern areas	合计 Both	64 510	25.43	6.97	14.33	14.16	1.65	6
	男性 Male	47 896	37.57	9.80	22.34	22.03	2.56	4
	女性 Female	16 614	13.16	3.81	6.56	6.52	0.75	7
中部地区 Central areas	合计 Both	39 370	26.19	9.27	16.78	16.53	1.94	4
	男性 Male	28 471	37.20	12.35	24.94	24.55	2.88	2
	女性 Female	10 899	14.77	5.61	8.72	8.64	1.00	7
西部地区 Western areas	合计 Both	65 729	29.29	11.61	18.99	18.50	2.13	2
	男性 Male	50 005	43.56	15.36	29.28	28.47	3.27	2
	女性 Female	15 724	14.35	6.54	8.55	8.41	0.96	5

表 5-6b 中国肿瘤登记地区肝癌死亡情况
Table 5-6b Mortality of liver cancer in registration areas of China

地区 Area	性别 Sex	死亡数 No. deaths	粗率 Crude rate/ 100 000⁻¹	构成比 Freq./%	中标率 ASR China/ 100 000⁻¹	世标率 ASR world/ 100 000⁻¹	累积率 Cum. Rate 0~74/%	顺位 Rank
合计 All	合计 Both	149 617	23.81	13.76	14.20	13.96	1.60	2
	男性 Male	110 868	34.77	15.87	21.88	21.47	2.46	2
	女性 Female	38 749	12.52	9.96	6.65	6.58	0.74	2
城市地区 Urban areas	合计 Both	60 262	22.45	12.62	12.90	12.72	1.44	2
	男性 Male	44 457	33.07	14.65	20.04	19.75	2.26	2
	女性 Female	15 805	11.79	9.09	6.00	5.94	0.64	3
农村地区 Rural areas	合计 Both	89 355	24.82	14.65	15.20	14.91	1.72	2
	男性 Male	66 411	36.02	16.81	23.26	22.76	2.62	2
	女性 Female	22 944	13.07	10.67	7.15	7.09	0.81	2
东部地区 Eastern areas	合计 Both	56 661	22.34	11.72	12.12	11.98	1.38	2
	男性 Male	41 675	32.69	13.65	18.88	18.65	2.16	2
	女性 Female	14 986	11.87	8.41	5.60	5.55	0.62	4
中部地区 Central areas	合计 Both	34 158	22.72	13.92	14.27	14.06	1.63	2
	男性 Male	24 581	32.11	15.68	21.26	20.89	2.42	2
	女性 Female	9 577	12.98	10.80	7.43	7.37	0.84	2
西部地区 Western areas	合计 Both	58 798	26.20	16.40	16.69	16.33	1.85	2
	男性 Male	44 612	38.86	18.87	25.83	25.21	2.87	2
	女性 Female	14 186	12.94	11.62	7.45	7.37	0.83	2

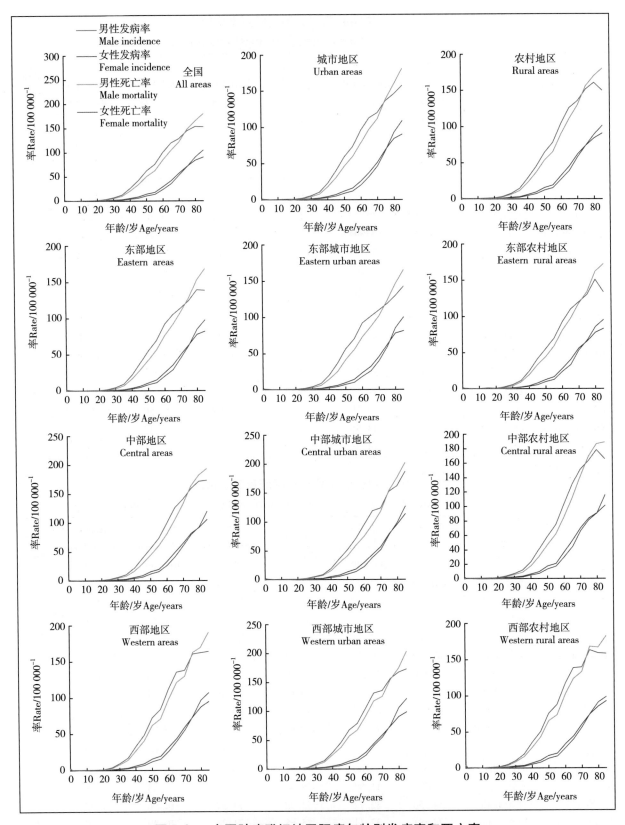

图 5-6a　中国肿瘤登记地区肝癌年龄别发病率和死亡率

Figure 5-6a　Age-specific incidence and mortality rates of liver cancer in the registration areas of China

中标率ASR China/100 000^{-1}

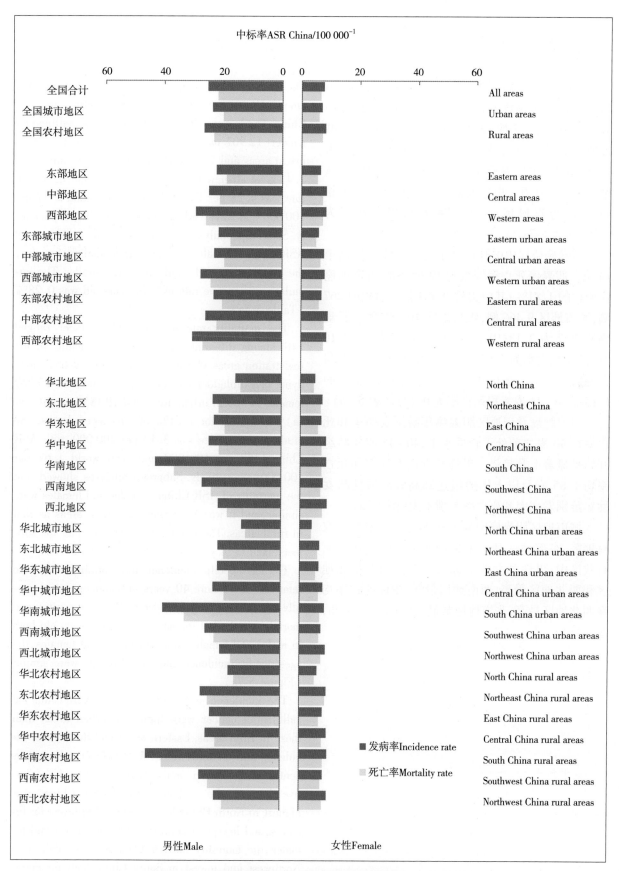

全国合计	All areas
全国城市地区	Urban areas
全国农村地区	Rural areas
东部地区	Eastern areas
中部地区	Central areas
西部地区	Western areas
东部城市地区	Eastern urban areas
中部城市地区	Central urban areas
西部城市地区	Western urban areas
东部农村地区	Eastern rural areas
中部农村地区	Central rural areas
西部农村地区	Western rural areas
华北地区	North China
东北地区	Northeast China
华东地区	East China
华中地区	Central China
华南地区	South China
西南地区	Southwest China
西北地区	Northwest China
华北城市地区	North China urban areas
东北城市地区	Northeast China urban areas
华东城市地区	East China urban areas
华中城市地区	Central China urban areas
华南城市地区	South China urban areas
西南城市地区	Southwest China urban areas
西北城市地区	Northwest China urban areas
华北农村地区	North China rural areas
东北农村地区	Northeast China rural areas
华东农村地区	East China rural areas
华中农村地区	Central China rural areas
华南农村地区	South China rural areas
西南农村地区	Southwest China rural areas
西北农村地区	Northwest China rural areas

■ 发病率Incidence rate
□ 死亡率Mortality rate

男性Male　　　　　　女性Female

图 5-6b　中国肿瘤登记不同地区肝癌发病率和死亡率
Figure 5-6b　Incidence and mortality rates of liver cancer in different
registration areas of China

7 胆囊

胆囊癌位居中国肿瘤登记地区癌症发病谱第18位。新发病例数为 26 923 例,占全部癌症发病的 1.41%;其中男性 12 907 例,女性 14 016 例,城市地区 12 785 例,农村地区 14 138 例。发病率为 4.28/10 万,中标发病率为 2.37/10 万,世标发病率为 2.36/10 万。中标发病率男性与女性基本相同,城市与农村接近。0~74 岁累积发病率为 0.28%(表 5-7a)。

胆囊癌位居中国肿瘤登记地区癌症死亡谱第14 位。胆囊癌死亡病例数为 19 651 例,占全部癌症死亡的 1.81%;其中男性 9 384 例,女性 10 267 例,城市地区 9 466 例,农村地区 10 185 例。胆囊癌死亡率为 3.13/10 万,中标死亡率为 1.67/10 万,世标死亡率为 1.67/10 万;女性中标死亡率与男性接近,城市地区中标死亡率为农村地区的 1.15 倍,0~74 岁累积死亡率为 0.19%(表 5-7b)。

中国肿瘤登记地区胆囊癌年龄别发病率和死亡率在 40 岁之前处于较低水平,40~44 岁年龄组开始呈显著上升趋势。男性和女性发病率和死亡率均于 85 岁及以上年龄组达到高峰。男性与女性年龄别发病率和死亡率差别不大(图 5-7a)。

城市地区胆囊癌中标发病率与死亡率高于农村地区,东部地区高于中部和西部地区。在七大行政区中,男性和女性中标发病率分别在华北地区和西北地区最高,西南地区最低,中标死亡率均在西北地区最高,华南地区最低(表 5-7a,表 5-7b,图 5-7b)。

7 Gallbladder

The incidence of gallbladder cancer ranked 18th among all cancer types in the registration areas of China. There were 26 923 new cases of gallbladder cancer(12 907 males and 14 016 females, 12 785 in urban areas and 14 138 in rural areas), accounting for 1.41% of all new cancer cases. The crude incidence rate was 4.28 per 100 000, with ASR China 2.37 per 100 000 and ASR world 2.36 per 100 000, respectively. Subgroup analyses showed that the incidence of ASR China in males was similar to that in females, the urban areas and rural areas was similar. The cumulative incidence rate of 0-74 years old was 0.28% (Table 5-7a).

The mortality rate of gallbladder cancer ranked 14th among different causes of cancer deaths in the registration areas of China. There were 19 651 cases dying of gallbladder cancer(9 384 males and 10 267 females, 9 466 in urban areas and 10 185 in rural areas), accounting for 1.81% of all cancer deaths. The crude mortality rate was 3.13 per 100 000, with ASR China 1.67 per 100 000 and ASR world 1.67 per 100 000, respectively. Subgroup analyses showed that the mortality of ASR China in males and females were similar, and it was 1.15 times in urban areas as that in rural areas. The cumulative mortality rate for subjects aged 0-74 years was 0.19% (Table 5-7b).

The age-specific incidence and mortality rates were relatively low before 40 years old, and increased rapidly since then. The age-specific incidence rates and mortality peaked at the age group of 85 years old both in males and females. Both for males and females, the age-specific incidence and mortality rate were similar (Figure 5-7a).

The incidence and mortality rates(ASR China) of gallbladder cancer were higher in urban areas than those in rural areas. Eastern areas had the highest incidence and mortality rates(ASR China), followed by central and western areas. Among seven administrative districts, the incidence rate (ASR China) was highest in North China for males and Northwest for females, and lowest in Southwest both for males and females, the mortality rate(ASR China) was highest in Northwest and lowest in South China both for males and females(Table 5-7a, Table 5-7b, Figure 5-7b).

表 5-7a 中国肿瘤登记地区胆囊癌发病情况
Table 5-7a Incidence of gallbladder cancer in registration areas of China

地区 Area	性别 Sex	发病数 No. cases	粗率 Crude rate/ 100 000⁻¹	构成比 Freq./%	中标率 ASR China/ 100 000⁻¹	世标率 ASR world/ 100 000⁻¹	累积率 Cum. rate 0~74/%	顺位 Rank
合计 All	合计 Both	26 923	4. 28	1. 41	2. 37	2. 36	0. 28	18
	男性 Male	12 907	4. 05	1. 24	2. 36	2. 37	0. 28	16
	女性 Female	14 016	4. 53	1. 61	2. 37	2. 35	0. 27	15
城市地区 Urban areas	合计 Both	12 785	4. 76	1. 43	2. 53	2. 53	0. 29	18
	男性 Male	6 076	4. 52	1. 28	2. 53	2. 54	0. 30	16
	女性 Female	6 709	5. 01	1. 61	2. 51	2. 50	0. 28	16
农村地区 Rural areas	合计 Both	14 138	3. 93	1. 38	2. 24	2. 23	0. 27	18
	男性 Male	6 831	3. 71	1. 20	2. 23	2. 23	0. 27	16
	女性 Female	7 307	4. 16	1. 61	2. 25	2. 24	0. 26	15
东部地区 Eastern areas	合计 Both	13 323	5. 25	1. 44	2. 60	2. 60	0. 31	18
	男性 Male	6 623	5. 20	1. 36	2. 73	2. 75	0. 33	16
	女性 Female	6 700	5. 31	1. 53	2. 48	2. 47	0. 28	16
中部地区 Central areas	合计 Both	5 858	3. 90	1. 38	2. 35	2. 34	0. 28	19
	男性 Male	2 676	3. 50	1. 16	2. 23	2. 23	0. 27	16
	女性 Female	3 182	4. 31	1. 64	2. 46	2. 45	0. 29	15
西部地区 Western areas	合计 Both	7 742	3. 45	1. 37	2. 05	2. 04	0. 24	19
	男性 Male	3 608	3. 14	1. 11	1. 96	1. 95	0. 23	16
	女性 Female	4 134	3. 77	1. 72	2. 14	2. 12	0. 25	15

表 5-7b 中国肿瘤登记地区胆囊癌死亡情况
Table 5-7b Mortality of gallbladder cancer inregistration areas of China

地区 Area	性别 Sex	死亡数 No. deaths	粗率 Crude rate/ 100 000⁻¹	构成比 Freq./%	中标率 ASR China/ 100 000⁻¹	世标率 ASR world/ 100 000⁻¹	累积率 Cum. rate 0~74/%	顺位 Rank
合计 All	合计 Both	19 651	3. 13	1. 81	1. 67	1. 67	0. 19	14
	男性 Male	9 384	2. 94	1. 34	1. 68	1. 68	0. 19	13
	女性 Female	10 267	3. 32	2. 64	1. 65	1. 65	0. 18	11
城市地区 Urban areas	合计 Both	9 466	3. 53	1. 98	1. 79	1. 79	0. 19	14
	男性 Male	4 475	3. 33	1. 47	1. 81	1. 82	0. 20	13
	女性 Female	4 991	3. 72	2. 87	1. 77	1. 77	0. 19	11
农村地区 Rural areas	合计 Both	10 185	2. 83	1. 67	1. 56	1. 56	0. 18	14
	男性 Male	4 909	2. 66	1. 24	1. 57	1. 57	0. 18	14
	女性 Female	5 276	3. 00	2. 45	1. 55	1. 55	0. 18	12
东部地区 Eastern areas	合计 Both	9 962	3. 93	2. 06	1. 86	1. 86	0. 21	14
	男性 Male	4 897	3. 84	1. 60	1. 96	1. 97	0. 22	12
	女性 Female	5 065	4. 01	2. 84	1. 76	1. 76	0. 19	11
中部地区 Central areas	合计 Both	4 325	2. 88	1. 76	1. 68	1. 68	0. 19	14
	男性 Male	2 004	2. 62	1. 28	1. 63	1. 64	0. 19	13
	女性 Female	2 321	3. 14	2. 62	1. 72	1. 72	0. 20	11
西部地区 Western areas	合计 Both	5 364	2. 39	1. 50	1. 39	1. 38	0. 16	15
	男性 Male	2 483	2. 16	1. 05	1. 33	1. 33	0. 15	14
	女性 Female	2 881	2. 63	2. 36	1. 44	1. 43	0. 16	13

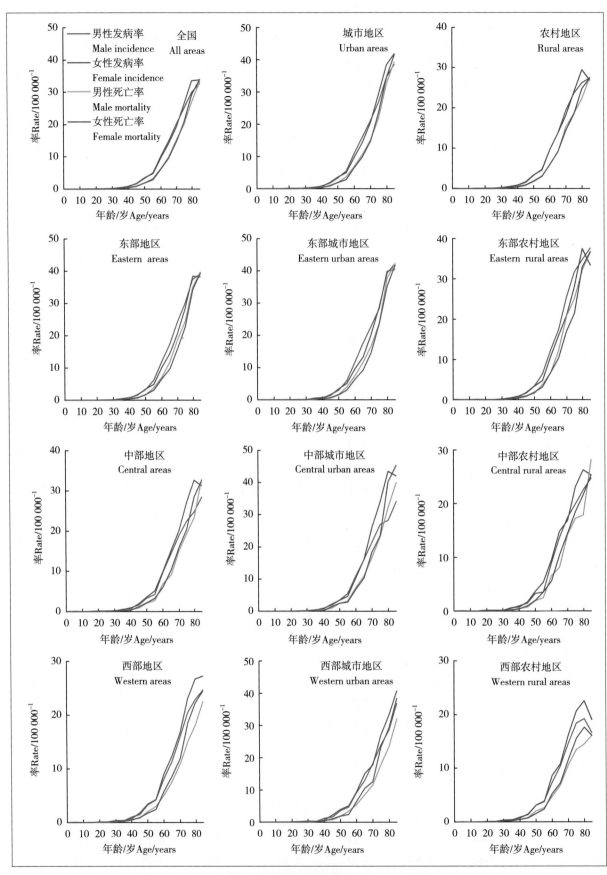

图 5-7a　中国肿瘤登记地区胆囊癌年龄别发病率和死亡率
Figure 5-7a　Age-specific incidence and mortality rates of gallbladder cancer in
registration areas of China

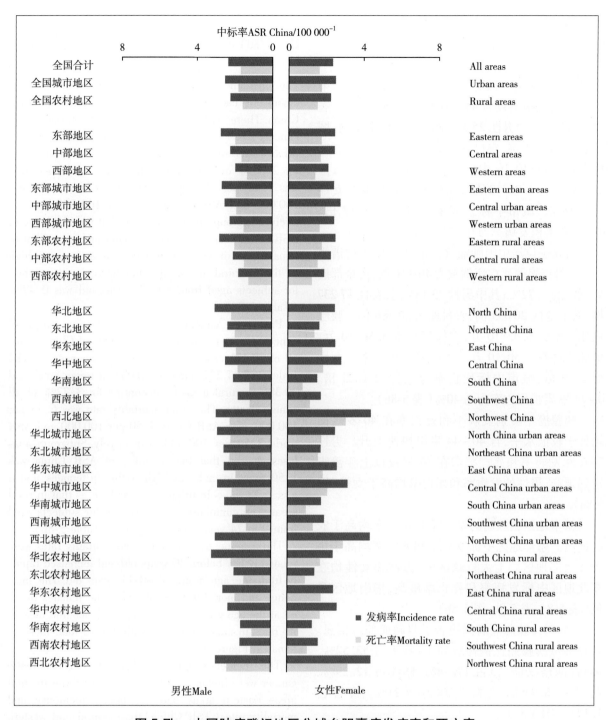

中标率ASR China/100 000⁻¹

	男性Male				女性Female			
	8	4	0	0	4	8		

全国合计 — All areas
全国城市地区 — Urban areas
全国农村地区 — Rural areas

东部地区 — Eastern areas
中部地区 — Central areas
西部地区 — Western areas
东部城市地区 — Eastern urban areas
中部城市地区 — Central urban areas
西部城市地区 — Western urban areas
东部农村地区 — Eastern rural areas
中部农村地区 — Central rural areas
西部农村地区 — Western rural areas

华北地区 — North China
东北地区 — Northeast China
华东地区 — East China
华中地区 — Central China
华南地区 — South China
西南地区 — Southwest China
西北地区 — Northwest China
华北城市地区 — North China urban areas
东北城市地区 — Northeast China urban areas
华东城市地区 — East China urban areas
华中城市地区 — Central China urban areas
华南城市地区 — South China urban areas
西南城市地区 — Southwest China urban areas
西北城市地区 — Northwest China urban areas
华北农村地区 — North China rural areas
东北农村地区 — Northeast China rural areas
华东农村地区 — East China rural areas
华中农村地区 — Central China rural areas
华南农村地区 — South China rural areas
西南农村地区 — Southwest China rural areas
西北农村地区 — Northwest China rural areas

发病率Incidence rate
死亡率Mortality rate

男性Male　　　女性Female

图 5-7b　中国肿瘤登记地区分城乡胆囊癌发病率和死亡率
Figure 5-7b　Incidence and mortality rates of gallbladder cancer in different
registration areas of China

8 胰腺

胰腺癌位居中国肿瘤登记地区癌症发病谱第13位。新发病例数为44 700例,占全部癌症发病的2.33%;其中男性25 541例,女性19 159例,城市地区21 551例,农村地区23 149例。胰腺癌发病率为7.11/10万,中标发病率为3.98/10万,世标发病率为3.96/10万。男性中标发病率为女性的1.45倍,城市中标发病率为农村的1.17倍。0~74岁累积发病率为0.47%(表5-8a)。

胰腺癌位居中国肿瘤登记地区癌症死亡谱第7位。因胰腺癌死亡病例数为40 421例,占全部癌症死亡的3.72%;其中男性23 184例,女性17 237例,城市地区20 035例,农村地区20 386例。胰腺癌死亡率为6.43/10万,中标死亡率3.50/10万,世标死亡率3.50/10万。男性中标死亡率为女性的1.50倍,城市中标死亡率为农村的1.23倍。0~74岁累积死亡率为0.40%(表5-8b)。

胰腺癌年龄别发病率和死亡率在40岁之前均处于较低水平,自40~44岁组快速上升。男性和女性发病率和死亡率均在85岁及以上年龄组达到顶峰,男性的发病率和死亡率均高于女性(图5-8a)。

城市地区胰腺癌的发病率和死亡率均高于农村地区。东部地区中标发病率和死亡率均高于中部和西部地区。七大行政区中,男性和女性均在东北地区中标发病率和死亡率最高,华南地区最低(表5-8a,表5-8b,图5-8b)。

34.50%胰腺癌病例报告了明确亚部位信息。各亚部位胰腺癌比例构成如下:胰头占52.52%、胰岛(朗格汉斯岛)占17.74%、胰体占12.29%、胰尾占8.94%、交搭跨越占5.21%,胰管占1.17%(图5-8c)。

8 Pancreas

The incidence of pancreatic cancer ranked 13th among all cancer types in the registration areas of China. There were 44 700 new cases of pancreatic cancer(25 541 males and 19 159 females, 21 551 in urban areas and 23 149 in rural areas.), accounting for 2.33% of new cases. The crude incidence rate was 7.11 per 100 000, with ASR China 3.98 per 100 000 and ASR world 3.96 per 100 000, respectively. Subgroup analyses showed that the incidence of ASR China was 1.45 times in males as high as that in females, and it was 1.17 times in urban areas as high as that in rural areas. The cumulative incidence rate for subjects aged from 0 to 74 years old was 0.47% (Table 5-8a).

Pancreatic cancer was the 7th leading cause of cancer deaths in the registration areas of China. A total of 40 421 cases died of pancreatic cancer(23 184 males and 17 237 females, 20 035 in urban areas and 20 386 in rural areas), accounting for 3.72% of all cancer deaths. The crude mortality rate was 6.43 per 100 000, with ASR China 3.50 per 100 000 and ASR world 3.50 per 100 000, respectively. Subgroup analyses showed that the mortality of ASR China was 1.50 times in males as high as that in females, and it was 1.23 times in urban areas as high as that in rural areas. The cumulative mortality rate for subjects aged from 0 to 74 years old was 0.40% (Table 5-8b).

The age-specific incidence and mortality rates were relatively low before 40 years old and increased rapidly from the age group of 40-44 years old. The incidence and mortality rates of males and females peaked at the age group of 85+. The incidence and mortality rates in males were generally higher than those in females(Figure 5-8a).

The incidence and mortality rates of pancreatic cancer were higher in urban areas than those in rural areas. Eastern areas had the higher incidence and mortality rates(ASR China) than central and western areas. Among the seven administrative districts, the highest pancreatic cancer incidence and mortality (ASR China) rates were shown in Northeast China, and the lowest rates in South China for both male and female(Table 5-8a, Table 5-8b, Figure 5-8b).

There were 34.50% of pancreatic cancer cases with specific subsite information. Among those, 52.52% of cases occurred in head, followed by islets of Langerhans (17.74%), body (12.29%), tail (8.94%), overlapping(5.21%) and pancreatic duct (1.17%) (Figure 5-8c).

表 5-8a 中国肿瘤登记地区胰腺癌发病情况

Table 5-8a Incidence of pancreatic cancer in the registration areas of China

地区 Area	性别 Sex	发病数 No. cases	粗率 Crude rate/ 100 000^{-1}	构成比 Freq./%	中标率 ASR China/ 100 000^{-1}	世标率 ASR world/ 100 000^{-1}	累积率 Cum. rate 0~74/%	顺位 Rank
合计 All	合计 Both	44 700	7.11	2.33	3.98	3.96	0.47	13
	男性 Male	25 541	8.01	2.44	4.72	4.72	0.56	9
	女性 Female	19 159	6.19	2.20	3.25	3.22	0.37	12
城市地区 Urban areas	合计 Both	21 551	8.03	2.41	4.32	4.32	0.50	14
	男性 Male	12 159	9.04	2.55	5.13	5.15	0.61	10
	女性 Female	9 392	7.01	2.25	3.55	3.52	0.40	12
农村地区 Rural areas	合计 Both	23 149	6.43	2.26	3.70	3.68	0.44	13
	男性 Male	13 382	7.26	2.35	4.41	4.39	0.52	8
	女性 Female	9 767	5.56	2.15	3.01	2.98	0.35	12
东部地区 Eastern areas	合计 Both	23 418	9.23	2.53	4.66	4.64	0.55	12
	男性 Male	13 150	10.32	2.69	5.53	5.53	0.66	9
	女性 Female	10 268	8.14	2.35	3.83	3.80	0.44	12
中部地区 Central areas	合计 Both	8 680	5.77	2.04	3.51	3.49	0.42	15
	男性 Male	4 874	6.37	2.11	4.06	4.05	0.48	12
	女性 Female	3 806	5.16	1.96	2.98	2.96	0.35	13
西部地区 Western areas	合计 Both	12 602	5.62	2.23	3.37	3.35	0.40	13
	男性 Male	7 517	6.55	2.31	4.11	4.11	0.49	8
	女性 Female	5 085	4.64	2.11	2.64	2.61	0.30	12

表 5-8b 中国肿瘤登记地区胰腺癌死亡情况

Table 5-8b Mortality of pancreatic cancer in the registration areas of China

地区 Area	性别 Sex	死亡数 No. deaths	粗率 Crude rate/ 100 000^{-1}	构成比 Freq./%	中标率 ASR China/ 100 000^{-1}	世标率 ASR world/ 100 000^{-1}	累积率 Cum. rate 0~74/%	顺位 Rank
合计地区 All	合计 Both	40 421	6.43	3.72	3.50	3.50	0.40	7
	男性 Male	23 184	7.27	3.32	4.22	4.22	0.49	6
	女性 Female	17 237	5.57	4.43	2.81	2.80	0.31	7
城市地区 Urban areas	合计 Both	20 035	7.46	4.20	3.91	3.91	0.44	7
	男性 Male	11 308	8.41	3.73	4.69	4.71	0.54	6
	女性 Female	8 727	6.51	5.02	3.18	3.15	0.35	6
农村地区 Rural areas	合计 Both	20 386	5.66	3.34	3.18	3.17	0.37	8
	男性 Male	11 876	6.44	3.01	3.85	3.84	0.45	6
	女性 Female	8 510	4.85	3.96	2.52	2.51	0.29	8
东部地区 Eastern areas	合计 Both	21 452	8.46	4.44	4.14	4.12	0.47	7
	男性 Male	12 057	9.46	3.95	4.97	4.98	0.58	6
	女性 Female	9 395	7.44	5.27	3.34	3.32	0.37	7
中部地区 Central areas	合计 Both	7 779	5.17	3.17	3.08	3.07	0.36	8
	男性 Male	4 513	5.90	2.88	3.71	3.70	0.43	6
	女性 Female	3 266	4.42	3.68	2.47	2.46	0.29	8
西部地区 Western areas	合计 Both	11 190	4.99	3.12	2.94	2.93	0.34	8
	男性 Male	6 614	5.76	2.80	3.57	3.57	0.41	6
	女性 Female	4 576	4.18	3.75	2.32	2.29	0.26	8

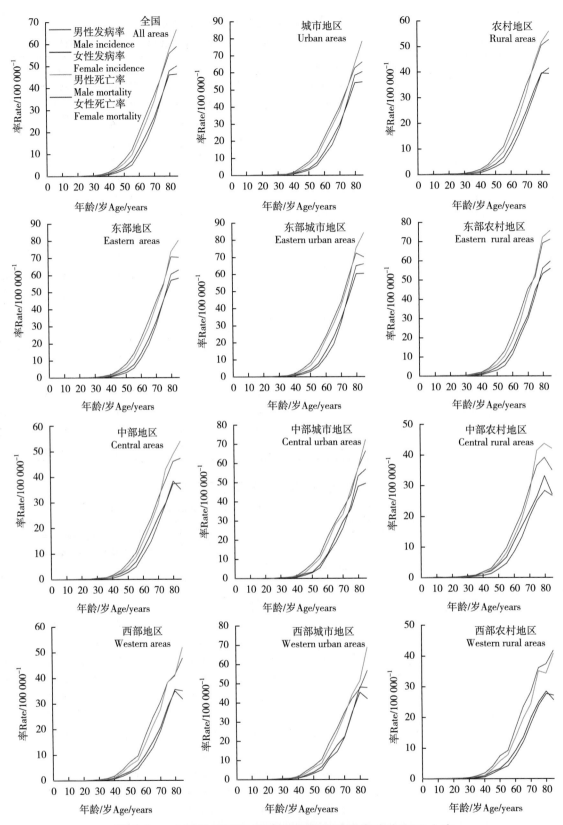

图 5-8a　中国肿瘤登记地区胰腺癌年龄别发病率和死亡率
Figure 5-8a　Age-specific incidence and mortality rates of pancreatic cancer in the registration areas of China

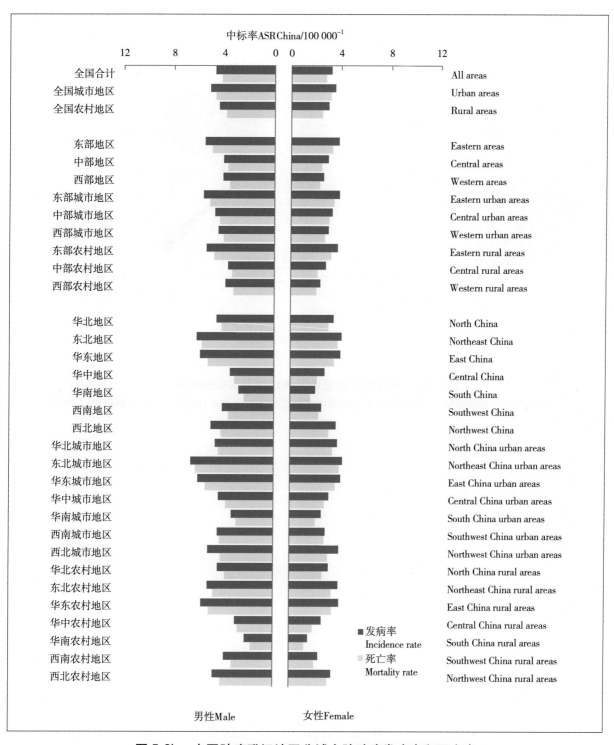

图 5-8b　中国肿瘤登记地区分城乡胰腺癌发病率和死亡率

Figure 5-8b　Incidence and mortality rates of pancreatic cancer in different registration areas of China

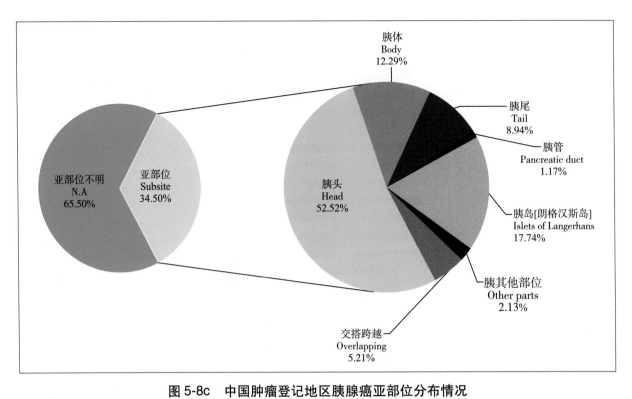

图 5-8c　中国肿瘤登记地区胰腺癌亚部位分布情况

Figure 5-8c　Subsite distribution of pancreatic cancer in the registration areas of China

9 喉

喉癌位居中国肿瘤登记地区癌症发病谱第21位。新发病例数为 11 637 例,占全部癌症发病的 0.61%;其中男性 10 548 例,女性 1 089 例,城市地区 5 701 例,农村地区 5 936 例。喉癌发病率为 1.85/10 万,中标发病率为 1.06/10 万,世标发病率为 1.08/10 万;男性中标发病率为女性的 10.32 倍,城市中标发病率为农村的 1.22 倍。0~74 岁累积发病率为 0.14%(表 5-9a)。

喉癌位居中国肿瘤登记地区癌症死亡谱第21位。喉癌死亡病例数为 6 789 例,占全部癌症死亡的 0.62%;其中男性 6 023 例,女性 766 例,城市地区 3 069 例,农村地区 3 720 例。喉癌死亡率为 1.08/10 万,中标死亡率和世标死亡率均为 0.59/10 万;男性中标死亡率为女性的 9.08 倍,城市中标死亡率稍高于农村。0~74 岁累积死亡率为 0.07%(表 5-9b)。

喉癌年龄别发病率、年龄别死亡率呈现性别差异。男性年龄别发病率和死亡率在 0~39 岁处于较低水平,40~44 岁组后显著上升;女性在 0~49 岁处于较低水平,50~54 岁组后上升。各年龄组男性发病率和死亡率一般高于女性(图 5-9a)。

城市地区喉癌中标发病率和死亡率均高于农村地区。中部地区中标发病率最高。七大行政区中,男性喉癌的中标发病率和死亡率最高的是东北地区和华南地区,西北地区最低;女性中标发病率和死亡率最高的是东北地区,最低的分别是华东地区和西北地区最低(表 5-9a,表 5-9b,图 5-9b)。

9 Larynx

The incidence of laryngeal cancer ranked 21st among all cancer types in cancer registration areas of China. There were 11 637 new cases diagnosed with laryngeal cancer (10 548 males and 1 089 females, 5 701 in urban areas and 5 936 in rural areas), accounting for 0.61% of new cancer cases. The crude incidence rate was 1.85 per 100 000, with ASR China and ASR world 1.06 per 100 000 and 1.08 per 100 000, respectively. The incidence rate of ASR China in males was 10.32 times as high as that in females. The incidence rate of ASR China in urban areas was 1.22 folds as high as that in rural areas. The cumulative incidence rate for subjects aged 0-74 years was 0.14% (Table 5-9a).

Laryngeal cancer ranked 21st among all causes of cancer deaths. A total of 6 789 cases died of laryngeal cancer(6 023 males and 766 females, 3 069 in urban areas and 3 720 in rural areas), accounting for 0.62% of all cancer deaths. The crude mortality rate was 1.08 per 100 000. The ASR China and ASR world were both 0.59 per 100 000. The mortality rate of ASR China in males was 9.08 times as high as that in females. The mortality rate of ASR China in urban areas was slightly higher than that in rural areas. The cumulative mortality rate for subjects aged 0-74 years was 0.07% (Table 5-9b).

The age-specific incidence and mortality rates showed differences between males and females. Theage-specific incidence and mortality rates for males were relatively low in 0-39 years old, and increased significantly after 40-44 years old. For females, the age-specific rates were relatively low in 0-49 years old, and increased after 50-54 years old. Age-specific incidence and mortality rates in males were generally higher than those in females (Figure 5-9a).

The incidence and mortality rates (ASR China) of laryngeal cancer in urban areas were higher than those in rural areas. Central areas had the highest incidence rate of ASR China. Among the seven administrative districts, for males, Northeast China and South China had the highest incidence and mortality rates (ASR China), while Northwest China had the lowest rates. For females, the highest incidence and mortality rates(ASR China) were in Northeast China, the lowest incidence and mortality rates (ASR China) were in East China and Northwest China (Table 5-9a, Table 5-9b, Figure 5-9b).

表 5-9a　中国肿瘤登记地区喉癌发病情况

Table 5-9a　Incidence of laryngeal cancer in registration areas of China

地区 Area	性别 Sex	发病数 No. cases	粗率 Crude rate/ 100 000^{-1}	构成比 Freq./%	中标率 ASR China/ 100 000^{-1}	世标率 ASR world/ 100 000^{-1}	累积率 Cum. rate 0~74/%	顺位 Rank
合计 All	合计 Both	11 637	1.85	0.61	1.06	1.08	0.14	21
	男性 Male	10 548	3.31	1.01	1.96	2.00	0.26	17
	女性 Female	1 089	0.35	0.13	0.19	0.19	0.02	23
城市地区 Urban areas	合计 Both	5 701	2.12	0.64	1.18	1.21	0.15	21
	男性 Male	5 230	3.89	1.10	2.23	2.28	0.29	17
	女性 Female	471	0.35	0.11	0.18	0.18	0.02	23
农村地区 Rural areas	合计 Both	5 936	1.65	0.58	0.97	0.98	0.13	22
	男性 Male	5 318	2.88	0.93	1.76	1.78	0.23	17
	女性 Female	618	0.35	0.14	0.20	0.20	0.02	23
东部地区 Eastern areas	合计 Both	5 306	2.09	0.57	1.11	1.13	0.15	21
	男性 Male	4 937	3.87	1.01	2.12	2.16	0.28	17
	女性 Female	369	0.29	0.08	0.14	0.14	0.01	23
中部地区 Central areas	合计 Both	2 782	1.85	0.65	1.14	1.16	0.15	21
	男性 Male	2 448	3.20	1.06	2.04	2.07	0.26	17
	女性 Female	334	0.45	0.17	0.27	0.27	0.03	23
西部地区 Western areas	合计 Both	3 549	1.58	0.63	0.96	0.97	0.12	22
	男性 Male	3 163	2.76	0.97	1.72	1.74	0.22	17
	女性 Female	386	0.35	0.16	0.21	0.21	0.02	23

表 5-9b　中国肿瘤登记地区喉癌死亡情况

Table 5-9b　Mortality of laryngeal cancer in registration areas of China

地区 Area	性别 Sex	死亡数 No. deaths	粗率 Crude rate/ 100 000^{-1}	构成比 Freq./%	中标率 ASR China/ 100 000^{-1}	世标率 ASR world/ 100 000^{-1}	累积率 Cum. Rate 0~74/%	顺位 Rank
合计 All	合计 Both	6 789	1.08	0.62	0.59	0.59	0.07	21
	男性 Male	6 023	1.89	0.86	1.09	1.09	0.13	16
	女性 Female	766	0.25	0.20	0.12	0.12	0.01	23
城市地区 Urban areas	合计 Both	3 069	1.14	0.64	0.60	0.60	0.07	20
	男性 Male	2 758	2.05	0.91	1.13	1.14	0.13	16
	女性 Female	311	0.23	0.18	0.10	0.10	0.01	23
农村地区 Rural areas	合计 Both	3 720	1.03	0.61	0.58	0.58	0.07	21
	男性 Male	3 265	1.77	0.83	1.05	1.05	0.12	16
	女性 Female	455	0.26	0.21	0.13	0.13	0.01	22
东部地区 Eastern areas	合计 Both	2 877	1.13	0.59	0.55	0.56	0.06	21
	男性 Male	2 578	2.02	0.84	1.05	1.05	0.12	16
	女性 Female	299	0.24	0.17	0.10	0.10	0.01	23
中部地区 Central areas	合计 Both	1 610	1.07	0.66	0.63	0.63	0.07	21
	男性 Male	1 405	1.84	0.90	1.15	1.14	0.14	16
	女性 Female	205	0.28	0.23	0.14	0.14	0.01	22
西部地区 Western areas	合计 Both	2 302	1.03	0.64	0.60	0.61	0.07	21
	男性 Male	2 040	1.78	0.86	1.09	1.10	0.13	15
	女性 Female	262	0.24	0.21	0.13	0.13	0.01	22

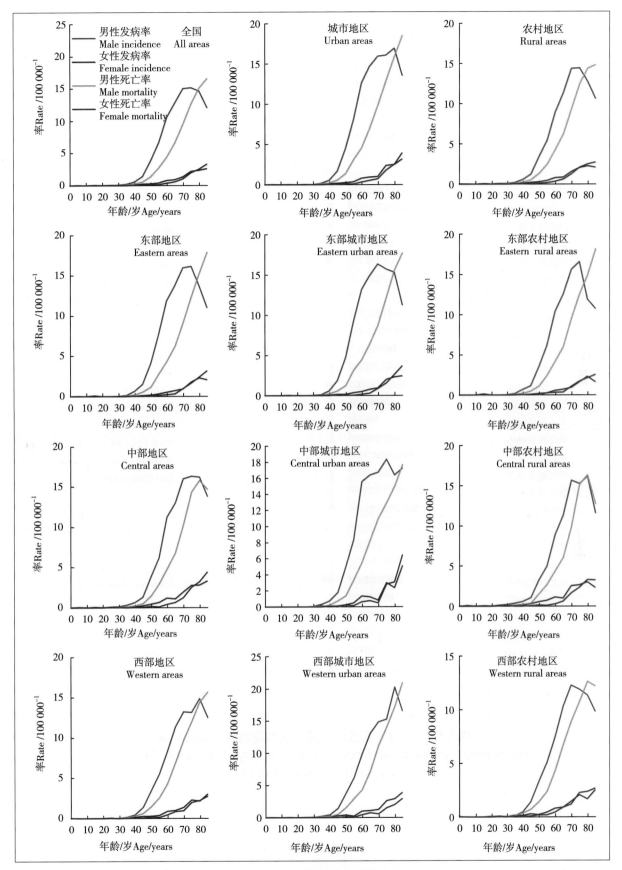

图 5-9a　中国肿瘤登记地区喉癌年龄别发病率和死亡率

Figure 5-9a　Age-specific incidence and mortality rates of laryngeal cancer in registration areas of China

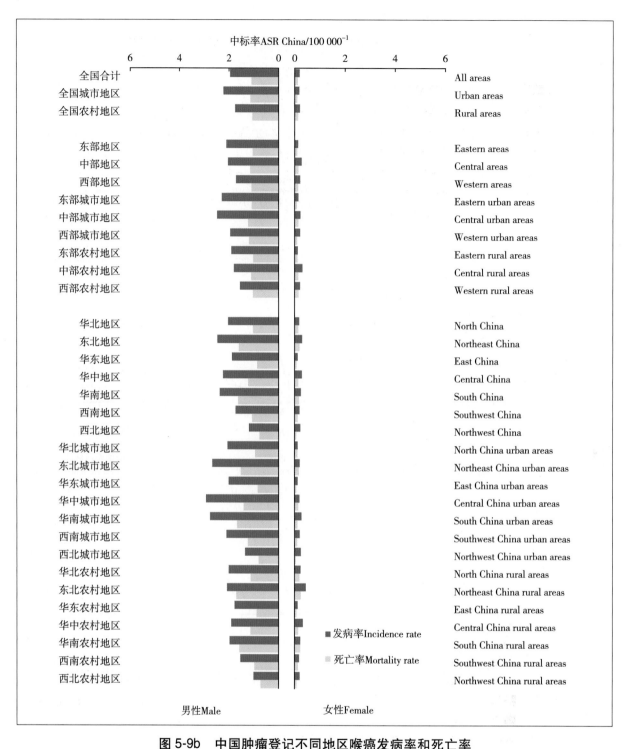

中标率ASR China/100 000⁻¹

全国合计	All areas
全国城市地区	Urban areas
全国农村地区	Rural areas
东部地区	Eastern areas
中部地区	Central areas
西部地区	Western areas
东部城市地区	Eastern urban areas
中部城市地区	Central urban areas
西部城市地区	Western urban areas
东部农村地区	Eastern rural areas
中部农村地区	Central rural areas
西部农村地区	Western rural areas
华北地区	North China
东北地区	Northeast China
华东地区	East China
华中地区	Central China
华南地区	South China
西南地区	Southwest China
西北地区	Northwest China
华北城市地区	North China urban areas
东北城市地区	Northeast China urban areas
华东城市地区	East China urban areas
华中城市地区	Central China urban areas
华南城市地区	South China urban areas
西南城市地区	Southwest China urban areas
西北城市地区	Northwest China urban areas
华北农村地区	North China rural areas
东北农村地区	Northeast China rural areas
华东农村地区	East China rural areas
华中农村地区	Central China rural areas
华南农村地区	South China rural areas
西南农村地区	Southwest China rural areas
西北农村地区	Northwest China rural areas

■ 发病率Incidence rate
■ 死亡率Mortality rate

男性Male   女性Female

图 5-9b　中国肿瘤登记不同地区喉癌发病率和死亡率
Figure 5-9b　Incidence and mortality rates of laryngeal cancer in different registration areas of China

10 肺

　　肺癌位居中国肿瘤登记地区癌症发病谱第 1 位。新发病例数为 422 442 例,占全部癌症发病的 22.05%;其中男性 270 953 例,女性 151 489 例,城市地区 194 266 例,农村地区 228 176 例。肺癌发病率为 67.22/10 万,中标发病率为 38.58/10 万,世标发病率为 38.45/10 万;男性中标发病率为女性的 1.81 倍,城市中标发病率为农村的 1.09 倍。0~74 岁累积发病率为 4.72%(表 5-10a)。

　　肺癌位居中国肿瘤登记地区癌症死亡谱第 1 位。肺癌死亡病例数为 303 211 例,占全部癌症死亡的 27.88%;其中男性 212 974 例,女性 90 237 例,城市地区 133 105 例,农村地区 170 106 例。肺癌死亡率为 48.25/10 万,中标死亡率为 26.23/10 万,世标死亡率为 26.19/10 万;男性中标死亡率为女性的 2.60 倍,城市中标死亡率与农村接近。0~74 岁累积死亡率为 3.06%(表 5-10b)。

　　肺癌年龄别发病率和死亡率在 40 岁之前均处于较低水平,自 40~44 岁组开始快速上升,男性和女性发病率均在 80~84 岁组达到高峰,男性死亡率在 80 岁及以上组达到高峰,女性死亡率在 85 岁及以上组达到高峰,男性上升速度快于女性。40~44 岁组后,男性各年龄别发病率和死亡率均明显高于女性(图 5-10a)。

10　Lung

Lung cancer was the most frequently diagnosed cancer in the cancer registration areas of China. There were 422 442 new cases diagnosed with lung cancer (270 953 males and 151 489 females, 194 266 in urban areas and 228 176 in rural areas), accounting for 22.05% of new cases of all cancers. The crude incidence rate was 67.22 per 100 000, with the ASR China and ASR world were 38.58 and 38.45 per 100 000, respectively. The incidence rate of ASR China was 1.81 and 1.09 folds in males and in urban areas as those in females and in rural areas, respectively. The cumulative incidence rate for subjects aged 0-74 years was 4.72% (Table 5-10a).

Lung cancer was the leading cause of cancer deaths. A total of 303 211 cases died of lung cancer (212 974 males and 90 237 females, 133 105 in urban areas and 170 106 in rural areas), accounting for 27.88% of all cancer deaths. The crude mortality rate was 48.25 per 100 000, with the ASR China and ASR world were 26.23 and 26.19 per 100 000, respectively. The mortality rate of ASR China was 2.60 folds in males as that in females, while the ASR China in urban areas was similar to that in rural areas. The cumulative mortality rate for subjects aged 0-74 years was 3.06% (Table 5-10b).

The age-specific incidence and mortality rates of lung cancer were relatively low before 40 years old and increased dramatically since then. The age-specific incidence rate for both males and females peaked in the age group of 80-84 years, while the age-specific mortality rate peaked in the age group of 80+ years for males and 85 years old for females, respectively. Incidence and mortality rates in males increased faster than those in females. Age-specific incidence and mortality rates in males were generally higher than those in females since the age group of 40-44 years (Figure 5-10a).

城市地区肺癌的发病率和死亡率高于农村地区。东部地区中标发病率高于中部地区和西部地区;中标死亡率以中部地区最高,其次是西部地区,东部地区最低。在七大行政区中,男性中标发病率、死亡率均华中地区最高,西北地区男性中标发病率和死亡率均最低;女性中标发病率和死亡率均东北地区最高,西北地区女性发病率和死亡率均最低(表5-10a,表5-10b,图5-10b)。

全部肺癌病例中有明确亚部位的病例占34.19%,其中主要在肺上叶,占51.57%,其次是肺下叶(30.47%)和肺中叶(9.76%),主支气管仅占5.13%(图5-10c)。

全部肺癌病例中有明确组织学类型的病例占56.77%,其中腺癌是主要的病理类型,占61.49%,其次是鳞状细胞癌(22.77%)和小细胞癌(10.02%)(图5-10d)。

The incidence and mortality rates of lung cancer in urban areas were higher than those in rural areas. The incidence rate of ASR China in eastern areas was slightly higher than central and western areas. Central areas had the highest mortality rate of ASR China, followed by western areas and eastern areas. Among the seven administrative districts, the incidence and mortality rates (ASR China) of lung cancer for males were highest in Central China and the lowest incidence and mortality rates (ASR China) for males were in Northwest China. While Northeast China had the highest incidence and mortality rates (ASR China) for females, and the lowest incidence and mortality rates (ASR China) for females were in Northwest China (Table 5-10a, Table 5-10b, Figure 5-10b).

About 34.19% cases of lung cancer had specified-subsites. Among those, lung cancer occurred more frequently in upper lobe (51.57%), followed by lower lobe (30.47%), middle lobe (9.76%) and main bronchus (5.13%) (Figure 5-10c).

About 56.77% cases of lung cancer had morphological verification. Among those, adenocarcinoma was the most common histological type, accounting for 61.49% of all cases, followed by squamous cell carcinoma (22.77%) and small cell carcinoma (10.02%) (Figure 5-10d).

表 5-10a 中国肿瘤登记地区肺癌发病情况
Table 5-10a Incidence of lung cancer in the registration areas of China

地区 Area	性别 Sex	发病数 No. cases	粗率 Crude rate/ 100 000⁻¹	构成比 Freq./%	中标率 ASR China/ 100 000⁻¹	世标率 ASR world/ 100 000⁻¹	累积率 Cum. Rate 0~74/%	顺位 Rank
合计 All	合计 Both	422 442	67.22	22.05	38.58	38.45	4.72	1
	男性 Male	270 953	84.99	25.93	50.14	50.28	6.26	1
	女性 Female	151 489	48.93	17.39	27.67	27.28	3.22	1
城市地区 Urban areas	合计 Both	194 266	72.36	21.73	40.53	40.39	4.92	1
	男性 Male	121 472	90.35	25.52	51.60	51.82	6.42	1
	女性 Female	72 794	54.31	17.42	30.28	29.79	3.48	1
农村地区 Rural areas	合计 Both	228 176	63.39	22.32	37.05	36.92	4.56	1
	男性 Male	149 481	81.08	26.27	48.99	49.05	6.13	1
	女性 Female	78 695	44.82	17.36	25.61	25.30	3.01	1
东部地区 Eastern areas	合计 Both	201 597	79.47	21.79	42.49	42.15	5.19	1
	男性 Male	121 428	95.26	24.84	51.62	51.64	6.47	1
	女性 Female	80 169	63.53	18.37	34.15	33.45	3.96	1
中部地区 Central areas	合计 Both	92 037	61.21	21.67	37.19	37.20	4.57	1
	男性 Male	63 004	82.31	27.32	52.06	52.17	6.47	1
	女性 Female	29 033	39.34	14.95	23.06	22.95	2.70	2
西部地区 Western areas	合计 Both	128 808	57.40	22.75	34.70	34.71	4.23	1
	男性 Male	86 521	75.37	26.58	47.00	47.29	5.84	1
	女性 Female	42 287	38.58	17.58	22.72	22.45	2.63	1

表 5-10b 中国肿瘤登记地区肺癌死亡情况
Table 5-10b Mortality of lung cancer in the registration areas of China

地区 Area	性别 Sex	死亡数 No. deaths	粗率 Crude rate/ 100 000⁻¹	构成比 Freq./%	中标率 ASR China/ 100 000⁻¹	世标率 ASR world/ 100 000⁻¹	累积率 Cum. rate 0~74/%	顺位 Rank
合计 All	合计 Both	303 211	48.25	27.88	26.23	26.19	3.06	1
	男性 Male	212 974	66.80	30.49	38.39	38.43	4.55	1
	女性 Female	90 237	29.15	23.19	14.77	14.65	1.60	1
城市地区 Urban areas	合计 Both	133 105	49.58	27.88	25.89	25.87	2.96	1
	男性 Male	93 230	69.34	30.72	38.25	38.37	4.50	1
	女性 Female	39 875	29.75	22.92	14.43	14.28	1.48	1
农村地区 Rural areas	合计 Both	170 106	47.26	27.88	26.48	26.40	3.14	1
	男性 Male	119 744	64.95	30.31	38.45	38.41	4.59	1
	女性 Female	50 362	28.68	23.41	15.03	14.93	1.69	1
东部地区 Eastern areas	合计 Both	132 246	52.13	27.35	25.40	25.27	2.93	1
	男性 Male	90 576	71.05	29.67	36.78	36.70	4.31	1
	女性 Female	41 670	33.02	23.38	14.91	14.74	1.59	1
中部地区 Central areas	合计 Both	69 211	46.03	28.20	27.08	27.04	3.18	1
	男性 Male	49 965	65.28	31.88	40.61	40.59	4.82	1
	女性 Female	19 246	26.08	21.70	14.34	14.28	1.57	1
西部地区 Western areas	合计 Both	101 754	45.34	28.38	26.63	26.70	3.15	1
	男性 Male	72 433	63.10	30.63	38.80	39.05	4.67	1
	女性 Female	29 321	26.75	24.01	14.81	14.71	1.63	1

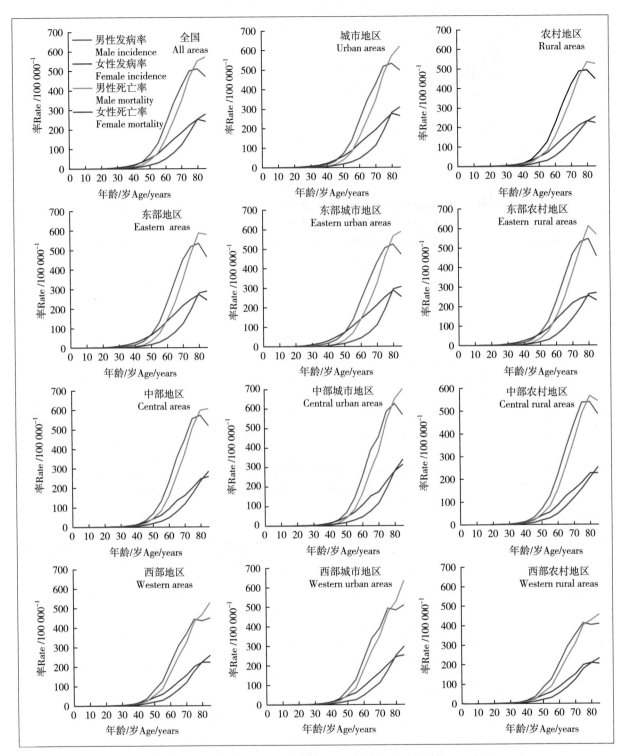

图 5-10a　中国肿瘤登记地区肺癌年龄别发病率和死亡率

Figure 5-10a　Age-specific incidence and mortality rates of lung cancer in the registration areas of China

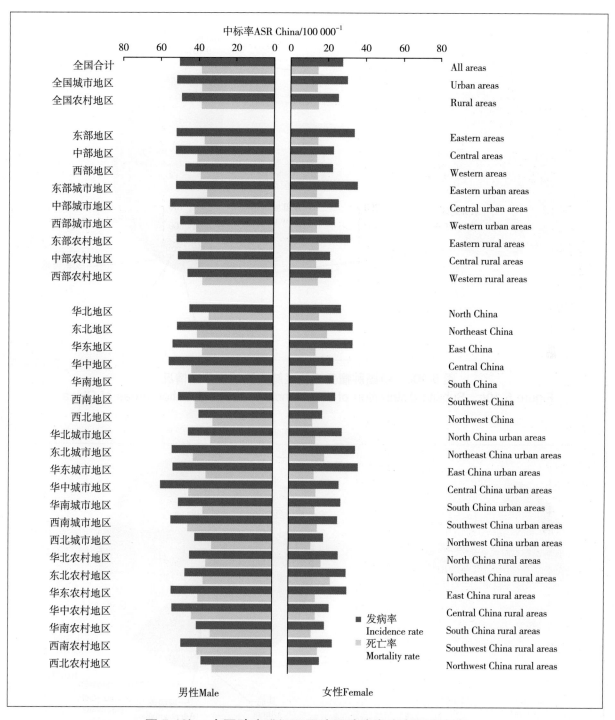

中标率ASR China/100 000⁻¹

全国合计		All areas
全国城市地区		Urban areas
全国农村地区		Rural areas
东部地区		Eastern areas
中部地区		Central areas
西部地区		Western areas
东部城市地区		Eastern urban areas
中部城市地区		Central urban areas
西部城市地区		Western urban areas
东部农村地区		Eastern rural areas
中部农村地区		Central rural areas
西部农村地区		Western rural areas
华北地区		North China
东北地区		Northeast China
华东地区		East China
华中地区		Central China
华南地区		South China
西南地区		Southwest China
西北地区		Northwest China
华北城市地区		North China urban areas
东北城市地区		Northeast China urban areas
华东城市地区		East China urban areas
华中城市地区		Central China urban areas
华南城市地区		South China urban areas
西南城市地区		Southwest China urban areas
西北城市地区		Northwest China urban areas
华北农村地区		North China rural areas
东北农村地区		Northeast China rural areas
华东农村地区		East China rural areas
华中农村地区		Central China rural areas
华南农村地区		South China rural areas
西南农村地区		Southwest China rural areas
西北农村地区		Northwest China rural areas

发病率 Incidence rate
死亡率 Mortality rate

男性Male　　　　女性Female

图 5-10b　中国肿瘤登记不同地区肺癌发病率和死亡率
Figure 5-10b　Incidence and mortality rates of lung cancer in the different registration areas of China

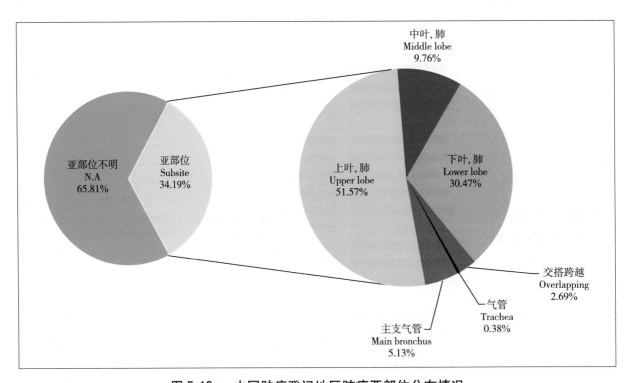

图 5-10c　中国肿瘤登记地区肺癌亚部位分布情况

Figure 5-10c　Subsite distribution of lung cancer in the registration areas of China

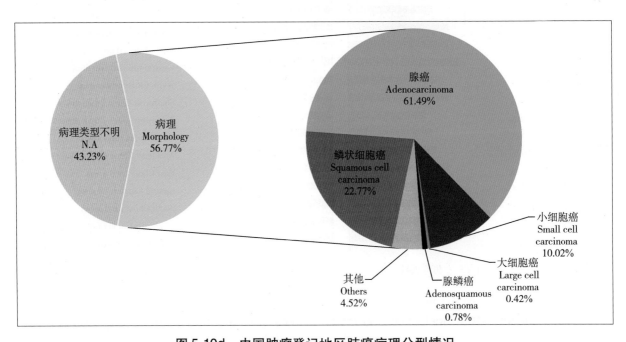

图 5-10d　中国肿瘤登记地区肺癌病理分型情况

Figure 5-10d　Morphological distribution of lung cancer in the registration areas of China

11 骨

骨癌位居中国肿瘤登记地区癌症发病谱第22位。新发病例数为10 803例,占全部癌症发病的0.56%;其中男性6 111例,女性4 692例,城市地区4 157例,农村地区6 646例。骨癌发病率为1.72/10万,中标发病率为1.25/10万,世标发病率为1.22/10万;男性中标发病率为女性的1.33倍,农村中标发病率为城市的1.25倍。0~74岁累积发病率为0.12%(表5-11a)。

骨癌位居中国肿瘤登记地区癌症死亡谱第20位。骨癌死亡病例数为7 859例,占全部癌症死亡的0.72%;其中男性4 777例,女性3 082例,城市地区2 909例,农村地区4 950例。骨癌死亡率为1.25/10万,中标死亡率为0.79/10万,世标死亡率为0.77/10万;男性中标死亡率为女性的1.65倍,农村中标死亡率为城市的1.31倍。0~74岁累积死亡率为0.08%(表5-11b)。

骨癌年龄别发病率和死亡率均在10~19岁组出现一个小高峰,但总体看骨癌年龄别发病率和死亡率在45岁之前处于较低水平,45岁之后迅速上升,呈现男性高于女性的分布特征,城乡和不同地区年龄别发病率、死亡率总体趋势基本相同(图5-11a)。

农村地区骨癌发病率和死亡率高于城市。中标发病率中部地区最高。中标死亡率西部地区最高,其次是中部地区,东部地区最低。在七大行政区中,华中地区中标发病率最高、华东地区最低,华北地区中标死亡率最低,西北地区中标死亡率最高(表5-11a,表5-11b,图5-11b)。

分亚部位比较,36.68%的骨癌发生在四肢的骨、关节和关节软骨,63.32%发生在其他及未特指部位的骨、关节和关节软骨(图5-11c)。

11 Bone

The incidence of bone cancer ranked 22nd among all cancer types in cancer registration areas of China. There were 10 803 new cases diagnosed with bone cancer(6 111 males and 4 692 females, 4 157 in urban areas and 6 646 in rural areas), accounting for 0.56% of all new cancer cases. The crude incidence rate was 1.72 per 100 000, with ASR China 1.25 per 100 000 and ASR world 1.22 per 100 000, respectively. The incidence rate of ASR China in males was 1.33 times of that in females. It was 1.25 times in rural areas of that in urban areas. The cumulative incidence rate for subjects aged 0-74 years was 0.12% (Table 5-11a).

The mortality of bone cancer ranked 20th among all causes of cancer deaths in cancer registration areas of China. A total of 7 859 cases died of bone cancer (4 777 males and 3 082 females, 2 909 in urban areas and 4 950 in rural areas), accounting for 0.72% of all cancer deaths. The crude mortality rate was 1.25 per 100 000, with ASR China 0.79 per 100 000 and ASR world 0.77 per 100 000, respectively. The mortality rate of ASR China in males was 1.65 times of that in females, and it was 1.31 times in rural areas of that in urban areas. The cumulative mortality rate for subjects aged 0-74 years was 0.08% (Table 5-11b).

Both the age-specific incidence and mortality of bone cancer showed a small peak in the age group of 10-19 years. The age-specific incidence and mortality rate of bone cancer were relatively low before 45 years old, but dramatically increased after then. The incidence and mortality rates in males were higher than those in females across all age groups. The age-specific incidence and mortality rates had slight variation among different areas, but showed similar trends (Figure 5-11a).

The incidence and mortality rates of bone cancer were higher in rural areas than those in urban areas. Central areas had the highest incidence of ASR China. Western areas had the highest mortality of ASR China, followed by central and eastern areas. Among the seven administrative districts, Central China had the highest incidence(ASR China), Northwest China had the highest mortality (ASR China), Eastern China and North China had the lowest incidence and mortality rate (ASR China), respectively (Table 5-11a, Table 5-11b, Figure 5-11b).

By subsite, 36.68% of bone cancer occurred in the bone and articular cartilage of limbs, whereas others occurred in other unspecific bone and articular cartilage sites (Figure 5-11c).

表 5-11a　中国肿瘤登记地区骨癌发病情况

表 5-11a　中国肿瘤登记地区骨癌发病情况
Table 5-11a　Incidence of bone cancer in registration areas of China

地区 Area	性别 Sex	发病数 No. cases	粗率 Crude rate/ 100 000⁻¹	构成比 Freq./%	中标率 ASR China/ 100 000⁻¹	世标率 ASR world/ 100 000⁻¹	累积率 Cum. rate 0~74/%	顺位 Rank
合计 All	合计 Both	10 803	1. 72	0. 56	1. 25	1. 22	0. 12	22
	男性 Male	6 111	1. 92	0. 58	1. 42	1. 40	0. 14	18
	女性 Female	4 692	1. 52	0. 54	1. 07	1. 04	0. 10	20
城市地区 Urban areas	合计 Both	4 157	1. 55	0. 47	1. 09	1. 06	0. 10	22
	男性 Male	2 330	1. 73	0. 49	1. 24	1. 22	0. 12	18
	女性 Female	1 827	1. 36	0. 44	0. 94	0. 91	0. 09	20
农村地区 Rural areas	合计 Both	6 646	1. 85	0. 65	1. 36	1. 34	0. 13	21
	男性 Male	3 781	2. 05	0. 66	1. 55	1. 52	0. 15	18
	女性 Female	2 865	1. 63	0. 63	1. 17	1. 15	0. 11	20
东部地区 Eastern areas	合计 Both	3 933	1. 55	0. 43	1. 09	1. 06	0. 10	22
	男性 Male	2 220	1. 74	0. 45	1. 26	1. 24	0. 12	18
	女性 Female	1 713	1. 36	0. 39	0. 92	0. 88	0. 08	20
中部地区 Central areas	合计 Both	2 714	1. 81	0. 64	1. 39	1. 37	0. 13	22
	男性 Male	1 486	1. 94	0. 64	1. 54	1. 52	0. 15	18
	女性 Female	1 228	1. 66	0. 63	1. 25	1. 24	0. 12	20
西部地区 Western areas	合计 Both	4 156	1. 85	0. 73	1. 34	1. 31	0. 13	21
	男性 Male	2 405	2. 10	0. 74	1. 54	1. 51	0. 15	18
	女性 Female	1 751	1. 60	0. 73	1. 14	1. 11	0. 11	20

表 5-11b　中国肿瘤登记地区骨癌死亡情况
Table 5-11b　Mortality of bone cancer in registration areas of China

地区 Area	性别 Sex	死亡数 No. deaths	粗率 Crude rate/ 100 000⁻¹	构成比 Freq./%	中标率 ASR China/ 100 000⁻¹	世标率 ASR world/ 100 000⁻¹	累积率 Cum. rate 0~74/%	顺位 Rank
合计 All	合计 Both	7 859	1. 25	0. 72	0. 79	0. 77	0. 08	20
	男性 Male	4 777	1. 50	0. 68	0. 99	0. 97	0. 10	17
	女性 Female	3 082	1. 00	0. 79	0. 60	0. 58	0. 06	19
城市地区 Urban areas	合计 Both	2 909	1. 08	0. 61	0. 67	0. 66	0. 07	21
	男性 Male	1 734	1. 29	0. 57	0. 83	0. 82	0. 08	17
	女性 Female	1 175	0. 88	0. 68	0. 52	0. 50	0. 05	19
农村地区 Rural areas	合计 Both	4 950	1. 38	0. 81	0. 88	0. 86	0. 10	20
	男性 Male	3 043	1. 65	0. 77	1. 10	1. 08	0. 12	17
	女性 Female	1 907	1. 09	0. 89	0. 66	0. 65	0. 07	15
东部地区 Eastern areas	合计 Both	2 988	1. 18	0. 62	0. 69	0. 68	0. 07	20
	男性 Male	1 770	1. 39	0. 58	0. 86	0. 84	0. 09	17
	女性 Female	1 218	0. 97	0. 68	0. 53	0. 52	0. 05	19
中部地区 Central areas	合计 Both	1 809	1. 20	0. 74	0. 82	0. 80	0. 09	20
	男性 Male	1 119	1. 46	0. 71	1. 05	1. 02	0. 12	17
	女性 Female	690	0. 93	0. 78	0. 60	0. 58	0. 07	17
西部地区 Western areas	合计 Both	3 062	1. 36	0. 85	0. 89	0. 88	0. 09	19
	男性 Male	1 888	1. 64	0. 80	1. 11	1. 10	0. 12	16
	女性 Female	1 174	1. 07	0. 96	0. 68	0. 67	0. 07	16

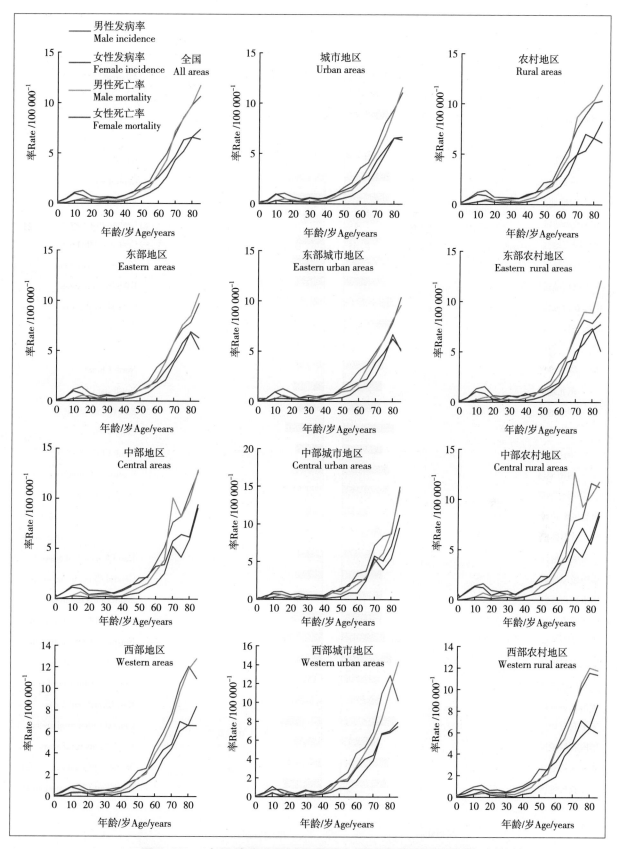

图 5-11a 中国肿瘤登记地区骨癌年龄别发病率和死亡率

Figure 5-11a Age-specific incidence and mortality rates of bone cancer in registration areas of China

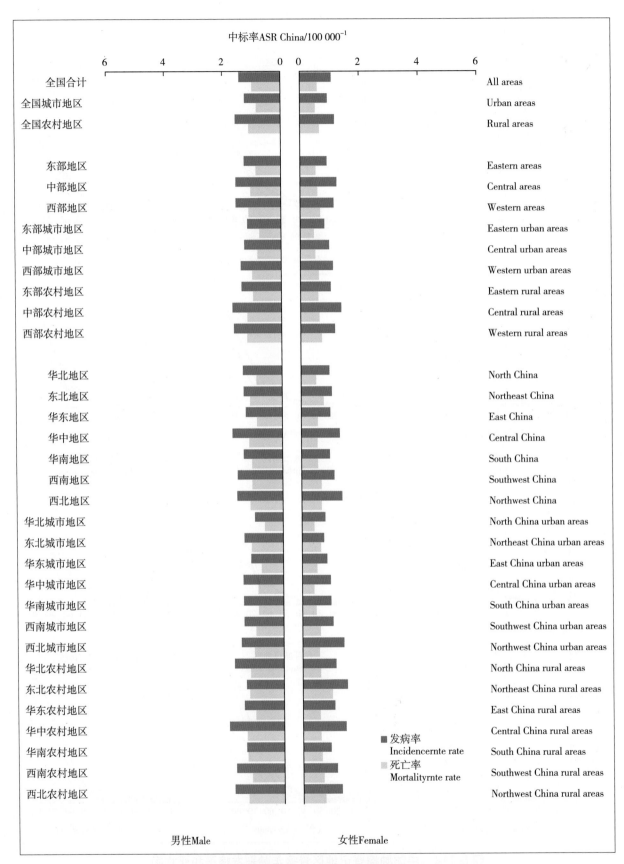

中标率ASR China/100 000⁻¹

	全国合计	All areas
全国城市地区		Urban areas
全国农村地区		Rural areas
东部地区		Eastern areas
中部地区		Central areas
西部地区		Western areas
东部城市地区		Eastern urban areas
中部城市地区		Central urban areas
西部城市地区		Western urban areas
东部农村地区		Eastern rural areas
中部农村地区		Central rural areas
西部农村地区		Western rural areas
华北地区		North China
东北地区		Northeast China
华东地区		East China
华中地区		Central China
华南地区		South China
西南地区		Southwest China
西北地区		Northwest China
华北城市地区		North China urban areas
东北城市地区		Northeast China urban areas
华东城市地区		East China urban areas
华中城市地区		Central China urban areas
华南城市地区		South China urban areas
西南城市地区		Southwest China urban areas
西北城市地区		Northwest China urban areas
华北农村地区		North China rural areas
东北农村地区		Northeast China rural areas
华东农村地区		East China rural areas
华中农村地区		Central China rural areas
华南农村地区		South China rural areas
西南农村地区		Southwest China rural areas
西北农村地区		Northwest China rural areas

发病率 Incidencernte rate
死亡率 Mortalityrnte rate

男性Male　　　　女性Female

图 5-11b　中国肿瘤登记不同地区骨癌发病率和死亡率
Figure 5-11b　Incidence and mortality rates of bone cancer in different
registration areas of China

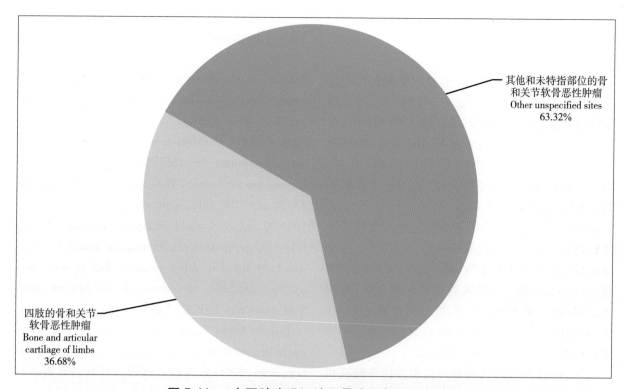

其他和未特指部位的骨
和关节软骨恶性肿瘤
Other unspecified sites
63.32%

四肢的骨和关节
软骨恶性肿瘤
Bone and articular
cartilage of limbs
36.68%

图 5-11c　中国肿瘤登记地区骨癌亚部位分布情况
Figure 5-11c　Subsite distribution of bone cancer in registration areas of China

12 女性乳腺

　　女性乳腺癌位居中国肿瘤登记地区女性癌症发病谱第 2 位。新发病例数为 133 447 例,占全部女性癌症发病的 15.32%;城市地区 69 616 例,农村地区 63 831 例。发病率为 43.10/10 万,中标发病率为 30.11/10 万,世标发病率为 28.08/10 万;城市中标发病率为农村的 1.34 倍。0~74 岁累积发病率为 3.01%(表 5-12a)。

　　女性乳腺癌位居中国肿瘤登记地区女性癌症死亡谱第 5 位。女性乳腺癌死亡 28 607 例,占全部女性癌症死亡的 7.35%;城市地区 14 338 例,农村地区 14 269 例。女性乳腺癌死亡率为 9.24/10 万,中标死亡率 5.57/10 万,世标死亡率 5.42/10 万;城市中标死亡率为农村的 1.22 倍。0~74 岁累积死亡率为 0.59%(表 5-12b)。

　　城市和农村女性乳腺癌年龄别发病率特征相似。女性乳腺癌发病率均自 20~24 岁组开始快速上升,城市地区至 60~64 岁组达到高峰,而农村地区至 45~50 岁组达到高峰,随后下降;女性乳腺癌死亡率从 25~29 岁组开始缓慢上升(图 5-12a)。

12 Female breast

Female breast cancer was the 2nd common cancer among females in the registration areas of China. There were 133 447 new cases of female breast cancer(69 616 in urban areas and 63 831 in rural areas), accounting for 15.32% of new cases of all cancers among females. The crude incidence rate was 43.10 per 100 000, with ASR China 30.11 per 100 000 and ASR world 28.08 per 100 000, respectively. Subgroup analyses showed that the ASR China was 1.34 times in urban areas as that in rural areas. The cumulative incidence rate for subjects aged 0-74 years was 3.01% (Table 5-12a).

Female breast cancer was the 5th most common cause of cancer deaths among females in the registration areas of China. A total of 28 607 women died of breast cancer(14 338 in urban areas and 14 269 in rural areas), accounting for 7.35% of all cancer deaths among females. The crude mortality rate was 9.24 per 100 000, with ASR China 5.57 per 100 000 and ASR world 5.42 per 100 000, respectively. Subgroup analyses showed that the mortality of ASR China was 1.22 times in urban areas as that in rural areas. The cumulative mortality rate for subjects aged 0-74 years was 0.59% (Table 5-12b).

Age-specific incidence rates took on almost the same pattern between urban areas and rural areas. The incidence rate increased rapidly from the age group of 20-24 years with the peak occurring in the age group of 60-64 years in urban areas and 45-50 years in rural areas, thereafter began to drop. Age-specific mortality rates increased slowly from the age group of 25-29 years(Figure 5-12a).

城市地区女性乳腺癌的中标发病率和死亡率均高于农村地区。东部地区中标发病率最高,其次是中部地区,西部地区最低;七大行政区中,华北地区、东北地区和华中地区中标发病率较高,西南地区中标发病率最低。东部地区中标死亡率最高,其次是中部地区,西部地区最低;东北地区、华中地区和华南地区中标死亡率较高,西南地区中标死亡率最低(表5-12a,表5-12b,图5-12b)。

全部女性乳腺癌病例中,33.92%的病例报告了明确的亚部位,其中外上象限是最主要的亚部位,占37.10%;其次是交搭跨越(22.41%)、内上象限(17.15%)、外下象限(8.15%)、内下象限(6.39%)、中央部(4.93%)、乳头和乳晕(3.44%)、腋尾部(0.43%)(图5-12c)。

全部女性乳腺癌病例中有明确组织学类型的病例占77.67%,其中导管癌是最主要的病理类型,占79.92%;其次是小叶癌,占3.90%;佩吉特病占1.45%;髓样癌占0.23%(图5-12d)。

Both the incidence and mortality rates of ASR China of female breast cancer were higher in urban areas than those in rural areas. Eastern areas had the highest incidence rate(ASR China), followed by central and western areas. Among the seven administrative districts, North China, Northeast China and Central China had the top three incidence rates(ASR China), and Southwest China had the lowest incidence rate(ASR China). Eastern areas had the highest mortality rate(ASR China), followed by central and western areas. Northeast China, Central China and South China had the top three mortality rates(ASR China), and Southwest China had the lowest mortality rate(ASR China)(Table 5-12a, Table 5-12b, Figure 5-12b).

About 33.92% female breast cancer cases reported specific subsites. Among them, 37.10% occurred in upper outer, 22.41% at overlapping, 17.15% in upper inner, 8.15% in lower outer, 6.39% in lower inner, 4.93% in central portion, 3.44% in nipple and areola, and 0.43% in axillary tail(Figure 5-12c).

About 77.67% cases of female breast cancer had morphological verification. Among them, ductal cancer was the most common histological type, accounting for 79.92%, followed by lobular carcinoma(3.90%), Paget's disease(1.45%), medullary carcinoma(0.23%)(Figure 5-12d).

表 5-12a 中国肿瘤登记地区女性乳腺癌发病情况

Table 5-12a Incidence of female breast cancer in the registration areas of China

地区 Area	发病数 No. cases	粗率 Crude rate/ 100 000^{-1}	构成比 Freq. /%	中标率 ASR China/ 100 000^{-1}	世标率 ASR world/ 100 000^{-1}	累积率 Cum. rate 0~74/%	顺位 Rank
合计 All	133 447	43. 10	15. 32	30. 11	28. 08	3. 01	2
城市地区 Urban areas	69 616	51. 94	16. 66	35. 04	32. 91	3. 58	2
农村地区 Rural areas	63 831	36. 35	14. 08	26. 23	24. 28	2. 57	2
东部地区 Eastern areas	71 099	56. 34	16. 29	37. 75	35. 25	3. 82	2
中部地区 Central areas	30 670	41. 55	15. 80	30. 11	28. 06	2. 98	1
西部地区 Western areas	31 678	28. 90	13. 17	20. 87	19. 33	2. 02	2

表 5-12b 中国肿瘤登记地区女性乳腺癌死亡情况

Table 5-12b Mortality of female breast cancer in the registration areas of China

地区 Area	死亡数 No. deaths	粗率 Crude rate/ 100 000^{-1}	构成比 Freq. /%	中标率 ASR China/ 100 000^{-1}	世标率 ASR world/ 100 000^{-1}	累积率 Cum. rate 0~74/%	顺位 Rank
合计 All	28 607	9. 24	7. 35	5. 57	5. 42	0. 59	5
城市地区 Urban areas	14 338	10. 70	8. 24	6. 19	6. 05	0. 66	5
农村地区 Rural areas	14 269	8. 13	6. 63	5. 07	4. 91	0. 54	6
东部地区 Eastern areas	14 184	11. 24	7. 96	6. 15	6. 00	0. 66	5
中部地区 Central areas	6 721	9. 11	7. 58	5. 83	5. 66	0. 63	5
西部地区 Western areas	7 702	7. 03	6. 31	4. 60	4. 44	0. 49	5

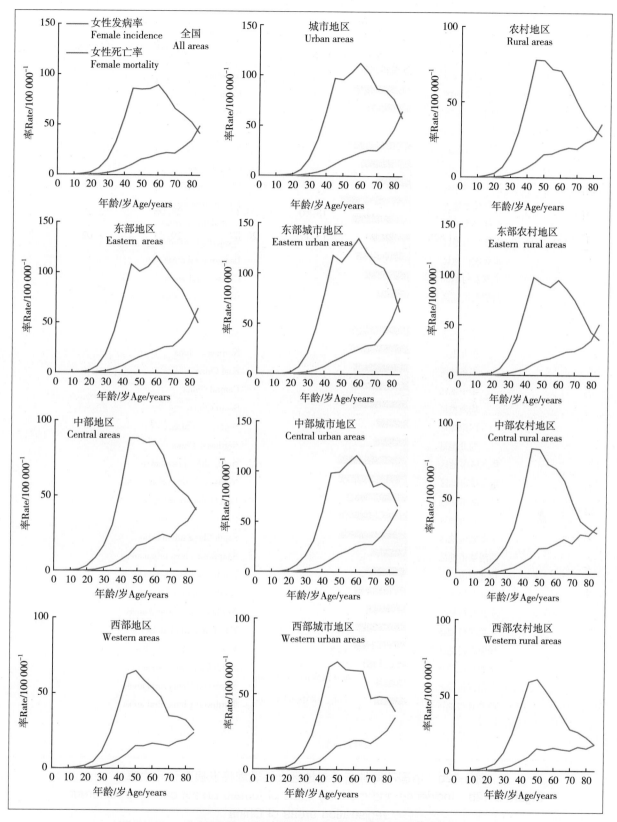

图 5-12a　中国肿瘤登记地区女性乳腺癌年龄别发病率和死亡率

Figure 5-12a　Age-specific incidence and mortality rates of female breast cancer in the registration areas of China

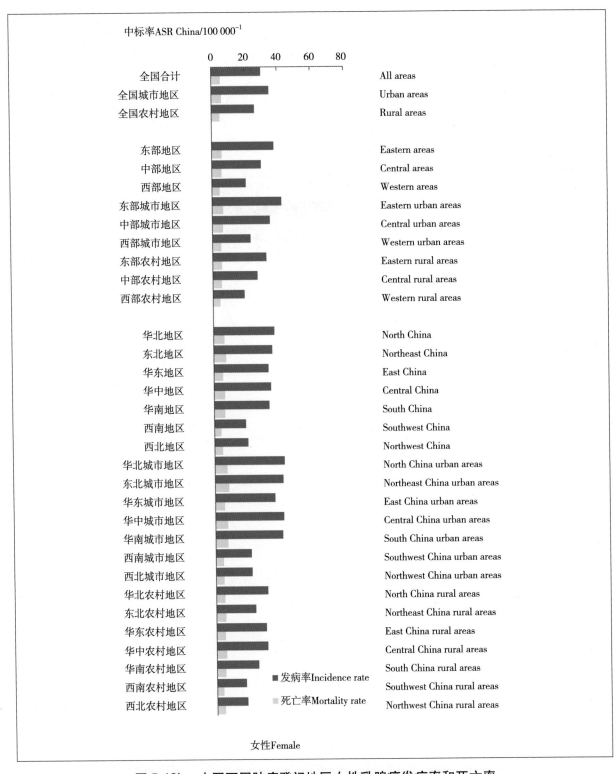

中标率ASR China/100 000⁻¹

全国合计	All areas
全国城市地区	Urban areas
全国农村地区	Rural areas
东部地区	Eastern areas
中部地区	Central areas
西部地区	Western areas
东部城市地区	Eastern urban areas
中部城市地区	Central urban areas
西部城市地区	Western urban areas
东部农村地区	Eastern rural areas
中部农村地区	Central rural areas
西部农村地区	Western rural areas
华北地区	North China
东北地区	Northeast China
华东地区	East China
华中地区	Central China
华南地区	South China
西南地区	Southwest China
西北地区	Northwest China
华北城市地区	North China urban areas
东北城市地区	Northeast China urban areas
华东城市地区	East China urban areas
华中城市地区	Central China urban areas
华南城市地区	South China urban areas
西南城市地区	Southwest China urban areas
西北城市地区	Northwest China urban areas
华北农村地区	North China rural areas
东北农村地区	Northeast China rural areas
华东农村地区	East China rural areas
华中农村地区	Central China rural areas
华南农村地区	South China rural areas
西南农村地区	Southwest China rural areas
西北农村地区	Northwest China rural areas

■发病率Incidence rate
死亡率Mortality rate

女性Female

图 5-12b　中国不同肿瘤登记地区女性乳腺癌发病率和死亡率
Figure 5-12b　Incidence and mortality rates of female breast cancer in different registration areas of China

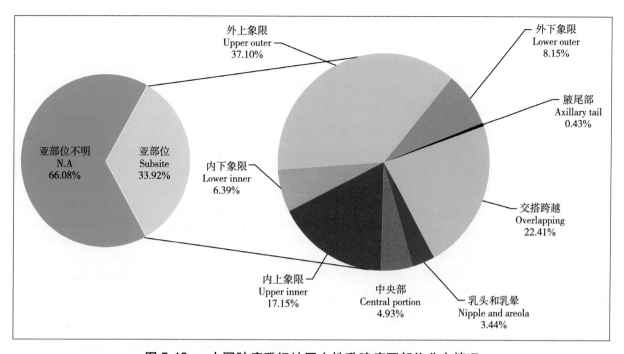

图 5-12c　中国肿瘤登记地区女性乳腺癌亚部位分布情况

Figure 5-12c　Subsite distribution of female breast cancer in the registration areas of China

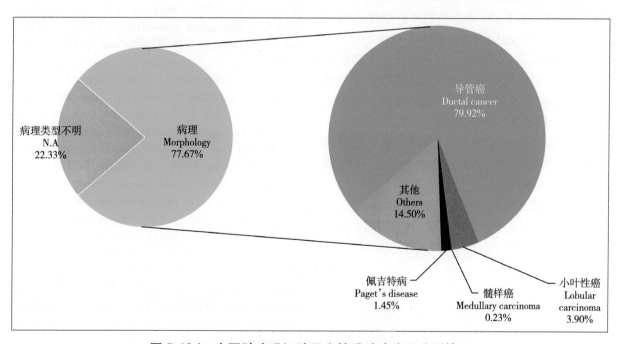

图 5-12d　中国肿瘤登记地区女性乳腺癌病理分型情况

Figure 5-12d　Morphological distribution of female breast cancer in the registration areas of China

13 子宫颈

子宫颈癌位居中国肿瘤登记地区女性癌症发病谱第 5 位。新发病例数为 56 231 例,占女性全部癌症发病的 6.45%;其中城市地区 22 850 例,农村地区 33 381 例。发病率为 18.16/10 万,中标发病率为 12.74/10 万,世标发病率为 11.80/10 万;农村中标发病率是城市的 1.14 倍。0~74 岁累积发病率为 1.27%(表 5-13a)。

子宫颈癌位居中国肿瘤登记地区女性癌症死亡谱第 8 位。死亡病例数为 17 198 例,占女性全部癌症死亡的 4.42%。其中城市地区 6 822 例,农村地区 10 376 例。子宫颈癌死亡率为 5.55/10 万,中标死亡率 3.39/10 万,世标死亡率 3.27/10 万,农村中标死亡率为城市的 1.17 倍。0~74 岁累积死亡率为 0.37%(表 5-13b)。

子宫颈癌年龄别发病率在 20 岁之前处于较低水平,自 20 岁以后快速上升,至 50~54 岁年龄组达高峰,之后逐渐下降。年龄别死亡率在 30 岁之前处于较低水平,30 岁以后随年龄增加逐渐升高,在 75~79 岁组达到高峰(图 5-13a)。

农村地区子宫颈癌的发病率和死亡率均高于城市地区。中标发病率及中标死亡率均以中部地区最高,其次是西部地区,东部地区最低。在七大行政区中,华中地区和西北地区中标发病率和死亡率显著高于全国平均水平,华北地区中标发病率和死亡率明显低于全国平均水平(表 5-13a,表 5-13b,图 5-13b)。

全部子宫颈癌病例中,10.89% 的病例报告了明确的亚部位,其中宫颈内膜癌、外宫颈癌和宫颈交界部位癌分别占 52.77%、35.72%、11.51%(图 5-13c)。

13 Cervix

Cervical cancer was the 5th most common female cancer in the registration areas of China. There were 56 231 new cases of cervical cancer(22 850 in urban areas and 33 381 in rural areas), accounting for 6.45% of new cases of all female cancers. The crude incidence rate was 18.16 per 100 000, with ASR China 12.74 per 100 000 and ASR world 11.80 per 100 000, respectively. Subgroup analyses showed that the incidence of ASR China was 1.14 times in rural areas as that in urban areas. The cumulative incidence rate for subjects aged 0-74 years was 1.27% (Table 5-13a).

Cervical cancer was the 8th common cause of cancer deaths among females in the registration areas of China. A total of 17 198 women died of cervical cancer(6 822 in urban areas and 10 376 in rural areas), accounting for 4.42% of all female cancer deaths. The crude mortality rate was 5.55 per 100 000, with ASR China 3.39 per 100 000 and ASR world 3.27 per 100 000, respectively. Subgroup analyses showed that the mortality of ASR China was 1.17 times in rural areas as that in urban areas. The cumulative mortality rate for subjects aged 0-74 years was 0.37% (Table 5-13b).

The age-specific incidence rate was low before age 20. It went up rapidly thereafter, with the peak occurring in age group 50-54 years and then decreased gradually. The age-specific mortality was low before age 30 and then increased gradually, reaching the peak in age group 75-79 years(Figure 5-13a).

Both the incidence and mortality rates of cervical cancer were higher in rural areas than in urban areas. Central areas had both the highest incidence and mortality rates(ASR China) while eastern areas had both the lowest incidence and mortality rates(ASR China), leaving western areas in between. Among the seven administrative districts, both the incidence and mortality rates(ASR China) of cervical cancer in Central China and Northwest China areas were markedly higher than the national average whereas both the incidence and mortality rates(ASR China) in North China were lower than the national average(Table 5-13a, Table 5-13b, Figure 5-13b).

There were 10.89% cases of cervical cancers reported to have occurred in specificsubsites, with endocervix, exocervix and overlapping parts comprising 52.77%, 35.72% and 11.51%, respectively(Figure 5-13c).

表 5-13a 中国肿瘤登记地区子宫颈癌发病情况
Table 5-13a Incidence of cervical cancer in the registration areas of China

地区 Area	发病数 No. cases	粗率 Crude rate/ 100 000^{-1}	构成比 Freq./%	中标率 ASR China/ 100 000^{-1}	世标率 ASR world/ 100 000^{-1}	累积率 Cum. rate 0~74/%	顺位 Rank
合计 All	56 231	18.16	6.45	12.74	11.80	1.27	5
城市地区 Urban areas	22 850	17.05	5.47	11.78	10.94	1.18	5
农村地区 Rural areas	33 381	19.01	7.36	13.48	12.48	1.34	5
东部地区 Eastern areas	20 363	16.14	4.66	11.05	10.20	1.09	6
中部地区 Central areas	16 051	21.75	8.27	15.49	14.45	1.58	5
西部地区 Western areas	19 817	18.08	8.24	12.94	11.99	1.29	4

表 5-13b 中国肿瘤登记地区子宫颈癌死亡情况
Table 5-13b Mortality of cervical cancer in the registration areas of China

地区 Area	死亡数 No. deaths	粗率 Crude rate/ 100 000^{-1}	构成比 Freq./%	中标率 ASR China/ 100 000^{-1}	世标率 ASR world/ 100 000^{-1}	累积率 Cum. rate 0~74/%	顺位 Rank
合计 All	17 198	5.55	4.42	3.39	3.27	0.37	8
城市地区 Urban areas	6 822	5.09	3.92	3.09	2.97	0.33	7
农村地区 Rural areas	10 376	5.91	4.82	3.63	3.51	0.40	7
东部地区 Eastern areas	5 813	4.61	3.26	2.65	2.55	0.28	8
中部地区 Central areas	4 768	6.46	5.37	4.07	3.96	0.46	7
西部地区 Western areas	6 617	6.04	5.42	3.87	3.73	0.43	6

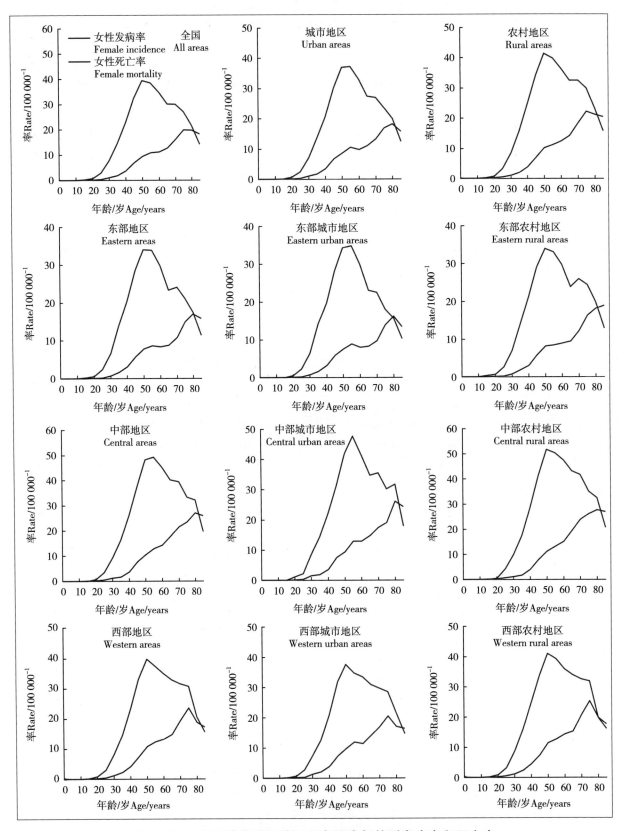

图 5-13a　中国肿瘤登记地区子宫颈癌年龄别发病率和死亡率

Figure 5-13a　Age-specific incidence and mortality rates of cervical cancer in the registration areas of China

中标率ASR China/100 000^{-1}

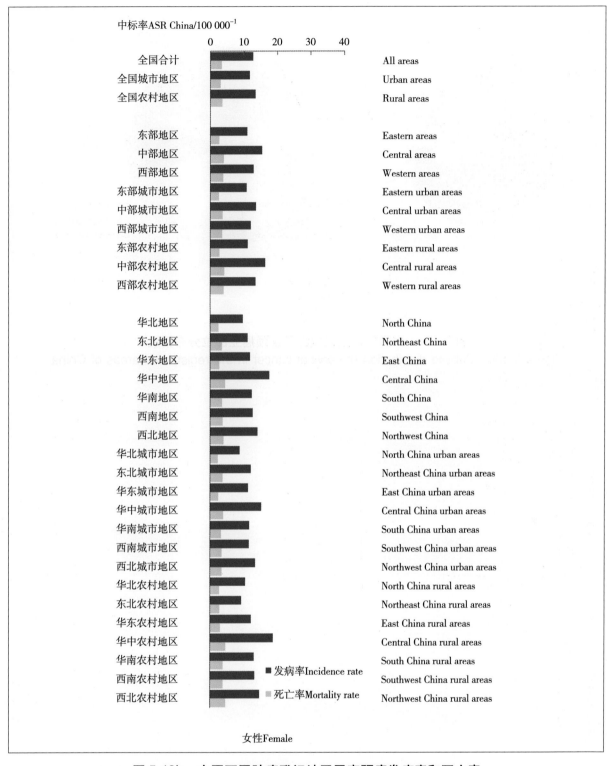

图 5-13b　中国不同肿瘤登记地区子宫颈癌发病率和死亡率
Figure 5-13b　Incidence and mortality rates of cervical cancer in different registration areas of China

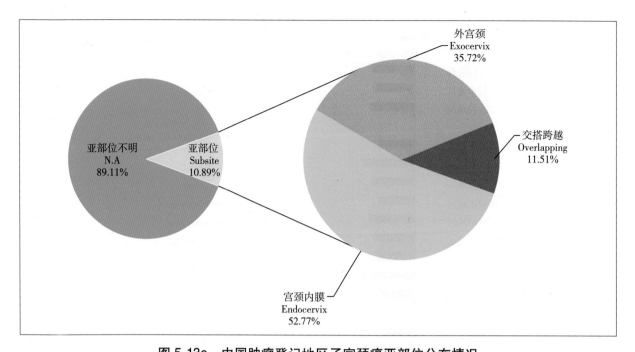

图 5-13c　中国肿瘤登记地区子宫颈癌亚部位分布情况

Figure 5-13c　Subsite distribution of cervical cancer in the registration areas of China

14　子宫体

子宫体癌位居中国肿瘤登记地区女性癌症发病谱第 8 位。新发病例数为 33 531 例,占女性全部癌症发病的 3.85%;其中城市地区 15 682 例,农村地区 17 849 例。子宫体癌发病率为 10.83/10 万,中标发病率为 7.08/10 万,世标发病率为 6.84/10 万;城市中标发病率为农村的 1.11 倍。0~74 岁累积发病率为 0.77%(表 5-14a)。

子宫体癌位居中国肿瘤登记地区女性癌症死亡谱第 14 位。子宫体癌死亡病例数为 8 385 例,占女性全部癌症死亡的 2.16%;其中城市地区 3 541 例,农村地区 4 844 例。子宫体癌死亡率为 2.71/10 万,中标死亡率 1.55/10 万,世标死亡率 1.54/10 万;农村中标死亡率为城市的 1.09 倍。0~74 岁累积死亡率为 0.18%(表 5-14b)。

子宫体癌年龄别发病率在 20 岁前处于较低水平,20 岁以后快速上升,至 55~59 岁组达高峰,之后逐渐下降。年龄别死亡率 30 岁前处于较低水平,30 岁以后迅速上升(图 5-14a)。

东部地区中标发病率最高,其次是中部地区,西部地区最低;西部地区中标死亡率最高,其次是中部地区,东部地区最低。在七大行政区中,华北、华南、华中地区子宫体癌中标发病率较高,西南地区最低。华南、华中、西南地区的中标死亡率较高,华东地区最低(表 5-14a,表 5-14b,图 5-14b)。

14　Uterus

Uterus cancer was the 8th most common female cancer in the registration areas of China. There were 33 531 new cases of uterus cancer(15 682 in urban areas and 17 849 in rural areas), accounting for 3.85% of all female cancer cases. The crude incidence rate was 10.83 per 100 000, with ASR China 7.08 per 100 000 and ASR world 6.84 per 100 000, respectively. The incidence of ASR China was 1.11 times in urban areas as that in rural areas. The cumulative incidence rate for persons aged 0-74 years was 0.77%(Table 5-14a).

Uterus cancer was the 14th most common cause of female cancer deaths in the registration areas of China. A total of 8 385 women died of uterus cancer(3 541 in urban areas and 4 844 in rural areas), accounting for 2.16% of all female cancer deaths. The crude mortality rate was 2.71 per 100 000, with ASR China 1.55 per 100 000 and ASR world 1.54 per 100 000, respectively. The mortality of ASR China was 1.09 times in rural areas as that in urban areas. The cumulative mortality rate for persons aged 0-74 years was 0.18%(Table 5-14b).

The age-specific incidence rate was low before age 20. It went up rapidly thereafter and reached the peak at age group 55-59, then started to go down gradually. The age-specific mortality was low before age 30, then gradually went up thereafter(Figure 5-14a).

Eastern areas had the highest incidence rate(ASR China), followed by central and western areas. Western areas had the highest mortality rate(ASR China), followed by central and eastern areas. Among the seven administrative districts, North China, South China and Central China had the top three incidence rates(ASR China), and Southwest China had the lowest incidence rate(ASR China). South China, Central China and Southwest China had the top three mortality rates, and East China had the lowest mortality rate(ASR China)(Table 5-14a, Table 5-14b, Figure 5-14b).

表 5-14a　中国肿瘤登记地区子宫体癌发病情况

Table 5-14a　Incidence of uterus cancer in the registration areas of China

地区 Area	发病数 No. cases	粗率 Crude rate/ 100 000^{-1}	构成比 Freq./%	中标率 ASR China/ 100 000^{-1}	世标率 ASR world/ 100 000^{-1}	累积率 Cum. Rate 0~74/%	顺位 Rank
合计 All	33 531	10.83	3.85	7.08	6.84	0.77	8
城市地区 Urban areas	15 682	11.70	3.75	7.50	7.28	0.83	8
农村地区 Rural areas	17 849	10.17	3.94	6.76	6.49	0.72	9
东部地区 Eastern areas	16 019	12.69	3.67	7.92	7.68	0.87	8
中部地区 Central areas	7 746	10.49	3.99	7.09	6.85	0.76	9
西部地区 Western areas	9 766	8.91	4.06	6.03	5.77	0.64	8

表 5-14b　中国肿瘤登记地区子宫体癌死亡情况

Table 5-14b　Mortality of uterus cancer in the registration areas of China

地区 Area	死亡数 No. deaths	粗率 Crude rate/ 100 000^{-1}	构成比 Freq./%	中标率 ASR China/ 100 000^{-1}	世标率 ASR world/ 100 000^{-1}	累积率 Cum. Rate 0~74/%	顺位 Rank
合计 All	8 385	2.71	2.16	1.55	1.54	0.18	14
城市地区 Urban areas	3 541	2.64	2.04	1.48	1.47	0.17	14
农村地区 Rural areas	4 844	2.76	2.25	1.61	1.59	0.19	13
东部地区 Eastern areas	3 470	2.75	1.95	1.44	1.42	0.17	14
中部地区 Central areas	1 890	2.56	2.13	1.54	1.53	0.18	14
西部地区 Western areas	3 025	2.76	2.48	1.70	1.68	0.20	11

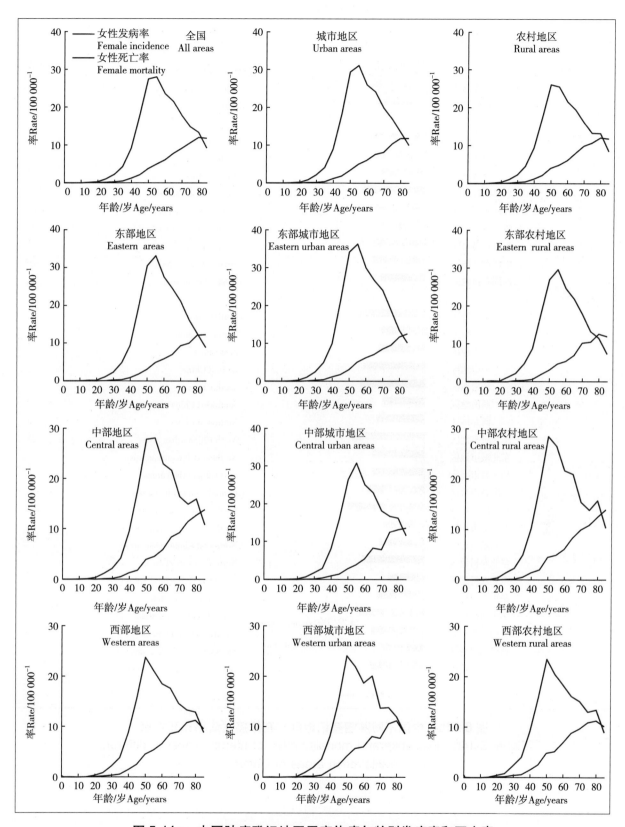

图 5-14a　中国肿瘤登记地区子宫体癌年龄别发病率和死亡率

Figure 5-14a　Age-specific incidence and mortality rates of uterus cancer in the registration areas of China

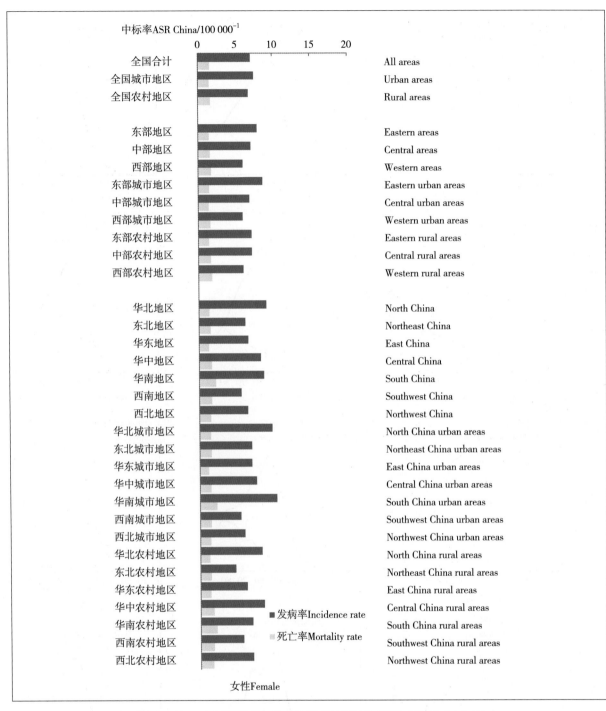

中标率ASR China/100 000⁻¹

全国合计	All areas	
全国城市地区	Urban areas	
全国农村地区	Rural areas	
东部地区	Eastern areas	
中部地区	Central areas	
西部地区	Western areas	
东部城市地区	Eastern urban areas	
中部城市地区	Central urban areas	
西部城市地区	Western urban areas	
东部农村地区	Eastern rural areas	
中部农村地区	Central rural areas	
西部农村地区	Western rural areas	
华北地区	North China	
东北地区	Northeast China	
华东地区	East China	
华中地区	Central China	
华南地区	South China	
西南地区	Southwest China	
西北地区	Northwest China	
华北城市地区	North China urban areas	
东北城市地区	Northeast China urban areas	
华东城市地区	East China urban areas	
华中城市地区	Central China urban areas	
华南城市地区	South China urban areas	
西南城市地区	Southwest China urban areas	
西北城市地区	Northwest China urban areas	
华北农村地区	North China rural areas	
东北农村地区	Northeast China rural areas	
华东农村地区	East China rural areas	
华中农村地区	Central China rural areas	
华南农村地区	South China rural areas	
西南农村地区	Southwest China rural areas	
西北农村地区	Northwest China rural areas	

■发病率Incidence rate
□死亡率Mortality rate

女性Female

图 5-14b　中国不同肿瘤登记地区子宫体癌发病率和死亡率
Figure 5-14b　Incidence and mortality rates of uterus cancer in different
registration areas of China

15 卵巢

卵巢癌位居中国肿瘤登记地区女性癌症发病谱第11位。新发病例数为24 265例,占女性癌症发病的2.79%;其中城市地区11 572例,农村地区12 693例。发病率为7.84/10万,中标发病率为5.48/10万,世标发病率为5.20/10万;城市中标发病率为农村的1.16倍。0~74岁累积发病率为0.56%(表5-15a)。

卵巢癌位居中国肿瘤登记地区女性癌症死亡谱第10位。死亡病例数为11 043例,占女性癌症死亡的2.84%;其中城市地区5 599例,农村地区5 444例。死亡率为3.57/10万,中标死亡率为2.12/10万,世标死亡率为2.09/10万;城市中标死亡率为农村的1.28倍。0~74岁累积死亡率为0.25%(表5-15b)。

卵巢癌年龄别发病率从35~39岁组开始快速上升,至65~69岁组达高峰。卵巢癌年龄别死亡率从35~39岁组开始逐渐上升,至80~84岁组达高峰(图5-15a)。

城市地区卵巢癌的发病率和死亡率均高于农村地区。中标发病率和中标死亡率均以东部地区最高,其次是中部地区,西部地区最低。在七大行政区中,中标发病率以华北地区最高,其次是东北地区和华中地区,西北地区最低;中标死亡率以东北地区最高,其次是华北地区和西北地区,西南地区最低(表5-15a,表5-15b,图5-15b)。

15 Ovary

Ovarian cancer was the 11th most common female cancer in the registration areas of China. There were 24 265 new ovarian cancer cases(11 572 in urban areas and 12 693 in rural areas), accounting for 2.79% of new female cancer cases of all sites. The crude incidence rate was 7.84 per 100 000, with ASR China 5.48 per 100 000 and ASR world 5.20 per 100 000, respectively. The incidence of ASR China was 1.16 times in urban areas as that in rural areas. The cumulative incidence rate for subjects aged 0-74 years was 0.56%(Table 5-15a).

Ovarian cancer was the 10th most common cause of female cancer deaths in the registration areas of China. A total of 11 043 cases died of ovarian cancer(5 599 in urban areas and 5 444 in rural areas), accounting for 2.84% of all female cancer deaths. The crude mortality rate was 3.57 per 100 000, with ASR China 2.12 per 100 000 and ASR world 2.09 per 100 000, respectively. The mortality of ASR China was 1.28 times in urban areas as that in rural areas. The cumulative mortality rate for subjects aged 0-74 years was 0.25%(Table 5-15b).

The age-specific incidence rates increased rapidly from the age group of 35-39 years and peaked at the age group of 65-69 years. The age-specific mortality rates increased from the age group of 35-39 years and peaked at the age group of 80-84 years(Figure 5-15a).

The incidence and mortality rates of ovarian cancer were higher in urban areas than in rural areas. Eastern areas had the highest incidence rate and mortality rate(ASR China), followed by central and western areas. Among the seven administrative districts, North China had the highest incidence(ASR China), followed by Northeast China and Central China, while the Northwest China had the lowest incidence rate(ASR China). Northeast China had the highest mortality(ASR China), followed by North China and Northwest China, Southwest China had the lowest mortality rate(ASR China)(Table 5-15a, Table 5-15b, Figure 5-15b).

表 5-15a 中国肿瘤登记地区卵巢癌发病情况

Table 5-15a Incidence of ovarian cancer in the registration areas of China

地区 Area	发病数 No. cases	粗率 Crude rate/ 100 000^{-1}	构成比 Freq. /%	中标率 ASR China/ 100 000^{-1}	世标率 ASR world/ 100 000^{-1}	累积率 Cum. Rate 0~74/%	顺位 Rank
合计 All	24 265	7. 84	2. 79	5. 48	5. 20	0. 56	11
城市地区 Urban areas	11 572	8. 63	2. 77	5. 93	5. 63	0. 61	10
农村地区 Rural areas	12 693	7. 23	2. 80	5. 13	4. 86	0. 52	11
东部地区 Eastern areas	11 039	8. 75	2. 53	5. 84	5. 54	0. 60	11
中部地区 Central areas	5 438	7. 37	2. 80	5. 30	5. 04	0. 55	11
西部地区 Western areas	7 788	7. 11	3. 24	5. 17	4. 88	0. 52	10

表 5-15b 中国肿瘤登记地区卵巢癌死亡情况

Table 5-15b Mortality of ovarian cancer in the registration areas of China

地区 Area	死亡数 No. deaths	粗率 Crude rate/ 100 000^{-1}	构成比 Freq. /%	中标率 ASR China/ 100 000^{-1}	世标率 ASR world/ 100 000^{-1}	累积率 Cum. Rate 0~74/%	顺位 Rank
合计 All	11 043	3. 57	2. 84	2. 12	2. 09	0. 25	10
城市地区 Urban areas	5 599	4. 18	3. 22	2. 42	2. 39	0. 28	9
农村地区 Rural areas	5 444	3. 10	2. 53	1. 89	1. 86	0. 22	11
东部地区 Eastern areas	5 260	4. 17	2. 95	2. 29	2. 26	0. 27	10
中部地区 Central areas	2 504	3. 39	2. 82	2. 13	2. 10	0. 25	10
西部地区 Western areas	3 279	2. 99	2. 68	1. 89	1. 86	0. 22	10

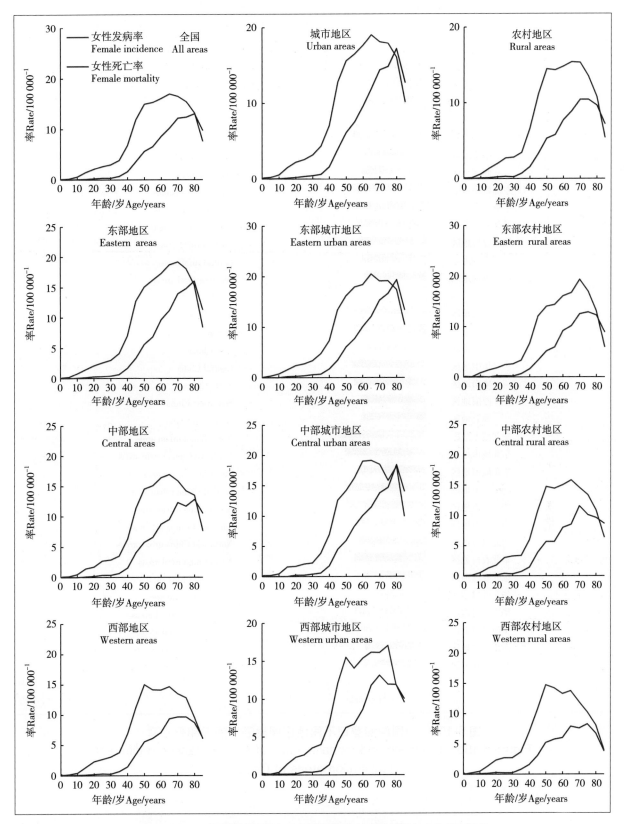

图 5-15a　中国肿瘤登记地区卵巢癌年龄别发病率和死亡率

Figure 5-15a　Age-specific incidence and mortality rates of ovarian cancer in the registration areas of China

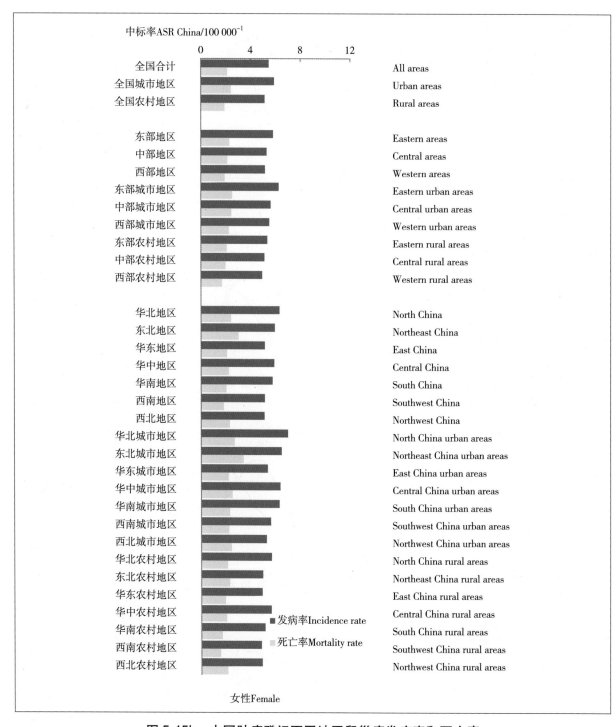

中标率ASR China/100 000⁻¹

全国合计	All areas
全国城市地区	Urban areas
全国农村地区	Rural areas
东部地区	Eastern areas
中部地区	Central areas
西部地区	Western areas
东部城市地区	Eastern urban areas
中部城市地区	Central urban areas
西部城市地区	Western urban areas
东部农村地区	Eastern rural areas
中部农村地区	Central rural areas
西部农村地区	Western rural areas
华北地区	North China
东北地区	Northeast China
华东地区	East China
华中地区	Central China
华南地区	South China
西南地区	Southwest China
西北地区	Northwest China
华北城市地区	North China urban areas
东北城市地区	Northeast China urban areas
华东城市地区	East China urban areas
华中城市地区	Central China urban areas
华南城市地区	South China urban areas
西南城市地区	Southwest China urban areas
西北城市地区	Northwest China urban areas
华北农村地区	North China rural areas
东北农村地区	Northeast China rural areas
华东农村地区	East China rural areas
华中农村地区	Central China rural areas
华南农村地区	South China rural areas
西南农村地区	Southwest China rural areas
西北农村地区	Northwest China rural areas

■发病率Incidence rate
■死亡率Mortality rate

女性Female

图 5-15b   中国肿瘤登记不同地区卵巢癌发病率和死亡率
Figure 5-15b   Incidence and mortality rates of ovarian cancer in different
registration areas of China

16 前列腺

前列腺癌位居中国肿瘤登记地区男性癌症发病谱第6位。新发病例数为43 416例,占全部癌症发病的4.15%;其中城市地区23 683例,农村地区19 733例。发病率为13.62/10万,中标发病率为7.53/10万,世标发病率为7.41/10万;城市中标发病率为农村的1.54倍。0~74岁累积发病率为0.81%(表5-16a)。

前列腺癌位居中国肿瘤登记地区男性癌症死亡谱第7位。死亡病例数为17 004例,占全部癌症死亡的2.43%;其中城市地区9 093例,农村地区7 911例。前列腺癌死亡率为5.33/10万,中标死亡率2.72/10万,世标死亡率2.77/10万;城市中标死亡率为农村的1.39倍。0~74岁累积死亡率为0.19%(表5-16b)。

前列腺癌年龄别发病率和死亡率在55岁之前处于较低水平,55岁开始呈上升趋势,60岁以后快速上升,在85岁及以上年龄组达到峰值(图5-16a)。

城市地区前列腺癌的发病率和死亡率均高于农村地区。中标发病率和死亡率均以东部地区最高。在七大行政区中,华东地区前列腺癌中标发病率最高,其次是华南地区和华北地区,东北地区最低;中标死亡率是华东地区最高,其次为华南地区和华中地区(表5-16a,表5-16b,图5-16b)。

16 Prostate

Prostate cancer was the 6th most common male cancer in the registration areas of China. There were 43 416 new cases of prostate cancer(23 683 in urban areas and 19 733 in rural areas), accounting for 4.15% of new cancer cases of all sites. The crude incidence rate was 13.62 per 100 000,with ASR China 7.53 per 100 000 and ASR world 7.41 per 100 000, respectively. Subgroup analyses showed that the incidence of ASR China in urban areas was 1.54 times as that in rural areas. The cumulative incidence rate for subjects aged 0-74 years was 0.81%(Table 5-16a).

Prostate cancer was the 7th most common male cause of cancer deaths. A total of 17 004 cases died of prostate cancer(9 093 in urban areas and 7 911 in rural areas), accounting for 2.43% of all cancer deaths. The crude mortality rate was 5.33 per 100 000,with ASR China 2.72 per 100 000 and ASR world 2.77 per 100 000, respectively. Subgroup analyses showed that the mortality of ASR China in urban areas was 1.39 times as that in rural areas. The cumulative mortality rate for subjects aged 0-74 years was 0.19% (Table 5-16b).

The age-specific incidence and mortality rates were low before 55 years old and increased constantly since then. The age-specific incidence and mortality rates dramatically increased over 60 years old. The incidence and mortality rate reached peak at the age group of 85 years old,respectively(Figure 5-16a).

The prostate cancer incidence rate and mortality rate were higher in urban areas than that in rural areas. The incidence and mortality rates(ASR China) were highest in eastern areas. Among the seven administrative districts,the incidence rate(ASR China) was highest in East China, followed by South China and North China,and was lowest in Northeast China. Mortality rate(ASR China) was highest in East China, followed by South China and Central China (Table 5-16a,Table 5-16b,Figure 5-16b).

表 5-16a　中国肿瘤登记地区前列腺癌发病情况

Table 5-16a　Incidence of prostate cancer in the registration areas of China

地区 Area	发病数 No. cases	粗率 Crude rate/ 100 000^{-1}	构成比 Freq. /%	中标率 ASR China/ 100 000^{-1}	世标率 ASR world/ 100 000^{-1}	累积率 Cum. Rate 0~74/%	顺位 Rank
合计 All	43 416	13. 62	4. 15	7. 53	7. 41	0. 81	6
城市地区 Urban areas	23 683	17. 62	4. 98	9. 37	9. 24	1. 02	6
农村地区 Rural areas	19 733	10. 70	3. 47	6. 10	5. 99	0. 66	6
东部地区 Eastern areas	24 833	19. 48	5. 08	9. 81	9. 65	1. 12	6
中部地区 Central areas	7 334	9. 58	3. 18	5. 78	5. 68	0. 59	6
西部地区 Western areas	11 249	9. 80	3. 46	5. 74	5. 63	0. 57	6

表 5-16b　中国肿瘤登记地区前列腺癌死亡情况

Table 5-16b　Mortality of prostate cancer in the registration areas of China

地区 Area	死亡数 No. deaths	粗率 Crude rate/ 100 000^{-1}	构成比 Freq. /%	中标率 ASR China/ 100 000^{-1}	世标率 ASR world/ 100 000^{-1}	累积率 Cum. Rate 0~74/%	顺位 Rank
合计 All	17 004	5. 33	2. 43	2. 72	2. 77	0. 19	7
城市地区 Urban areas	9 093	6. 76	3. 00	3. 22	3. 29	0. 22	7
农村地区 Rural areas	7 911	4. 29	2. 00	2. 31	2. 34	0. 17	8
东部地区 Eastern areas	8 684	6. 81	2. 84	3. 00	3. 08	0. 20	7
中部地区 Central areas	3 293	4. 30	2. 10	2. 47	2. 49	0. 18	8
西部地区 Western areas	5 027	4. 38	2. 13	2. 47	2. 49	0. 19	8

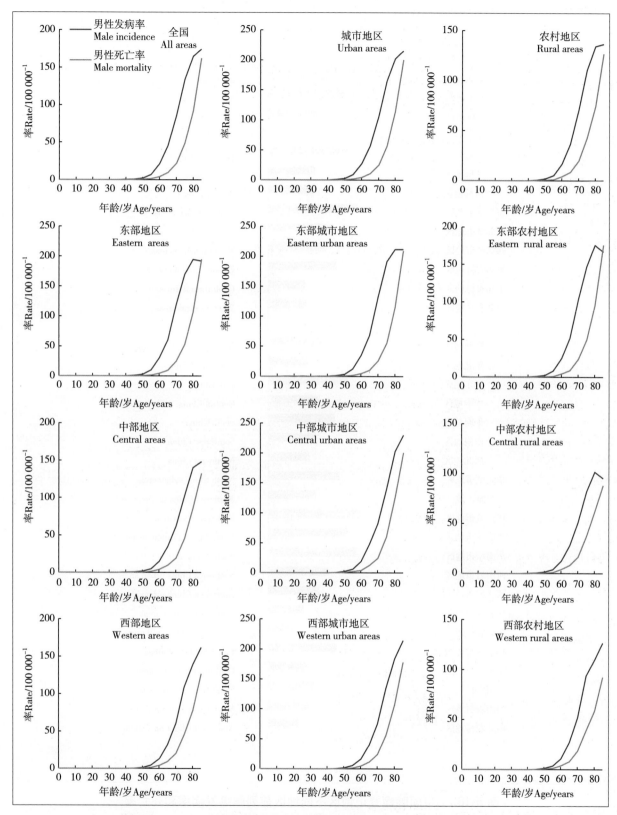

图 5-16a　中国肿瘤登记地区前列腺癌年龄别发病率和死亡率

Figure 5-16a　Age-specific incidence and mortality rates of prostate cancer in the registration areas of China

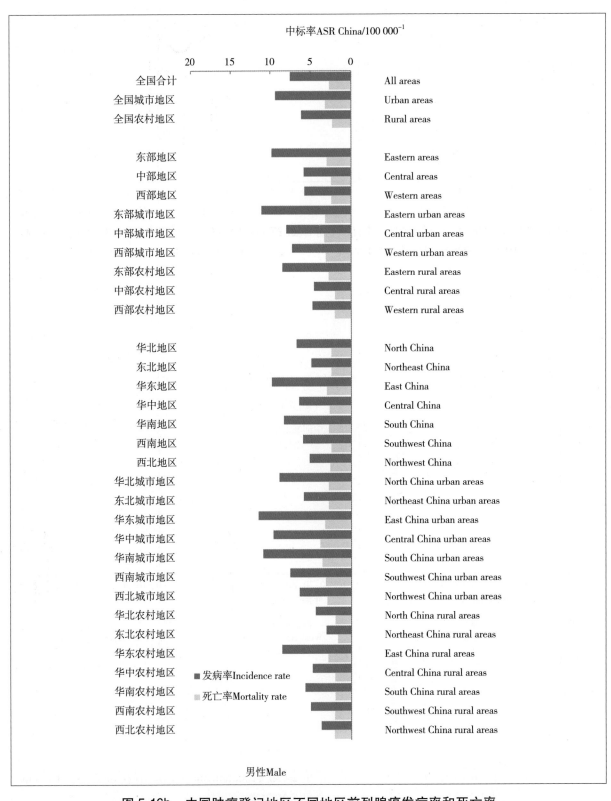

中标率ASR China/100 000⁻¹

全国合计	All areas
全国城市地区	Urban areas
全国农村地区	Rural areas
东部地区	Eastern areas
中部地区	Central areas
西部地区	Western areas
东部城市地区	Eastern urban areas
中部城市地区	Central urban areas
西部城市地区	Western urban areas
东部农村地区	Eastern rural areas
中部农村地区	Central rural areas
西部农村地区	Western rural areas
华北地区	North China
东北地区	Northeast China
华东地区	East China
华中地区	Central China
华南地区	South China
西南地区	Southwest China
西北地区	Northwest China
华北城市地区	North China urban areas
东北城市地区	Northeast China urban areas
华东城市地区	East China urban areas
华中城市地区	Central China urban areas
华南城市地区	South China urban areas
西南城市地区	Southwest China urban areas
西北城市地区	Northwest China urban areas
华北农村地区	North China rural areas
东北农村地区	Northeast China rural areas
华东农村地区	East China rural areas
华中农村地区	Central China rural areas
华南农村地区	South China rural areas
西南农村地区	Southwest China rural areas
西北农村地区	Northwest China rural areas

■ 发病率Incidence rate
■ 死亡率Mortality rate

男性Male

图 5-16b 中国肿瘤登记地区不同地区前列腺癌发病率和死亡率
Figure 5-16b Incidence and mortality rates of prostate cancer in different registration areas of China

17 肾及泌尿系统不明

中国肿瘤登记地区肾及泌尿系统不明癌位居癌症发病谱第17位。新发病例数为33 300例，占全部癌症发病的1.74%；其中男性21 105例，女性12 195例，城市地区18 699例，农村地区14 601例。发病率为5.30/10万，中标发病率为3.27/10万，世标发病率3.25/10万；男性中标发病率为女性的1.80倍，城市中标发病率为农村的1.61倍；0~74岁累积发病率为0.38%（表5-17a）。

中国肿瘤登记地区肾及泌尿系统不明癌位居癌症死亡谱第19位，死亡病例数为11 972例，占全部癌症死亡的1.10%；其中男性7 593例，女性4 379例，城市地区6 688例，农村地区5 284例。死亡率为1.91/10万，中标死亡率1.04/10万，世标死亡率1.04/10万；男性中标死亡率为女性的1.92倍，城市中标死亡率为农村的1.52倍。0~74岁累积死亡率为0.11%（表5-17b）。

按部位划分，肾癌发病率为4.09/10万，中标发病率为2.60/10万；肾癌死亡率为1.37/10万，中标死亡率为0.76/10万。肾盂癌发病率为0.51/10万，中标发病率为0.29/10万；肾盂癌死亡率为0.23/10万，中标死亡率为0.12/10万。输尿管癌发病率为0.57/10万，中标发病率为0.31/10万；输尿管癌死亡率为0.26/10万，中标死亡率为0.13/10万（表5-17c~表5-17h）。

17 Kidney & unspecified urinary organs

Cancer of the kidney & unspecified urinary organs was the 17th most common cancer in the registration areas of China. There were 33 300 new cancer cases (21 105 males and 12 195 females, 18 699 in urban areas and 14 601 in rural areas), accounting for 1.74% of new cases of all cancers. The crude incidence rate was 5.30 per 100 000, with ASR China 3.27 per 100 000 and ASR world 3.25 per 100 000, respectively. The incidence of ASR China was 1.80 times in males as that in females, and it was 1.61 times in urban areas as that in rural areas. The cumulative incidence rate for subjects aged 0-74 years was 0.38% (Table 5-17a).

Cancer of the kidney & unspecified urinary organs was the 19th most common cause of cancer deaths in the registration areas of China. A total of 11 972 cases died of cancer of kidney & unspecified urinary organs (7 593 males and 4 379 females, 6 688 in urban areas and 5 284 in rural areas.), accounting for 1.10% of all cancer deaths. The crude mortality rate was 1.91 per 100 000, with ASR China 1.04 per 100 000 and ASR world 1.04 per 100 000, respectively. The mortality of ASR China was 1.92 times in males as that in females, and it was 1.52 times in urban areas as that in rural areas. The cumulative mortality rate for subjects aged 0-74 years was 0.11% (Table 5-17b).

By subsite, the renal cancer incidence rate was 4.09 per 100 000 with ASR China 2.60 per 100 000; and the mortality rate was 1.37 per 100 000, with ASR China 0.76 per 100 000. The cancer incidence rate of renal pelvis was 0.51 per 100 000, with ASR China 0.29 per 100 000; and the mortality rate was 0.23 per 100 000, with ASR China 0.12 per 100 000. The ureter cancer incidence rate was 0.57 per 100 000, with ASR China 0.31 per 100 000; and the mortality rate was 0.26 per 100 000, with ASR China 0.13 per 100 000 (Table 5-17c~ Table 5-17h).

肾及泌尿系统不明癌年龄别发病率在20岁之前均处于较低水平,自20~24岁组开始快速上升,至80~84岁组达高峰,85岁以后降低;年龄别死亡率从40~44岁组开始迅速上升(图5-17a)。

城市地区肾及泌尿系统不明癌的发病率和死亡率均高于农村地区。中标发病率和中标死亡率均以东部地区最高,其次是中部地区,西部地区最低。在七大行政区中,华北地区中标发病率最高,东北地区中标死亡率最高,西南地区中标发病率和死亡率最低(表5-17a,表5-17b,图5-17b)。

肾(除外肾盂)是肾及泌尿系统不明癌发生的最主要亚部位,占全部病例的77.20%,其次为输尿管,占10.70%;肾盂占9.61%;其他泌尿器官占2.49%(图5-17c)。

全部肾及泌尿系统不明癌病例中有明确组织学类型的病例占67.69%,其中透明细胞腺癌是最主要的病理类型,占77.01%;其次是乳头状腺癌,占3.99%;肾嫌色细胞癌占3.58%;肾集合管癌占0.44%;其他类型癌占14.97%(图5-17d)。

The age-specific incidence of cancer of kidney and unspecified urinary organs was low before 20 years old. It increased rapidly from the age group of 20-24 years and peaked at the age group of 80-84 years, and then it decreased at the age group of 85 years old. Age-specific mortality rates increased rapidly from the age group of 40-44 years (Figure 5-17a).

The incidence and mortality rates of cancer in kidney & unspecified urinary organs were higher in urban areas than in rural areas. Eastern areas had the highest incidence and mortality (ASR China), followed by central and western areas. Among the seven administrative districts, North China had the highest incidence (ASR China) and Northeast China had the highest mortality (ASR China). Southwest China had the lowest incidence and mortality (ASR China) (Table 5-17a, Table 5-17b, Figure 5-17b).

Kidney (except for the renal pelvis) was the most common subsite of cancer in kidney & unspecified urinary organs, accounting for 77.20% of total cases, followed by ureter (10.70%), renal pelvis (9.61%), and other urinary organs (2.49%) (Figure 5-17c).

About 67.69% cases of cancer in kidney and unspecified urinary organs had morphological verification. Among those, clear cell adenocarcinoma was the most common histological type, accounting for 77.01% of all cases, followed by papillary adenocarcinoma (3.99%), chromophobe renal cell carcinoma (3.58%), collecting duct carcinoma (0.44%), and others (14.97%) (Figure 5-17d).

表 5-17a　中国肿瘤登记地区肾及泌尿系统不明癌发病情况

Table 5-17a　Incidence of cancer of kidney & unspecified urinary organs in the registration areas of China

地区 Area	性别 Sex	发病数 No. cases	粗率 Crude rate/ 100 000^{-1}	构成比 Freq./%	中标率 ASR China/ 100 000^{-1}	世标率 ASR world/ 100 000^{-1}	累积率 Cum. Rate 0~74/%	顺位 Rank
合计	合计 Both	33 300	5.30	1.74	3.27	3.25	0.38	17
All	男性 Male	21 105	6.62	2.02	4.22	4.18	0.49	13
	女性 Female	12 195	3.94	1.40	2.34	2.33	0.27	16
城市地区	合计 Both	18 699	6.96	2.09	4.16	4.12	0.48	16
Urban areas	男性 Male	11 966	8.90	2.51	5.49	5.44	0.64	11
	女性 Female	6 733	5.02	1.61	2.88	2.85	0.33	15
农村地区	合计 Both	14 601	4.06	1.43	2.58	2.56	0.30	17
Rural areas	男性 Male	9 139	4.96	1.61	3.25	3.22	0.38	15
	女性 Female	5 462	3.11	1.20	1.92	1.92	0.22	16
东部地区	合计 Both	19 543	7.70	2.11	4.47	4.43	0.52	16
Eastern areas	男性 Male	12 660	9.93	2.59	5.95	5.89	0.70	11
	女性 Female	6 883	5.45	1.58	3.04	3.02	0.35	15
中部地区	合计 Both	6 799	4.52	1.60	2.96	2.94	0.34	17
Central areas	男性 Male	4 241	5.54	1.84	3.75	3.71	0.43	14
	女性 Female	2 558	3.47	1.32	2.19	2.19	0.25	16
西部地区	合计 Both	6 958	3.10	1.23	1.99	1.97	0.23	20
Western areas	男性 Male	4 204	3.66	1.29	2.42	2.40	0.28	15
	女性 Female	2 754	2.51	1.15	1.56	1.55	0.17	16

表 5-17b　中国肿瘤登记地区肾及泌尿系统不明癌死亡情况

Table 5-17b　Mortality of cancer of kidney & unspecified urinary organs in the registration areas of China

地区 Area	性别 Sex	死亡数 No. deaths	粗率 Crude rate/ 100 000^{-1}	构成比 Freq./%	中标率 ASR China/ 100 000^{-1}	世标率 ASR world/ 100 000^{-1}	累积率 Cum. Rate 0~74/%	顺位 Rank
合计	合计 Both	11 972	1.91	1.10	1.04	1.04	0.11	19
All	男性 Male	7 593	2.38	1.09	1.38	1.39	0.15	15
	女性 Female	4 379	1.41	1.13	0.72	0.72	0.07	15
城市地区	合计 Both	6 688	2.49	1.40	1.28	1.29	0.13	17
Urban areas	男性 Male	4 199	3.12	1.38	1.71	1.73	0.19	14
	女性 Female	2 489	1.86	1.43	0.88	0.88	0.09	15
农村地区	合计 Both	5 284	1.47	0.87	0.84	0.84	0.09	19
Rural areas	男性 Male	3 394	1.84	0.86	1.12	1.12	0.13	15
	女性 Female	1 890	1.08	0.88	0.58	0.58	0.06	16
东部地区	合计 Both	6 533	2.58	1.35	1.25	1.25	0.13	17
Eastern areas	男性 Male	4 218	3.31	1.38	1.72	1.73	0.19	13
	女性 Female	2 315	1.83	1.30	0.81	0.81	0.08	15
中部地区	合计 Both	2 565	1.71	1.05	1.03	1.02	0.11	18
Central areas	男性 Male	1 619	2.12	1.03	1.35	1.34	0.15	15
	女性 Female	946	1.28	1.07	0.72	0.72	0.08	15
西部地区	合计 Both	2 874	1.28	0.80	0.77	0.77	0.08	20
Western areas	男性 Male	1 756	1.53	0.74	0.96	0.97	0.11	17
	女性 Female	1 118	1.02	0.92	0.57	0.57	0.06	18

表 5-17c　中国肿瘤登记地区肾癌发病情况

Table 5-17c　Incidence of kidney cancer in the registration areas of China

地区 Area	性别 Sex	病例数 No. cases	粗率 Crude rate/ 100 000^{-1}	构成比 Freq./%	中标率 ASR China/ 100 000^{-1}	世标率 ASR world/ 100 000^{-1}	累积率 Cum. Rate 0~74/%
合计 All	合计 Both	25 707	4.09	1.34	2.60	2.58	0.30
	男性 Male	16 701	5.24	1.60	3.41	3.37	0.40
	女性 Female	9 006	2.91	1.03	1.80	1.80	0.20
城市地区 Urban areas	合计 Both	14 386	5.36	1.61	3.30	3.27	0.38
	男性 Male	9 497	7.06	2.00	4.45	4.41	0.52
	女性 Female	4 889	3.65	1.17	2.19	2.18	0.25
农村地区 Rural areas	合计 Both	11 321	3.15	1.11	2.06	2.04	0.23
	男性 Male	7 204	3.91	1.27	2.61	2.58	0.30
	女性 Female	4 117	2.34	0.91	1.50	1.50	0.17
东部地区 Eastern areas	合计 Both	15 208	6.00	1.64	3.62	3.57	0.42
	男性 Male	10 158	7.97	2.08	4.92	4.85	0.57
	女性 Female	5 050	4.00	1.16	2.36	2.34	0.27
中部地区 Central areas	合计 Both	5 314	3.53	1.25	2.36	2.34	0.27
	男性 Male	3 336	4.36	1.45	2.99	2.95	0.34
	女性 Female	1 978	2.68	1.02	1.75	1.75	0.20
西部地区 Western areas	合计 Both	5 185	2.31	0.92	1.52	1.51	0.17
	男性 Male	3 207	2.79	0.99	1.88	1.86	0.21
	女性 Female	1 978	1.80	0.82	1.16	1.16	0.13

表 5-17d　中国肿瘤登记地区肾癌死亡情况

Table 5-17d　Mortality of kidney cancer in the registration areas of China

地区 Area	性别 Sex	死亡数 No. deaths	粗率 Crude rate/ 100 000^{-1}	构成比 Freq./%	中标率 ASR China/ 100 000^{-1}	世标率 ASR world/ 100 000^{-1}	累积率 Cum. Rate 0~74/%
合计 All	合计 Both	8 583	1.37	0.79	0.76	0.76	0.08
	男性 Male	5 676	1.78	0.81	1.04	1.05	0.12
	女性 Female	2 907	0.94	0.75	0.49	0.49	0.05
城市地区 Urban areas	合计 Both	4 675	1.74	0.98	0.92	0.92	0.10
	男性 Male	3 093	2.30	1.02	1.28	1.29	0.14
	女性 Female	1 582	1.18	0.91	0.59	0.58	0.06
农村地区 Rural areas	合计 Both	3 908	1.09	0.64	0.64	0.64	0.07
	男性 Male	2 583	1.40	0.65	0.86	0.86	0.10
	女性 Female	1 325	0.75	0.62	0.42	0.42	0.05
东部地区 Eastern areas	合计 Both	4 623	1.82	0.96	0.91	0.91	0.10
	男性 Male	3 141	2.46	1.03	1.30	1.31	0.14
	女性 Female	1 482	1.17	0.83	0.55	0.55	0.06
中部地区 Central areas	合计 Both	1 887	1.26	0.77	0.77	0.76	0.09
	男性 Male	1 220	1.59	0.78	1.03	1.02	0.12
	女性 Female	667	0.90	0.75	0.52	0.52	0.06
西部地区 Western areas	合计 Both	2 073	0.92	0.58	0.56	0.56	0.06
	男性 Male	1 315	1.15	0.56	0.72	0.73	0.08
	女性 Female	758	0.69	0.62	0.40	0.40	0.04

表 5-17e　中国肿瘤登记地区肾盂癌发病情况
Table 5-17e　Incidence of cancer of renal pelvis in the registration areas of China

地区 Area	性别 Sex	发病数 No. cases	粗率 Crude rate/ 100 000⁻¹	构成比 Freq. /%	中标率 ASR China/ 100 000⁻¹	世标率 ASR world/ 100 000⁻¹	累积率 Cum. Rate 0~74/%
合计 All	合计 Both	3 199	0.51	0.17	0.29	0.28	0.03
	男性 Male	1 914	0.60	0.18	0.35	0.36	0.04
	女性 Female	1 285	0.42	0.15	0.22	0.22	0.03
城市地区 Urban areas	合计 Both	1 832	0.68	0.20	0.37	0.37	0.04
	男性 Male	1 069	0.80	0.22	0.46	0.45	0.05
	女性 Female	763	0.57	0.18	0.29	0.28	0.03
农村地区 Rural areas	合计 Both	1 367	0.38	0.13	0.22	0.22	0.03
	男性 Male	845	0.46	0.15	0.28	0.28	0.03
	女性 Female	522	0.30	0.12	0.16	0.16	0.02
东部地区 Eastern areas	合计 Both	1 840	0.73	0.20	0.37	0.37	0.04
	男性 Male	1 083	0.85	0.22	0.46	0.46	0.05
	女性 Female	757	0.60	0.17	0.29	0.28	0.03
中部地区 Central areas	合计 Both	610	0.41	0.14	0.25	0.25	0.03
	男性 Male	389	0.51	0.17	0.32	0.33	0.04
	女性 Female	221	0.30	0.11	0.17	0.17	0.02
西部地区 Western areas	合计 Both	749	0.33	0.13	0.20	0.20	0.02
	男性 Male	442	0.39	0.14	0.24	0.24	0.03
	女性 Female	307	0.28	0.13	0.16	0.15	0.02

表 5-17f　中国肿瘤登记地区肾盂癌死亡情况
Table 5-17f　Mortality of cancer of renal pelvis in the registration areas of China

地区 Area	性别 Sex	死亡数 No. deaths	粗率 Crude rate/ 100 000⁻¹	构成比 Freq. /%	中标率 ASR China/ 100 000⁻¹	世标率 ASR world/ 100 000⁻¹	累积率 Cum. Rate 0~74/%
合计 All	合计 Both	1 416	0.23	0.13	0.12	0.12	0.01
	男性 Male	840	0.26	0.12	0.15	0.15	0.02
	女性 Female	576	0.19	0.15	0.09	0.09	0.01
城市地区 Urban areas	合计 Both	828	0.31	0.17	0.15	0.15	0.02
	男性 Male	477	0.35	0.16	0.19	0.19	0.02
	女性 Female	351	0.26	0.20	0.11	0.12	0.01
农村地区 Rural areas	合计 Both	588	0.16	0.10	0.09	0.09	0.01
	男性 Male	363	0.20	0.09	0.12	0.12	0.01
	女性 Female	225	0.13	0.10	0.06	0.06	0.01
东部地区 Eastern areas	合计 Both	768	0.30	0.16	0.14	0.14	0.01
	男性 Male	441	0.35	0.14	0.17	0.18	0.02
	女性 Female	327	0.26	0.18	0.10	0.10	0.01
中部地区 Central areas	合计 Both	280	0.19	0.11	0.11	0.11	0.01
	男性 Male	178	0.23	0.11	0.14	0.14	0.01
	女性 Female	102	0.14	0.11	0.07	0.08	0.01
西部地区 Western areas	合计 Both	368	0.16	0.10	0.10	0.10	0.01
	男性 Male	221	0.19	0.09	0.12	0.12	0.01
	女性 Female	147	0.13	0.12	0.07	0.07	0.01

表 5-17g 中国肿瘤登记地区输尿管癌发病情况

Table 5-17g Incidence of ureter cancer in the registration areas of China

地区 Area	性别 Sex	发病数 No. cases	粗率 Crude rate/ 100 000^{-1}	构成比 Freq./%	中标率 ASR China/ 100 000^{-1}	世标率 ASR world/ 100 000^{-1}	累积率 Cum. Rate 0~74/%
合计	合计 Both	3 564	0.57	0.19	0.31	0.31	0.04
All	男性 Male	1 999	0.63	0.19	0.36	0.36	0.04
	女性 Female	1 565	0.51	0.18	0.26	0.26	0.03
城市地区	合计 Both	2 068	0.77	0.23	0.40	0.40	0.05
Urban areas	男性 Male	1 156	0.86	0.24	0.47	0.48	0.06
	女性 Female	912	0.68	0.22	0.34	0.33	0.04
农村地区	合计 Both	1 496	0.42	0.15	0.24	0.23	0.03
Rural areas	男性 Male	843	0.46	0.15	0.27	0.27	0.03
	女性 Female	653	0.37	0.14	0.20	0.20	0.02
东部地区	合计 Both	2 094	0.83	0.23	0.41	0.41	0.05
Eastern areas	男性 Male	1 182	0.93	0.24	0.48	0.49	0.06
	女性 Female	912	0.72	0.21	0.34	0.33	0.04
中部地区	合计 Both	692	0.46	0.16	0.28	0.27	0.03
Central areas	男性 Male	403	0.53	0.17	0.33	0.33	0.04
	女性 Female	289	0.39	0.15	0.22	0.22	0.03
西部地区	合计 Both	778	0.35	0.14	0.20	0.20	0.02
Western areas	男性 Male	414	0.36	0.13	0.22	0.22	0.03
	女性 Female	364	0.33	0.15	0.19	0.18	0.02

表 5-17h 中国肿瘤登记地区输尿管癌死亡情况

Table 5-17h Mortality of ureter cancer in the registration areas of China

地区 Area	性别 Sex	死亡数 No. deaths	粗率 Crude rate/ 100 000^{-1}	构成比 Freq./%	中标率 ASR China/ 100 000^{-1}	世标率 ASR world/ 100 000^{-1}	累积率 Cum. Rate 0~74/%
合计	合计 Both	1 615	0.26	0.15	0.13	0.13	0.01
All	男性 Male	867	0.27	0.12	0.15	0.15	0.02
	女性 Female	748	0.24	0.19	0.11	0.11	0.01
城市地区	合计 Both	987	0.37	0.21	0.18	0.18	0.02
Urban areas	男性 Male	518	0.39	0.17	0.20	0.21	0.02
	女性 Female	469	0.35	0.27	0.16	0.16	0.02
农村地区	合计 Both	628	0.17	0.10	0.09	0.09	0.01
Rural areas	男性 Male	349	0.19	0.09	0.11	0.11	0.01
	女性 Female	279	0.16	0.13	0.08	0.08	0.01
东部地区	合计 Both	949	0.37	0.20	0.17	0.17	0.02
Eastern areas	男性 Male	522	0.41	0.17	0.20	0.21	0.02
	女性 Female	427	0.34	0.24	0.14	0.14	0.01
中部地区	合计 Both	321	0.21	0.13	0.12	0.12	0.01
Central areas	男性 Male	176	0.23	0.11	0.14	0.14	0.02
	女性 Female	145	0.20	0.16	0.10	0.10	0.01
西部地区	合计 Both	345	0.15	0.10	0.09	0.09	0.01
Western areas	男性 Male	169	0.15	0.07	0.09	0.09	0.01
	女性 Female	176	0.16	0.14	0.08	0.08	0.01

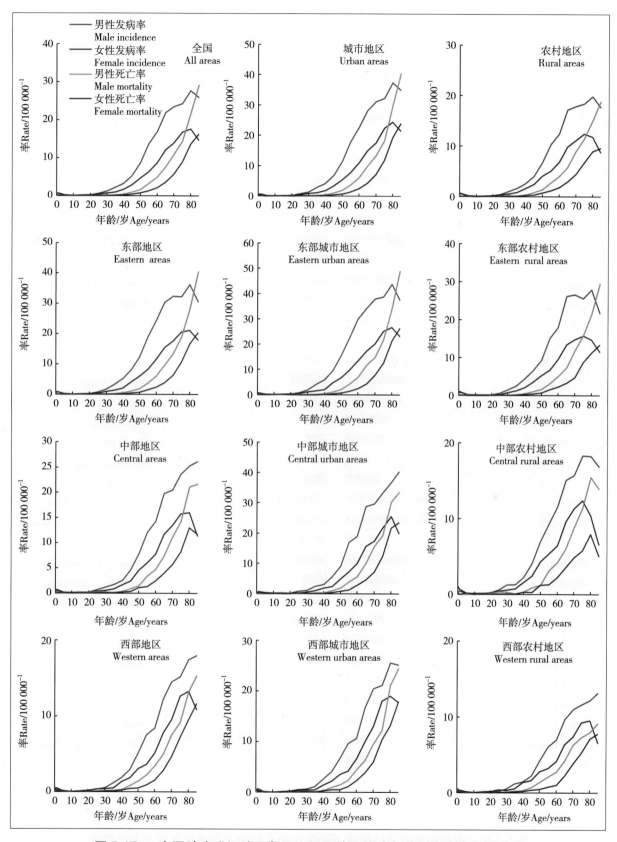

图 5-17a　中国肿瘤登记地区肾及泌尿系统不明癌年龄别发病率和死亡率

Figure 5-17a　Age-specific incidence and mortality rates of cancer of kidney & unspecified urinary organs in the registration areas of China

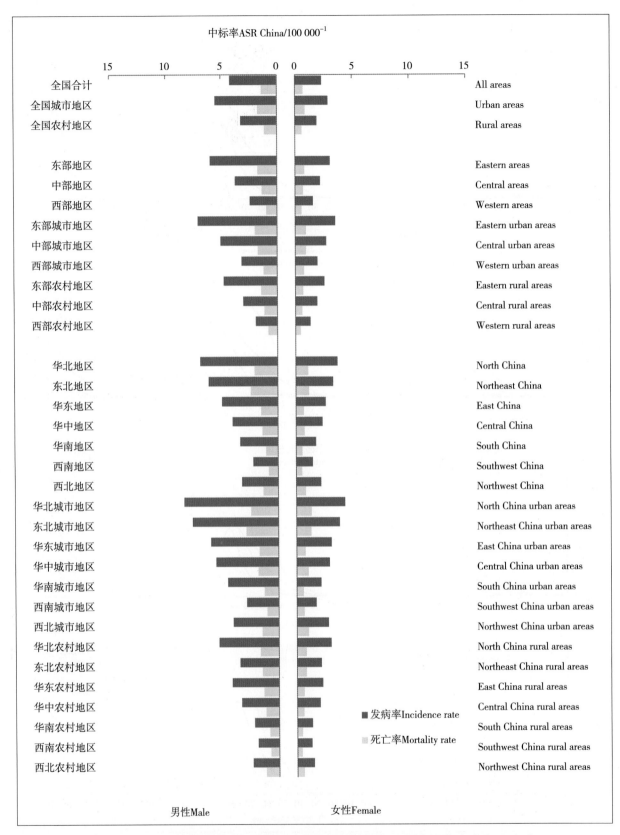

图 5-17b　中国肿瘤登记地区肾及泌尿系统不明癌不同地区发病率和死亡率

Figure 5-17b　Incidence and mortality rates of cancer of kidney & unspecified urinary organs in different registration areas of China

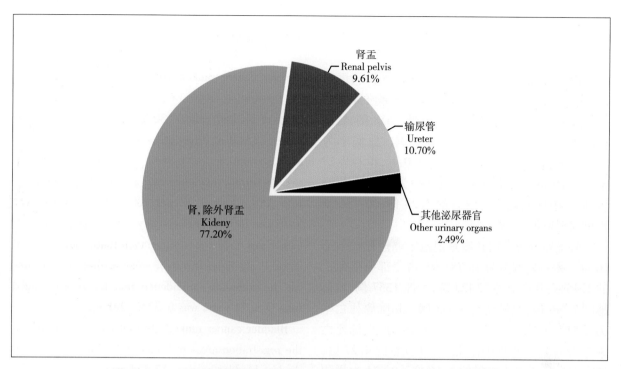

图 5-17c　中国肿瘤登记地区肾及泌尿系统不明癌亚部位分布情况
Figure 5-17c　Subsite distribution of cancer of kidney & unspecified urinary organs
in the registration areas of China

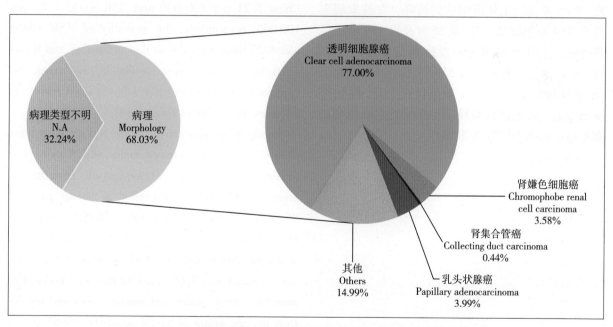

图 5-17d　中国肿瘤登记地区肾及泌尿系统不明癌病理分型情况
Figure 5-17d　Morphological distribution of cancer of kidney & unspecified urinary organs
in the registration areas of China

18 膀胱

膀胱癌位居中国肿瘤登记地区癌症发病谱第16位。新发病例数为 37 624 例,占全部癌症发病的 1.96%;其中男性 30 006 例,女性 7 618 例,城市地区 18 980 例,农村地区 18 644 例。发病率为 5.99/10 万,中标发病率为 3.32/10 万,世标发病率为 3.29/10 万;男性中标发病率为女性的 4.22 倍,城市中标发病率为农村的 1.28 倍。0~74 岁累积发病率为 0.37%(表 5-18a)。

膀胱癌位居中国肿瘤登记地区癌症死亡谱第16位。死亡病例数为 15 781 例,占全部癌症死亡的 1.45%;其中男性 12 424 例,女性 3 357 例,城市地区 7 746 例,农村地区 8 035 例。膀胱癌死亡率为 2.51/10 万,中标死亡率 1.21/10 万,世标死亡率 1.22/10 万;男性中标死亡率为女性的 4.27 倍,城市中标死亡率为农村的 1.16 倍。0~74 岁累积死亡率为 0.10%(表 5-18b)。

膀胱癌的年龄别发病率和死亡率呈明显的性别差异。男性发病率自 40~45 岁组开始快速上升,至 85 岁及以上年龄组达到高峰。女性发病率自 50~54 岁组缓慢上升,至 85 岁及以上年龄组达到高峰。男性年龄别峰值发病率是女性的 4.65 倍。男性膀胱癌死亡率自 55~59 岁组开始快速上升,女性死亡率自 60~64 岁组快速上升,均至 85 岁及以上年龄组达到高峰。男性年龄别峰值死亡率是女性的 4.56 倍(图 5-18a)。

18 Bladder

Bladder cancer ranked 16th for cancer incidence in the registration areas of China. There were 37 624 new cases of bladder cancer(30 006 males and 7 618 females,18 980 in urban areas and 18 644 in rural areas),accounting for 1.96% of all new cancer cases. The crude incidence rate was 5.99 per 100 000, with ASR China 3.32 per 100 000 and ASR world 3.29 per 100 000,respectively. The incidence of ASR China was 4.22 times in males as that in females,and it was 1.28 times in urban areas as that in rural areas. The cumulative incidence rate for subjects aged from 0 to 74 years was 0.37%(Table 5-18a).

Bladder cancer ranked 16th for cancer mortality in the registration areas of China. A total of 15 781 cases died of bladder cancer(12 424 males and 3 357 females,7 746 in urban areas and 8 035 in rural areas),accounting for 1.45% of all cancer deaths. The crude mortality rate was 2.51 per 100 000,with ASR China 1.21 per 100 000 and ASR world 1.22 per 100 000,respectively. The mortality of ASR China was 4.27 times in males as that in females,and it was 1.16 times in urban areas as that in rural areas. The cumulative mortality rate for subjects aged from 0 to 74 years was 0.10%(Table 5-18b).

Trends of age-specific incidence and mortality rates showed differences between males and females. The incidence rate in males increased rapidly from the age group of 40-45 years and peaked at the age group of 85 years old. The incidence rate in females increased slowly from the age group of 50-54 years and peaked at the age group of 85 years old. The peak incidence rate in males was 4.65 times as that in females. The mortality rate in males and females increased rapidly from the age group of 55-59 years and 60-64 years, and both peaked at the age group of 85 years old. The peak mortality rate in males was 4.56 times as that in females(Figure 5-18a).

膀胱癌的中标发病率和死亡率呈现地域差异。东部地区的中标发病率和死亡率高于中部和西部地区,中部和西部地区中标发病率和死亡率水平接近。七大行政区中,男性中标发病率为东北地区最高,西南地区最低,中标死亡率为东北地区最高,华南地区最低;女性中标发病率最高的为华北地区,最低为华南地区,中标死亡率最高的为东北地区,最低为华南地区(表 5-18a,表 5-18b,图5-18b)。

约 20.20% 的膀胱癌新发病例具有明确的亚部位信息,其中膀胱侧壁的比例最高,占 37.68%,其次是膀胱三角区(16.18%)、膀胱后壁(12.58%)、交搭跨越(8.95%)、膀胱前壁(7.08%)、膀胱顶(6.39%)、膀胱颈(4.97%)、输尿管口(4.93%)和脐尿管(1.24%)(图 5-18c)。

全部膀胱癌病例中有明确组织学类型的病例占 66.04%,其中移行细胞癌是最主要的病理类型,占 77.35%;其次是其他类型(9.77%)、鳞状细胞癌(7.37%)和腺癌(5.51%)(图 5-18d)。

The incidence and mortality of ASR China of bladder cancer varied geographically. Eastern areas had the highest incidence and mortality rates of ASR China, and the incidence and mortality of ASR China in central and western areas were similar. Among the seven administrative districts, Northeast China had the highest incidence rate of ASR China and Southwest China had the lowest incidence rate of ASR China for males. Northeast China had the highest mortality rate of ASR China and South China had the lowest mortality rate of ASR China for males. North China had the highest incidence rate of ASR China and South China had the lowest incidence rate of ASR China for females. Northeast China had the highest mortality rate of ASR China and South China had the lowest mortality rate of ASR China for females(Table 5-18a, Table 5-18b, Figure 5-18b).

About 20.20% of the bladder cancer cases had complete information on subsite. Among them, lateral wall was the most common subsite(37.68%), followed by trigone(16.18%), posterior wall(12.58%), overlapping(8.95%), anterior wall(7.08%), dome(6.39%), bladder neck(4.97%), ureteric orifice(4.93%) and urachus(1.24%)(Figure 5-18c).

About 66.04% of the bladder cancer cases could be morphologically classified. Transitional cell carcinoma was the most common histological type, accounting for 77.35% of all cases, followed by other types(9.77%), squamous cell carcinoma(7.37%) and adenocarcinoma(5.51%)(Figure 5-18d).

表 5-18a　中国肿瘤登记地区膀胱癌发病情况

Table 5-18a　Incidence of bladder cancer in the registration areas of China

地区 Area	性别 Sex	发病数 No. cases	粗率 Crude rate/ 100 000^{-1}	构成比 Freq./%	中标率 ASR China/ 100 000^{-1}	世标率 ASR world/ 100 000^{-1}	累积率 Cum. rate 0~74/%	顺位 Rank
合计 All	合计 Both	37 624	5.99	1.96	3.32	3.29	0.37	16
	男性 Male	30 006	9.41	2.87	5.48	5.45	0.61	7
	女性 Female	7 618	2.46	0.87	1.30	1.27	0.14	18
城市地区 Urban areas	合计 Both	18 980	7.07	2.12	3.78	3.75	0.42	15
	男性 Male	15 048	11.19	3.16	6.26	6.24	0.70	8
	女性 Female	3 932	2.93	0.94	1.49	1.47	0.16	17
农村地区 Rural areas	合计 Both	18 644	5.18	1.82	2.96	2.93	0.33	16
	男性 Male	14 958	8.11	2.63	4.88	4.84	0.54	7
	女性 Female	3 686	2.10	0.81	1.15	1.12	0.13	19
东部地区 Eastern areas	合计 Both	19 381	7.64	2.09	3.88	3.84	0.44	17
	男性 Male	15 510	12.17	3.17	6.49	6.45	0.74	8
	女性 Female	3 871	3.07	0.89	1.47	1.44	0.16	17
中部地区 Central areas	合计 Both	7 579	5.04	1.78	3.03	3.01	0.34	16
	男性 Male	6 036	7.89	2.62	4.97	4.96	0.56	7
	女性 Female	1 543	2.09	0.79	1.21	1.18	0.13	18
西部地区 Western areas	合计 Both	10 664	4.75	1.88	2.80	2.76	0.30	16
	男性 Male	8 460	7.37	2.60	4.54	4.50	0.48	7
	女性 Female	2 204	2.01	0.92	1.14	1.11	0.12	19

表 5-18b　中国肿瘤登记地区膀胱癌死亡情况

Table 5-18b　Mortality of bladder cancer in the registration areas of China

地区 Area	性别 Sex	死亡数 No. deaths	粗率 Crude rate/ 100 000^{-1}	构成比 Freq./%	中标率 ASR China/ 100 000^{-1}	世标率 ASR world/ 100 000^{-1}	累积率 Cum. Rate 0~74/%	顺位 Rank
合计 All	合计 Both	15 781	2.51	1.45	1.21	1.22	0.10	16
	男性 Male	12 424	3.90	1.78	2.05	2.09	0.17	11
	女性 Female	3 357	1.08	0.86	0.48	0.48	0.04	16
城市地区 Urban areas	合计 Both	7 746	2.89	1.62	1.31	1.34	0.11	15
	男性 Male	6 024	4.48	1.99	2.21	2.27	0.18	11
	女性 Female	1 722	1.28	0.99	0.53	0.54	0.04	16
农村地区 Rural areas	合计 Both	8 035	2.23	1.32	1.13	1.13	0.10	16
	男性 Male	6 400	3.47	1.62	1.92	1.94	0.16	11
	女性 Female	1 635	0.93	0.76	0.44	0.44	0.04	19
东部地区 Eastern areas	合计 Both	7 895	3.11	1.63	1.29	1.31	0.11	15
	男性 Male	6 179	4.85	2.02	2.22	2.27	0.18	10
	女性 Female	1 716	1.36	0.96	0.50	0.51	0.04	16
中部地区 Central areas	合计 Both	3 125	2.08	1.27	1.13	1.13	0.10	16
	男性 Male	2 479	3.24	1.58	1.91	1.93	0.17	11
	女性 Female	646	0.88	0.73	0.44	0.43	0.04	18
西部地区 Western areas	合计 Both	4 761	2.12	1.33	1.14	1.15	0.10	16
	男性 Male	3 766	3.28	1.59	1.90	1.92	0.16	11
	女性 Female	995	0.91	0.81	0.46	0.46	0.04	19

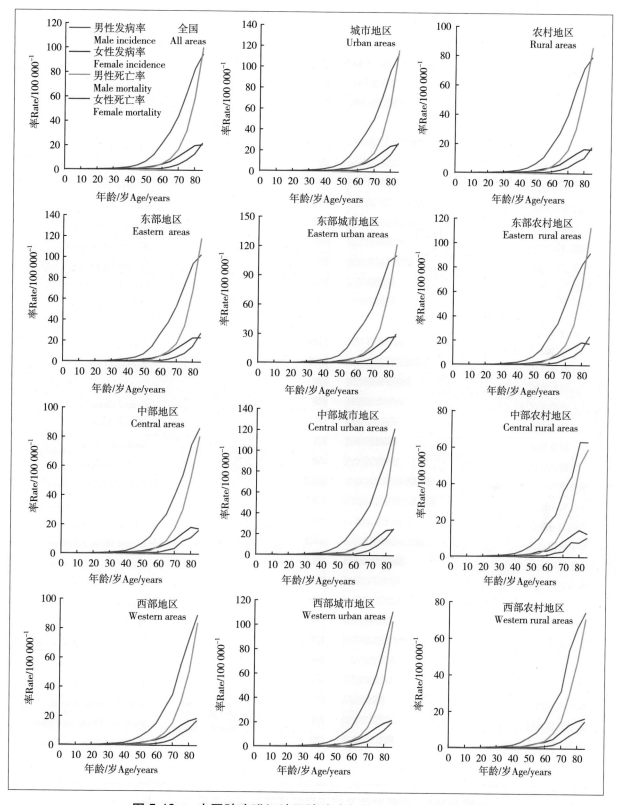

图 5-18a　中国肿瘤登记地区膀胱癌年龄别发病率和死亡率

Figure 5-18a　Age-specific incidence and mortality rates of bladder cancer in the registration areas of China

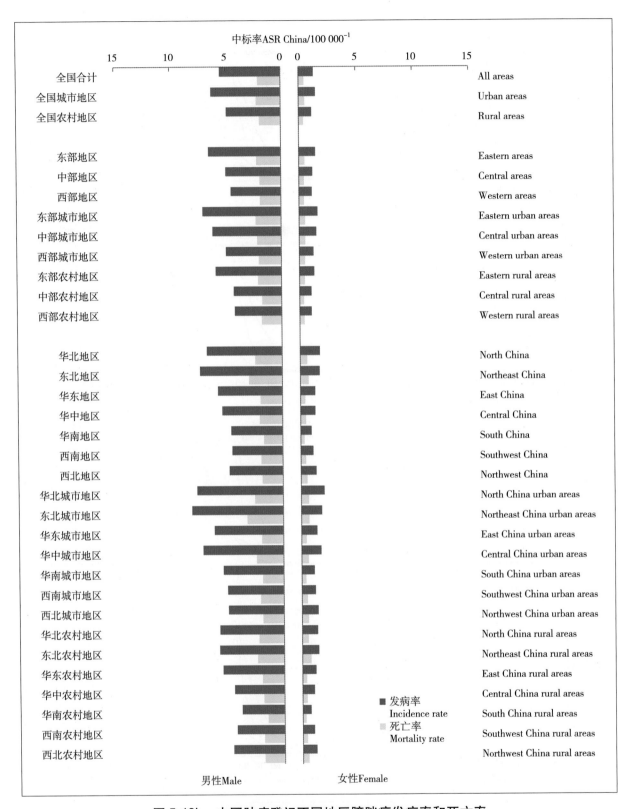

中标率ASR China/100 000⁻¹

15	10	5	0	5	10	15

全国合计 — All areas
全国城市地区 — Urban areas
全国农村地区 — Rural areas

东部地区 — Eastern areas
中部地区 — Central areas
西部地区 — Western areas
东部城市地区 — Eastern urban areas
中部城市地区 — Central urban areas
西部城市地区 — Western urban areas
东部农村地区 — Eastern rural areas
中部农村地区 — Central rural areas
西部农村地区 — Western rural areas

华北地区 — North China
东北地区 — Northeast China
华东地区 — East China
华中地区 — Central China
华南地区 — South China
西南地区 — Southwest China
西北地区 — Northwest China
华北城市地区 — North China urban areas
东北城市地区 — Northeast China urban areas
华东城市地区 — East China urban areas
华中城市地区 — Central China urban areas
华南城市地区 — South China urban areas
西南城市地区 — Southwest China urban areas
西北城市地区 — Northwest China urban areas
华北农村地区 — North China rural areas
东北农村地区 — Northeast China rural areas
华东农村地区 — East China rural areas
华中农村地区 — Central China rural areas
华南农村地区 — South China rural areas
西南农村地区 — Southwest China rural areas
西北农村地区 — Northwest China rural areas

■ 发病率 Incidence rate
■ 死亡率 Mortality rate

男性Male　　　女性Female

图 5-18b　中国肿瘤登记不同地区膀胱癌发病率和死亡率
Figure 5-18b　Incidence and mortality rates of bladder cancer in different registration areas of China

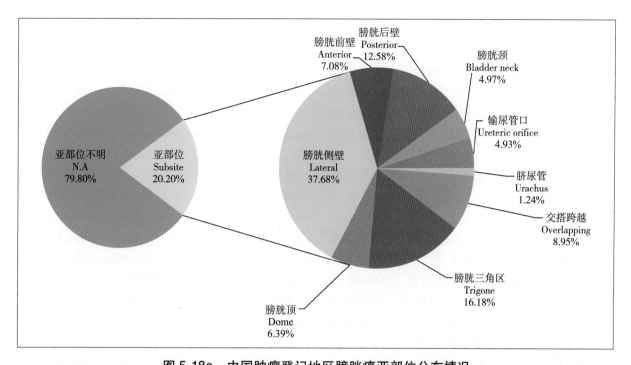

图 5-18c　中国肿瘤登记地区膀胱癌亚部位分布情况
Figure 5-18c　Subsite distribution of bladder cancer in the registration areas of China

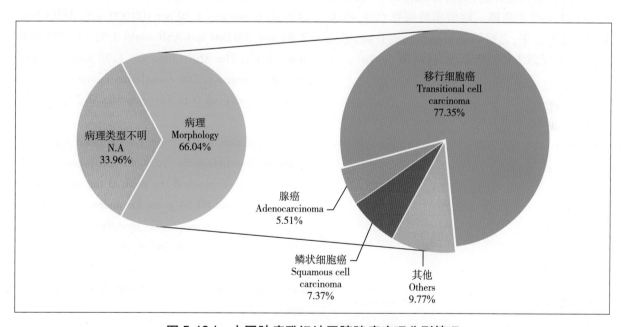

图 5-18d　中国肿瘤登记地区膀胱癌病理分型情况
Figure 5-18d　Morphological distribution of bladder cancer in the
registration areas of China

19 脑

脑瘤位居中国肿瘤登记地区癌症发病谱的第
11 位。新发病例数为 52 104 例,占全部癌症发病
的 2.72%;其中男性 23 572 例,女性 28 532 例,城
市地区 23 374 例,农村地区 28 730 例。脑瘤发病
率为 8.29/10 万,中标发病率为 5.79/10 万,世标
发病率为 5.70/10 万;女性中标发病率为男性的
1.15 倍。0~74 岁累积发病率为 0.59%(表 5-
19a)。

脑瘤位居中国肿瘤登记地区癌症死亡谱的第
10 位。死亡病例数为 27 014 例,占全部癌症死亡
的 2.48%;其中男性 14 845 例,女性 12 169 例,城
市地区 11 164 例,农村地区 15 850 例。脑瘤死亡
率为 4.30/10 万,中标死亡率 2.81/10 万,世标死
亡率 2.81/10 万;男性中标死亡率为女性的 1.30
倍。0~74 岁累积死亡率为 0.29%(表 5-19b)。

脑瘤年龄别发病率 20 岁前处于较低水平,之
后均随年龄增长而升高,男女分别在 85 岁及以上
和 80~84 岁组达高峰。脑瘤年龄别死亡率 40 岁
前处于较低水平,之后均随年龄增长而升高,男女
均在 85 岁及以上年龄组达到高峰(图 5-19a)。

19 Brain

Brain tumor ranked 11th for cancer incidence in the
registration areas of China. There were 52 104 new
cases of brain tumor(23 572 males and 28 532 females,23 374 in urban areas and 28 730 in rural areas), accounting for 2.72% of all cancer cases. The
crude incidence rate of brain tumor was 8.29 per
100 000,with ASR China 5.79 per 100 000 and ASR
world 5.70 per 100 000,respectively. The ASR China
was 1.15 times in females as that in males. The cumulative incidence rate for subjects aged from 0 to 74
years was 0.59%(Table 5-19a).

Brain tumor was the 10th most common cause of
cancer deaths in the registration areas of China. The
number of deaths due to brain tumor was 27 014
(14 845 males and 12 169 females,11 164 in urban
areas and 15 850 in rural areas), accounting for
2.48% of all cancer deaths. The crude mortality rate
of brain tumor was 4.30 per 100 000,with ASR China
2.81 per 100 000 and ASR world 2.81 per 100 000,
respectively. The ASR China was 1.30 times in males
as that in females. The cumulative mortality rate for
subjects aged from 0 to 74 years was 0.29%(Table
5-19b).

The age-specific incidence rate of brain tumor was
relatively low before 20 years old and increased with
age after that. It reached the peak at the age group of
85 years old and 80-84 years for males and females,
respectively. The age-specific mortality rate of brain
tumor was relatively low before 40 years old and increased with age after that. It reached the peak at the
age group of 85 years old for both sexes(Figure 5-
19a).

脑瘤的中标发病率城市地区均高于农村地区,中标死亡率农村地区高于城市地区。中标发病率以东部地区最高,其次为中部地区,西部地区最低。中标死亡率以中部地区最高,其次为西部地区,东部地区最低。在七大行政区中,华中地区男性和华南地区女性的中标发病率最高,东北地区男性和女性的中标发病率最低;华中地区男性和女性的中标死亡率最高,华北地区男性和女性的中标死亡率最低(表5-19a,表5-19b,图5-19b)。

约39.37%的脑瘤新发病例具有明确的亚部位信息,其中大脑占24.16%,额叶占21.23%,颞叶占13.84%,小脑占10.77%,交搭跨越占10.72%,脑干占6.52%,脑室占5.74%,顶叶占4.32%,枕叶占2.70%(图5-19c)。

The incidence rates(ASR China)of brain tumor were higher in urban areas than in rural areas while the mortality rates(ASR China)of brain tumor were higher in rural areas than in urban areas. The incidence rate(ASR China)was highest in eastern areas, followed by central and western areas. The mortality rate(ASR China)was highest in central areas, followed by western and eastern areas. Among the seven administrative districts, the highest incidence rates(ASR China)were shown in Central China for males and South China for females, respectively, while Northeast China had the lowest incidence rates(ASR China)for both sexes. The highest mortality rates(ASR China)were found in Central China for both sexes while North China had the lowest mortality rates(ASR China)for both sexes(Table 5-19a, Table 5-19b, Figure 5-19b).

About 39.37% of brain tumor cases had specified sub categorical information. Among those, 24.16% of cases occurred in cerebrum, followed by frontal lobe(21.23%), temporal lobe(13.84%), cerebellum(10.77%), overlapping(10.72%), brain stem(6.52%), cerebral ventricle(5.74%), parietal lobe(4.32%) and occipital lobe(2.70%)(Figure 5-19c).

表 5-19a 中国肿瘤登记地区脑瘤发病情况

Table 5-19a Incidence of brain tumor in the registration areas of China

地区 Area	性别 Sex	发病数 No. cases	粗率 Crude rate/ 100 000^{-1}	构成比 Freq. /%	中标率 ASR China/ 100 000^{-1}	世标率 ASR world/ 100 000^{-1}	累积率 Cum. Rate 0~74/%	顺位 Rank
合计 All	合计 Both	52 104	8.29	2.72	5.79	5.70	0.59	11
	男性 Male	23 572	7.39	2.26	5.38	5.31	0.54	11
	女性 Female	28 532	9.22	3.28	6.18	6.09	0.64	9
城市地区 Urban areas	合计 Both	23 374	8.71	2.62	5.92	5.84	0.61	11
	男性 Male	10 263	7.63	2.16	5.41	5.35	0.54	13
	女性 Female	13 111	9.78	3.14	6.41	6.32	0.67	9
农村地区 Rural areas	合计 Both	28 730	7.98	2.81	5.68	5.59	0.58	11
	男性 Male	13 309	7.22	2.34	5.36	5.27	0.54	9
	女性 Female	15 421	8.78	3.40	6.00	5.90	0.62	10
东部地区 Eastern areas	合计 Both	24 996	9.85	2.70	6.50	6.38	0.67	11
	男性 Male	10 753	8.44	2.20	5.85	5.75	0.59	13
	女性 Female	14 243	11.29	3.26	7.13	7.00	0.75	9
中部地区 Central areas	合计 Both	11 979	7.97	2.82	5.81	5.77	0.59	11
	男性 Male	5 661	7.40	2.45	5.63	5.59	0.57	8
	女性 Female	6 318	8.56	3.25	5.99	5.93	0.62	10
西部地区 Western areas	合计 Both	15 129	6.74	2.67	4.90	4.82	0.50	12
	男性 Male	7 158	6.24	2.20	4.67	4.60	0.47	9
	女性 Female	7 971	7.27	3.31	5.13	5.04	0.52	9

表 5-19b 中国肿瘤登记地区脑瘤死亡情况

Table 5-19b Mortality of brain tumor in the registration areas of China

地区 Area	性别 Sex	死亡数 No. deaths	粗率 Crude rate/ 100 000^{-1}	构成比 Freq. /%	中标率 ASR China/ 100 000^{-1}	世标率 ASR world/ 100 000^{-1}	累积率 Cum. rate 0~74/%	顺位 Rank
合计 All	合计 Both	27 014	4.30	2.48	2.81	2.81	0.29	10
	男性 Male	14 845	4.66	2.13	3.18	3.16	0.33	8
	女性 Female	12 169	3.93	3.13	2.45	2.45	0.25	9
城市地区 Urban areas	合计 Both	11 164	4.16	2.34	2.64	2.65	0.27	12
	男性 Male	6 072	4.52	2.00	2.99	2.99	0.31	10
	女性 Female	5 092	3.80	2.93	2.31	2.32	0.23	10
农村地区 Rural areas	合计 Both	15 850	4.40	2.60	2.95	2.93	0.31	9
	男性 Male	8 773	4.76	2.22	3.33	3.29	0.35	7
	女性 Female	7 077	4.03	3.29	2.56	2.56	0.27	9
东部地区 Eastern areas	合计 Both	11 478	4.52	2.37	2.73	2.72	0.28	12
	男性 Male	6 162	4.83	2.02	3.06	3.04	0.32	11
	女性 Female	5 316	4.21	2.98	2.40	2.39	0.24	9
中部地区 Central areas	合计 Both	6 598	4.39	2.69	3.02	3.02	0.32	9
	男性 Male	3 602	4.71	2.30	3.37	3.35	0.35	7
	女性 Female	2 996	4.06	3.38	2.67	2.70	0.28	9
西部地区 Western areas	合计 Both	8 938	3.98	2.49	2.77	2.77	0.29	10
	男性 Male	5 081	4.43	2.15	3.19	3.17	0.33	7
	女性 Female	3 857	3.52	3.16	2.35	2.35	0.24	9

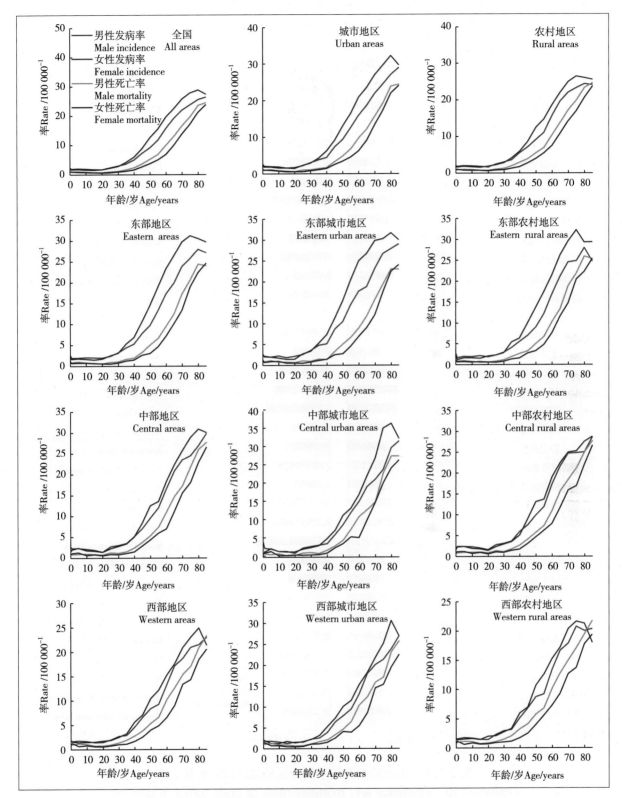

图 5-19a　中国肿瘤登记地区脑瘤年龄别发病率和死亡率

Figure 5-19a　Age-specific incidence and mortality rates of brain tumor
in the registration areas of China

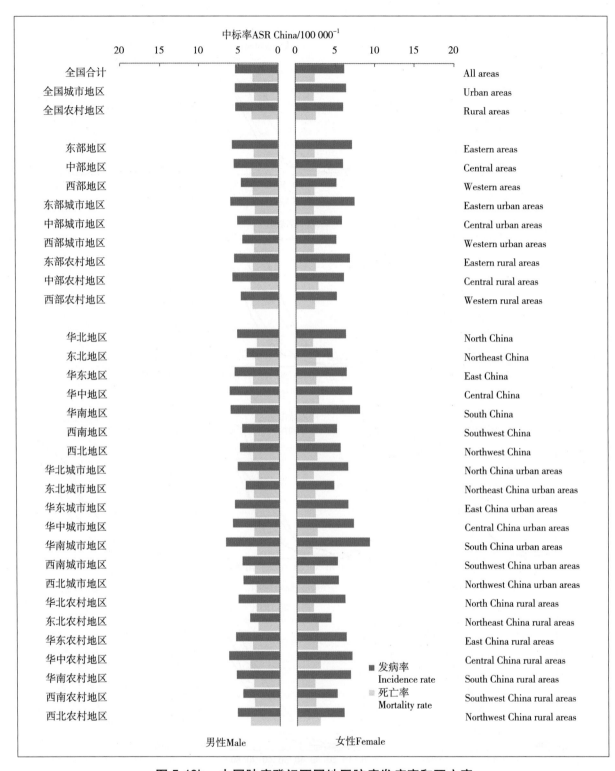

中标率ASR China/100 000⁻¹

	男性Male		女性Female	

全国合计 — All areas
全国城市地区 — Urban areas
全国农村地区 — Rural areas

东部地区 — Eastern areas
中部地区 — Central areas
西部地区 — Western areas
东部城市地区 — Eastern urban areas
中部城市地区 — Central urban areas
西部城市地区 — Western urban areas
东部农村地区 — Eastern rural areas
中部农村地区 — Central rural areas
西部农村地区 — Western rural areas

华北地区 — North China
东北地区 — Northeast China
华东地区 — East China
华中地区 — Central China
华南地区 — South China
西南地区 — Southwest China
西北地区 — Northwest China
华北城市地区 — North China urban areas
东北城市地区 — Northeast China urban areas
华东城市地区 — East China urban areas
华中城市地区 — Central China urban areas
华南城市地区 — South China urban areas
西南城市地区 — Southwest China urban areas
西北城市地区 — Northwest China urban areas
华北农村地区 — North China rural areas
东北农村地区 — Northeast China rural areas
华东农村地区 — East China rural areas
华中农村地区 — Central China rural areas
华南农村地区 — South China rural areas
西南农村地区 — Southwest China rural areas
西北农村地区 — Northwest China rural areas

■ 发病率 Incidence rate
□ 死亡率 Mortality rate

图 5-19b　中国肿瘤登记不同地区脑瘤发病率和死亡率
Figure 5-19b　Incidence and mortality rates of brain tumor in different registration areas of China

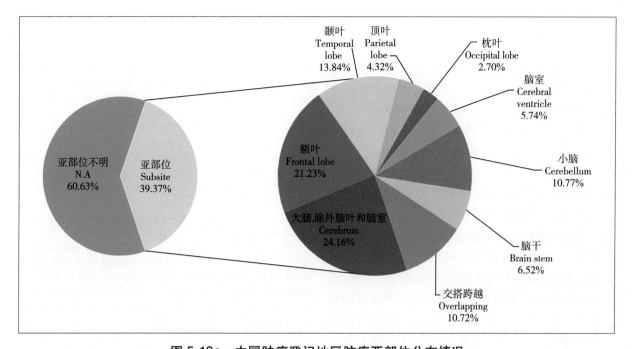

图 5-19c　中国肿瘤登记地区脑瘤亚部位分布情况

Figure 5-19c　Subsite distribution of brain tumor in the registration areas of China

20 甲状腺

甲状腺癌位居中国肿瘤登记地区癌症发病谱第 6 位。新发病例数为 119 157 例,占全部癌症发病的 6.22%;其中男性 29 427 例,女性 89 730 例,城市地区 67 990 例,农村地区 51 167 例。发病率为 18.96/10 万,中标发病率为 16.46/10 万,世标发病率为 14.09/10 万。女性中标发病率为男性的 2.98 倍,城市中标发病率为农村的 1.78 倍。0~74 岁累积发病率为 1.32%(表 5-20a)。

甲状腺癌位居中国肿瘤登记地区癌症死亡谱第 22 位。死亡病例数为 4 193 例,占全部癌症死亡的 0.39%;其中男性 1 579 例,女性 2 614 例,城市地区 1 908 例,农村地区 2 285 例。甲状腺癌死亡率为 0.67/10 万,中标死亡率为 0.39/10 万,世标死亡率为 0.38/10 万;女性中标死亡率为男性的 1.60 倍,城市中标死亡率为农村的 1.08 倍。0~74 岁累积死亡率为 0.04%(表 5-20b)。

甲状腺癌年龄别发病率呈明显的性别差异。女性自 15~19 岁组开始快速上升,至 50~54 岁组达到高峰;而男性从 20~24 岁组开始呈缓慢上升趋势。女性各年龄别发病率均明显高于男性。甲状腺癌年龄别死亡率从 40~44 岁组开始缓慢上升,至 85 岁及以上组到达高峰(图 5-20a)。

城市地区的甲状腺癌中标发病率和死亡率均高于农村地区。中标发病率以东部地区最高,其次是中部地区,西部地区最低;中标死亡率以中部地区最高,其次是东部地区,西部地区最低。七大行政区中,华东地区男性和女性中标发病率最高,西北地区男性和女性的中标发病率最低;东北地区男性和女性中标死亡率最高,华北地区男性和女性的中标死亡率最低(表 5-20a,表 5-20b,图 5-20b)。

全部甲状腺癌病例中有明确组织学类型的病例占 87.31%,其中乳头状腺癌是最主要的病理类型,占 94.22%;其次是其他类型、滤泡性腺癌和髓样癌,分别占 4.53%、1.10% 和 0.15%(图 5-20c)。

20 Thyroid

Thyroid cancer was the 6th most common cancer in the registration areas of China. There were 119 157 new cases of thyroid cancer(29 427 males and 89 730 females,67 990 in urban areas and 51 167 in rural areas),accounting for 6.22% of new cases of all cancers. The crude incidence rate was 18.96 per 100 000, with ASR China 16.46 per 100 000 and ASR world 14.09 per 100 000, respectively. The incidence of ASR China was 2.98 times more in females than in males,and 1.78 times more in urban areas than in rural areas. The cumulative incidence rate for subjects aged from 0 to 74 years was 1.32% (Table 5-20a).

Thyroid cancer ranked 22nd for cancer mortality in the registration areas of China. A total of 4 193 cases died of thyroid cancer (1 579 males and 2 614 females,1 908 in urban areas and 2 285 in rural areas),accounting for 0.39% of all cancer deaths. The crude mortality rate was 0.67 per 100 000, with ASR China 0.39 per 100 000 and ASR world 0.38 per 100 000, respectively. The mortality of ASR China was 1.60 times more in females than in males,and it was 1.08 times more in urban areas than in rural areas. The cumulative mortality rate for subjects aged from 0 to 74 years was 0.04% (Table 5-20b).

The age-specific incidence rate of thyroid cancer showed differences between males and females. The incidence rate in females increased rapidly from the age group of 15-19 years and peaked at the age group of 50-54 years,while the incidence rate in males increased from the age group of 20-24 years with a slow speed. The age-specific incidence rates in females were generally higher than those in males. The age-specific mortality rate of thyroid cancer increased slowly from the age group of 40-44 years and peaked at the age group of over 85 years(Figure 5-20a).

The incidence and mortality rates(ASR China) of thyroid cancer were higher in urban areas than those in rural areas. Eastern areas had the highest incidence rate(ASR China),followed by central and western areas. Central areas had the highest mortality rate (ASR China),followed by eastern and western areas. Among the seven administrative districts,the highest incidence rates(ASR China) were shown in East China for both sexes,while the lowest incidence rates (ASR China)were shown in Northwest China for both sexes. The highest mortality rates(ASR China) were shown in Northeast China for both sexes,while the lowest mortality rates(ASR China) were shown in North China for both sexes(Table 5-20a,Table 5-20b,Figure 5-20b).

About 87.31% cases of thyroid cancer had morphological verification. Among those,papillary thyroid cancer was the most common histological type,accounting for 94.22% of all cases,followed by other types(4.53%),follicular adenoma(1.10%) and medullary thyroid cancer(0.15%)(Figure 5-20c).

表 5-20a　中国肿瘤登记地区甲状腺癌发病情况

Table 5-20a　Incidence of thyroid cancer in the registration areas of China

地区 Area	性别 Sex	发病数 No. cases	粗率 Crude rate/ 100 000^{-1}	构成比 Freq./%	中标率 ASR China/ 100 000^{-1}	世标率 ASR world/ 100 000^{-1}	累积率 Cum. Rate 0~74/%	顺位 Rank
合计 All	合计 Both	119 157	18.96	6.22	16.46	14.09	1.32	6
	男性 Male	29 427	9.23	2.82	8.31	6.99	0.65	8
	女性 Female	89 730	28.98	10.30	24.77	21.33	2.01	3
城市地区 Urban areas	合计 Both	67 990	25.32	7.61	21.85	18.56	1.73	5
	男性 Male	17 655	13.13	3.71	11.77	9.81	0.90	7
	女性 Female	50 335	37.55	12.05	31.83	27.25	2.56	3
农村地区 Rural areas	合计 Both	51 167	14.22	5.00	12.26	10.63	1.01	8
	男性 Male	11 772	6.38	2.07	5.68	4.86	0.46	12
	女性 Female	39 395	22.44	8.69	19.11	16.63	1.57	4
东部地区 Eastern areas	合计 Both	76 260	30.06	8.24	26.14	22.28	2.07	5
	男性 Male	19 586	15.36	4.01	13.91	11.64	1.06	7
	女性 Female	56 674	44.91	12.98	38.36	32.94	3.08	3
中部地区 Central areas	合计 Both	23 400	15.56	5.51	13.27	11.55	1.10	8
	男性 Male	5 361	7.00	2.32	6.23	5.34	0.50	9
	女性 Female	18 039	24.44	9.29	20.43	17.86	1.70	3
西部地区 Western areas	合计 Both	19 497	8.69	3.44	7.58	6.50	0.60	10
	男性 Male	4 480	3.90	1.38	3.45	2.94	0.28	14
	女性 Female	15 017	13.70	6.24	11.91	10.22	0.95	6

表 5-20b　中国肿瘤登记地区甲状腺癌死亡情况

Table 5-20b　Mortality of thyroid cancer in the registration areas of China

地区 Area	性别 Sex	死亡数 No. deaths	粗率 Crude rate/ 100 000^{-1}	构成比 Freq./%	中标率 ASR China/ 100 000^{-1}	世标率 ASR world/ 100 000^{-1}	累积率 Cum. Rate 0~74/%	顺位 Rank
合计 All	合计 Both	4 193	0.67	0.39	0.39	0.38	0.04	22
	男性 Male	1 579	0.50	0.23	0.30	0.30	0.03	19
	女性 Female	2 614	0.84	0.67	0.48	0.46	0.05	20
城市地区 Urban areas	合计 Both	1 908	0.71	0.40	0.41	0.39	0.04	22
	男性 Male	741	0.55	0.24	0.33	0.32	0.04	19
	女性 Female	1 167	0.87	0.67	0.48	0.46	0.05	20
农村地区 Rural areas	合计 Both	2 285	0.63	0.37	0.38	0.37	0.04	22
	男性 Male	838	0.45	0.21	0.29	0.28	0.03	19
	女性 Female	1 447	0.82	0.67	0.48	0.46	0.05	20
东部地区 Eastern areas	合计 Both	1 869	0.74	0.39	0.39	0.38	0.04	22
	男性 Male	734	0.58	0.24	0.32	0.32	0.04	19
	女性 Female	1 135	0.90	0.64	0.45	0.44	0.05	20
中部地区 Central areas	合计 Both	1 083	0.72	0.44	0.45	0.44	0.05	22
	男性 Male	357	0.47	0.23	0.31	0.30	0.03	19
	女性 Female	726	0.98	0.82	0.60	0.58	0.06	16
西部地区 Western areas	合计 Both	1 241	0.55	0.35	0.35	0.34	0.04	22
	男性 Male	488	0.43	0.21	0.28	0.28	0.03	19
	女性 Female	753	0.69	0.62	0.43	0.41	0.05	20

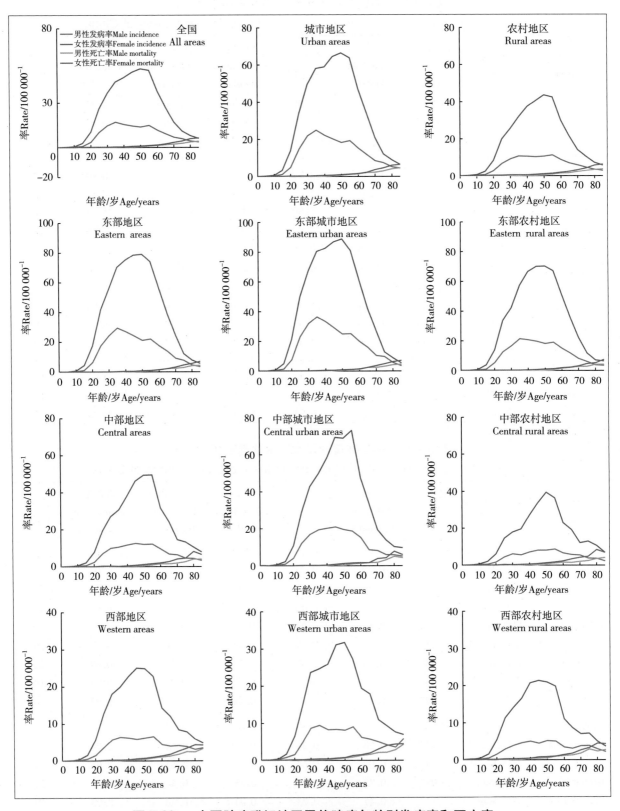

图 5-20a　中国肿瘤登记地区甲状腺癌年龄别发病率和死亡率

Figure 5-20a　Age-specific incidence and mortality rates of thyroid cancer in the registration areas of China

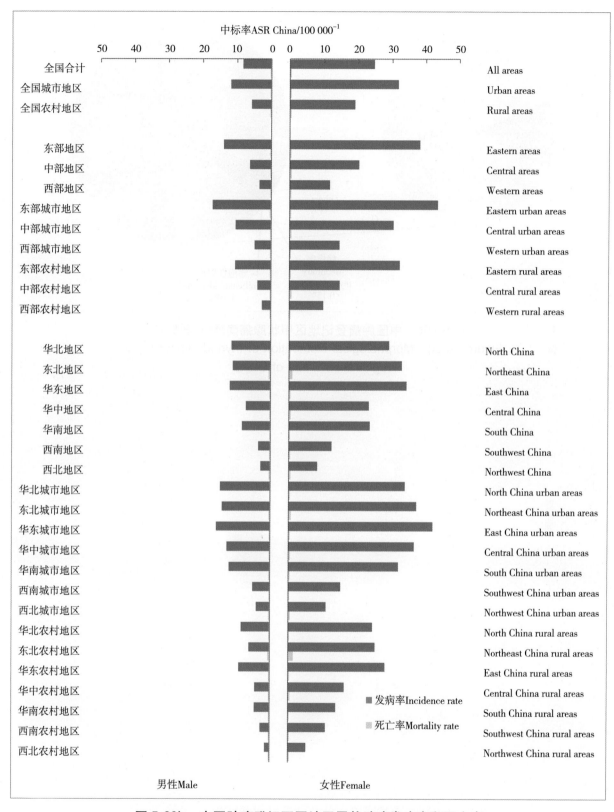

中标率ASR China/100 000⁻¹

全国合计	All areas
全国城市地区	Urban areas
全国农村地区	Rural areas
东部地区	Eastern areas
中部地区	Central areas
西部地区	Western areas
东部城市地区	Eastern urban areas
中部城市地区	Central urban areas
西部城市地区	Western urban areas
东部农村地区	Eastern rural areas
中部农村地区	Central rural areas
西部农村地区	Western rural areas
华北地区	North China
东北地区	Northeast China
华东地区	East China
华中地区	Central China
华南地区	South China
西南地区	Southwest China
西北地区	Northwest China
华北城市地区	North China urban areas
东北城市地区	Northeast China urban areas
华东城市地区	East China urban areas
华中城市地区	Central China urban areas
华南城市地区	South China urban areas
西南城市地区	Southwest China urban areas
西北城市地区	Northwest China urban areas
华北农村地区	North China rural areas
东北农村地区	Northeast China rural areas
华东农村地区	East China rural areas
华中农村地区	Central China rural areas
华南农村地区	South China rural areas
西南农村地区	Southwest China rural areas
西北农村地区	Northwest China rural areas

■ 发病率Incidence rate
□ 死亡率Mortality rate

男性Male　　　　　　女性Female

图 5-20b　中国肿瘤登记不同地区甲状腺癌发病率和死亡率
Figure 5-20b　Incidence and mortality rates of thyroid cancer in different
registration areas of China

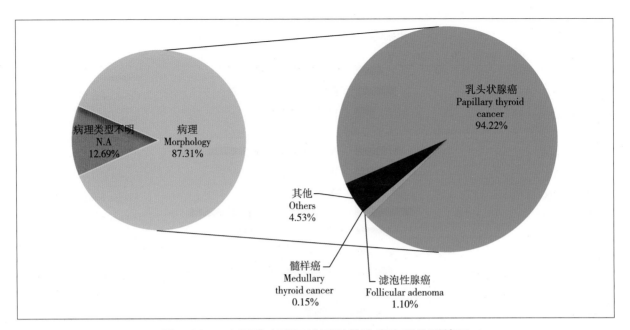

图 5-20c 中国肿瘤登记地区甲状腺癌病理分型情况
Figure 5-20c   Morphological distribution of thyroid cancer in the
registration areas of China

21 淋巴瘤

淋巴瘤位居中国肿瘤登记地区癌症发病谱第14位。新发病例数为42 394例，占全部癌症发病的2.21%；其中男性24 340例，女性18 054例，城市地区21 667例，农村地区20 727例。发病率为6.75/10万，中标发病率为4.38/10万，世标发病率为4.28/10万；男性中标发病率是女性的1.38倍，城市中标发病率是农村的1.34倍。0~74岁累积发病率为0.48%（表5-21a）。

淋巴瘤位居中国肿瘤登记地区癌症死亡谱第12位。死亡病例数为22 648例，占全部癌症死亡的2.08%；其中男性13 735例，女性8 913例，城市地区11 284例，农村地区11 364例。淋巴瘤死亡率为3.60/10万，中标死亡率2.12/10万，世标死亡率2.09/10万；男性中标死亡率为女性的1.65倍，城市中标死亡率为农村的1.22倍。0~74岁累积死亡率为0.24%（表5-21b）。

淋巴瘤年龄别发病率和死亡率从40~44岁组开始快速上升，男女均于80~84岁组达到高峰。总体上，男性年龄别发病率和死亡率均高于女性（图5-21a）。

城市地区淋巴瘤的中标发病率和死亡率均高于农村地区。中标发病率和死亡率均为东部地区最高，其次是中部地区，西部地区最低。七大行政区中，华南地区男性和女性的中标发病率最高，西北地区男性和女性的中标发病率最低；华中地区男性和华东地区女性的中标死亡率最高，西北地区男性和女性的中标死亡率最低（表5-21a，表5-21b，图5-21b）。

全部淋巴瘤病例中，非霍奇金淋巴瘤的其他和未特指类型（ICD-10：C85）是最主要的病理类型，占37.57%；其次是多发性骨髓瘤和恶性浆细胞性肿瘤（C90），占24.94%；弥漫性非霍奇金淋巴瘤（C83），占21.52%；霍奇金淋巴瘤（C81），占4.75%；周围和皮肤的T细胞淋巴瘤（C84），占4.14%；滤泡性非霍奇金淋巴瘤（C82），占4.11%；其他和未特指的淋巴、造血和有关组织的恶性肿瘤（C96），占1.59%；以及恶性免疫增生性疾病（C88），占1.38%（图5-21c）。

21 Lymphoma

Lymphoma ranked 14th for cancer incidence in the registration areas of China. There were 42 394 new cases of lymphoma (24 340 males and 18 054 females, 21 667 in urban areas and 20 727 in rural areas), accounting for 2.21% of all new cancer cases. The crude incidence rate was 6.75 per 100 000, with ASR China 4.38 per 100 000 and ASR world 4.28 per 100 000, respectively. The incidence of the ASR China was 1.38 times more in males than in females, and 1.34 times more in urban areas than in rural areas. The cumulative incidence rate for subjects aged from 0 to 74 years was 0.48% (Table 5-21a).

Lymphoma ranked 12th for cancer mortality in the registration areas of China. A total of 22 648 cases died of lymphoma (13 735 males and 8 913 females, 11 284 in urban areas and 11 364 in rural areas), accounting for 2.08% of all cancer deaths. The crude mortality rate was 3.60 per 100 000, with ASR China 2.12 per 100 000 and ASR world 2.09 per 100 000, respectively. The mortality rate of the ASR China was 1.65 times in males as that in females, and it was 1.22 times in the urban areas as that in rural areas. The cumulative mortality rate for subjects aged from 0 to 74 years was 0.24% (Table 5-21b).

The age-specific incidence and mortality rates of lymphoma increased rapidly from the age group of 40-44 years and then peaked at the age group of 80-84 years for both sexed. The age-specific incidence and mortality rates of lymphoma were generally higher in males than those in females (Figure 5-21a).

The incidence and mortality rates (ASR China) of lymphoma were higher in urban areas than those in rural areas. Eastern areas had the highest incidence and mortality rates (ASR China), followed by the central and western areas. Among the seven administrative districts, the highest incidence rates (ASR China) were shown in South China for both sexes, while the lowest incidence rates (ASR China) were shown in Northwest China for both sexes. The highest mortality rates (ASR China) were shown in Central China for males and East China for females, respectively, while Northwest China had the lowest mortality rates (ASR China) for both sexes (Table 5-21a, Table 5-21b, Figure 5-21b).

Among all lymphoma cases, other and unspecified types of non-Hodgkin lymphoma (ICD-10：C85) were the most common histological type, accounting for 37.57% of all cases, followed by multiple myeloma & malignant plasma cell neoplasms (C90, 24.94%), diffuse non-Hodgkin lymphoma (C83, 21.52%), Hodgkin lymphoma (C81, 4.75%), peripheral & cutaneous T-cell lymphoma (C84, 4.14%), follicular non-Hodgkin lymphoma (C82, 4.11%), other and unspecified malignant neoplasms of lymphoid, hematopoietic and related tissue (C96, 1.59%), and malignant immunoproliferative disease (C88, 1.38%) (Figure 5-21c).

表 5-21a　中国肿瘤登记地区淋巴瘤发病情况

Table 5-21a　Incidence of lymphoma in the registration areas of China

地区 Area	性别 Sex	发病数 No. cases	粗率 Crude rate/ 100 000^{-1}	构成比 Freq./%	中标率 ASR China/ 100 000^{-1}	世标率 ASR world/ 100 000^{-1}	累积率 Cum. Rate 0~74/%	顺位 Rank
合计 All	合计 Both	42 394	6.75	2.21	4.38	4.28	0.48	14
	男性 Male	24 340	7.63	2.33	5.09	4.99	0.56	10
	女性 Female	18 054	5.83	2.07	3.69	3.60	0.41	13
城市地区 Urban areas	合计 Both	21 667	8.07	2.42	5.11	4.98	0.56	13
	男性 Male	12 204	9.08	2.56	5.88	5.75	0.64	9
	女性 Female	9 463	7.06	2.26	4.38	4.25	0.48	11
农村地区 Rural areas	合计 Both	20 727	5.76	2.03	3.82	3.74	0.43	15
	男性 Male	12 136	6.58	2.13	4.49	4.41	0.50	11
	女性 Female	8 591	4.89	1.90	3.15	3.08	0.35	14
东部地区 Eastern areas	合计 Both	22 369	8.82	2.42	5.33	5.19	0.59	13
	男性 Male	12 742	10.00	2.61	6.21	6.06	0.68	10
	女性 Female	9 627	7.63	2.21	4.50	4.37	0.50	13
中部地区 Central areas	合计 Both	9 076	6.04	2.14	4.15	4.10	0.46	13
	男性 Male	5 219	6.82	2.26	4.83	4.78	0.54	10
	女性 Female	3 857	5.23	1.99	3.49	3.43	0.38	12
西部地区 Western areas	合计 Both	10 949	4.88	1.93	3.34	3.26	0.37	15
	男性 Male	6 379	5.56	1.96	3.89	3.79	0.42	11
	女性 Female	4 570	4.17	1.90	2.79	2.73	0.31	14

表 5-21b　中国肿瘤登记地区淋巴瘤死亡情况

Table 5-21b　Mortality of lymphoma in the registration areas of China

地区 Area	性别 Sex	死亡数 No. deaths	粗率 Crude rate/ 100 000^{-1}	构成比 Freq./%	中标率 ASR China/ 100 000^{-1}	世标率 ASR world/ 100 000^{-1}	累积率 Cum. rate 0~74/%	顺位 Rank
合计 All	合计 Both	22 648	3.60	2.08	2.12	2.09	0.24	12
	男性 Male	13 735	4.31	1.97	2.65	2.61	0.29	10
	女性 Female	8 913	2.88	2.29	1.61	1.59	0.18	13
城市地区 Urban areas	合计 Both	11 284	4.20	2.36	2.36	2.32	0.26	10
	男性 Male	6 788	5.05	2.24	2.96	2.92	0.32	8
	女性 Female	4 496	3.35	2.58	1.80	1.77	0.20	12
农村地区 Rural areas	合计 Both	11 364	3.16	1.86	1.93	1.90	0.22	12
	男性 Male	6 947	3.77	1.76	2.40	2.37	0.28	10
	女性 Female	4 417	2.52	2.05	1.47	1.45	0.16	14
东部地区 Eastern areas	合计 Both	11 728	4.62	2.43	2.46	2.41	0.27	9
	男性 Male	7 000	5.49	2.29	3.06	3.01	0.34	8
	女性 Female	4 728	3.75	2.65	1.90	1.87	0.21	13
中部地区 Central areas	合计 Both	4 871	3.24	1.98	2.05	2.02	0.23	13
	男性 Male	2 947	3.85	1.88	2.56	2.52	0.29	10
	女性 Female	1 924	2.61	2.17	1.56	1.54	0.17	13
西部地区 Western areas	合计 Both	6 049	2.70	1.69	1.71	1.70	0.19	14
	男性 Male	3 788	3.30	1.60	2.16	2.15	0.24	10
	女性 Female	2 261	2.06	1.85	1.27	1.26	0.15	14

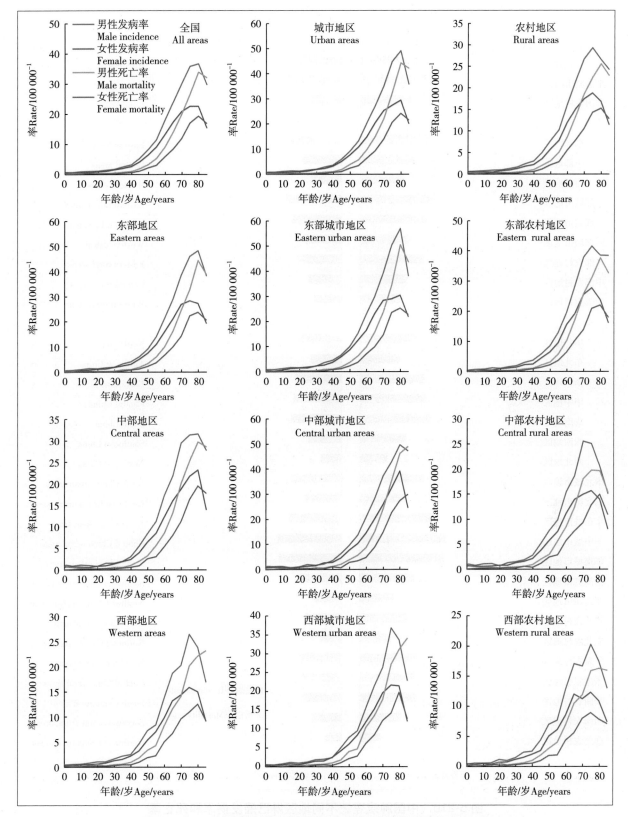

图 5-21a　中国肿瘤登记地区淋巴瘤年龄别发病率和死亡率

Figure 5-21a　Age-specific incidence and mortality rates of lymphoma in the registration areas of China

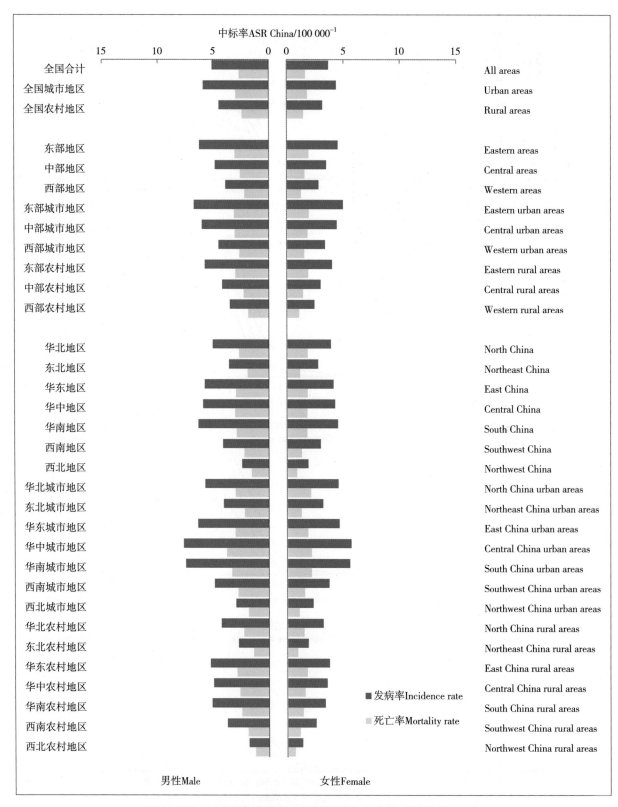

中标率ASR China/100 000⁻¹

全国合计		All areas
全国城市地区		Urban areas
全国农村地区		Rural areas
东部地区		Eastern areas
中部地区		Central areas
西部地区		Western areas
东部城市地区		Eastern urban areas
中部城市地区		Central urban areas
西部城市地区		Western urban areas
东部农村地区		Eastern rural areas
中部农村地区		Central rural areas
西部农村地区		Western rural areas
华北地区		North China
东北地区		Northeast China
华东地区		East China
华中地区		Central China
华南地区		South China
西南地区		Southwest China
西北地区		Northwest China
华北城市地区		North China urban areas
东北城市地区		Northeast China urban areas
华东城市地区		East China urban areas
华中城市地区		Central China urban areas
华南城市地区		South China urban areas
西南城市地区		Southwest China urban areas
西北城市地区		Northwest China urban areas
华北农村地区		North China rural areas
东北农村地区		Northeast China rural areas
华东农村地区		East China rural areas
华中农村地区		Central China rural areas
华南农村地区		South China rural areas
西南农村地区		Southwest China rural areas
西北农村地区		Northwest China rural areas

■ 发病率Incidence rate
□ 死亡率Mortality rate

男性Male   女性Female

图 5-21b　中国肿瘤登记不同地区淋巴瘤发病率和死亡率
Figure 5-21b　Incidence and mortality rates of lymphoma in different
registration areas of China

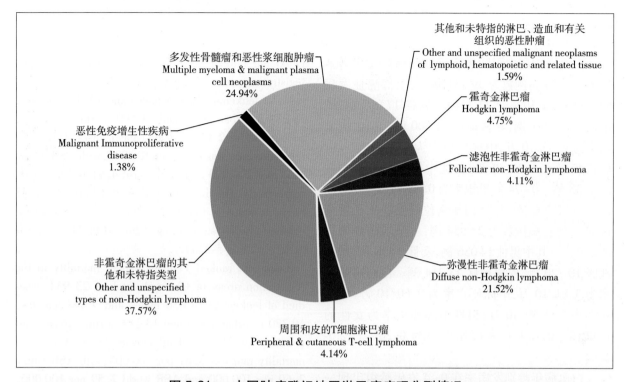

图 5-21c　中国肿瘤登记地区淋巴瘤病理分型情况

Figure 5-21c　Morphological distribution of lymphoma in the registration areas of China

22 白血病

白血病位居中国肿瘤登记地区癌症发病谱第15位。新发病例数为 39 781 例，占全部癌症发病的 2.08%；其中男性 22 774 例，女性 17 007 例，城市地区 18 281 例，农村地区 21 500 例。白血病发病率为 6.33/10 万，中标发病率为 4.77/10 万，世标发病率为 4.91/10 万；男性中标发病率为女性的 1.33 倍。0~74 岁累积率为 0.45%（表 5-22a）。

中国肿瘤登记地区白血病位居癌症死亡谱第11 位。死亡病例数为 23 934 例，占全部癌症死亡的 2.20%；其中男性 14 036 例，女性 9 898 例，城市地区 10 720 例，农村地区 13 214 例。白血病死亡率为 3.81/10 万，中标死亡率为 2.60/10 万，世标死亡率为 2.59/10 万；男性中标死亡率为女性的 1.44 倍。0~74 岁累积死亡率为 0.26%（表 5-22b）。

白血病年龄别发病率在 0~4 岁年龄组出现一个小高峰，在 5~39 岁趋于平缓，40 岁后开始快速上升，至 80~84 岁年龄组达到高峰。白血病年龄别死亡率从 40~44 岁组开始快速上升，男性死亡率至 85 岁及以上年龄组达到高峰，女性死亡率至 80~84 岁组达到高峰（图 5-22a）。

城市地区白血病发病率和死亡率与农村地区接近。东部地区的中标发病率和死亡率最高，其次是中部地区和西部地区。七大行政区中，华南地区男女的中标发病率最高，西北地区男女的中标发病率最低；华南地区男性和华中地区女性的中标死亡率最高，西北地区男女的中标死亡率最低（表 5-22a，表 5-22b，图 5-22b）。

22 Leukemia

Leukemia ranked 15th for cancer incidence in the registration areas of China. There were 39 781 new cases of leukemia(22 774 males and 17 007 females, 18 281 in urban areas and 21 500 in rural areas.), accounting for 2. 08% of all cancer cases. The crude incidence rate was 6. 33 per 100 000,with ASR China 4. 77 per 100 000 and ASR world 4. 91 per 100 000, respectively. The incidence of ASR China was 1. 33 times in males as that in females. The cumulative incidence rate for subjects aged from 0 to 74 years was 0. 45% (Table 5-22a).

Leukemia ranked 11th for cancer mortality in the registration areas of China. A total of 23 934 cases died of leukemia(14 036 males and 9 898 females, 10 720 in urban areas and 13 214 in rural areas) ,accounting for 2. 20% of all cancer deaths. The crude mortality rate was 3. 81 per 100 000,with ASR China 2. 60 per 100 000 and ASR world 2. 59 per 100 000, respectively. The mortality of ASR China was 1. 44 times in males as that in females. The cumulative mortality rate for subjects aged from 0 to 74 years was 0. 26% (Table 5-22b).

The first peak of the age-specific incidence rate of leukemia occurred in the age group of 0-4 years. Age-specific incidence rates were relatively stable at 5-39 years and dramatically increased after the age of 40, and peaked at the age group of 80-84 years. The age-specific mortality rate of leukemia increased rapidly from the age group of 40-44 years and peaked at the age group of 85 years and above and 80-84 years for males and females,respectively(Figure 5-22a).

The incidence and mortality rates of leukemia in urban areas were close to those in rural areas. Eastern areas had the highest incidenceand mortality rates (ASR China) ,followed by central and western areas. Among the seven administrative districts, South China had the highest incidence rates (ASR China) for both sexes while Northwest China had the lowest incidence rates (ASR China) for both sexes. The highest mortality rates (ASR China) were shown in South China for males and Central China for females, respectively ,while Northwest China had the lowest mortality rates (ASR China) for both sexes (Table 5-22a, Table 5-22b, Figure 5-22b).

全部白血病新发病例中,髓系白血病(ICD-10:C92)是最主要的病理类型,占 36.24%;其次是未特指细胞类型的白血病(C95),占 32.92%;淋巴细胞白血病(C91),占 22.09%;单核细胞白血病(C93),占 4.40%;以及特指细胞类型的其他白血病(C94),占 4.35%(图 5-22c)。

中国肿瘤登记地区淋巴细胞白血病新发病例为 7 460 例,发病率为 1.19/10 万(中标发病率为 1.01/10 万,世标发病率为 1.16/10 万),占全部癌症发病的 0.39%。淋巴细胞白血病死亡病例为 4 409 例,死亡率为 0.70/10 万(中标发病率和世标发病率均为 0.53/10 万),占全部癌症死亡的 0.41%(表 5-22c,表 5-22d)。

中国肿瘤登记地区髓系白血病新发病例为 21 200 例,发病率为 3.37/10 万(中标发病率为 2.43/10 万,世标率为 2.37/10 万),占全部癌症发病的 1.11%。髓系白血病死亡病例为 10 090 例,死亡率为 1.61/10 万(中标死亡率为 1.03/10 万,世标死亡率为 1.01/10 万),占全部癌症死亡的 0.93%(表 5-22e,表 5-22f)。

Among all leukemia cases, myeloid leukemia(ICD-10:C92) was the most common histological type, accounting for 36.24% of all cases, followed by leukemia of unspecified cell type(C95, 32.92%), lymphocytic leukemia(C91, 22.09%), monocytic leukemia (C93, 4.40%) and other leukemias of specified cell type(C94, 4.35%) (Figure 5-22c).

There were 7 460 new cases diagnosed as lymphocytic leukemia in the registration areas of China, accounting for 0.39% of all cancer cases. The crude incidence rate was 1.19 per 100 000, with ASR China 1.01 per 100 000 and ASR world 1.16 per 100 000, respectively. A total of 4 409 cases died of lymphocytic leukemia, accounting for 0.41% of all cancer deaths. The crude mortality rate was 0.70 per 100 000, with ASR China and ASR world both 0.53 per 100 000(Table 5-22c, Table 5-22d).

There were 21 200 new cases diagnosed as myeloid leukemia in the registration areas of China, accounting for 1.11% of all cancer cases. The crude incidence rate was 3.37 per 100 000, with ASR China 2.43 per 100 000 and ASR world 2.37 per 100 000, respectively. A total of 10 090 cases died of myeloid leukemia, accounting for 0.93% of all cancer deaths. The crude mortality rate of myeloid leukemia was 1.61 per 100 000, with ASR China 1.03 per 100 000 and ASR world 1.01 per 100 000, respectively (Table 5-22e, Table 5-22f).

表 5-22a　中国肿瘤登记地区白血病发病情况
Table 5-22a　Incidence of leukemia in the registration areas of China

地区 Area	性别 Sex	发病数 No. cases	粗率 Crude rate/ 100 000^{-1}	构成比 Freq. /%	中标率 ASR China/ 100 000^{-1}	世标率 ASR world/ 100 000^{-1}	累积率 Cum. Rate 0~74/%	顺位 Rank
合计 All	合计 Both	39 781	6. 33	2. 08	4. 77	4. 91	0. 45	15
	男性 Male	22 774	7. 14	2. 18	5. 45	5. 59	0. 52	12
	女性 Female	17 007	5. 49	1. 95	4. 10	4. 24	0. 39	14
城市地区 Urban areas	合计 Both	18 281	6. 81	2. 05	4. 92	5. 10	0. 47	17
	男性 Male	10 526	7. 83	2. 21	5. 73	5. 91	0. 55	12
	女性 Female	7 755	5. 79	1. 86	4. 14	4. 32	0. 40	14
农村地区 Rural areas	合计 Both	21 500	5. 97	2. 10	4. 64	4. 76	0. 44	14
	男性 Male	12 248	6. 64	2. 15	5. 22	5. 34	0. 49	10
	女性 Female	9 252	5. 27	2. 04	4. 05	4. 17	0. 38	13
东部地区 Eastern areas	合计 Both	20 095	7. 92	2. 17	5. 58	5. 76	0. 53	15
	男性 Male	11 534	9. 05	2. 36	6. 44	6. 62	0. 61	12
	女性 Female	8 561	6. 78	1. 96	4. 74	4. 94	0. 45	14
中部地区 Central areas	合计 Both	8 695	5. 78	2. 05	4. 59	4. 71	0. 43	14
	男性 Male	5 050	6. 60	2. 19	5. 31	5. 41	0. 50	11
	女性 Female	3 645	4. 94	1. 88	3. 87	4. 02	0. 36	14
西部地区 Western areas	合计 Both	10 991	4. 90	1. 94	3. 89	3. 99	0. 36	14
	男性 Male	6 190	5. 39	1. 90	4. 34	4. 45	0. 41	12
	女性 Female	4 801	4. 38	2. 00	3. 45	3. 53	0. 32	13

表 5-22b　中国肿瘤登记地区白血病死亡情况
Table 5-22b　Mortality of leukemia in the registration areas of China

地区 Area	性别 Sex	死亡数 No. deaths	粗率 Crude rate/ 100 000^{-1}	构成比 Freq. /%	中标率 ASR China/ 100 000^{-1}	世标率 ASR world/ 100 000^{-1}	累积率 Cum. Rate 0~74/%	顺位 Rank
合计 All	合计 Both	23 934	3. 81	2. 20	2. 60	2. 59	0. 26	11
	男性 Male	14 036	4. 40	2. 01	3. 08	3. 06	0. 30	9
	女性 Female	9 898	3. 20	2. 54	2. 14	2. 14	0. 21	12
城市地区 Urban areas	合计 Both	10 720	3. 99	2. 25	2. 58	2. 57	0. 25	13
	男性 Male	6 295	4. 68	2. 07	3. 10	3. 08	0. 30	9
	女性 Female	4 425	3. 30	2. 54	2. 09	2. 10	0. 20	13
农村地区 Rural areas	合计 Both	13 214	3. 67	2. 17	2. 61	2. 59	0. 26	11
	男性 Male	7 741	4. 20	1. 96	3. 07	3. 03	0. 30	9
	女性 Female	5 473	3. 12	2. 54	2. 17	2. 17	0. 21	10
东部地区 Eastern areas	合计 Both	11 679	4. 60	2. 42	2. 82	2. 79	0. 28	11
	男性 Male	6 946	5. 45	2. 27	3. 42	3. 38	0. 33	9
	女性 Female	4 733	3. 75	2. 66	2. 25	2. 25	0. 22	12
中部地区 Central areas	合计 Both	5 159	3. 43	2. 10	2. 52	2. 50	0. 25	11
	男性 Male	3 009	3. 93	1. 92	2. 97	2. 91	0. 29	9
	女性 Female	2 150	2. 91	2. 42	2. 09	2. 10	0. 21	12
西部地区 Western areas	合计 Both	7 096	3. 16	1. 98	2. 35	2. 35	0. 23	11
	男性 Male	4 081	3. 55	1. 73	2. 70	2. 69	0. 26	9
	女性 Female	3 015	2. 75	2. 47	2. 01	2. 01	0. 19	12

表 5-22c　中国肿瘤登记地区淋巴细胞白血病发病情况

Table 5-22c　Incidence of lymphocytic leukemia in the registration areas of China

地区 Area	性别 Sex	发病数 No. cases	粗率 Crude rate/ 100 000^{-1}	构成比 Freq. /%	中标率 ASR China/ 100 000^{-1}	世标率 ASR world/ 100 000^{-1}	累积率 Cum. rate 0~74/%
合计	合计 Both	7 460	1.19	0.39	1.01	1.16	0.09
All	男性 Male	4 426	1.39	0.42	1.18	1.34	0.11
	女性 Female	3 034	0.98	0.35	0.84	0.98	0.08
城市地区	合计 Both	3 550	1.32	0.40	1.12	1.32	0.10
Urban areas	男性 Male	2 128	1.58	0.45	1.34	1.54	0.12
	女性 Female	1 422	1.06	0.34	0.90	1.09	0.08
农村地区	合计 Both	3 910	1.09	0.38	0.93	1.05	0.08
Rural areas	男性 Male	2 298	1.25	0.40	1.07	1.20	0.10
	女性 Female	1 612	0.92	0.36	0.79	0.90	0.07
东部地区	合计 Both	3 964	1.56	0.43	1.30	1.54	0.12
Eastern areas	男性 Male	2 350	1.84	0.48	1.53	1.77	0.13
	女性 Female	1 614	1.28	0.37	1.08	1.30	0.10
中部地区	合计 Both	1 567	1.04	0.37	0.90	1.02	0.08
Central areas	男性 Male	948	1.24	0.41	1.07	1.19	0.10
	女性 Female	619	0.84	0.32	0.73	0.86	0.06
西部地区	合计 Both	1 929	0.86	0.34	0.75	0.83	0.07
Western areas	男性 Male	1 128	0.98	0.35	0.86	0.95	0.08
	女性 Female	801	0.73	0.33	0.63	0.70	0.06

表 5-22d　中国肿瘤登记地区淋巴细胞白血病死亡情况

Table 5-22d　Mortality of lymphocytic leukemia in the registration areas of China

地区 Area	性别 Sex	死亡数 No. deaths	粗率 Crude rate/ 100 000^{-1}	构成比 Freq. /%	中标率 ASR China/ 100 000^{-1}	世标率 ASR world/ 100 000^{-1}	累积率 Cum. rate 0~74/%
合计	合计 Both	4 409	0.70	0.41	0.53	0.53	0.05
All	男性 Male	2 580	0.81	0.37	0.62	0.62	0.06
	女性 Female	1 829	0.59	0.47	0.44	0.45	0.04
城市地区	合计 Both	2 035	0.76	0.43	0.55	0.56	0.05
Urban areas	男性 Male	1 192	0.89	0.39	0.65	0.65	0.06
	女性 Female	843	0.63	0.48	0.45	0.47	0.04
农村地区	合计 Both	2 374	0.66	0.39	0.51	0.51	0.05
Rural areas	男性 Male	1 388	0.75	0.35	0.60	0.59	0.05
	女性 Female	986	0.56	0.46	0.43	0.44	0.04
东部地区	合计 Both	2 134	0.84	0.44	0.59	0.60	0.05
Eastern areas	男性 Male	1 266	0.99	0.41	0.70	0.71	0.06
	女性 Female	868	0.69	0.49	0.49	0.50	0.04
中部地区	合计 Both	931	0.62	0.38	0.49	0.49	0.05
Central areas	男性 Male	549	0.72	0.35	0.59	0.57	0.05
	女性 Female	382	0.52	0.43	0.39	0.41	0.04
西部地区	合计 Both	1 344	0.60	0.37	0.48	0.48	0.04
Western areas	男性 Male	765	0.67	0.32	0.54	0.54	0.05
	女性 Female	579	0.53	0.47	0.42	0.42	0.04

表 5-22e　中国肿瘤登记地区髓系白血病发病情况

Table 5-22e　Incidence of myeloid leukemia in the registration areas of China

地区 Area	性别 Sex	发病数 No. cases	粗率 Crude rate/ 100 000^{-1}	构成比 Freq. /%	中标率 ASR China/ 100 000^{-1}	世标率 ASR world/ 100 000^{-1}	累积率 Cum. Rate 0~74/%
合计 All	合计 Both	21 200	3. 37	1. 11	2. 43	2. 37	0. 24
	男性 Male	12 035	3. 77	1. 15	2. 76	2. 69	0. 27
	女性 Female	9 165	2. 96	1. 05	2. 11	2. 06	0. 20
城市地区 Urban areas	合计 Both	10 732	4. 00	1. 20	2. 75	2. 68	0. 27
	男性 Male	6 116	4. 55	1. 29	3. 18	3. 10	0. 32
	女性 Female	4 616	3. 44	1. 10	2. 35	2. 29	0. 23
农村地区 Rural areas	合计 Both	10 468	2. 91	1. 02	2. 18	2. 13	0. 21
	男性 Male	5 919	3. 21	1. 04	2. 44	2. 38	0. 24
	女性 Female	4 549	2. 59	1. 00	1. 92	1. 88	0. 19
东部地区 Eastern areas	合计 Both	12 367	4. 88	1. 34	3. 29	3. 22	0. 33
	男性 Male	7 057	5. 54	1. 44	3. 79	3. 70	0. 38
	女性 Female	5 310	4. 21	1. 22	2. 81	2. 76	0. 28
中部地区 Central areas	合计 Both	3 943	2. 62	0. 93	2. 00	1. 95	0. 19
	男性 Male	2 267	2. 96	0. 98	2. 30	2. 24	0. 22
	女性 Female	1 676	2. 27	0. 86	1. 70	1. 66	0. 16
西部地区 Western areas	合计 Both	4 890	2. 18	0. 86	1. 68	1. 63	0. 16
	男性 Male	2 711	2. 36	0. 83	1. 84	1. 79	0. 17
	女性 Female	2 179	1. 99	0. 91	1. 52	1. 47	0. 14

表 5-22f　中国肿瘤登记地区髓系白血病死亡情况

Table 5-22f　Mortality of myeloid leukemia in the registration areas of China

地区 Area	性别 Sex	死亡数 No. deaths	粗率 Crude rate/ 100 000^{-1}	构成比 Freq. /%	中标率 ASR China/ 100 000^{-1}	世标率 ASR world/ 100 000^{-1}	累积率 Cum. rate 0~74/%
合计 All	合计 Both	10 090	1. 61	0. 93	1. 03	1. 01	0. 11
	男性 Male	5 996	1. 88	0. 86	1. 24	1. 22	0. 13
	女性 Female	4 094	1. 32	1. 05	0. 83	0. 82	0. 09
城市地区 Urban areas	合计 Both	5 188	1. 93	1. 09	1. 18	1. 16	0. 12
	男性 Male	3 089	2. 30	1. 02	1. 44	1. 42	0. 15
	女性 Female	2 099	1. 57	1. 21	0. 94	0. 92	0. 09
农村地区 Rural areas	合计 Both	4 902	1. 36	0. 80	0. 92	0. 90	0. 10
	男性 Male	2 907	1. 58	0. 74	1. 09	1. 07	0. 11
	女性 Female	1 995	1. 14	0. 93	0. 75	0. 73	0. 08
东部地区 Eastern areas	合计 Both	5 735	2. 26	1. 19	1. 30	1. 27	0. 13
	男性 Male	3 459	2. 71	1. 13	1. 59	1. 56	0. 16
	女性 Female	2 276	1. 80	1. 28	1. 02	1. 01	0. 11
中部地区 Central areas	合计 Both	1 882	1. 25	0. 77	0. 88	0. 86	0. 09
	男性 Male	1 115	1. 46	0. 71	1. 05	1. 03	0. 11
	女性 Female	767	1. 04	0. 86	0. 72	0. 69	0. 07
西部地区 Western areas	合计 Both	2 473	1. 10	0. 69	0. 79	0. 77	0. 08
	男性 Male	1 422	1. 24	0. 60	0. 91	0. 90	0. 09
	女性 Female	1 051	0. 96	0. 86	0. 66	0. 65	0. 07

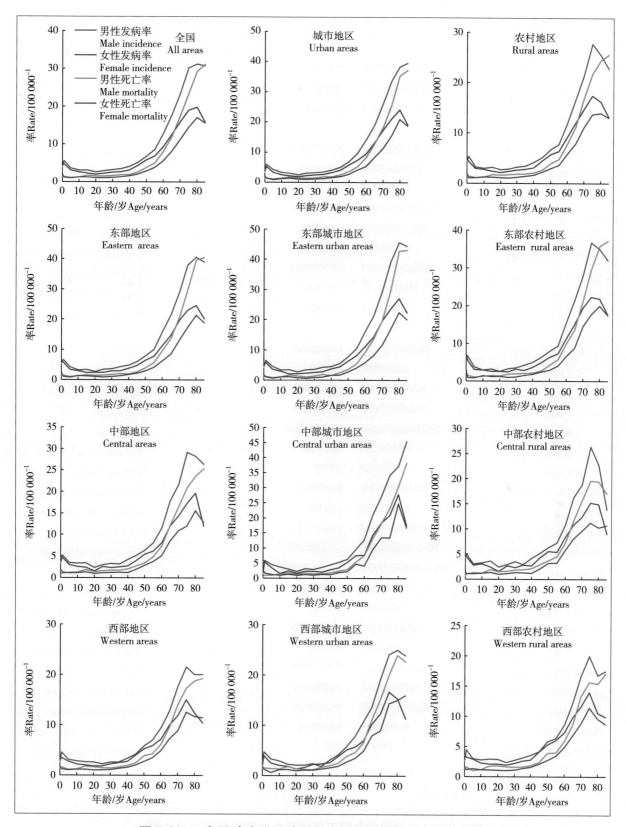

图 5-22a 中国肿瘤登记地区白血病年龄别发病率和死亡率

Figure 5-22a Age-specific incidence and mortality rates of leukemia in the registration areas of China

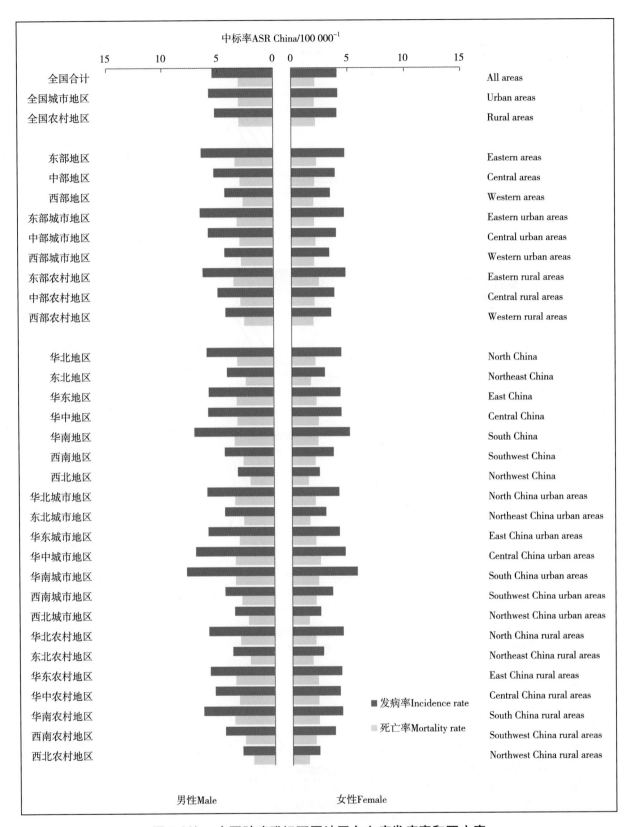

中标率ASR China/100 000⁻¹

全国合计		All areas
全国城市地区		Urban areas
全国农村地区		Rural areas
东部地区		Eastern areas
中部地区		Central areas
西部地区		Western areas
东部城市地区		Eastern urban areas
中部城市地区		Central urban areas
西部城市地区		Western urban areas
东部农村地区		Eastern rural areas
中部农村地区		Central rural areas
西部农村地区		Western rural areas
华北地区		North China
东北地区		Northeast China
华东地区		East China
华中地区		Central China
华南地区		South China
西南地区		Southwest China
西北地区		Northwest China
华北城市地区		North China urban areas
东北城市地区		Northeast China urban areas
华东城市地区		East China urban areas
华中城市地区		Central China urban areas
华南城市地区		South China urban areas
西南城市地区		Southwest China urban areas
西北城市地区		Northwest China urban areas
华北农村地区		North China rural areas
东北农村地区		Northeast China rural areas
华东农村地区		East China rural areas
华中农村地区		Central China rural areas
华南农村地区		South China rural areas
西南农村地区		Southwest China rural areas
西北农村地区		Northwest China rural areas

■ 发病率Incidence rate
死亡率Mortality rate

男性Male   女性Female

图 5-22b   中国肿瘤登记不同地区白血病发病率和死亡率
Figure 5-22b   Incidence and mortality rates of leukemia in different
registration areas of China

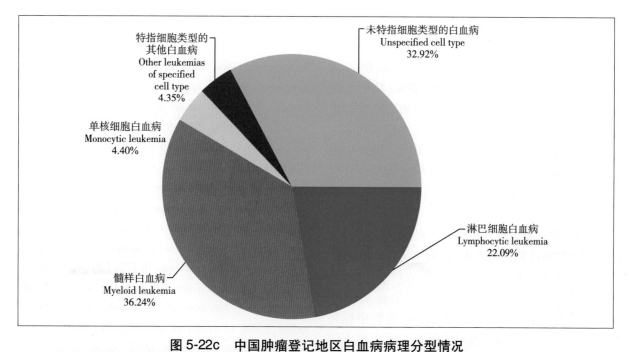

图 5-22c　中国肿瘤登记地区白血病病理分型情况

Figure 5-22c　Morphological distribution of leukemia in the registration areas of China

23 皮肤

中国肿瘤登记地区皮肤癌新发病例数为18 157例,占全部癌症发病的0.95%;其中男性9 059例,女性9 098例,城市地区8 567例,农村地区9 590例。发病率为2.89/10万,中标发病率为1.65/10万,世标发病率为1.62/10万;男性中标发病率为女性的1.11倍,城市中标发病率为农村的1.14倍。0~74岁累积发病率为0.17%(表5-23a)。

中国肿瘤登记地区皮肤癌死亡病例数为5 309例,占全部癌症死亡的0.49%;其中男性2 924例,女性2 385例,城市地区2 096例,农村地区3 213例。皮肤癌死亡率为0.84/10万,中标死亡率0.41/10万,世标死亡率0.43/10万;男性中标死亡率为女性的1.52倍,农村中标死亡率为城市的1.28倍。0~74岁累积死亡率为0.03%(表5-23b)。

皮肤癌年龄别发病率和死亡率在男性和女性中均随年龄呈上升趋势,发病率在30~34岁组开始上升明显,死亡率在50~54岁组开始上升明显,发病率和死亡率在85岁及以上年龄组达到高峰(图5-23a)。

城市地区皮肤癌的发病率高于农村地区,农村地区皮肤癌的死亡率高于城市地区。男性和女性的中标发病率均以东部地区最高,中标死亡率均以西部地区最高。在七大行政区中,华南地区皮肤癌中标发病率最高,其次是华东地区;男性中标死亡率是华中地区最高,其次为西南地区和华南地区;女性中标死亡率是西南地区最高,其次为华东地区和华中地区(表5-23a,表5-23b,图5-23b)。

23 Skin

In the registration areas of China, there were 18 157 new cases of skin cancer (9 059 males and 9 098 females, 8 567 in urban areas and 9 590 in rural areas), accounting for 0.95% of new cancer cases of all sites. The crude incidence rate was 2.89 per 100 000, with ASR China 1.65 per 100 000 and ASR world 1.62 per 100 000, respectively. The incidence of ASR China was 1.11 times in males as that in females, and was 1.14 times in urban areas as that in rural areas. The cumulative incidence rate for subjects aged from 0 to 74 years was 0.17% (Table 5-23a).

In the registration areas of China, a total of 5 309 cases died of skin cancer (2 924 males and 2 385 females, 2 096 in urban areas and 3 213 in rural areas), accounting for 0.49% of all cancer deaths. The crude mortality rate was 0.84 per 100 000, with ASR China 0.41 per 100 000 and ASR world 0.43 per 100 000, respectively. The mortality of ASR China was 1.52 times in males as that in females, and was 1.28 times in rural areas as that in urban areas. The cumulative mortality rate for subjects aged from 0 to 74 years was 0.03% (Table 5-23b).

The age-specific incidence and mortality rates increased with age in both sexes, especially after age group of 30-34 yearsfor incidence rates and age group of 50-54 years for mortality rates, and reached the peak at the age group of 85 years old (Figure 5-23a).

The skin cancer incidence rate was higher in urban areas than that in rural areas. The skin cancer mortality rate was higher in rural areas than that in urban areas. In both males and females, the incidence rate (ASR China) was highest in eastern areas, and the mortality rate (ASR China) was highest in western areas. Among the seven administrative districts, the incidence rate (ASR China) was highest in South China, followed by East China. The mortality rate (ASR China) in males was highest in Central China, followed by Southwest China and South China. The mortality rate (ASR China) in females was highest in Southwest China, followed by East China and Central China (Table 5-23a, Table 5-23b, Figure 5-23b).

表 5-23a　中国肿瘤登记地区皮肤癌发病情况

Table 5-23a　Incidence of skin cancer in the registration areas of China

地区 Area	性别 Sex	发病数 No. cases	粗率 Crude rate/ 100 000^{-1}	构成比 Freq. /%	中标率 ASR China/ 100 000^{-1}	世标率 ASR world/ 100 000^{-1}	累积率 Cum. rate 0~74/%
合计 All	合计 Both	18 157	2.89	0.95	1.65	1.62	0.17
	男性 Male	9 059	2.84	0.87	1.73	1.71	0.18
	女性 Female	9 098	2.94	1.04	1.56	1.54	0.16
城市地区 Urban areas	合计 Both	8 567	3.19	0.96	1.77	1.74	0.18
	男性 Male	4 318	3.21	0.91	1.88	1.85	0.19
	女性 Female	4 249	3.17	1.02	1.66	1.63	0.17
农村地区 Rural areas	合计 Both	9 590	2.66	0.94	1.55	1.54	0.16
	男性 Male	4 741	2.57	0.83	1.61	1.59	0.17
	女性 Female	4 849	2.76	1.07	1.49	1.48	0.15
东部地区 Eastern areas	合计 Both	9 335	3.68	1.01	1.88	1.85	0.19
	男性 Male	4 570	3.59	0.93	1.97	1.94	0.20
	女性 Female	4 765	3.78	1.09	1.79	1.77	0.18
中部地区 Central areas	合计 Both	3 399	2.26	0.80	1.40	1.38	0.14
	男性 Male	1 788	2.34	0.78	1.54	1.52	0.16
	女性 Female	1 611	2.18	0.83	1.27	1.24	0.13
西部地区 Western areas	合计 Both	5 423	2.42	0.96	1.49	1.47	0.15
	男性 Male	2 701	2.35	0.83	1.54	1.51	0.16
	女性 Female	2 722	2.48	1.13	1.45	1.43	0.14

表 5-23b　中国肿瘤登记地区皮肤癌死亡情况

Table 5-23b　Mortality of skin cancer in the registration areas of China

地区 Area	性别 Sex	死亡数 No. deaths	粗率 Crude rate/ 100 000^{-1}	构成比 Freq. /%	中标率 ASR China/ 100 000^{-1}	世标率 ASR world/ 100 000^{-1}	累积率 Cum. rate 0~74/%
合计 All	合计 Both	5 309	0.84	0.49	0.41	0.43	0.03
	男性 Male	2 924	0.92	0.42	0.50	0.52	0.04
	女性 Female	2 385	0.77	0.61	0.33	0.35	0.02
城市地区 Urban areas	合计 Both	2 096	0.78	0.44	0.36	0.38	0.03
	男性 Male	1 208	0.90	0.40	0.46	0.48	0.04
	女性 Female	888	0.66	0.51	0.27	0.28	0.02
农村地区 Rural areas	合计 Both	3 213	0.89	0.53	0.46	0.47	0.04
	男性 Male	1 716	0.93	0.43	0.54	0.54	0.05
	女性 Female	1 497	0.85	0.70	0.37	0.40	0.03
东部地区 Eastern areas	合计 Both	2 228	0.88	0.46	0.34	0.37	0.02
	男性 Male	1 150	0.90	0.38	0.42	0.44	0.03
	女性 Female	1 078	0.85	0.60	0.28	0.30	0.02
中部地区 Central areas	合计 Both	1 220	0.81	0.50	0.44	0.45	0.03
	男性 Male	715	0.93	0.46	0.56	0.56	0.04
	女性 Female	505	0.68	0.57	0.33	0.35	0.02
西部地区 Western areas	合计 Both	1 861	0.83	0.52	0.47	0.48	0.04
	男性 Male	1 059	0.92	0.45	0.57	0.58	0.05
	女性 Female	802	0.73	0.66	0.38	0.38	0.03

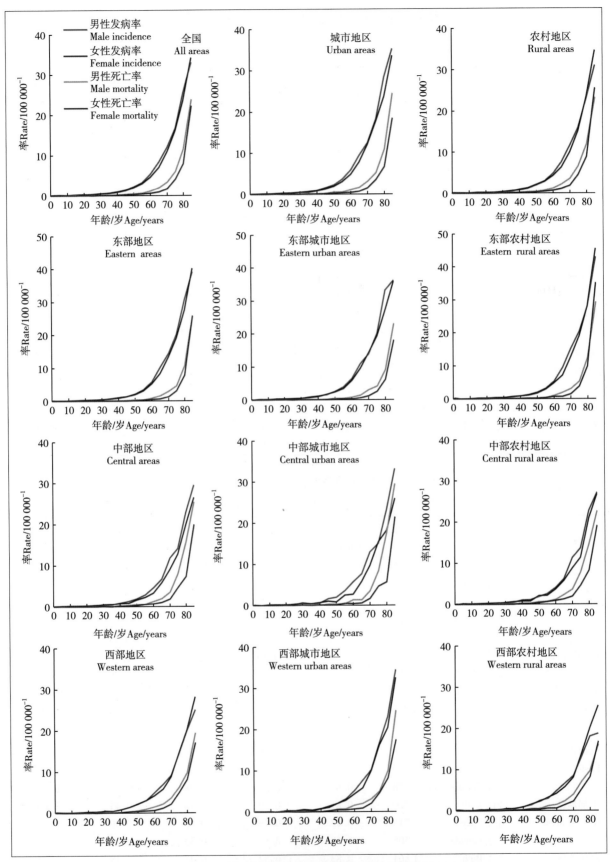

图 5-23a　中国肿瘤登记地区皮肤癌年龄别发病率和死亡率
Figure 5-23a　Age-specific incidence and mortality rates of skin cancer in
the registration areas of China

中标率ASR China/100 000^{-1}

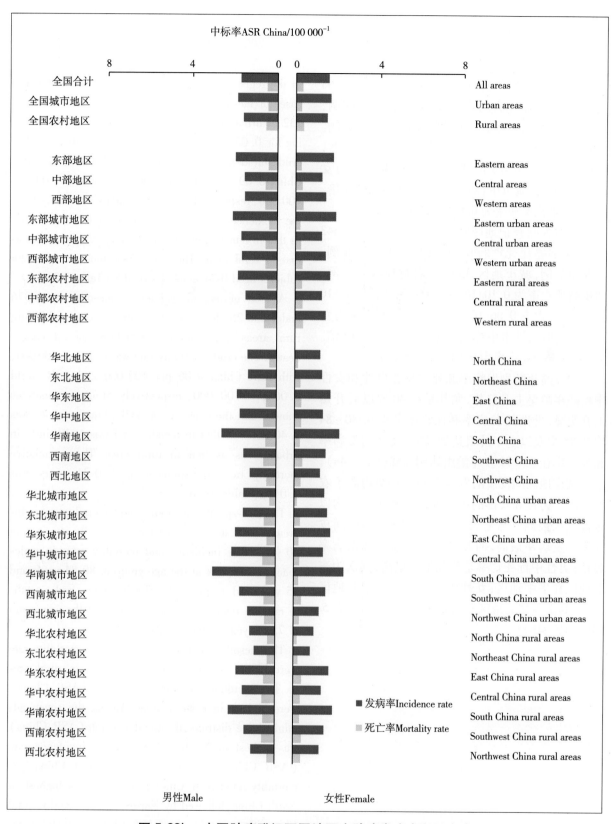

图 5-23b　中国肿瘤登记不同地区皮肤癌发病率和死亡率
Figure 5-23b　Incidence and mortality rates of skin cancer in different
Registration areas of China

24 间皮瘤

24 Mesothelioma

中国肿瘤登记地区间皮瘤新发病例数为 968 例,占全部癌症发病的 0.05%;其中男性 538 例,女性 430 例,城市地区 532 例,农村地区 436 例。发病率为 0.15/10 万,中标发病率为 0.09/10 万,世标发病率为 0.09/10 万;男性中标发病率为女性的 1.11 倍,城市中标发病率为农村的 1.50 倍。0~74 岁累积发病率为 0.01%(表 5-24a)。

中国肿瘤登记地区间皮瘤死亡病例数为 643 例,占全部癌症死亡的 0.06%;其中男性 376 例,女性 267 例,城市地区 350 例,农村地区 293 例。间皮瘤死亡率为 0.10/10 万,中标死亡率 0.06/10 万,世标死亡率 0.06/10 万;男性中标死亡率为女性的 1.40 倍,城市中标死亡率为农村的 1.40 倍。0~74 岁累积死亡率为 0.01%(表 5-24b)。

间皮瘤年龄别发病率和死亡率在男性和女性中均随年龄呈上升趋势,尤其是在 40 岁以后开始上升明显,男性的发病率和死亡率分别在 80~84 岁和 85 岁及以上年龄组达到高峰,女性的发病率和死亡率在 75~79 岁年龄组达到高峰(图 5-24a)。

城市地区间皮瘤的发病率和死亡率均高于农村地区。男性和女性的中标发病率和死亡率均以东部地区最高。在七大行政区中,华北地区间皮瘤中标发病率最高,西北地区间皮瘤中标发病率最低;男性中标死亡率是华北地区最高,其次为东北地区和华中地区;女性中标死亡率是东北地区最高,其次为华北地区和华东地区(表 5-24a,表 5-24b,图 5-24b)。

In the registration areas of China, there were 968 new cases of mesothelioma (538 males and 430 females, 532 in urban areas and 436 in rural areas), accounting for 0.05% of new cancer cases of all sites. The crude incidence rate was 0.15 per 100 000, with ASR China 0.09 per 100 000 and ASR world 0.09 per 100 000, respectively. Subgroup analyses showed that the incidence of ASR China in males was 1.11 times as that in females, and was 1.50 times in urban areas as that in rural areas. The cumulative incidence rate for subjects aged 0-74 years was 0.01% (Table 5-24a).

A total of 643 cases died of mesothelioma (376 males and 267 females, 350 in urban areas and 293 in rural areas), accounting for 0.06% of all cancer deaths. The crude mortality rate was 0.10 per 100 000, with ASR China 0.06 per 100 000 and ASR world 0.06 per 100 000, respectively. Subgroup analyses showed that the mortality of ASR China in males was 1.40 times as that in females, and was 1.40 times in urban areas as that in rural areas. The cumulative mortality rate for subjects aged 0-74 years was 0.01% (Table 5-24b).

The age-specific incidence and mortality rates increased with age in both sexes, especially after age of 40 years. The incidence and mortality rates in males reached the peak at the age group of 80-84 years and 85 years old, respectively. The incidence and mortality rates in females reached the peak at the age group of 75-79 years (Figure 5-24a).

The mesothelioma incidence rate and mortality rate were higher in urban areas than that in rural areas. The incidence and mortality rates (ASR China) were highest in eastern areas. Among the seven administrative districts, the incidence rate (ASR China) was highest in North China, and the incidence rate (ASR China) was lowest in Northwest China. The mortality rate (ASR China) in males was highest in North China, followed by Northeast China and Central China. The mortality rate (ASR China) in females was highest in Northeast China, followed by North China and East China (Table 5-24a, Table 5-24b, Figure 5-24b).

地区 Area	性别 Sex	发病数 No. cases	粗率 Crude rate/ 100 000^{-1}	构成比 Freq. /%	中标率 ASR China/ 100 000^{-1}	世标率 ASR world/ 100 000^{-1}	累积率 Cum. rate 0~74/%
合计 All	合计 Both	968	0.15	0.05	0.09	0.09	0.01
	男性 Male	538	0.17	0.05	0.10	0.10	0.01
	女性 Female	430	0.14	0.05	0.09	0.08	0.01
城市地区 Urban areas	合计 Both	532	0.20	0.06	0.12	0.12	0.01
	男性 Male	299	0.22	0.06	0.13	0.13	0.02
	女性 Female	233	0.17	0.06	0.10	0.10	0.01
农村地区 Rural areas	合计 Both	436	0.12	0.04	0.08	0.07	0.01
	男性 Male	239	0.13	0.04	0.08	0.08	0.01
	女性 Female	197	0.11	0.04	0.07	0.07	0.01
东部地区 Eastern areas	合计 Both	572	0.23	0.06	0.13	0.13	0.02
	男性 Male	313	0.25	0.06	0.14	0.14	0.02
	女性 Female	259	0.21	0.06	0.12	0.11	0.01
中部地区 Central areas	合计 Both	158	0.11	0.04	0.07	0.07	0.01
	男性 Male	94	0.12	0.04	0.08	0.08	0.01
	女性 Female	64	0.09	0.03	0.05	0.05	0.01
西部地区 Western areas	合计 Both	238	0.11	0.04	0.07	0.07	0.01
	男性 Male	131	0.11	0.04	0.07	0.07	0.01
	女性 Female	107	0.10	0.04	0.06	0.06	0.01

地区 Area	性别 Sex	死亡数 No. deaths	粗率 Crude rate/ 100 000^{-1}	构成比 Freq. /%	中标率 ASR China/ 100 000^{-1}	世标率 ASR world/ 100 000^{-1}	累积率 Cum. rate 0~74/%
合计 All	合计 Both	643	0.10	0.06	0.06	0.06	0.01
	男性 Male	376	0.12	0.05	0.07	0.07	0.01
	女性 Female	267	0.09	0.07	0.05	0.05	0.01
城市地区 Urban areas	合计 Both	350	0.13	0.07	0.07	0.07	0.01
	男性 Male	217	0.16	0.07	0.09	0.10	0.01
	女性 Female	133	0.10	0.08	0.05	0.05	0.01
农村地区 Rural areas	合计 Both	293	0.08	0.05	0.05	0.05	0.01
	男性 Male	159	0.09	0.04	0.05	0.05	0.01
	女性 Female	134	0.08	0.06	0.05	0.04	0.00
东部地区 Eastern areas	合计 Both	356	0.14	0.07	0.07	0.07	0.01
	男性 Male	208	0.16	0.07	0.09	0.09	0.01
	女性 Female	148	0.12	0.08	0.06	0.06	0.01
中部地区 Central areas	合计 Both	117	0.08	0.05	0.05	0.05	0.01
	男性 Male	74	0.10	0.05	0.06	0.06	0.01
	女性 Female	43	0.06	0.05	0.04	0.04	0.00
西部地区 Western areas	合计 Both	170	0.08	0.05	0.05	0.05	0.01
	男性 Male	94	0.08	0.04	0.05	0.06	0.01
	女性 Female	76	0.07	0.06	0.04	0.04	0.00

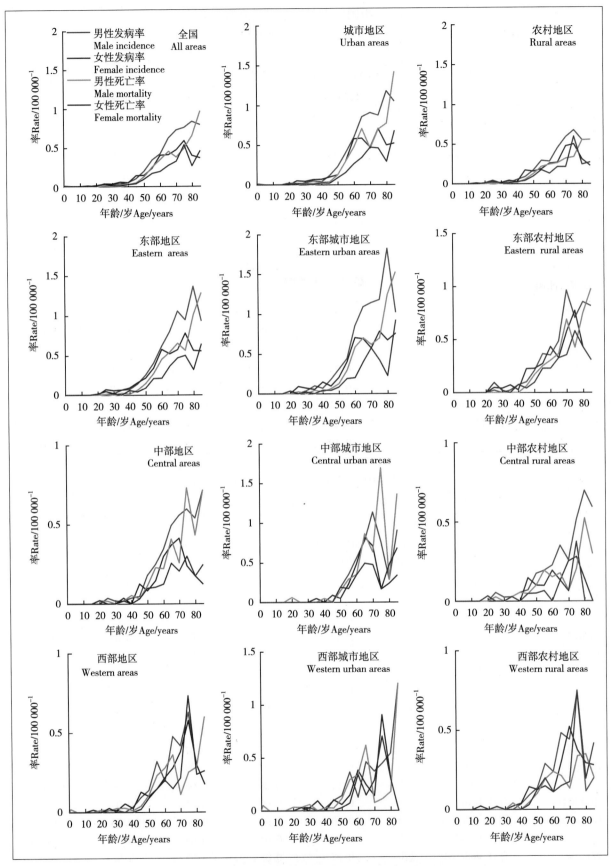

图 5-24a 中国肿瘤登记地区间皮瘤年龄别发病率和死亡率
Figure 5-24a Age-specific incidence and mortality rates of mesothelioma
in the registration areas of China

中标率ASR China/100 000⁻¹

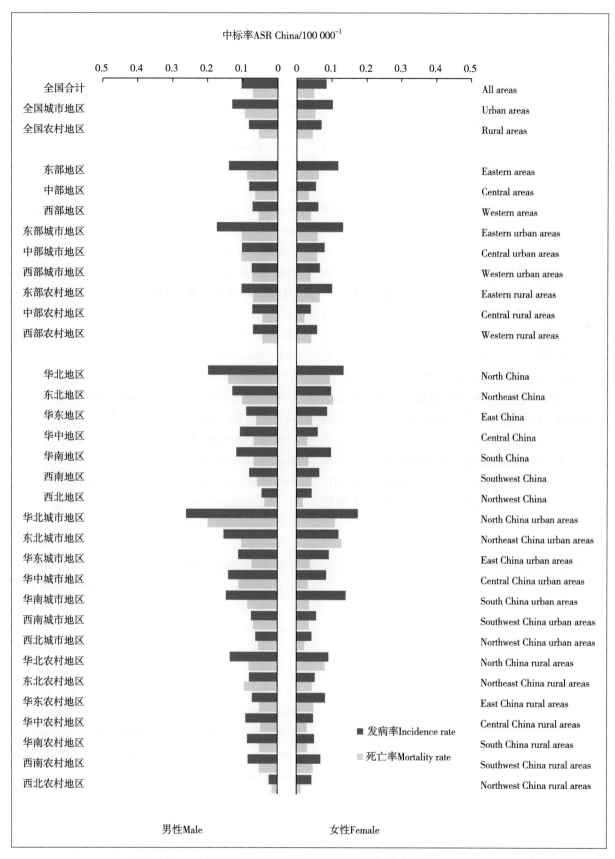

图 5-24b 中国肿瘤登记地区不同地区间皮瘤发病率和死亡率
Figure 5-24b Incidence and mortality rates of mesothelioma in different
registration areas of China

25 阴茎

中国肿瘤登记地区阴茎癌新发病例数为 2 445 例,占全部癌症发病的 0.23%;其中城市地区 1 037 例,农村地区 1 408 例。发病率为 0.77/10 万,中标发病率为 0.47/10 万,世标发病率为 0.46/10 万。0~74 岁累积发病率为 0.05%(表 5-25a)。

中国肿瘤登记地区阴茎癌死亡病例数为 878 例,占全部癌症死亡的 0.13%;其中城市地区 384 例,农村地区 494 例。阴茎癌死亡率为 0.28/10 万,中标死亡率 0.16/10 万,世标死亡率 0.16/10 万。0~74 岁累积死亡率为 0.02%(表 5-25b)。

阴茎癌年龄别发病率和死亡率在 30 岁之前处于较低水平,35 岁开始呈上升趋势,60 岁以后快速上升,发病率在 80~84 岁年龄组达到峰值,死亡率在 85 岁及以上年龄组达到峰值(图 5-25a)。

阴茎癌中标发病率以西部地区最高,其次是东部地区,中部地区最低。中标死亡率以中部地区最高,其次是西部地区,东部地区最低。在七大行政区中,西南地区阴茎癌中标发病率最高,其次是华中地区和华东地区,东北地区最低;中标死亡率是华中地区最高,其次为西南地区和华东地区(表 5-25a,表 5-25b,图 5-25b)。

25 Penis

In the registration areas of China, there were 2 445 new cases of penis cancer(1 037 in urban areas and 1 408 in rural areas), accounting for 0.23% of new cancer cases of all sites. The crude incidence rate was 0.77 per 100 000, with ASR China 0.47 per 100 000 and ASR world 0.46 per 100 000, respectively. The cumulative incidence rate for subjects aged 0-74 years was 0.05% (Table 5-25a).

A total of 878 cases died of penis cancer(384 in urban areas and 494 in rural areas), accounting for 0.13% of all cancer deaths. The crude mortality rate was 0.28 per 100 000, with ASR China 0.16 per 100 000 and ASR world 0.16 per 100 000, respectively. The cumulative mortality rate for subjects aged 0-74 years was 0.02% (Table 5-25b).

The age-specific incidence and mortality rates were low before 30 years old and increased constantly since then. The age-specific incidence and mortality rates dramatically increased over 60 years old. The incidence reached peak at the age group of 80-84 years, and the mortality rate reached peak at the age group of 85 years old(Figure 5-25a).

The incidence rates(ASR China) were the highest in western areas, followed by eastern areas, and the lowest in central areas. The mortality rates(ASR China) were the highest in central areas, followed by western areas, and the lowest in eastern areas. Among the seven administrative districts, the incidence rate (ASR China) was the highest in Southwest China, followed by Central China and East China, and was the lowest in Northeast China. The mortality rate (ASR China) was the highest in Central China, followed by Southwest China and East China(Table 5-25a, Table 5-25b, Figure 5-25b).

表 5-25a 中国肿瘤登记地区阴茎癌发病情况

Table 5-25a Incidence of penis cancer in the registration areas of China

地区 Area	发病数 No. cases	粗率 Crude rate/ 100 000^{-1}	构成比 Freq. /%	中标率 ASR China/ 100 000^{-1}	世标率 ASR world/ 100 000^{-1}	累积率 Cum. Rate 0~74/%
合计 All	2 445	0. 77	0. 23	0. 47	0. 46	0. 05
城市地区 Urban areas	1 037	0. 77	0. 22	0. 45	0. 45	0. 05
农村地区 Rural areas	1 408	0. 76	0. 25	0. 48	0. 47	0. 05
东部地区 Eastern areas	1 089	0. 85	0. 22	0. 47	0. 46	0. 05
中部地区 Central areas	520	0. 68	0. 23	0. 44	0. 44	0. 05
西部地区 Western areas	836	0. 73	0. 26	0. 48	0. 47	0. 05

表 5-25b 中国肿瘤登记地区阴茎癌死亡情况

Table 5-25b Mortality of penis cancer in the registration areas of China

地区 Area	死亡数 No. deaths	粗率 Crude rate/ 100 000^{-1}	构成比 Freq. /%	中标率 ASR China/ 100 000^{-1}	世标率 ASR world/ 100 000^{-1}	累积率 Cum. rate 0~74/%
合计 All	878	0. 28	0. 13	0. 16	0. 16	0. 02
城市地区 Urban areas	384	0. 29	0. 13	0. 15	0. 16	0. 02
农村地区 Rural areas	494	0. 27	0. 13	0. 16	0. 16	0. 02
东部地区 Eastern areas	374	0. 29	0. 12	0. 15	0. 15	0. 01
中部地区 Central areas	221	0. 29	0. 14	0. 18	0. 18	0. 02
西部地区 Western areas	283	0. 25	0. 12	0. 16	0. 16	0. 02

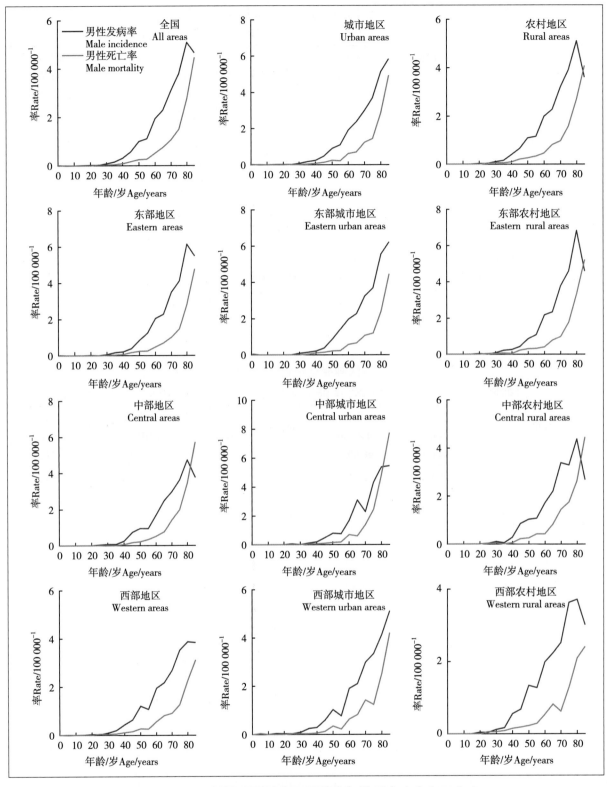

图 5-25a 中国肿瘤登记地区阴茎癌年龄别发病率和死亡率
Figure 5-25a Age-specific incidence and mortality rates of penis cancer in
the registration areas of China

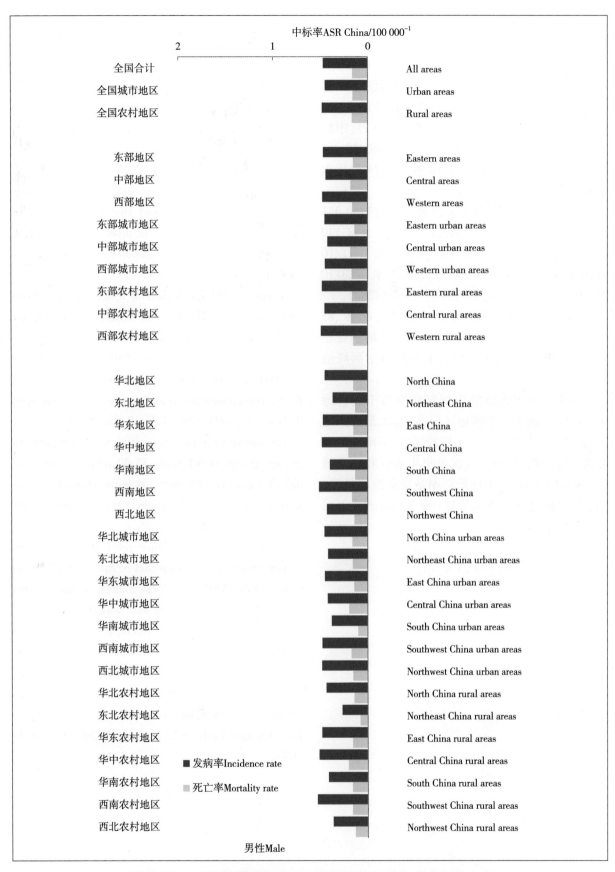

中标率ASR China/100 000^{-1}

全国合计	All areas
全国城市地区	Urban areas
全国农村地区	Rural areas
东部地区	Eastern areas
中部地区	Central areas
西部地区	Western areas
东部城市地区	Eastern urban areas
中部城市地区	Central urban areas
西部城市地区	Western urban areas
东部农村地区	Eastern rural areas
中部农村地区	Central rural areas
西部农村地区	Western rural areas
华北地区	North China
东北地区	Northeast China
华东地区	East China
华中地区	Central China
华南地区	South China
西南地区	Southwest China
西北地区	Northwest China
华北城市地区	North China urban areas
东北城市地区	Northeast China urban areas
华东城市地区	East China urban areas
华中城市地区	Central China urban areas
华南城市地区	South China urban areas
西南城市地区	Southwest China urban areas
西北城市地区	Northwest China urban areas
华北农村地区	North China rural areas
东北农村地区	Northeast China rural areas
华东农村地区	East China rural areas
华中农村地区	Central China rural areas
华南农村地区	South China rural areas
西南农村地区	Southwest China rural areas
西北农村地区	Northwest China rural areas

■ 发病率Incidence rate
■ 死亡率Mortality rate

男性Male

图 5-25b 中国肿瘤登记地区不同地区阴茎癌发病率和死亡率
Figure 5-25b Incidence and mortality rates of penis cancer in different registration areas of China

26 睾丸

中国肿瘤登记地区睾丸癌新发病例数为1 454例,占全部癌症发病的0.14%;其中城市地区666例,农村地区788例。发病率为0.46/10万,中标发病率为0.43/10万,世标发病率为0.40/10万;城市中标发病率为农村的1.18倍。0~74岁累积发病率为0.03%(表5-26a)。

中国肿瘤登记地区睾丸癌死亡病例数为351例,占全部癌症死亡的0.05%;其中城市地区140例,农村地区211例。睾丸癌死亡率为0.11/10万,中标死亡率0.08/10万,世标死亡率0.08/10万。0~74岁累积死亡率为0.01%(表5-26b)。

睾丸癌年龄别发病率在0~1岁、35~40岁、85岁及以上年龄组有三个高峰,睾丸癌年龄别死亡率呈上升趋势,在85岁及以上年龄组达到峰值(图5-26a)。

城市地区睾丸癌的中标发病率高于农村地区。中标发病率以东部地区最高,其次是西部地区,中部地区最低。在七大行政区中,华南地区睾丸癌中标发病率最高,其次是华东地区和华北地区,西北地区最低;中标死亡率是华南地区最高,其次为西南地区和华东地区(表5-26a,表5-26b,图5-26b)。

26 Testis

In the registration areas of China, there were 1 454 new cases of testis cancer (666 in urban areas and 788 in rural areas), accounting for 0.14% of new cancer cases of all sites. The crude incidence rate was 0.46 per 100 000, with ASR China 0.43 per 100 000 and ASR world 0.40 per 100 000, respectively. Subgroup analyses showed that the incidence of ASR China was 1.18 times in urban areas as that in rural areas. The cumulative incidence rate for subjects aged 0-74 years was 0.03% (Table 5-26a).

A total of 351 cases died of testis cancer (140 in urban areas and 211 in rural areas), accounting for 0.05% of all cancer deaths. The crude mortality rate was 0.11 per 100 000, with ASR China 0.08 per 100 000 and ASR world 0.08 per 100 000, respectively. The cumulative mortality rate for subjects aged 0-74 years was 0.01% (Table 5-26b).

The age-specific incidence rates had three peaks in the age groups of 0-1 years, 35-40 years and 85 years old. The age-specific mortality rates showed an upward trend, reaching the peak at the age group of 85 years old (Figure 5-26a).

The testis cancer incidence rate (ASR China) was higher in urban areas than that in rural areas. The incidence rate (ASR China) was highest in eastern areas, and followed by western and central areas. Among the seven administrative districts, the incidence rate (ASR China) was highest in South China, followed by East China and North China, and was lowest in Northwest China. The mortality rate (ASR China) was highest in South China, followed by Southwest China and East China (Table 5-26a, Table 5-26b, Figure 5-26b).

表 5-26a　中国肿瘤登记地区睾丸癌发病情况

Table 5-26a　Incidence of testis cancer in the registration areas of China

地区 Area	发病数 No. cases	粗率 Crude rate/ 100 000^{-1}	构成比 Freq./%	中标率 ASR China/ 100 000^{-1}	世标率 ASR world/ 100 000^{-1}	累积率 Cum. rate 0~74/%
合计 All	1 454	0.46	0.14	0.43	0.40	0.03
城市地区 Urban areas	666	0.50	0.14	0.47	0.43	0.03
农村地区 Rural areas	788	0.43	0.14	0.40	0.38	0.03
东部地区 Eastern areas	704	0.55	0.14	0.54	0.50	0.04
中部地区 Central areas	297	0.39	0.13	0.35	0.34	0.03
西部地区 Western areas	453	0.39	0.14	0.37	0.34	0.03

表 5-26b　中国肿瘤登记地区睾丸癌死亡情况

Table 5-26b　Mortality of testis cancer in the registration areas of China

地区 Area	死亡数 No. deaths	粗率 Crude rate/ 100 000^{-1}	构成比 Freq./%	中标率 ASR China/ 100 000^{-1}	世标率 ASR world/ 100 000^{-1}	累积率 Cum. rate 0~74/%
合计 All	351	0.11	0.05	0.08	0.08	0.01
城市地区 Urban areas	140	0.10	0.05	0.08	0.07	0.01
农村地区 Rural areas	211	0.11	0.05	0.08	0.08	0.01
东部地区 Eastern areas	148	0.12	0.05	0.08	0.08	0.01
中部地区 Central areas	82	0.11	0.05	0.08	0.08	0.01
西部地区 Western areas	121	0.11	0.05	0.09	0.08	0.01

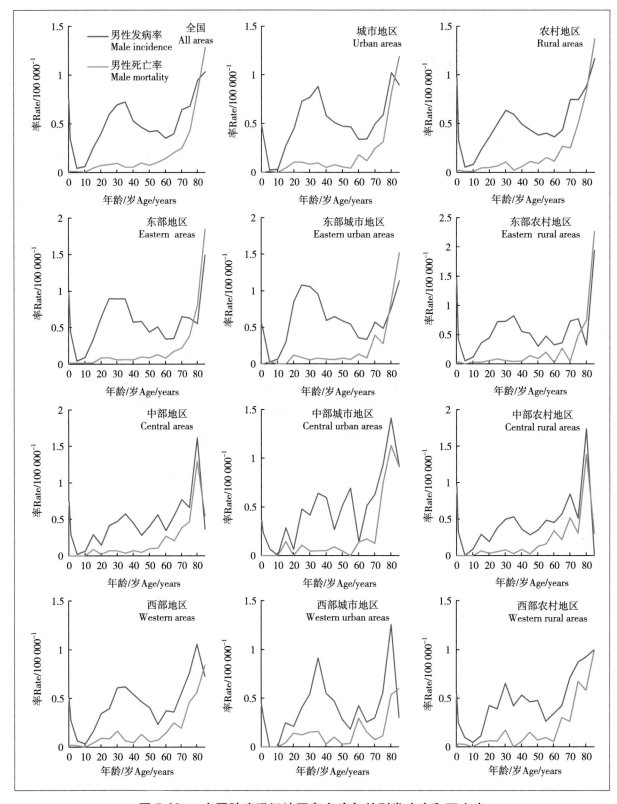

图 5-26a 中国肿瘤登记地区睾丸癌年龄别发病率和死亡率

Figure 5-26a Age-specific incidence and mortality rates of testis cancer in the registration areas of China

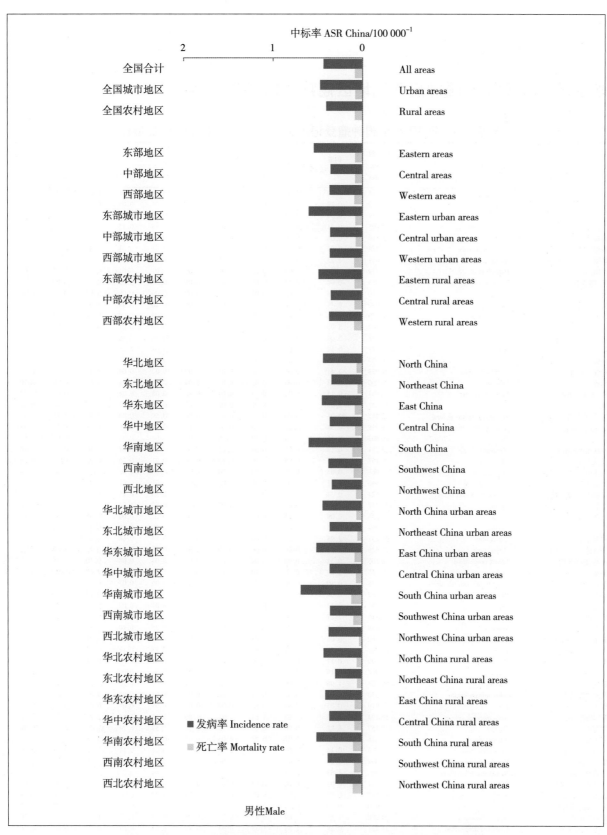

图 5-26b　中国肿瘤登记地区不同地区睾丸癌发病率和死亡率

Figure 5-26b　Incidence and mortality rates of testis cancer in different registration areas of China

附录

附录 1　2019 年全国肿瘤登记地区癌症发病与死亡结果

附表 1-1　2019 年全国肿瘤登记地区男女合计癌症发病主要指标

部位 Site		病例数 No. cases	构成 Freq. /%	年龄组								
				0~	1~4	5~9	10~14	15~19	20~24	25~29	30~34	35~39
唇	Lip	1 765	0.09	0.03	0.02	0.01	0.01	0.01	0.03	0.03	0.04	0.05
舌	Tongue	5 599	0.29	0.02	0.01	0.01	0.01	0.03	0.05	0.10	0.25	0.36
口	Mouth	7 359	0.38	0.03	0.02	0.04	0.07	0.05	0.08	0.08	0.16	0.28
唾液腺	Salivary gland	3 995	0.21	0.00	0.01	0.03	0.06	0.13	0.15	0.27	0.36	0.36
扁桃体	Tonsil	1 110	0.06	0.00	0.00	0.02	0.01	0.02	0.01	0.03	0.04	0.05
其他口咽	Other oropharynx	1 748	0.09	0.00	0.01	0.01	0.01	0.01	0.01	0.02	0.04	0.07
鼻咽	Nasopharynx	23 651	1.23	0.03	0.03	0.04	0.16	0.40	0.43	0.99	1.88	2.93
下咽	Hypopharynx	3 279	0.17	0.00	0.00	0.01	0.00	0.01	0.01	0.01	0.02	0.05
咽,部位不明	Pharynx unspecified	1 483	0.08	0.02	0.01	0.00	0.01	0.01	0.02	0.02	0.01	0.02
食管	Esophagus	105 070	5.48	0.03	0.01	0.01	0.02	0.09	0.08	0.13	0.20	0.40
胃	Stomach	162 680	8.49	0.06	0.02	0.02	0.05	0.26	0.44	1.07	1.99	3.25
小肠	Small intestine	8 179	0.43	0.03	0.01	0.00	0.00	0.03	0.04	0.08	0.15	0.30
结肠	Colon	96 967	5.06	0.00	0.02	0.01	0.05	0.18	0.37	0.97	1.90	3.05
直肠	Rectum	97 038	5.06	0.00	0.01	0.01	0.02	0.16	0.30	0.82	1.53	2.31
肛门	Anus	2 273	0.12	0.00	0.00	0.00	0.00	0.01	0.01	0.02	0.06	0.09
肝脏	Liver	169 609	8.85	1.01	0.49	0.13	0.16	0.39	0.57	1.79	3.97	7.25
胆囊及其他	Gallbladder etc.	26 923	1.41	0.03	0.01	0.01	0.00	0.02	0.04	0.08	0.18	0.36
胰腺	Pancreas	44 700	2.33	0.03	0.01	0.02	0.04	0.05	0.11	0.19	0.38	0.70
鼻、鼻窦及其他	Nose, sinuses etc.	2 904	0.15	0.02	0.03	0.04	0.06	0.05	0.08	0.08	0.12	0.22
喉	Larynx	11 637	0.61	0.02	0.01	0.02	0.00	0.04	0.02	0.04	0.06	0.13
气管、支气管、肺	Trachea, bronchus & lung	422 442	22.05	0.06	0.07	0.05	0.06	0.59	0.84	2.08	4.51	8.71
其他胸腔器官	Other thoracic organs	6 538	0.34	0.27	0.16	0.05	0.10	0.17	0.16	0.28	0.34	0.41
骨	Bone	10 803	0.56	0.14	0.19	0.46	1.05	1.04	0.55	0.51	0.61	0.54
皮肤黑色素瘤	Melanoma of skin	3 281	0.17	0.05	0.03	0.03	0.01	0.05	0.04	0.10	0.12	0.16
皮肤其他	Other skin	18 157	0.95	0.05	0.10	0.10	0.09	0.21	0.25	0.28	0.46	0.58
间皮瘤	Mesothelioma	968	0.05	0.00	0.00	0.00	0.00	0.00	0.00	0.02	0.02	0.04
卡波西肉瘤	Kaposi sarcoma	146	0.01	0.02	0.01	0.00	0.00	0.01	0.01	0.01	0.01	0.02
结缔组织、软组织	Connective & soft tissue	6 421	0.34	0.51	0.41	0.25	0.23	0.36	0.25	0.46	0.57	0.57
乳腺	Breast	133 447	7.06	0.00	0.01	0.00	0.06	0.65	1.94	6.24	15.63	32.41
外阴	Vulva	1 638	0.09	0.01	0.01	0.01	0.01	0.01	0.02	0.04	0.05	0.08	0.19
阴道	Vagina	964	0.05	0.07	0.04	0.00	0.01	0.00	0.02	0.02	0.04	0.07
子宫颈	Cervix uteri	56 231	2.93	0.00	0.00	0.00	0.00	0.14	0.68	2.88	7.76	14.68
子宫体	Corpus uteri	27 426	1.43	0.00	0.00	0.00	0.01	0.07	0.21	0.73	1.59	3.27
子宫,部位不明	Uterus unspecified	6 105	0.32	0.00	0.00	0.01	0.00	0.04	0.08	0.30	0.65	1.07
卵巢	Ovary	24 265	1.27	0.10	0.10	0.15	0.56	1.40	2.08	2.62	2.96	3.84
其他女性生殖器官	Other female genital organs	1 928	0.10	0.02	0.01	0.03	0.06	0.07	0.10	0.12	0.26
胎盘	Placenta	232	0.01	0.00	0.00	0.00	0.00	0.05	0.11	0.24	0.13	0.12
阴茎	Penis	2 445	0.13	0.00	0.01	0.00	0.00	0.01	0.02	0.02	0.08	0.16
前列腺	Prostate	43 416	2.27	0.00	0.01	0.01	0.01	0.01	0.06	0.02	0.06	0.09
睾丸	Testis	1 454	0.08	0.76	0.34	0.04	0.06	0.25	0.40	0.60	0.69	0.72
其他男性生殖器官	Other male genital organs	569	0.03	0.00	0.03	0.02	0.01	0.06	0.02	0.01	0.01	0.03
肾	Kidney	25 707	1.34	0.51	0.60	0.18	0.08	0.13	0.18	0.47	0.89	1.51
肾盂	Renal pelvis	3 199	0.17	0.00	0.01	0.00	0.00	0.01	0.00	0.01	0.02	0.03
输尿管	Ureter	3 564	0.19	0.00	0.00	0.00	0.00	0.00	0.00	0.00	0.02	0.03
膀胱	Bladder	37 624	1.96	0.00	0.04	0.00	0.01	0.07	0.12	0.25	0.46	0.79
其他泌尿器官	Other urinary organs	830	0.04	0.02	0.01	0.00	0.00	0.01	0.01	0.00	0.01	0.03
眼	Eye	979	0.05	0.85	0.51	0.06	0.02	0.01	0.03	0.02	0.05	0.04
脑、神经系统	Brain, nervous system	52 104	2.72	2.23	1.84	1.92	1.80	1.65	1.66	2.28	2.92	3.92
甲状腺	Thyroid	119 157	6.22	0.00	0.01	0.06	0.36	1.57	6.74	17.64	25.28	30.26
肾上腺	Adrenal gland	1 845	0.10	0.27	0.23	0.06	0.02	0.03	0.04	0.08	0.09	0.11
其他内分泌腺	Other endocrine	2 773	0.14	0.03	0.07	0.08	0.13	0.14	0.14	0.22	0.27	0.40
霍奇金淋巴瘤	Hodgkin lymphoma	1 998	0.10	0.02	0.02	0.09	0.18	0.19	0.26	0.26	0.28	0.25
非霍奇金淋巴瘤	Non-Hodgkin lymphoma	29 303	1.53	0.35	0.60	0.48	0.56	0.64	0.72	0.97	1.33	1.89
免疫增生性疾病	Immunoproliferative diseases	581	0.03	0.00	0.02	0.00	0.01	0.01	0.01	0.01	0.00	0.02
多发性骨髓瘤	Multiple myeloma	10 512	0.55	0.05	0.01	0.03	0.06	0.07	0.07	0.07	0.12	0.21
淋巴细胞白血病	Lymphoid leukemia	7 460	0.39	0.91	2.76	1.58	1.02	0.68	0.48	0.45	0.47	0.47
髓系白血病	Myeloid leukemia	21 200	1.11	1.69	0.89	0.71	0.85	1.03	1.07	1.31	1.60	1.70
白血病,未特指	Leukemia unspecified	11 121	0.58	1.53	1.35	0.93	0.84	0.84	0.59	0.67	0.65	0.76
其他或未指明部位	Other and unspecified	37 447	1.95	1.44	1.07	0.64	0.67	0.74	0.72	0.93	1.26	1.79
所有部位合计	All sites	1 916 152	100.00	12.93	12.03	8.33	9.26	13.53	20.55	43.02	70.59	105.79
所有部位除外 C44	All sites except C44	1 897 995	99.05	12.88	11.93	8.23	9.17	13.32	20.30	42.73	70.13	105.21

Appendix 1   Cancer incidence and mortality in registration areas of China,2019

Appendix Table 1-1   Cancer incidence in registration areas of China,both sexes in 2019

Age group										粗率 Crude rate/ 100 000⁻¹	中标率 ASR China/ 100 000⁻¹	世标率 ASR world/ 100 000⁻¹	累积率 Cum. Rate/%		ICD-10
40~44	45~49	50~54	55~59	60~64	65~69	70~74	75~79	80~84	85+				0~64	0~74	
0.09	0.18	0.28	0.34	0.59	0.86	1.12	1.67	1.52	1.84	0.28	0.17	0.17	0.01	0.02	C00
0.63	0.86	1.31	1.61	2.28	2.61	2.76	3.01	2.72	2.29	0.89	0.57	0.55	0.04	0.06	C01-C02
0.45	0.80	1.46	1.95	2.71	3.60	4.63	5.20	5.47	5.77	1.17	0.71	0.70	0.04	0.08	C03-C06
0.49	0.62	0.93	1.12	1.29	1.64	1.61	1.58	1.89	1.91	0.64	0.45	0.42	0.03	0.05	C07-C08
0.09	0.21	0.28	0.43	0.46	0.41	0.48	0.52	0.48	0.47	0.18	0.11	0.11	0.01	0.01	C09
0.11	0.23	0.33	0.50	0.60	0.93	0.95	1.00	1.04	0.91	0.28	0.17	0.17	0.01	0.02	C10
4.17	5.84	6.98	7.56	7.88	7.45	7.40	6.56	6.04	4.80	3.76	2.71	2.52	0.20	0.27	C11
0.12	0.33	0.78	1.36	1.72	1.78	1.84	1.50	1.50	0.95	0.52	0.31	0.31	0.02	0.04	C12-C13
0.05	0.13	0.25	0.43	0.60	0.73	1.05	0.99	1.38	1.31	0.24	0.14	0.14	0.01	0.02	C14
1.36	4.35	11.96	20.69	41.90	64.61	86.85	104.07	107.65	98.29	16.72	9.20	9.25	0.41	1.16	C15
5.82	11.57	21.96	35.93	63.02	92.10	121.30	145.34	155.34	138.68	25.89	14.79	14.68	0.73	1.79	C16
0.49	0.87	1.59	2.07	3.19	4.33	4.98	5.89	6.40	6.26	1.30	0.77	0.76	0.04	0.09	C17
5.17	8.72	14.50	22.99	36.07	49.53	64.15	79.43	94.35	91.89	15.43	8.98	8.84	0.47	1.04	C18
4.81	9.30	16.00	23.98	38.57	52.56	65.43	76.21	82.35	75.05	15.44	9.00	8.92	0.49	1.08	C19-C20
0.16	0.26	0.41	0.51	0.91	1.09	1.37	1.77	2.36	2.27	0.36	0.21	0.21	0.02	0.03	C21
15.50	25.36	37.78	46.17	64.60	79.83	91.56	105.72	114.77	115.32	26.99	16.50	16.20	1.02	1.88	C22
0.80	1.65	3.36	4.90	9.96	14.32	19.62	25.69	32.00	33.45	4.28	2.37	2.36	0.11	0.28	C23-C24
1.42	3.22	5.74	9.42	16.36	23.77	31.74	40.73	50.49	51.46	7.11	3.98	3.96	0.19	0.47	C25
0.28	0.47	0.65	0.74	1.04	1.26	1.44	1.49	1.66	1.73	0.46	0.31	0.30	0.02	0.03	C30-C31
0.33	0.81	2.06	3.53	5.70	6.73	8.03	8.32	7.87	6.36	1.85	1.06	1.08	0.06	0.14	C32
16.62	33.09	62.96	103.42	171.37	240.80	298.96	352.70	367.21	333.27	67.22	38.58	38.45	2.02	4.72	C33-C34
0.67	0.95	1.38	1.95	2.49	3.02	2.95	3.28	3.00	2.88	1.04	0.70	0.69	0.05	0.08	C37-C38
0.80	1.11	1.69	2.10	3.23	4.27	5.78	7.40	8.03	8.11	1.72	1.25	1.22	0.07	0.12	C40-C41
0.28	0.38	0.53	0.72	1.16	1.57	1.87	2.42	2.66	3.01	0.52	0.32	0.32	0.02	0.04	C43
0.90	1.34	2.07	3.09	4.93	7.63	11.43	16.47	24.50	33.76	2.89	1.65	1.62	0.07	0.17	C44
0.05	0.12	0.17	0.28	0.41	0.51	0.59	0.67	0.60	0.53	0.15	0.09	0.09	0.01	0.01	C45
0.01	0.02	0.04	0.02	0.05	0.04	0.08	0.06	0.07	0.13	0.02	0.02	0.02	0.00	0.00	C46
0.71	0.93	1.24	1.41	1.90	2.29	2.64	3.30	3.57	3.93	1.02	0.75	0.74	0.05	0.07	C47,C49
56.80	85.50	84.68	85.29	89.03	78.78	65.52	59.45	52.24	40.88	43.10	30.11	28.08	2.29	3.01	C50
0.27	0.43	0.59	0.70	1.15	1.37	1.95	2.36	2.52	2.72	0.53	0.31	0.31	0.02	0.03	C51
0.26	0.36	0.45	0.61	0.65	0.80	1.04	1.04	1.06	0.65	0.31	0.19	0.19	0.01	0.02	C52
22.73	32.32	39.45	38.59	34.73	30.08	29.97	27.00	21.55	14.08	18.16	12.74	11.80	0.97	1.27	C53
7.07	14.35	23.36	24.26	19.91	17.84	14.09	10.89	9.00	5.85	8.86	5.76	5.59	0.47	0.63	C54
2.13	3.38	4.13	3.82	3.74	3.71	3.73	4.05	4.41	3.34	1.97	1.32	1.24	0.10	0.13	C55
6.77	11.84	14.93	15.27	16.07	16.95	16.50	15.41	13.20	7.56	7.84	5.48	5.20	0.39	0.56	C56
0.53	0.91	1.15	1.29	1.41	1.69	1.40	1.20	1.05	0.87	0.62	0.41	0.40	0.03	0.05	C57
0.15	0.11	0.08	0.02	0.01	0.00	0.01	0.01	0.00	0.02	0.07	0.08	0.07	0.01	0.01	C58
0.31	0.57	1.00	1.12	1.95	2.29	3.10	3.79	5.09	4.65	0.77	0.47	0.46	0.03	0.05	C60
0.18	0.66	2.06	7.01	21.20	45.20	85.76	133.66	165.07	174.64	13.62	7.53	7.41	0.16	0.81	C61
0.53	0.47	0.42	0.43	0.35	0.40	0.64	0.68	0.94	1.04	0.46	0.43	0.40	0.03	0.03	C62
0.06	0.08	0.16	0.27	0.38	0.59	0.80	1.08	1.20	1.00	0.18	0.11	0.11	0.01	0.01	C63
2.28	3.68	5.86	8.41	10.04	12.58	12.93	12.65	13.28	11.30	4.09	2.60	2.58	0.17	0.30	C64
0.12	0.19	0.43	0.73	1.10	1.81	2.30	3.11	3.49	3.08	0.51	0.29	0.28	0.01	0.03	C65
0.07	0.15	0.28	0.64	1.39	2.07	2.75	3.89	4.52	3.65	0.57	0.31	0.31	0.01	0.04	C66
1.22	2.20	4.08	7.31	12.81	18.55	26.74	37.68	47.91	50.38	5.99	3.32	3.29	0.15	0.37	C67
0.03	0.04	0.07	0.18	0.28	0.47	0.61	0.73	0.91	1.09	0.13	0.07	0.07	0.00	0.01	C68
0.06	0.11	0.14	0.15	0.27	0.27	0.42	0.51	0.74	0.59	0.16	0.11	0.15	0.01	0.01	C69
5.49	7.97	10.90	13.60	17.71	20.92	23.90	25.94	27.42	27.10	8.29	5.79	5.70	0.37	0.59	C70-C72,D32-D33,D42-D43
30.81	32.14	32.91	33.04	24.28	17.83	11.83	8.37	6.08	4.82	18.96	16.46	14.09	1.18	1.32	C73
0.17	0.28	0.41	0.49	0.60	0.78	0.77	0.88	1.04	1.09	0.29	0.20	0.21	0.01	0.02	C74
0.39	0.46	0.61	0.77	0.89	0.93	1.02	0.89	0.88	0.62	0.44	0.34	0.32	0.02	0.03	C75
0.19	0.25	0.37	0.36	0.54	0.58	0.76	0.93	0.79	0.78	0.32	0.27	0.25	0.02	0.02	C81
2.36	3.62	5.32	7.27	10.48	13.59	17.07	18.70	20.04	14.47	4.66	3.07	2.99	0.18	0.33	C82-C86,C96
0.04	0.06	0.09	0.11	0.23	0.35	0.41	0.46	0.37	0.30	0.09	0.06	0.06	0.00	0.01	C88
0.40	0.93	1.69	2.67	4.41	6.20	7.21	8.86	7.78	5.68	1.67	0.98	0.98	0.05	0.12	C90
0.49	0.72	0.98	1.18	1.77	2.39	3.02	3.31	3.40	2.60	1.19	1.01	1.16	0.06	0.09	C91
2.07	2.71	3.58	4.47	6.30	8.40	10.60	13.16	13.61	11.43	3.37	2.43	2.37	0.14	0.24	C92-C94,D45-D47
0.92	1.12	1.56	1.87	2.80	4.13	5.72	7.65	7.74	7.64	1.77	1.33	1.37	0.07	0.12	C95
2.65	4.22	6.40	8.14	11.90	16.34	21.67	26.80	32.87	39.52	5.96	3.75	3.73	0.21	0.40	O & U
160.59	249.54	360.20	480.13	688.36	900.04	1 106.13	1 308.37	1 416.08	1 332.04	304.91	190.66	185.32	11.11	21.14	C00-C97,D32-D33, D42-D43,D45-D47
159.69	248.20	358.12	477.04	683.43	892.41	1 094.70	1 291.90	1 391.58	1 298.29	302.02	189.02	183.70	11.04	20.97	C00-C97,D32-D33, D42-D43,D45-D47 exc.C44

部位 Site		病例数 No. cases	构成 Freq. /%	年龄组								
				0~	1~4	5~9	10~14	15~19	20~24	25~29	30~34	35~39
唇	Lip	1 027	0.10	0.03	0.01	0.02	0.02	0.02	0.02	0.03	0.04	0.03
舌	Tongue	3 764	0.36	0.03	0.01	0.01	0.02	0.04	0.06	0.13	0.34	0.49
口	Mouth	4 862	0.47	0.03	0.02	0.04	0.08	0.06	0.07	0.07	0.20	0.33
唾液腺	Salivary gland	2 255	0.22	0.00	0.02	0.03	0.06	0.11	0.15	0.22	0.32	0.38
扁桃体	Tonsil	806	0.08	0.00	0.01	0.03	0.01	0.01	0.00	0.02	0.04	0.10
其他口咽	Other oropharynx	1 466	0.14	0.00	0.01	0.01	0.01	0.02	0.02	0.01	0.06	0.08
鼻咽	Nasopharynx	16 823	1.61	0.03	0.04	0.04	0.22	0.56	0.52	1.18	2.50	4.00
下咽	Hypopharynx	3 049	0.29	0.00	0.00	0.00	0.00	0.01	0.02	0.01	0.02	0.08
咽,部位不明	Pharynx unspecified	1 184	0.11	0.00	0.01	0.01	0.02	0.01	0.02	0.02	0.02	0.02
食管	Esophagus	78 494	7.51	0.06	0.01	0.01	0.02	0.16	0.05	0.14	0.26	0.53
胃	Stomach	113 418	10.85	0.09	0.03	0.02	0.07	0.36	0.39	0.89	1.77	3.14
小肠	Small intestine	4 655	0.45	0.00	0.01	0.00	0.00	0.00	0.04	0.08	0.14	0.38
结肠	Colon	55 155	5.28	0.00	0.03	0.01	0.06	0.25	0.46	1.05	2.07	3.13
直肠	Rectum	59 391	5.68	0.00	0.02	0.01	0.02	0.22	0.34	0.93	1.62	2.44
肛门	Anus	1 278	0.12	0.00	0.01	0.01	0.00	0.01	0.03	0.03	0.05	0.09
肝脏	Liver	126 372	12.09	1.13	0.54	0.17	0.18	0.54	0.83	2.72	6.48	12.17
胆囊及其他	Gallbladder etc.	12 907	1.24	0.06	0.02	0.01	0.00	0.04	0.01	0.07	0.17	0.29
胰腺	Pancreas	25 541	2.44	0.06	0.01	0.02	0.00	0.03	0.07	0.18	0.40	0.81
鼻、鼻窦及其他	Nose, sinuses etc.	1 805	0.17	0.03	0.03	0.06	0.04	0.09	0.09	0.13	0.23	
喉	Larynx	10 548	1.01	0.03	0.01	0.04	0.01	0.05	0.02	0.04	0.08	0.20
气管、支气管、肺	Trachea, bronchus & lung	270 953	25.93	0.06	0.07	0.05	0.07	0.73	0.81	1.63	3.67	7.39
其他胸腔器官	Other thoracic organs	3 931	0.38	0.27	0.18	0.05	0.16	0.23	0.23	0.36	0.44	0.48
骨	Bone	6 111	0.58	0.12	0.21	0.48	1.10	1.28	0.73	0.60	0.66	0.58
皮肤黑色素瘤	Melanoma of skin	1 661	0.16	0.03	0.04	0.01	0.02	0.03	0.02	0.09	0.07	0.12
皮肤其他	Other skin	9 059	0.87	0.06	0.09	0.13	0.08	0.23	0.24	0.33	0.46	0.60
间皮瘤	Mesothelioma	538	0.05	0.00	0.01	0.00	0.00	0.00	0.00	0.02	0.02	0.03
卡波西肉瘤	Kaposi sarcoma	103	0.01	0.03	0.00	0.00	0.00	0.02	0.01	0.02	0.02	0.03
结缔组织、软组织	Connective & soft tissue	3 518	0.34	0.43	0.36	0.25	0.26	0.35	0.27	0.50	0.60	0.56
乳腺	Breast	1 903	0.18	0.06	0.01	0.01	0.01	0.01	0.03	0.08	0.11	0.19
外阴	Vulva	—	—	—	—	—	—	—	—	—	—	—
阴道	Vagina	—	—	—	—	—	—	—	—	—	—	—
子宫颈	Cervix uteri	—	—	—	—	—	—	—	—	—	—	—
子宫体	Corpus uteri	—	—	—	—	—	—	—	—	—	—	—
子宫,部位不明	Uterus unspecified	—	—	—	—	—	—	—	—	—	—	—
卵巢	Ovary	—	—	—	—	—	—	—	—	—	—	—
其他女性生殖器官	Other female genital organs	—	—	—	—	—	—	—	—	—	—	—
胎盘	Placenta	—	—	—	—	—	—	—	—	—	—	—
阴茎	Penis	2 445	0.23	0.00	0.01	0.00	0.00	0.01	0.02	0.02	0.08	0.16
前列腺	Prostate	43 416	4.15	0.00	0.01	0.01	0.01	0.06	0.02	0.06	0.06	0.09
睾丸	Testis	1 454	0.14	0.76	0.34	0.04	0.06	0.25	0.40	0.60	0.69	0.72
其他男性生殖器官	Other male genital organs	569	0.05	0.00	0.03	0.02	0.01	0.06	0.02	0.01	0.01	0.03
肾	Kidney	16 701	1.60	0.49	0.57	0.15	0.07	0.15	0.18	0.57	1.14	2.12
肾盂	Renal pelvis	1 914	0.18	0.00	0.01	0.01	0.00	0.01	0.03	0.01	0.03	0.03
输尿管	Ureter	1 999	0.19	0.00	0.00	0.00	0.00	0.01	0.00	0.00	0.03	0.02
膀胱	Bladder	30 006	2.87	0.00	0.05	0.02	0.02	0.11	0.17	0.35	0.68	1.17
其他泌尿器官	Other urinary organs	491	0.05	0.03	0.01	0.00	0.01	0.01	0.00	0.00	0.01	0.05
眼	Eye	543	0.05	0.91	0.54	0.06	0.01	0.01	0.04	0.02	0.06	0.05
脑、神经系统	Brain, nervous system	23 572	2.26	2.40	1.95	2.01	1.93	1.73	1.65	2.33	3.01	3.69
甲状腺	Thyroid	29 427	2.82	0.00	0.01	0.07	0.22	0.67	3.40	9.86	14.39	16.83
肾上腺	Adrenal gland	1 045	0.10	0.43	0.23	0.06	0.03	0.04	0.03	0.08	0.06	0.13
其他内分泌腺	Other endocrine	1 324	0.13	0.06	0.09	0.12	0.20	0.15	0.15	0.16	0.23	0.35
霍奇金淋巴瘤	Hodgkin lymphoma	1 198	0.11	0.00	0.03	0.13	0.18	0.21	0.26	0.28	0.25	0.30
非霍奇金淋巴瘤	Non-Hodgkin lymphoma	16 845	1.61	0.40	0.71	0.62	0.72	0.83	0.83	1.13	1.44	2.07
免疫增生性疾病	Immunoproliferative diseases	364	0.03	0.00	0.02	0.00	0.00	0.01	0.02	0.01	0.00	0.03
多发性骨髓瘤	Multiple myeloma	5 933	0.57	0.06	0.02	0.03	0.06	0.08	0.07	0.08	0.15	0.26
淋巴细胞白血病	Lymphoid leukemia	4 426	0.42	0.79	3.04	1.71	1.18	0.76	0.60	0.55	0.60	0.54
髓系白血病	Myeloid leukemia	12 035	1.15	1.67	0.90	0.80	0.87	1.24	1.14	1.48	1.72	1.92
白血病,未特指	Leukemia unspecified	6 313	0.60	1.37	1.46	0.98	0.90	0.96	0.68	0.72	0.72	0.84
其他或未指明部位	Other and unspecified	20 362	1.95	1.49	1.11	0.70	0.69	0.74	0.68	0.89	1.25	1.71
所有部位合计	All sites	104 4959	100.00	13.48	12.95	9.03	9.76	13.44	15.90	30.77	49.36	72.00
所有部位除外 C44	All sites except C44	1 035 900	99.13	13.42	12.85	8.90	9.67	13.21	15.65	30.44	48.90	71.40

Appendix Table 1-2　Cancer incidence in registration areas of China, male in 2019

40~44	45~49	50~54	55~59	60~64	65~69	70~74	75~79	80~84	85+	粗率 Crude rate/ 100 000⁻¹	中标率 ASR China/ 100 000⁻¹	世标率 ASR world/ 100 000⁻¹	累积率 Cum. Rate/% 0~64	0~74	ICD-10
0.10	0.19	0.30	0.43	0.80	1.05	1.45	2.14	1.66	2.07	0.32	0.20	0.20	0.01	0.02	C00
0.87	1.17	1.93	2.31	3.18	3.55	3.62	3.85	3.34	2.29	1.18	0.78	0.76	0.05	0.09	C01-C02
0.66	1.15	2.10	2.76	3.88	4.93	5.98	6.91	6.31	7.47	1.53	0.96	0.95	0.06	0.11	C03-C06
0.39	0.61	1.12	1.33	1.55	2.11	1.98	2.13	2.47	2.32	0.71	0.49	0.47	0.03	0.05	C07-C08
0.13	0.31	0.39	0.62	0.71	0.64	0.75	0.77	0.62	0.72	0.25	0.17	0.16	0.01	0.02	C09
0.15	0.39	0.53	1.02	1.34	1.71	1.64	1.71	1.80	1.64	0.46	0.28	0.29	0.02	0.03	C10
5.94	8.22	9.84	11.15	11.52	10.98	10.85	9.42	8.92	6.69	5.28	3.82	3.57	0.28	0.39	C11
0.21	0.61	1.42	2.59	3.27	3.42	3.50	2.83	2.90	1.93	0.96	0.58	0.59	0.04	0.08	C12-C13
0.06	0.23	0.41	0.75	1.04	1.25	1.69	1.61	2.00	2.07	0.37	0.22	0.23	0.01	0.03	C14
2.02	7.34	20.18	35.16	69.07	101.76	130.40	149.74	154.25	135.28	24.62	14.28	14.43	0.67	1.84	C15
6.36	13.86	29.36	52.10	95.10	139.50	180.45	213.70	221.20	194.63	35.57	21.02	21.02	1.02	2.62	C16
0.58	0.96	1.89	2.41	3.74	5.13	5.79	6.60	7.49	8.26	1.46	0.90	0.89	0.05	0.11	C17
5.70	9.56	16.28	27.27	43.96	59.39	76.52	91.51	109.50	112.40	17.30	10.48	10.38	0.55	1.23	C18
5.45	10.60	19.10	30.32	49.83	68.63	83.23	97.15	104.50	96.49	18.63	11.24	11.19	0.60	1.36	C19-C20
0.14	0.24	0.42	0.58	0.88	1.42	1.67	2.11	2.74	2.79	0.40	0.24	0.24	0.01	0.03	C21
25.90	42.38	61.53	74.82	100.00	119.69	128.03	144.31	153.46	152.80	39.64	25.37	24.86	1.64	2.88	C22
0.85	1.60	3.28	5.07	10.21	14.70	20.08	24.91	29.90	32.78	4.05	2.36	2.37	0.11	0.28	C23-C24
1.83	4.08	7.50	11.86	20.08	28.31	36.80	45.51	55.89	59.10	8.01	4.72	4.72	0.23	0.56	C25
0.28	0.55	0.88	0.93	1.45	1.62	1.86	2.07	2.05	2.25	0.57	0.38	0.37	0.02	0.04	C30-C31
0.56	1.41	3.81	6.64	10.57	12.77	15.06	15.16	14.68	11.98	3.31	1.96	2.00	0.12	0.26	C32
15.21	33.66	73.52	130.11	229.23	334.89	420.21	499.35	510.59	470.99	84.99	50.14	50.28	2.48	6.26	C33-C34
0.72	1.03	1.58	2.38	3.11	3.79	3.64	4.12	3.89	3.90	1.23	0.85	0.84	0.05	0.09	C37-C38
0.81	1.09	1.96	2.25	3.82	4.97	6.88	8.59	9.84	10.69	1.92	1.42	1.40	0.08	0.14	C40-C41
0.32	0.39	0.53	0.70	1.23	1.63	1.99	2.79	2.95	3.43	0.52	0.33	0.32	0.02	0.04	C43
0.96	1.41	2.17	3.24	5.32	8.35	12.03	16.82	25.60	33.07	2.84	1.73	1.71	0.08	0.18	C44
0.05	0.10	0.19	0.34	0.42	0.62	0.73	0.77	0.85	0.79	0.17	0.10	0.10	0.01	0.01	C45
0.02	0.03	0.05	0.02	0.06	0.07	0.13	0.09	0.12	0.11	0.03	0.03	0.02	0.00	0.00	C46
0.75	0.98	1.38	1.46	2.08	2.59	3.17	4.22	4.49	4.93	1.10	0.82	0.80	0.05	0.08	C47,C49
0.32	0.68	0.83	1.07	1.39	1.92	2.12	2.14	2.49	2.29	0.60	0.39	0.38	0.02	0.04	C50
—	—	—	—	—	—	—	—	—	—	—	—	—	—	—	C51
—	—	—	—	—	—	—	—	—	—	—	—	—	—	—	C52
—	—	—	—	—	—	—	—	—	—	—	—	—	—	—	C53
—	—	—	—	—	—	—	—	—	—	—	—	—	—	—	C54
—	—	—	—	—	—	—	—	—	—	—	—	—	—	—	C55
—	—	—	—	—	—	—	—	—	—	—	—	—	—	—	C56
—	—	—	—	—	—	—	—	—	—	—	—	—	—	—	C57
—	—	—	—	—	—	—	—	—	—	—	—	—	—	—	C58
0.31	0.57	1.00	1.12	1.95	2.29	3.10	3.79	5.09	4.65	0.77	0.47	0.46	0.03	0.05	C60
0.18	0.66	2.06	7.01	21.20	45.20	85.76	133.66	165.07	174.64	13.62	7.53	7.41	0.16	0.81	C61
0.53	0.47	0.42	0.43	0.35	0.40	0.64	0.68	0.94	1.04	0.46	0.43	0.40	0.03	0.03	C62
0.06	0.08	0.16	0.27	0.38	0.59	0.80	1.08	1.20	1.00	0.18	0.11	0.11	0.01	0.01	C63
2.99	4.72	7.64	11.51	13.41	16.86	17.12	15.64	17.51	15.80	5.24	3.41	3.37	0.23	0.40	C64
0.17	0.29	0.58	0.98	1.50	2.17	2.63	3.39	4.19	3.79	0.60	0.35	0.36	0.02	0.04	C65
0.08	0.17	0.34	0.88	1.76	2.37	3.04	4.25	4.84	4.72	0.63	0.36	0.36	0.02	0.04	C66
1.90	3.50	6.42	11.84	21.19	30.94	43.66	62.67	82.69	94.88	9.41	5.48	5.45	0.24	0.61	C67
0.05	0.05	0.07	0.25	0.25	0.54	0.70	1.06	1.29	1.61	0.15	0.09	0.09	0.00	0.01	C68
0.08	0.12	0.14	0.20	0.29	0.28	0.47	0.55	0.88	0.79	0.17	0.13	0.16	0.01	0.01	C69
5.02	7.17	9.23	11.75	15.83	19.20	21.96	23.77	25.57	26.53	7.39	5.38	5.31	0.34	0.54	C70-C72,D32-D33,D42-D43
15.27	14.19	13.48	14.55	11.41	8.83	6.70	5.58	4.01	3.32	9.23	8.31	6.99	0.57	0.65	C73
0.19	0.28	0.45	0.57	0.72	0.93	0.87	1.00	1.36	1.64	0.33	0.22	0.24	0.01	0.02	C74
0.24	0.37	0.48	0.79	0.88	0.96	1.20	0.97	0.92	1.00	0.42	0.32	0.31	0.02	0.03	C75
0.24	0.27	0.44	0.41	0.76	0.75	1.00	1.20	1.06	1.18	0.38	0.31	0.30	0.02	0.03	C81
2.62	4.13	5.98	8.20	12.11	15.87	20.35	22.65	25.23	19.84	5.28	3.57	3.50	0.21	0.39	C82-C86,C96
0.03	0.05	0.10	0.09	0.31	0.45	0.59	0.69	0.62	0.46	0.11	0.07	0.07	0.00	0.01	C88
0.41	1.02	1.85	2.90	4.85	6.99	8.29	11.39	9.84	8.37	1.86	1.13	1.12	0.06	0.14	C90
0.58	0.80	1.09	1.32	2.21	2.89	3.64	4.40	4.31	4.15	1.39	1.18	1.34	0.07	0.11	C91
2.26	2.87	3.87	4.99	7.22	9.96	12.60	16.37	17.33	15.73	3.77	2.76	2.69	0.16	0.27	C92-C94,D45-D47
1.13	1.28	1.66	2.07	3.19	4.66	6.91	9.25	9.47	10.80	1.98	1.51	1.55	0.08	0.14	C95
2.51	4.00	6.44	9.01	13.79	19.60	25.74	31.65	38.52	47.08	6.39	4.11	4.12	0.22	0.44	O & U
114.15	191.89	328.37	502.83	814.43	1 134.14	1 430.02	1 718.70	1 868.43	1 809.19	327.76	203.52	201.24	10.82	23.65	C00-C97,D32-D33, D42-D43,D45-D47
113.20	190.48	326.20	499.59	809.11	1 125.79	1 417.99	1 701.88	1 842.83	1 776.12	324.92	201.80	199.54	10.75	23.47	C00-C97,D32-D33, D42-D43,D45-D47 exc. C44

附表 1-3　2019 年全国肿瘤登记地区女性癌症发病主要指标

部位 Site		病例数 No. cases	构成 Freq. /%	年龄组								
				0~	1~4	5~9	10~14	15~19	20~24	25~29	30~34	35~39
唇	Lip	738	0.08	0.03	0.02	0.01	0.01	0.00	0.04	0.02	0.05	0.06
舌	Tongue	1 835	0.21	0.00	0.00	0.01	0.01	0.03	0.03	0.05	0.16	0.24
口	Mouth	2 497	0.29	0.03	0.02	0.04	0.06	0.03	0.09	0.10	0.13	0.22
唾液腺	Salivary gland	1 740	0.20	0.00	0.01	0.02	0.06	0.14	0.16	0.32	0.40	0.34
扁桃体	Tonsil	304	0.03	0.00	0.00	0.01	0.01	0.02	0.02	0.04	0.04	0.00
其他口咽	Other oropharynx	282	0.03	0.00	0.01	0.01	0.01	0.00	0.01	0.02	0.01	0.05
鼻咽	Nasopharynx	6 828	0.78	0.03	0.01	0.04	0.09	0.22	0.33	0.79	1.25	1.85
下咽	Hypopharynx	230	0.03	0.00	0.00	0.01	0.00	0.00	0.01	0.00	0.03	0.02
咽,部位不明	Pharynx unspecified	299	0.03	0.03	0.01	0.01	0.00	0.01	0.02	0.01	0.01	0.01
食管	Esophagus	26 576	3.05	0.00	0.00	0.01	0.02	0.02	0.12	0.12	0.14	0.27
胃	Stomach	49 262	5.65	0.03	0.01	0.02	0.03	0.16	0.48	1.27	2.21	3.35
小肠	Small intestine	3 524	0.40	0.07	0.01	0.00	0.01	0.06	0.03	0.09	0.16	0.22
结肠	Colon	41 812	4.80	0.00	0.01	0.02	0.05	0.11	0.28	0.88	1.73	2.98
直肠	Rectum	37 647	4.32	0.00	0.00	0.01	0.01	0.11	0.26	0.71	1.45	2.17
肛门	Anus	995	0.11	0.00	0.00	0.01	0.01	0.01	0.00	0.01	0.07	0.09
肝脏	Liver	43 237	4.96	0.87	0.43	0.09	0.13	0.22	0.28	0.80	1.44	2.25
胆囊及其他	Gallbladder etc.	14 016	1.61	0.00	0.00	0.01	0.00	0.01	0.08	0.10	0.19	0.44
胰腺	Pancreas	19 159	2.20	0.00	0.01	0.01	0.06	0.07	0.15	0.20	0.36	0.59
鼻、鼻窦及其他	Nose, sinuses etc.	1 099	0.13	0.03	0.03	0.04	0.05	0.06	0.07	0.07	0.12	0.21
喉	Larynx	1 089	0.13	0.00	0.01	0.01	0.00	0.03	0.01	0.04	0.04	0.06
气管、支气管、肺	Trachea, bronchus & lung	151 489	17.39	0.07	0.07	0.04	0.05	0.43	0.88	2.55	5.35	10.05
其他胸腔器官	Other thoracic organs	2 607	0.30	0.27	0.15	0.05	0.04	0.11	0.09	0.21	0.24	0.33
骨	Bone	4 692	0.54	0.17	0.17	0.44	0.99	0.76	0.35	0.41	0.55	0.51
皮肤黑色素瘤	Melanoma of skin	1 620	0.19	0.07	0.03	0.04	0.01	0.07	0.07	0.11	0.16	0.20
皮肤其他	Other skin	9 098	1.04	0.03	0.10	0.06	0.10	0.18	0.25	0.24	0.46	0.57
间皮瘤	Mesothelioma	430	0.05	0.00	0.00	0.00	0.00	0.01	0.00	0.03	0.03	0.05
卡波西肉瘤	Kaposi sarcoma	43	0.00	0.00	0.01	0.00	0.00	0.00	0.01	0.00	0.00	0.01
结缔组织、软组织	Connective & soft tissue	2 903	0.33	0.60	0.46	0.25	0.20	0.36	0.24	0.41	0.53	0.59
乳腺	Breast	133 447	15.32	0.00	0.01	0.00	0.06	0.65	1.94	6.24	15.63	32.41
外阴	Vulva	1 638	0.19	0.13	0.01	0.01	0.01	0.02	0.04	0.05	0.08	0.19
阴道	Vagina	964	0.11	0.07	0.04	0.00	0.01	0.00	0.02	0.02	0.04	0.07
子宫颈	Cervix uteri	56 231	6.45	0.00	0.00	0.00	0.00	0.14	0.68	2.88	7.76	14.68
子宫体	Corpus uteri	27 426	3.15	0.00	0.00	0.00	0.01	0.07	0.21	0.73	1.59	3.27
子宫,部位不明	Uterus unspecified	6 105	0.70	0.00	0.00	0.01	0.00	0.01	0.08	0.30	0.65	1.07
卵巢	Ovary	24 265	2.79	0.10	0.10	0.15	0.56	1.40	2.08	2.62	2.96	3.84
其他女性生殖器官	Other female genital organs	1 928	0.22	0.00	0.00	0.01	0.03	0.06	0.07	0.10	0.12	0.26
胎盘	Placenta	232	0.03	0.00	0.00	0.00	0.00	0.05	0.11	0.24	0.13	0.12
阴茎	Penis	—	—	—	—	—	—	—	—	—	—	—
前列腺	Prostate	—	—	—	—	—	—	—	—	—	—	—
睾丸	Testis	—	—	—	—	—	—	—	—	—	—	—
其他男性生殖器官	Other male genital organs	—	—	—	—	—	—	—	—	—	—	—
肾	Kidney	9 006	1.03	0.54	0.64	0.20	0.08	0.12	0.18	0.37	0.64	0.89
肾盂	Renal pelvis	1 285	0.15	0.00	0.01	0.01	0.00	0.01	0.01	0.00	0.02	0.04
输尿管	Ureter	1 565	0.18	0.00	0.00	0.00	0.00	0.00	0.01	0.00	0.02	0.02
膀胱	Bladder	7 618	0.87	0.00	0.03	0.01	0.01	0.03	0.07	0.15	0.23	0.39
其他泌尿器官	Other urinary organs	339	0.04	0.00	0.00	0.00	0.00	0.01	0.01	0.00	0.00	0.02
眼	Eye	436	0.05	0.77	0.48	0.05	0.03	0.00	0.02	0.01	0.03	0.04
脑、神经系统	Brain, nervous system	28 532	3.28	2.05	1.72	1.81	1.64	1.55	1.67	2.22	2.83	4.15
甲状腺	Thyroid	89 730	10.30	0.00	0.01	0.05	0.53	2.59	10.34	25.81	36.27	43.91
肾上腺	Adrenal gland	800	0.09	0.10	0.23	0.05	0.01	0.02	0.04	0.08	0.11	0.09
其他内分泌腺	Other endocrine	1 449	0.17	0.00	0.04	0.04	0.06	0.13	0.13	0.29	0.31	0.44
霍奇金淋巴瘤	Hodgkin lymphoma	800	0.09	0.03	0.02	0.05	0.17	0.16	0.26	0.24	0.30	0.20
非霍奇金淋巴瘤	Non-Hodgkin lymphoma	12 458	1.43	0.30	0.47	0.33	0.37	0.43	0.60	0.80	1.22	1.71
免疫增生性疾病	Immunoproliferative diseases	217	0.02	0.00	0.02	0.01	0.01	0.01	0.01	0.02	0.01	0.01
多发性骨髓瘤	Multiple myeloma	4 579	0.53	0.03	0.01	0.01	0.04	0.06	0.07	0.03	0.05	0.16
淋巴细胞白血病	Lymphoid leukemia	3 034	0.35	1.04	2.44	1.42	0.83	0.59	0.35	0.35	0.33	0.39
髓系白血病	Myeloid leukemia	9 165	1.05	1.71	0.87	0.61	0.82	0.80	0.99	1.14	1.47	1.48
白血病,未特指	Leukemia unspecified	4 808	0.55	1.71	1.22	0.89	0.77	0.70	0.48	0.61	0.58	0.67
其他或未指明部位	Other and unspecified	17 085	1.96	1.38	1.03	0.57	0.64	0.75	0.76	0.96	1.26	1.87
所有部位合计	All sites	871 193	100.00	12.32	11.02	7.54	8.68	13.63	25.58	55.88	92.00	140.13
所有部位除外 C44	All sites except C44	862 095	98.96	12.28	10.91	7.48	8.59	13.45	25.33	55.64	91.54	139.57

Appendix Table 1-3　Cancer incidence in registration areas of China, female in 2019

40~44	45~49	50~54	55~59	60~64	65~69	70~74	75~79	80~84	85+	粗率 Crude rate/ 100 000⁻¹	中标率 ASR China/ 100 000⁻¹	世标率 ASR world/ 100 000⁻¹	累积率 Cum. Rate/% 0~64	累积率 Cum. Rate/% 0~74	ICD-10
0.08	0.17	0.26	0.25	0.38	0.68	0.82	1.25	1.40	1.68	0.24	0.14	0.13	0.01	0.01	C00
0.38	0.55	0.69	0.90	1.37	1.70	1.93	2.24	2.22	2.29	0.59	0.36	0.35	0.02	0.04	C01-C02
0.23	0.44	0.81	1.12	1.53	2.31	3.33	3.67	4.78	4.62	0.81	0.47	0.46	0.02	0.05	C03-C06
0.60	0.64	0.74	0.91	1.03	1.18	1.26	1.09	1.42	1.64	0.56	0.41	0.38	0.03	0.04	C07-C08
0.04	0.11	0.16	0.24	0.19	0.19	0.23	0.29	0.37	0.31	0.10	0.06	0.06	0.00	0.01	C09
0.08	0.07	0.12	0.16	0.15	0.18	0.29	0.36	0.43	0.41	0.09	0.06	0.06	0.00	0.01	C10
2.35	3.39	4.06	3.93	4.21	4.02	4.09	3.98	3.72	3.54	2.21	1.59	1.46	0.11	0.15	C11
0.03	0.04	0.13	0.12	0.15	0.19	0.25	0.31	0.35	0.29	0.07	0.05	0.04	0.00	0.00	C12-C13
0.04	0.03	0.08	0.11	0.16	0.23	0.44	0.43	0.88	0.79	0.10	0.05	0.05	0.00	0.01	C14
0.68	1.29	3.58	6.06	14.47	28.56	45.14	62.97	69.89	73.39	8.58	4.31	4.27	0.13	0.50	C15
5.27	9.22	14.41	19.59	30.64	46.10	64.66	83.81	101.97	101.02	15.91	8.85	8.62	0.43	0.99	C16
0.40	0.77	1.29	1.73	2.63	3.55	4.21	5.26	5.53	4.91	1.14	0.65	0.64	0.04	0.08	C17
4.62	7.87	12.68	18.67	28.11	39.97	52.30	68.55	82.06	78.08	13.50	7.54	7.38	0.39	0.85	C18
4.15	7.97	12.85	17.56	27.21	36.97	48.39	57.37	64.40	60.61	12.16	6.85	6.74	0.37	0.80	C19-C20
0.19	0.27	0.40	0.44	0.53	0.77	1.09	1.46	2.05	1.93	0.32	0.19	0.18	0.01	0.02	C21
4.84	7.94	13.57	17.22	28.86	41.15	56.64	71.00	83.41	90.09	13.96	7.73	7.64	0.39	0.88	C22
0.75	1.71	3.44	4.72	9.71	13.96	19.18	26.39	33.70	33.90	4.53	2.37	2.35	0.11	0.27	C23-C24
1.01	2.35	3.94	6.95	12.61	19.37	26.89	36.43	46.12	46.32	6.19	3.25	3.22	0.14	0.37	C25
0.29	0.38	0.41	0.55	0.62	0.92	1.05	0.97	1.34	1.37	0.35	0.24	0.23	0.01	0.02	C30-C31
0.10	0.19	0.27	0.39	0.77	0.88	1.29	2.17	2.35	2.57	0.35	0.19	0.19	0.01	0.01	C32
18.06	32.52	52.19	76.44	112.96	149.50	182.88	220.70	251.01	240.58	48.93	27.67	27.28	1.56	3.22	C33-C34
0.62	0.86	1.17	1.51	1.88	2.28	2.28	2.52	2.28	2.19	0.84	0.55	0.54	0.04	0.06	C37-C38
0.78	1.14	1.41	1.94	2.63	3.58	4.71	6.34	6.57	6.38	1.52	1.07	1.04	0.06	0.10	C40-C41
0.23	0.37	0.53	0.73	1.09	1.51	1.76	2.09	2.43	2.72	0.52	0.32	0.31	0.02	0.03	C43
0.84	1.26	1.97	2.94	4.53	6.94	10.86	16.15	23.62	34.22	2.94	1.56	1.54	0.07	0.16	C44
0.04	0.14	0.15	0.23	0.40	0.40	0.47	0.58	0.39	0.36	0.14	0.09	0.08	0.01	0.01	C45
0.01	0.01	0.03	0.02	0.03	0.01	0.04	0.03	0.04	0.14	0.01	0.01	0.01	0.00	0.00	C46
0.66	0.88	1.11	1.36	1.71	2.01	2.14	2.47	2.82	3.25	0.94	0.69	0.68	0.04	0.06	C47,C49
56.80	85.50	84.68	85.29	89.03	78.78	65.52	59.45	52.24	40.88	43.10	30.11	28.08	2.29	3.01	C50
0.27	0.43	0.59	0.70	1.15	1.37	1.95	2.36	2.52	2.72	0.53	0.31	0.31	0.02	0.03	C51
0.26	0.36	0.45	0.61	0.65	0.80	1.04	1.04	1.06	0.65	0.31	0.19	0.19	0.01	0.02	C52
22.73	32.32	39.45	38.59	34.73	30.08	29.97	27.00	21.55	14.08	18.16	12.74	11.80	0.97	1.27	C53
7.07	14.35	23.36	24.26	19.91	17.84	14.09	10.89	9.00	5.85	8.86	5.76	5.59	0.47	0.63	C54
2.13	3.38	4.13	3.82	3.74	3.71	3.73	4.05	4.41	3.34	1.97	1.32	1.24	0.10	0.13	C55
6.77	11.84	14.93	15.27	16.07	16.95	16.50	15.41	13.20	7.56	7.84	5.48	5.20	0.39	0.56	C56
0.53	0.91	1.15	1.29	1.41	1.69	1.40	1.20	1.05	0.87	0.62	0.41	0.40	0.03	0.05	C57
0.15	0.11	0.08	0.02	0.01	0.00	0.01	0.01	0.00	0.02	0.07	0.08	0.07	0.01	0.01	C58
—	—	—	—	—	—	—	—	—	—	—	—	—		—	C60
—	—	—	—	—	—	—	—	—	—	—	—	—		—	C61
—	—	—	—	—	—	—	—	—	—	—	—	—		—	C62
—	—	—	—	—	—	—	—	—	—	—	—	—		—	C63
1.56	2.62	4.04	5.28	6.64	8.43	8.91	9.95	9.86	8.28	2.91	1.80	1.80	0.12	0.20	C64
0.07	0.09	0.26	0.48	0.69	1.46	1.98	2.86	2.91	2.60	0.42	0.22	0.22	0.01	0.03	C65
0.06	0.13	0.23	0.39	1.02	1.78	2.48	3.57	4.26	2.94	0.51	0.26	0.26	0.01	0.03	C66
0.53	0.88	1.69	2.73	4.35	6.54	10.55	15.18	19.72	20.43	2.46	1.30	1.27	0.06	0.14	C67
0.01	0.03	0.08	0.11	0.31	0.40	0.52	0.44	0.60	0.75	0.11	0.06	0.06	0.00	0.01	C68
0.04	0.10	0.15	0.09	0.24	0.27	0.38	0.48	0.63	0.46	0.14	0.10	0.13	0.01	0.01	C69
5.98	8.78	12.60	15.48	19.61	22.58	25.76	27.89	28.92	27.48	9.22	6.18	6.09	0.40	0.64	C70-C72,D32-D33,D42-D43
46.75	50.52	52.72	51.73	37.28	26.56	16.74	10.88	7.77	5.82	28.98	24.77	21.33	1.79	2.01	C73
0.15	0.27	0.36	0.42	0.48	0.63	0.67	0.77	0.78	0.72	0.26	0.17	0.18	0.01	0.02	C74
0.54	0.56	0.76	0.74	0.90	0.90	0.84	0.81	0.84	0.36	0.47	0.36	0.33	0.02	0.03	C75
0.15	0.23	0.29	0.30	0.32	0.42	0.54	0.69	0.58	0.51	0.26	0.22	0.20	0.01	0.02	C81
2.09	3.10	4.66	6.32	8.84	11.37	13.94	15.14	15.83	10.85	4.02	2.57	2.50	0.15	0.28	C82-C86,C96
0.05	0.06	0.07	0.13	0.15	0.25	0.24	0.25	0.17	0.19	0.07	0.04	0.05	0.00	0.01	C88
0.39	0.83	1.52	2.44	3.96	5.44	6.17	6.57	6.11	3.87	1.48	0.85	0.85	0.05	0.11	C90
0.40	0.63	0.88	1.04	1.32	1.91	2.42	2.34	2.67	1.56	0.98	0.84	0.98	0.05	0.08	C91
1.88	2.55	3.28	3.93	5.37	6.89	8.69	10.28	10.61	8.54	2.96	2.11	2.06	0.13	0.20	C92-C94,D45-D47
0.72	0.96	1.45	1.67	2.41	3.61	4.58	6.20	6.33	5.51	1.55	1.15	1.20	0.07	0.11	C95
2.79	4.45	6.36	7.27	10.00	13.17	17.77	22.43	28.29	34.43	5.52	3.41	3.37	0.19	0.35	O & U
208.21	308.56	392.65	457.18	561.11	672.90	796.02	939.04	1 049.47	1 010.89	281.38	180.15	171.73	11.41	18.76	C00-C97,D32-D33,D42-D43,D45-D47
207.36	307.30	390.67	454.24	556.58	665.97	785.17	922.88	1 025.85	976.67	278.44	178.59	170.19	11.34	18.60	C00-C97,D32-D33,D42-D43, D45-D47 exc. C44

附表 1-4　2019 年全国城市肿瘤登记地区男女合计癌症发病主要指标

部位 Site		病例数 No. cases	构成 Freq. /%	年龄组								
				0~	1~4	5~9	10~14	15~19	20~24	25~29	30~34	35~39
唇	Lip	546	0.06	0.04	0.02	0.00	0.02	0.01	0.01	0.01	0.03	0.01
舌	Tongue	2 851	0.32	0.00	0.01	0.00	0.01	0.03	0.09	0.10	0.28	0.37
口	Mouth	3 427	0.38	0.00	0.02	0.02	0.06	0.05	0.11	0.11	0.15	0.28
唾液腺	Salivary gland	1 841	0.21	0.00	0.00	0.00	0.07	0.14	0.17	0.26	0.42	0.37
扁桃体	Tonsil	567	0.06	0.00	0.00	0.02	0.01	0.01	0.01	0.03	0.03	0.03
其他口咽	Other oropharynx	807	0.09	0.00	0.00	0.01	0.01	0.00	0.01	0.01	0.05	0.07
鼻咽	Nasopharynx	10 041	1.12	0.00	0.02	0.02	0.14	0.34	0.48	1.13	2.02	2.91
下咽	Hypopharynx	1724	0.19	0.00	0.00	0.01	0.00	0.00	0.01	0.01	0.03	0.04
咽, 部位不明	Pharynx unspecified	646	0.07	0.00	0.01	0.00	0.01	0.00	0.01	0.03	0.00	0.01
食管	Esophagus	36 693	4.11	0.04	0.02	0.01	0.02	0.11	0.04	0.07	0.14	0.30
胃	Stomach	67 192	7.52	0.00	0.00	0.02	0.07	0.17	0.40	1.02	2.03	3.32
小肠	Small intestine	3 926	0.44	0.04	0.01	0.00	0.00	0.02	0.01	0.07	0.16	0.33
结肠	Colon	53 311	5.96	0.00	0.02	0.03	0.06	0.19	0.32	1.02	2.00	3.23
直肠	Rectum	45 625	5.10	0.00	0.01	0.01	0.02	0.22	0.28	0.73	1.56	2.38
肛门	Anus	873	0.10	0.00	0.00	0.01	0.00	0.00	0.00	0.02	0.03	0.08
肝脏	Liver	69 156	7.74	1.16	0.61	0.15	0.17	0.39	0.48	1.41	3.30	5.97
胆囊及其他	Gallbladder etc.	12 785	1.43	0.07	0.02	0.00	0.00	0.02	0.03	0.09	0.16	0.32
胰腺	Pancreas	21 551	2.41	0.04	0.02	0.03	0.03	0.05	0.09	0.19	0.36	0.62
鼻、鼻窦及其他	Nose, sinuses etc.	1 283	0.14	0.00	0.03	0.01	0.05	0.06	0.05	0.09	0.13	0.21
喉	Larynx	5 701	0.64	0.00	0.01	0.01	0.00	0.02	0.00	0.02	0.04	0.11
气管、支气管、肺	Trachea, bronchus & lung	194 266	21.73	0.11	0.07	0.05	0.07	0.51	0.81	2.35	5.15	9.58
其他胸腔器官	Other thoracic organs	3 200	0.36	0.40	0.22	0.03	0.10	0.21	0.21	0.31	0.33	0.44
骨	Bone	4 157	0.47	0.07	0.16	0.32	0.93	0.82	0.48	0.38	0.59	0.47
皮肤黑色素瘤	Melanoma of skin	1 538	0.17	0.00	0.02	0.02	0.00	0.03	0.05	0.14	0.12	0.16
皮肤其他	Other skin	8 567	0.96	0.07	0.03	0.10	0.09	0.21	0.28	0.33	0.52	0.61
间皮瘤	Mesothelioma	532	0.06	0.00	0.01	0.00	0.00	0.00	0.00	0.03	0.04	0.06
卡波西肉瘤	Kaposi sarcoma	73	0.01	0.04	0.01	0.00	0.00	0.00	0.01	0.03	0.02	0.01
结缔组织、软组织	Connective & soft tissue	3 097	0.35	0.69	0.48	0.23	0.17	0.43	0.28	0.48	0.66	0.59
乳腺	Breast	69 616	7.88	0.00	0.00	0.00	0.03	0.42	1.30	5.89	16.44	35.34
外阴	Vulva	817	0.09	0.23	0.02	0.00	0.00	0.03	0.03	0.06	0.10	0.17
阴道	Vagina	464	0.05	0.15	0.02	0.00	0.02	0.00	0.03	0.01	0.06	0.06
子宫颈	Cervix uteri	22 850	2.56	0.00	0.00	0.00	0.00	0.08	0.69	2.39	7.10	13.66
子宫体	Corpus uteri	13 474	1.51	0.00	0.00	0.00	0.00	0.03	0.16	0.75	1.73	3.41
子宫, 部位不明	Uterus unspecified	2 208	0.25	0.00	0.00	0.01	0.00	0.05	0.04	0.17	0.45	0.73
卵巢	Ovary	11 572	1.29	0.08	0.14	0.21	0.53	1.50	2.21	2.54	3.16	4.32
其他女性生殖器官	Other female genital organs	954	0.11	0.00	0.00	0.00	0.02	0.02	0.04	0.09	0.08	0.27
胎盘	Placenta	99	0.01	0.00	0.00	0.00	0.00	0.05	0.09	0.27	0.09	0.12
阴茎	Penis	1 037	0.12	0.00	0.00	0.00	0.00	0.02	0.01	0.02	0.06	0.16
前列腺	Prostate	23 683	2.65	0.00	0.00	0.00	0.00	0.11	0.03	0.08	0.06	0.11
睾丸	Testis	666	0.07	0.49	0.37	0.03	0.03	0.28	0.45	0.74	0.77	0.88
其他男性生殖器官	Other male genital organs	313	0.04	0.00	0.03	0.04	0.01	0.06	0.03	0.01	0.01	0.03
肾	Kidney	14 386	1.61	0.36	0.64	0.18	0.06	0.16	0.20	0.56	1.03	1.87
肾盂	Renal pelvis	1 832	0.20	0.00	0.00	0.00	0.00	0.00	0.02	0.01	0.03	0.05
输尿管	Ureter	2 068	0.23	0.00	0.00	0.00	0.00	0.00	0.00	0.01	0.02	0.03
膀胱	Bladder	18 980	2.12	0.00	0.03	0.01	0.02	0.07	0.11	0.24	0.54	0.82
其他泌尿器官	Other urinary organs	413	0.05	0.00	0.00	0.00	0.00	0.00	0.00	0.01	0.01	0.03
眼	Eye	368	0.04	1.20	0.46	0.08	0.01	0.01	0.01	0.01	0.04	0.03
脑、神经系统	Brain, nervous system	23 374	2.62	2.58	2.01	1.91	1.73	1.56	1.57	2.23	2.94	4.01
甲状腺	Thyroid	67 990	7.61	0.00	0.01	0.05	0.41	1.94	8.92	24.10	35.74	41.43
肾上腺	Adrenal gland	839	0.09	0.29	0.30	0.04	0.03	0.02	0.05	0.07	0.07	0.10
其他内分泌腺	Other endocrine	1 233	0.14	0.07	0.10	0.12	0.16	0.16	0.15	0.26	0.27	0.38
霍奇金淋巴瘤	Hodgkin lymphoma	959	0.11	0.00	0.02	0.08	0.25	0.27	0.32	0.40	0.35	0.28
非霍奇金淋巴瘤	Non-Hodgkin lymphoma	14 943	1.67	0.51	0.64	0.53	0.61	0.78	0.82	1.04	1.52	2.10
免疫增生性疾病	Immunoproliferative diseases	387	0.04	0.00	0.03	0.01	0.02	0.03	0.02	0.02	0.01	0.03
多发性骨髓瘤	Multiple myeloma	5 378	0.60	0.04	0.02	0.05	0.09	0.09	0.09	0.09	0.12	0.22
淋巴细胞白血病	Lymphoid leukemia	3 550	0.40	1.09	3.34	2.03	1.09	0.72	0.49	0.47	0.42	0.48
髓系白血病	Myeloid leukemia	10 732	1.20	1.42	0.90	0.78	0.95	0.96	1.08	1.46	1.72	1.86
白血病, 未特指	Leukemia unspecified	3 999	0.45	0.98	1.13	0.75	0.60	0.65	0.36	0.44	0.44	0.48
其他或未指明部位	Other and unspecified	17 872	2.00	1.60	0.98	0.47	0.57	0.63	0.63	0.88	1.28	1.81
所有部位合计	All sites	893 818	100.00	13.39	12.74	8.34	9.04	13.38	21.99	49.26	82.29	119.06
所有部位除外 C44	All sites except C44	885 251	99.04	13.32	12.71	8.24	8.95	13.17	21.71	48.93	81.76	118.45

Appendix Table 1-4　Cancer incidence in urban registration areas of China, both sexes in 2019

Age group										粗率 Crude rate/ 100 000⁻¹	中标率 ASR China/ 100 000⁻¹	世标率 ASR world/ 100 000⁻¹	累积率 Cum. Rate/%		ICD-10
40~44	45~49	50~54	55~59	60~64	65~69	70~74	75~79	80~84	85+				0~64	0~74	
0.06	0.14	0.15	0.26	0.45	0.58	0.83	1.25	1.12	1.41	0.20	0.12	0.12	0.01	0.01	C00
0.71	0.97	1.37	1.88	2.67	3.06	3.35	3.89	3.51	3.03	1.06	0.66	0.64	0.04	0.07	C01-C02
0.44	0.78	1.44	2.19	2.97	3.96	4.69	5.57	6.22	6.39	1.28	0.75	0.74	0.04	0.09	C03-C06
0.53	0.57	0.95	1.19	1.30	1.73	1.76	1.80	2.37	2.29	0.69	0.47	0.44	0.03	0.05	C07-C08
0.13	0.28	0.36	0.54	0.61	0.42	0.57	0.42	0.52	0.46	0.21	0.13	0.13	0.01	0.02	C09
0.11	0.24	0.35	0.69	0.84	1.01	0.91	0.91	1.05	0.95	0.30	0.18	0.18	0.01	0.02	C10
3.94	5.75	6.80	7.54	7.65	7.13	7.03	6.27	5.19	4.74	3.74	2.66	2.47	0.19	0.26	C11
0.18	0.41	0.91	1.80	2.03	2.20	2.03	1.65	1.82	1.16	0.64	0.37	0.38	0.03	0.05	C12-C13
0.05	0.14	0.29	0.46	0.61	0.66	0.98	1.12	1.18	1.28	0.24	0.14	0.14	0.01	0.02	C14
0.92	3.94	10.91	18.19	34.79	50.22	65.99	78.71	83.17	76.10	13.67	7.35	7.42	0.35	0.93	C15
5.67	11.31	20.90	35.03	59.31	85.34	112.12	133.02	148.22	135.13	25.03	13.95	13.84	0.70	1.68	C16
0.47	0.83	1.67	2.22	3.29	4.63	5.49	7.11	8.18	8.07	1.46	0.83	0.82	0.05	0.10	C17
5.70	9.74	17.09	28.52	45.06	62.55	80.53	102.95	127.15	126.44	19.86	11.08	10.96	0.56	1.28	C18
4.76	9.31	16.84	26.76	42.28	57.17	68.94	80.83	89.36	84.51	16.99	9.61	9.56	0.53	1.16	C19-C20
0.19	0.21	0.34	0.46	0.60	0.89	1.31	1.52	2.35	1.84	0.33	0.19	0.18	0.01	0.02	C21
13.40	23.19	35.35	44.13	60.55	73.82	84.15	100.23	111.62	117.73	25.76	15.26	15.06	0.95	1.74	C22
0.77	1.78	3.44	5.22	10.31	15.05	20.83	28.16	36.90	40.68	4.76	2.53	2.53	0.11	0.29	C23-C24
1.29	3.45	5.84	10.28	17.95	26.00	34.67	45.75	58.04	59.31	8.03	4.32	4.32	0.20	0.50	C25
0.26	0.46	0.69	0.75	1.09	1.31	1.42	1.31	1.87	2.08	0.48	0.31	0.30	0.02	0.03	C30-C31
0.33	0.92	2.37	4.25	6.67	7.60	8.26	8.78	8.97	7.40	2.12	1.18	1.21	0.07	0.15	C32
18.04	35.45	65.30	111.16	182.17	250.08	303.38	366.46	390.14	359.02	72.36	40.53	40.39	2.15	4.92	C33-C34
0.75	1.04	1.52	2.18	2.85	3.21	3.26	3.92	3.69	3.76	1.19	0.78	0.77	0.05	0.08	C37-C38
0.60	0.97	1.47	1.93	2.95	3.48	5.14	6.71	7.86	8.47	1.55	1.09	1.06	0.06	0.10	C40-C41
0.25	0.38	0.51	0.78	1.23	1.61	2.07	2.62	3.14	3.85	0.57	0.34	0.33	0.02	0.04	C43
0.91	1.46	2.10	3.36	5.39	8.58	12.29	17.85	25.95	34.35	3.19	1.77	1.74	0.08	0.18	C44
0.06	0.10	0.18	0.35	0.58	0.71	0.69	0.79	0.82	0.73	0.20	0.12	0.12	0.01	0.01	C45
0.00	0.01	0.05	0.03	0.06	0.05	0.13	0.02	0.09	0.12	0.03	0.02	0.02	0.00	0.00	C46
0.77	0.87	1.35	1.46	2.14	2.64	3.03	4.03	4.44	4.65	1.15	0.82	0.81	0.05	0.08	C47,C49
62.60	96.45	95.52	102.87	111.72	101.47	86.18	84.49	76.30	56.82	51.94	35.04	32.91	2.64	3.58	C50
0.32	0.49	0.63	0.71	1.28	1.65	1.97	2.77	3.01	3.68	0.61	0.35	0.34	0.02	0.04	C51
0.22	0.39	0.46	0.76	0.67	0.93	1.16	1.10	1.28	0.78	0.35	0.21	0.21	0.01	0.02	C52
20.53	29.98	37.01	37.27	32.87	27.26	26.93	23.40	19.97	12.40	17.05	11.78	10.94	0.91	1.18	C53
7.36	15.53	25.88	27.67	22.90	20.87	16.99	13.57	10.25	6.85	10.05	6.43	6.26	0.53	0.72	C54
1.62	2.69	3.57	3.47	3.12	3.25	2.90	3.53	3.38	3.17	1.65	1.07	1.02	0.08	0.11	C55
7.03	12.82	15.63	16.48	17.67	18.99	18.07	17.92	16.14	10.12	8.63	5.93	5.63	0.42	0.61	C56
0.52	0.93	1.33	1.47	1.68	2.10	1.54	1.49	1.24	1.30	0.71	0.45	0.44	0.03	0.05	C57
0.15	0.10	0.09	0.03	0.01	0.00	0.02	0.00	0.00	0.00	0.07	0.08	0.07	0.01	0.01	C58
0.23	0.47	0.90	1.10	1.91	2.35	3.00	3.67	5.10	5.81	0.77	0.45	0.45	0.02	0.05	C60
0.24	0.87	2.52	9.17	26.96	56.54	106.43	164.87	202.83	216.12	17.62	9.37	9.24	0.20	1.02	C61
0.58	0.51	0.47	0.46	0.34	0.36	0.50	0.59	1.02	0.89	0.50	0.47	0.43	0.03	0.03	C62
0.06	0.05	0.12	0.33	0.55	0.77	1.10	1.35	1.73	1.49	0.23	0.14	0.14	0.01	0.02	C63
2.72	4.73	7.37	10.88	13.22	16.10	16.74	16.51	17.70	15.63	5.36	3.30	3.27	0.22	0.38	C64
0.15	0.24	0.55	0.83	1.37	2.29	3.03	4.37	5.03	4.34	0.68	0.37	0.37	0.02	0.04	C65
0.08	0.15	0.37	0.84	1.82	2.54	3.60	5.31	6.42	5.41	0.77	0.40	0.40	0.02	0.05	C66
1.37	2.39	4.39	8.27	14.73	21.59	30.17	42.76	56.36	61.26	7.07	3.78	3.75	0.16	0.42	C67
0.03	0.04	0.08	0.18	0.29	0.46	0.69	0.91	1.25	1.53	0.15	0.08	0.08	0.00	0.01	C68
0.06	0.07	0.12	0.14	0.21	0.23	0.33	0.34	0.66	0.55	0.14	0.10	0.14	0.01	0.01	C69
5.28	8.25	11.14	14.52	18.44	21.11	24.42	27.33	30.05	29.48	8.71	5.92	5.84	0.38	0.61	C70-C72,D32-D33,D42-D43
40.31	42.11	42.00	41.28	31.01	22.75	14.60	9.67	7.02	5.41	25.32	21.85	18.56	1.55	1.73	C73
0.14	0.24	0.36	0.53	0.60	0.86	0.85	1.07	1.41	1.32	0.31	0.20	0.22	0.01	0.02	C74
0.34	0.40	0.59	0.73	0.94	1.01	1.16	1.04	0.96	0.61	0.46	0.35	0.34	0.02	0.03	C75
0.19	0.28	0.40	0.38	0.49	0.57	0.85	0.92	0.82	0.89	0.36	0.31	0.29	0.02	0.03	C81
2.73	4.15	6.01	8.50	11.99	15.65	19.84	23.19	26.51	17.53	5.57	3.56	3.47	0.21	0.38	C82-C86,C96
0.06	0.10	0.14	0.16	0.33	0.51	0.65	0.63	0.55	0.49	0.14	0.09	0.09	0.00	0.01	C88
0.46	1.04	1.92	3.06	4.82	6.95	8.67	10.94	10.48	7.65	2.00	1.14	1.14	0.06	0.14	C90
0.50	0.69	1.10	1.38	1.96	2.41	3.37	3.69	4.03	3.27	1.32	1.12	1.32	0.07	0.10	C91
2.31	2.84	3.85	5.24	7.20	10.08	13.10	16.25	18.20	15.75	4.00	2.75	2.68	0.16	0.27	C92-C94,D45-D47
0.66	0.85	1.19	1.66	2.31	3.39	4.88	6.77	8.06	8.26	1.49	1.05	1.10	0.06	0.10	C95
2.79	4.34	6.75	8.90	12.84	17.22	23.73	30.33	39.09	50.19	6.66	3.99	3.97	0.21	0.42	O & U
172.52	268.35	380.75	522.20	734.99	942.11	1 141.71	1 375.54	1 537.69	1 474.91	332.92	204.00	197.87	11.98	22.39	C00-C97,D32-D33, D42-D43
171.61	266.89	378.65	518.84	729.60	933.53	1 129.41	1 357.68	1 511.74	1 440.56	329.72	202.23	196.13	11.90	22.21	C00-C97,D32-D33, D42-D43,D45-D47 exc. C44

附表 1-5　2019 年全国城市肿瘤登记地区男性癌症发病主要指标

部位	Site	病例数 No. cases	构成 Freq./%	0~	1~4	5~9	10~14	15~19	20~24	25~29	30~34	35~39
唇	Lip	310	0.07	0.00	0.00	0.00	0.03	0.02	0.00	0.01	0.03	0.02
舌	Tongue	1 850	0.39	0.00	0.02	0.00	0.01	0.03	0.12	0.16	0.41	0.51
口	Mouth	2 258	0.47	0.00	0.02	0.01	0.07	0.08	0.08	0.07	0.19	0.33
唾液腺	Salivary gland	1 052	0.22	0.00	0.00	0.00	0.09	0.14	0.18	0.22	0.39	0.41
扁桃体	Tonsil	414	0.09	0.00	0.00	0.04	0.01	0.01	0.00	0.02	0.04	0.05
其他口咽	Other oropharynx	691	0.15	0.00	0.00	0.00	0.01	0.00	0.01	0.01	0.09	0.08
鼻咽	Nasopharynx	7 148	1.50	0.00	0.03	0.00	0.22	0.40	0.57	1.33	2.74	4.00
下咽	Hypopharynx	1 617	0.34	0.00	0.00	0.00	0.00	0.00	0.01	0.01	0.02	0.08
咽,部位不明	Pharynx unspecified	528	0.11	0.00	0.00	0.00	0.01	0.00	0.01	0.02	0.00	0.02
食管	Esophagus	28 526	5.99	0.07	0.03	0.01	0.01	0.18	0.04	0.09	0.19	0.38
胃	Stomach	46 471	9.76	0.00	0.00	0.01	0.09	0.24	0.33	0.84	1.71	3.13
小肠	Small intestine	2 221	0.47	0.00	0.02	0.00	0.00	0.00	0.01	0.03	0.13	0.42
结肠	Colon	30 283	6.36	0.00	0.03	0.03	0.06	0.23	0.40	1.11	2.12	3.23
直肠	Rectum	28 234	5.93	0.00	0.02	0.01	0.01	0.29	0.32	0.85	1.72	2.60
肛门	Anus	488	0.10	0.00	0.00	0.01	0.00	0.00	0.00	0.03	0.02	0.08
肝脏	Liver	51 559	10.83	1.25	0.70	0.16	0.19	0.58	0.63	2.05	5.52	10.07
胆囊及其他	Gallbladder etc.	6 076	1.28	0.14	0.00	0.00	0.00	0.03	0.00	0.09	0.16	0.22
胰腺	Pancreas	12 159	2.55	0.07	0.03	0.04	0.00	0.02	0.06	0.18	0.41	0.64
鼻、鼻窦及其他	Nose, sinuses etc.	792	0.17	0.00	0.03	0.01	0.06	0.03	0.06	0.11	0.15	0.22
喉	Larynx	5 230	1.10	0.00	0.02	0.03	0.00	0.03	0.00	0.02	0.05	0.18
气管、支气管、肺	Trachea, bronchus & lung	121 472	25.52	0.07	0.05	0.05	0.12	0.67	0.76	1.83	3.68	7.40
其他胸腔器官	Other thoracic organs	1 899	0.40	0.35	0.25	0.03	0.15	0.32	0.32	0.44	0.39	0.54
骨	Bone	2 330	0.49	0.07	0.22	0.90	0.29	1.06	0.71	0.45	0.63	0.52
皮肤黑色素瘤	Melanoma of skin	783	0.16	0.00	0.03	0.01	0.03	0.02	0.00	0.15	0.04	0.10
皮肤其他	Other skin	4 318	0.91	0.07	0.05	0.11	0.06	0.24	0.30	0.37	0.52	0.70
间皮瘤	Mesothelioma	299	0.06	0.00	0.02	0.00	0.00	0.00	0.00	0.00	0.03	0.05
卡波西肉瘤	Kaposi sarcoma	53	0.01	0.07	0.00	0.00	0.00	0.00	0.01	0.04	0.04	0.03
结缔组织、软组织	Connective & soft tissue	1 738	0.37	0.56	0.48	0.20	0.16	0.47	0.27	0.58	0.77	0.57
乳腺	Breast	786	0.17	0.00	0.02	0.00	0.00	0.00	0.04	0.08	0.08	0.16
外阴	Vulva	—	—	—	—	—	—	—	—	—	—	—
阴道	Vagina	—	—	—	—	—	—	—	—	—	—	—
子宫颈	Cervix uteri	—	—	—	—	—	—	—	—	—	—	—
子宫体	Corpus uteri	—	—	—	—	—	—	—	—	—	—	—
子宫,部位不明	Uterus unspecified	—	—	—	—	—	—	—	—	—	—	—
卵巢	Ovary	—	—	—	—	—	—	—	—	—	—	—
其他女性生殖器官	Other female genital organs	—	—	—	—	—	—	—	—	—	—	—
胎盘	Placenta	—	—	—	—	—	—	—	—	—	—	—
阴茎	Penis	1 037	0.22	0.00	0.02	0.00	0.00	0.02	0.01	0.02	0.06	0.16
前列腺	Prostate	23 683	4.98	0.00	0.00	0.00	0.01	0.11	0.03	0.08	0.06	0.11
睾丸	Testis	666	0.14	0.49	0.37	0.03	0.03	0.28	0.45	0.74	0.77	0.88
其他男性生殖器官	Other male genital organs	313	0.07	0.00	0.03	0.04	0.01	0.06	0.03	0.01	0.01	0.03
肾	Kidney	9 497	2.00	0.49	0.61	0.16	0.04	0.20	0.19	0.72	1.27	2.74
肾盂	Renal pelvis	1 069	0.22	0.00	0.00	0.00	0.00	0.00	0.01	0.01	0.05	0.05
输尿管	Ureter	1 156	0.24	0.00	0.00	0.00	0.00	0.00	0.00	0.00	0.03	0.03
膀胱	Bladder	15 048	3.16	0.00	0.03	0.00	0.01	0.11	0.14	0.26	0.82	1.30
其他泌尿器官	Other urinary organs	244	0.05	0.00	0.00	0.00	0.00	0.00	0.00	0.01	0.02	0.05
眼	Eye	209	0.04	1.39	0.53	0.05	0.01	0.02	0.01	0.01	0.05	0.04
脑、神经系统	Brain, nervous system	10 263	2.16	2.79	2.14	1.99	1.90	1.58	1.70	2.21	3.05	3.80
甲状腺	Thyroid	17 655	3.71	0.00	0.00	0.04	0.27	0.93	4.58	14.57	21.56	24.57
肾上腺	Adrenal gland	481	0.10	0.42	0.33	0.04	0.06	0.03	0.03	0.04	0.07	0.12
其他内分泌腺	Other endocrine	599	0.13	0.14	0.12	0.18	0.27	0.20	0.18	0.18	0.17	0.32
霍奇金淋巴瘤	Hodgkin lymphoma	539	0.11	0.00	0.05	0.12	0.24	0.28	0.28	0.39	0.29	0.30
非霍奇金淋巴瘤	Non-Hodgkin lymphoma	8 406	1.77	0.70	0.79	0.71	0.86	0.99	0.98	1.24	1.62	2.32
免疫增生性疾病	Immunoproliferative diseases	249	0.05	0.00	0.03	0.00	0.01	0.05	0.01	0.03	0.00	0.05
多发性骨髓瘤	Multiple myeloma	3 010	0.63	0.00	0.05	0.05	0.07	0.08	0.06	0.10	0.15	0.25
淋巴细胞白血病	Lymphoid leukemia	2 128	0.45	0.84	3.66	2.28	1.35	0.76	0.64	0.60	0.63	0.59
髓系白血病	Myeloid leukemia	6 116	1.29	1.39	0.86	0.86	1.02	1.21	1.18	1.76	1.80	2.10
白血病,未特指	Leukemia unspecified	2 282	0.48	0.91	1.17	0.86	0.71	0.76	0.41	0.43	0.50	0.56
其他或未指明部位	Other and unspecified	9 697	2.04	1.74	1.00	0.49	0.58	0.58	0.53	0.91	1.28	1.83
所有部位合计	All sites	475 932	100.00	14.00	13.82	8.97	9.80	13.32	16.71	35.52	56.48	78.92
所有部位除外 C44	All sites except C44	471 614	99.09	13.93	13.78	8.86	9.74	13.07	16.41	35.15	55.96	78.21

Appendix Table 1-5　Cancer incidence in urban registration areas of China, male in 2019

Age group										粗率 Crude rate/ 100 000⁻¹	中标率 ASR China/ 100 000⁻¹	世标率 ASR world/ 100 000⁻¹	累积率 Cum. Rate/%		ICD-10
40~44	45~49	50~54	55~59	60~64	65~69	70~74	75~79	80~84	85+				0~64	0~74	
0.06	0.18	0.17	0.36	0.55	0.68	1.10	1.56	1.27	0.89	0.23	0.14	0.14	0.01	0.02	C00
0.92	1.29	2.05	2.70	3.63	4.10	4.15	4.82	4.08	2.61	1.38	0.89	0.86	0.06	0.10	C01-C02
0.68	1.17	2.19	3.39	4.38	5.32	5.68	7.52	6.78	7.75	1.68	1.02	1.01	0.06	0.12	C03-C06
0.46	0.58	1.22	1.36	1.68	2.23	2.16	2.29	3.11	2.68	0.78	0.53	0.51	0.03	0.06	C07-C08
0.19	0.42	0.49	0.76	0.93	0.67	0.97	0.66	0.71	0.74	0.31	0.20	0.20	0.01	0.02	C09
0.15	0.42	0.58	1.22	1.54	1.89	1.65	1.56	1.84	1.79	0.51	0.31	0.31	0.02	0.04	C10
5.70	8.09	9.90	11.12	11.29	10.84	10.46	8.94	7.90	6.70	5.32	3.79	3.53	0.28	0.38	C11
0.32	0.78	1.69	3.51	3.92	4.31	3.88	3.12	3.52	2.38	1.20	0.70	0.72	0.05	0.09	C12-C13
0.07	0.25	0.54	0.85	1.03	1.22	1.65	1.73	1.68	1.94	0.39	0.23	0.23	0.01	0.03	C14
1.44	6.81	19.25	32.71	60.28	83.11	103.50	116.10	123.29	109.06	21.22	11.96	12.13	0.61	1.54	C15
5.90	13.29	27.29	51.03	90.08	130.51	167.23	195.29	212.41	192.50	34.56	19.79	19.81	0.97	2.46	C16
0.52	0.92	1.95	2.65	3.97	5.66	6.54	7.80	9.18	10.58	1.65	0.97	0.96	0.05	0.11	C17
5.96	10.57	19.33	34.39	55.62	76.54	97.15	119.43	147.00	155.25	22.52	13.03	12.98	0.67	1.53	C18
5.45	10.83	20.17	35.15	56.15	76.06	89.21	103.45	113.04	112.19	21.00	12.24	12.25	0.67	1.49	C19-C20
0.16	0.17	0.35	0.48	0.79	1.13	1.65	2.01	2.60	2.38	0.36	0.21	0.21	0.01	0.02	C21
22.72	39.60	58.92	72.35	95.90	112.55	119.30	136.20	145.82	157.19	38.35	23.74	23.39	1.55	2.71	C22
0.85	1.71	3.30	5.52	10.91	15.92	21.11	26.65	34.47	38.59	4.52	2.53	2.54	0.11	0.30	C23-C24
1.71	4.52	7.79	13.24	22.17	30.96	39.77	50.63	62.82	66.23	9.04	5.13	5.15	0.25	0.61	C25
0.24	0.60	0.96	0.94	1.53	1.58	1.71	1.87	2.50	2.53	0.59	0.38	0.37	0.02	0.04	C30-C31
0.56	1.67	4.46	8.14	12.63	14.61	16.00	16.12	17.03	13.48	3.89	2.23	2.28	0.14	0.29	C32
15.06	33.41	72.69	136.57	242.22	346.84	422.82	516.67	532.62	496.75	90.35	51.60	51.82	2.57	6.42	C33-C34
0.76	1.15	1.67	2.65	3.55	3.89	4.21	5.16	4.79	4.77	1.41	0.95	0.94	0.06	0.10	C37-C38
0.56	0.94	1.61	2.15	3.56	4.15	5.95	8.11	9.48	11.10	1.73	1.24	1.22	0.07	0.12	C40-C41
0.33	0.40	0.60	0.75	1.33	1.80	2.05	2.98	3.31	4.62	0.58	0.35	0.35	0.02	0.04	C43
0.96	1.58	2.25	3.63	5.95	9.42	12.55	18.13	28.60	35.31	3.21	1.88	1.85	0.08	0.19	C44
0.05	0.11	0.23	0.40	0.59	0.85	0.92	0.90	1.22	1.04	0.22	0.13	0.13	0.01	0.02	C45
0.01	0.02	0.07	0.03	0.07	0.09	0.18	0.03	0.20	0.15	0.04	0.03	0.03	0.00	0.00	C46
0.87	0.94	1.65	1.51	2.48	3.08	3.74	4.99	5.40	6.18	1.29	0.93	0.91	0.05	0.09	C47,C49
0.18	0.56	0.59	0.97	1.46	1.87	2.23	2.53	2.75	2.98	0.58	0.36	0.35	0.02	0.04	C50
—	—	—	—	—	—	—	—	—	—	—	—	—	—	—	C51
—	—	—	—	—	—	—	—	—	—	—	—	—	—	—	C52
—	—	—	—	—	—	—	—	—	—	—	—	—	—	—	C53
—	—	—	—	—	—	—	—	—	—	—	—	—	—	—	C54
—	—	—	—	—	—	—	—	—	—	—	—	—	—	—	C55
—	—	—	—	—	—	—	—	—	—	—	—	—	—	—	C56
—	—	—	—	—	—	—	—	—	—	—	—	—	—	—	C57
—	—	—	—	—	—	—	—	—	—	—	—	—	—	—	C58
0.23	0.47	0.90	1.10	1.91	2.35	3.00	3.67	5.10	5.81	0.77	0.45	0.45	0.02	0.05	C60
0.24	0.87	2.52	9.17	26.96	56.54	106.43	164.87	202.83	216.12	17.62	9.37	9.24	0.20	1.02	C61
0.58	0.51	0.47	0.46	0.34	0.36	0.50	0.59	1.02	0.89	0.50	0.47	0.43	0.03	0.03	C62
0.06	0.05	0.12	0.33	0.55	0.77	1.10	1.35	1.73	1.49	0.23	0.14	0.14	0.01	0.02	C63
3.85	6.29	10.03	15.27	18.12	21.81	22.74	20.59	23.40	21.38	7.06	4.45	4.41	0.30	0.52	C64
0.21	0.38	0.80	1.12	1.83	2.79	3.49	4.51	5.66	4.99	0.80	0.46	0.45	0.02	0.05	C65
0.08	0.16	0.43	1.13	2.35	3.11	4.03	5.86	6.83	6.48	0.86	0.47	0.48	0.02	0.06	C66
2.19	3.84	6.92	13.74	24.44	36.25	49.40	70.87	96.37	112.27	11.19	6.26	6.24	0.27	0.70	C67
0.06	0.05	0.07	0.23	0.31	0.51	0.79	1.42	1.63	2.09	0.18	0.10	0.10	0.00	0.01	C68
0.09	0.09	0.15	0.18	0.22	0.27	0.36	0.42	0.76	0.52	0.16	0.12	0.16	0.01	0.01	C69
4.39	7.34	9.38	12.61	15.98	18.64	21.84	24.54	27.13	29.13	7.63	5.41	5.35	0.34	0.54	C70-C72,D32-D33,D42-D43
21.76	19.98	18.10	18.99	15.11	11.56	8.18	7.17	4.95	4.17	13.13	11.77	9.81	0.80	0.90	C73
0.17	0.24	0.41	0.61	0.81	1.03	0.95	1.32	1.78	1.64	0.36	0.23	0.25	0.01	0.03	C74
0.12	0.35	0.54	0.69	0.95	1.04	1.46	1.32	1.22	0.97	0.45	0.34	0.34	0.02	0.03	C75
0.26	0.31	0.45	0.39	0.67	0.64	1.22	1.18	0.97	1.42	0.40	0.34	0.32	0.02	0.03	C81
2.83	4.52	6.59	9.41	13.84	18.16	22.80	28.35	33.96	23.17	6.25	4.11	4.02	0.23	0.44	C82-C86,C96
0.05	0.10	0.16	0.16	0.49	0.68	0.99	1.01	0.87	0.67	0.19	0.12	0.12	0.01	0.01	C88
0.53	1.08	2.05	3.35	5.42	7.70	9.98	14.38	13.31	10.65	2.24	1.32	1.30	0.07	0.15	C90
0.59	0.80	1.33	1.60	2.54	2.81	3.74	4.82	5.76	5.29	1.58	1.34	1.54	0.08	0.12	C91
2.49	3.09	4.16	5.90	8.56	12.13	15.91	20.14	22.89	21.98	4.55	3.18	3.10	0.18	0.32	C92-C94,D45-D47
0.79	0.96	1.21	1.86	2.71	3.92	6.13	8.42	9.53	12.22	1.70	1.22	1.26	0.06	0.11	C95
2.77	3.89	7.10	9.76	15.30	21.08	27.74	36.42	44.51	60.05	7.21	4.42	4.42	0.23	0.47	O & U
117.15	198.37	337.85	538.56	859.62	1 176.03	1 462.29	1 790.37	2 001.67	1 993.78	353.99	213.59	211.10	11.43	24.62	C00-C97,D32-D33, D42-D43
116.19	196.79	335.59	534.94	853.67	1 166.61	1 449.74	1 772.24	1 973.07	1 958.47	350.78	211.71	209.25	11.34	24.42	C00-C97,D32-D33, D42-D43,D45-D47 exc. C44

部位	Site	病例数 No. cases	构成 Freq./%	年龄组								
				0~	1~4	5~9	10~14	15~19	20~24	25~29	30~34	35~39
唇	Lip	236	0.06	0.08	0.03	0.00	0.00	0.00	0.03	0.01	0.03	0.01
舌	Tongue	1 001	0.24	0.00	0.00	0.00	0.00	0.03	0.05	0.05	0.16	0.24
口	Mouth	1 169	0.28	0.00	0.02	0.03	0.05	0.02	0.14	0.16	0.11	0.23
唾液腺	Salivary gland	789	0.19	0.00	0.00	0.00	0.05	0.14	0.16	0.29	0.45	0.34
扁桃体	Tonsil	153	0.04	0.00	0.00	0.00	0.00	0.00	0.01	0.04	0.02	0.01
其他口咽	Other oropharynx	116	0.03	0.00	0.00	0.01	0.00	0.00	0.00	0.01	0.02	0.06
鼻咽	Nasopharynx	2 893	0.69	0.00	0.02	0.04	0.05	0.29	0.39	0.94	1.33	1.85
下咽	Hypopharynx	107	0.03	0.00	0.00	0.01	0.00	0.00	0.00	0.00	0.04	0.01
咽,部位不明	Pharynx unspecified	118	0.03	0.00	0.02	0.00	0.00	0.00	0.00	0.03	0.01	0.01
食管	Esophagus	8 167	1.95	0.00	0.00	0.01	0.02	0.03	0.04	0.05	0.08	0.22
胃	Stomach	20 721	4.96	0.00	0.00	0.03	0.05	0.08	0.46	1.21	2.33	3.51
小肠	Small intestine	1 705	0.41	0.08	0.00	0.00	0.00	0.03	0.00	0.11	0.19	0.24
结肠	Colon	23 028	5.51	0.00	0.02	0.03	0.07	0.15	0.24	0.93	1.89	3.24
直肠	Rectum	17 391	4.16	0.00	0.00	0.00	0.02	0.15	0.24	0.60	1.41	2.16
肛门	Anus	385	0.09	0.00	0.00	0.00	0.00	0.00	0.00	0.01	0.04	0.07
肝脏	Liver	17 597	4.21	1.07	0.51	0.13	0.15	0.17	0.33	0.77	1.18	2.00
胆囊及其他	Gallbladder etc.	6 709	1.61	0.00	0.00	0.00	0.00	0.00	0.05	0.09	0.16	0.41
胰腺	Pancreas	9 392	2.25	0.00	0.00	0.03	0.07	0.08	0.12	0.20	0.32	0.60
鼻、鼻窦及其他	Nose,sinuses etc.	491	0.12	0.00	0.03	0.01	0.03	0.10	0.03	0.06	0.11	0.20
喉	Larynx	471	0.11	0.00	0.00	0.00	0.00	0.02	0.00	0.01	0.03	0.04
气管、支气管、肺	Trachea,bronchus & lung	72 794	17.42	0.15	0.10	0.04	0.02	0.34	0.87	2.88	6.56	11.70
其他胸腔器官	Other thoracic organs	1 301	0.31	0.46	0.19	0.04	0.05	0.09	0.09	0.19	0.27	0.34
骨	Bone	1 827	0.44	0.08	0.10	0.35	0.96	0.56	0.23	0.32	0.55	0.42
皮肤黑色素瘤	Melanoma of skin	755	0.18	0.00	0.00	0.03	0.00	0.05	0.09	0.13	0.19	0.21
皮肤其他	Other skin	4 249	1.02	0.08	0.02	0.09	0.12	0.17	0.26	0.28	0.53	0.51
间皮瘤	Mesothelioma	233	0.06	0.00	0.00	0.00	0.00	0.00	0.00	0.05	0.04	0.07
卡波西肉瘤	Kaposi sarcoma	20	0.00	0.00	0.02	0.00	0.00	0.00	0.00	0.01	0.00	0.00
结缔组织、软组织	Connective & soft tissue	1 359	0.33	0.84	0.48	0.26	0.18	0.37	0.28	0.38	0.57	0.62
乳腺	Breast	69 616	16.66	0.00	0.02	0.00	0.03	0.42	1.30	5.89	16.44	35.34
外阴	Vulva	817	0.20	0.23	0.02	0.00	0.00	0.03	0.03	0.06	0.10	0.17
阴道	Vagina	464	0.11	0.15	0.02	0.00	0.02	0.00	0.03	0.01	0.06	0.06
子宫颈	Cervix uteri	22 850	5.47	0.00	0.00	0.00	0.00	0.08	0.69	2.39	7.10	13.66
子宫体	Corpus uteri	13 474	3.22	0.00	0.00	0.00	0.00	0.03	0.16	0.75	1.73	3.41
子宫,部位不明	Uterus unspecified	2 208	0.53	0.00	0.00	0.01	0.00	0.05	0.04	0.17	0.45	0.73
卵巢	Ovary	11 572	2.77	0.08	0.14	0.21	0.53	1.50	2.21	2.54	3.16	4.32
其他女性生殖器官	Other female genital organs	954	0.23	0.00	0.00	0.00	0.02	0.02	0.04	0.09	0.08	0.27
胎盘	Placenta	99	0.02	0.00	0.00	0.00	0.00	0.05	0.09	0.27	0.09	0.12
阴茎	Penis	—	—	—	—	—	—	—	—	—	—	—
前列腺	Prostate	—	—	—	—	—	—	—	—	—	—	—
睾丸	Testis	—	—	—	—	—	—	—	—	—	—	—
其他男性生殖器官	Other male genital organs	—	—	—	—	—	—	—	—	—	—	—
肾	Kidney	4 889	1.17	0.23	0.68	0.21	0.08	0.12	0.22	0.40	0.80	1.02
肾盂	Renal pelvis	763	0.18	0.00	0.00	0.00	0.00	0.00	0.03	0.00	0.02	0.06
输尿管	Ureter	912	0.22	0.00	0.00	0.00	0.00	0.00	0.00	0.01	0.02	0.03
膀胱	Bladder	3 932	0.94	0.00	0.03	0.03	0.02	0.03	0.08	0.21	0.27	0.36
其他泌尿器官	Other urinary organs	169	0.04	0.00	0.00	0.00	0.00	0.00	0.00	0.00	0.00	0.02
眼	Eye	159	0.04	0.99	0.38	0.12	0.00	0.00	0.00	0.01	0.04	0.02
脑、神经系统	Brain,nervous system	13 111	3.14	2.36	1.86	1.81	1.54	1.54	1.44	2.25	2.85	4.21
甲状腺	Thyroid	50 335	12.05	0.00	0.02	0.06	0.58	3.06	13.49	33.76	49.32	57.77
肾上腺	Adrenal gland	358	0.09	0.15	0.27	0.04	0.00	0.02	0.07	0.09	0.06	0.08
其他内分泌腺	Other endocrine	634	0.15	0.00	0.07	0.04	0.05	0.12	0.11	0.35	0.36	0.44
霍奇金淋巴瘤	Hodgkin lymphoma	420	0.10	0.00	0.00	0.04	0.26	0.27	0.35	0.40	0.42	0.26
非霍奇金淋巴瘤	Non-Hodgkin lymphoma	6 537	1.56	0.30	0.46	0.32	0.33	0.54	0.66	0.84	1.41	1.89
免疫增生性疾病	Immunoproliferative diseases	138	0.03	0.00	0.03	0.01	0.03	0.02	0.03	0.00	0.02	0.02
多发性骨髓瘤	Multiple myeloma	2 368	0.57	0.08	0.00	0.04	0.10	0.10	0.00	0.08	0.09	0.19
淋巴细胞白血病	Lymphoid leukemia	1 422	0.34	1.37	2.99	1.74	0.81	0.68	0.34	0.33	0.23	0.37
髓系白血病	Myeloid leukemia	4 616	1.10	1.45	0.94	0.69	0.88	0.69	0.96	1.17	1.63	1.62
白血病,未特指	Leukemia unspecified	1 717	0.41	1.07	1.10	0.63	0.48	0.52	0.31	0.45	0.38	0.41
其他或未指明部位	Other and unspecified	8 175	1.96	1.45	0.96	0.44	0.56	0.69	0.75	0.84	1.27	1.79
所有部位合计	All sites	417 886	100.00	12.73	11.55	7.64	8.18	13.45	27.55	63.17	106.99	157.95
所有部位除外 C44	All sites except C44	413 637	98.98	12.65	11.53	7.55	8.07	13.28	27.30	62.89	106.46	157.43

40~44	45~49	50~54	55~59	60~64	65~69	70~74	75~79	80~84	85+	粗率 Crude rate/ 100 000⁻¹	中标率 ASR China/ 100 000⁻¹	世标率 ASR world/ 100 000⁻¹	累积率 Cum. Rate/% 0~64	0~74	ICD-10
0.06	0.10	0.13	0.16	0.35	0.48	0.57	0.97	0.99	1.76	0.18	0.09	0.10	0.00	0.01	C00
0.50	0.65	0.69	1.05	1.71	2.06	2.60	3.07	3.05	3.32	0.75	0.44	0.43	0.03	0.05	C01-C02
0.21	0.39	0.69	0.97	1.57	2.67	3.76	3.86	5.76	5.45	0.87	0.49	0.48	0.02	0.06	C03-C06
0.61	0.56	0.69	1.02	0.93	1.26	1.37	1.37	1.77	2.02	0.59	0.41	0.38	0.03	0.04	C07-C08
0.07	0.15	0.22	0.32	0.30	0.18	0.19	0.21	0.37	0.26	0.11	0.07	0.07	0.01	0.01	C09
0.08	0.06	0.12	0.16	0.15	0.17	0.21	0.33	0.41	0.36	0.09	0.05	0.05	0.00	0.01	C10
2.19	3.39	3.66	3.94	4.05	3.61	3.83	3.92	3.01	3.37	2.16	1.56	1.43	0.11	0.15	C11
0.05	0.04	0.13	0.09	0.15	0.20	0.30	0.37	0.45	0.31	0.08	0.05	0.04	0.00	0.01	C12-C13
0.03	0.03	0.04	0.06	0.19	0.13	0.36	0.58	0.78	0.83	0.09	0.05	0.05	0.00	0.00	C14
0.40	1.05	2.47	3.58	9.58	18.98	30.80	45.88	50.77	53.14	6.09	2.97	2.93	0.09	0.34	C15
5.44	9.31	14.43	18.94	28.86	42.44	60.43	78.35	96.39	95.17	15.46	8.48	8.24	0.42	0.94	C16
0.42	0.74	1.38	1.80	2.62	3.64	4.50	6.51	7.37	6.33	1.27	0.70	0.69	0.04	0.08	C17
5.45	8.92	14.82	22.62	34.61	49.27	64.93	88.48	111.13	106.37	17.18	9.24	9.07	0.46	1.04	C18
4.07	7.78	13.47	18.32	28.55	39.22	49.93	60.97	70.24	65.23	12.97	7.12	7.02	0.38	0.83	C19-C20
0.23	0.25	0.33	0.44	0.40	0.66	0.99	1.10	2.14	1.45	0.29	0.16	0.16	0.01	0.02	C21
4.17	6.69	11.52	15.75	25.58	37.03	51.17	68.64	84.00	90.24	13.13	7.03	6.97	0.35	0.79	C22
0.69	1.85	3.57	4.92	9.72	14.23	20.57	29.48	38.87	42.13	5.01	2.51	2.50	0.11	0.28	C23-C24
0.87	2.38	3.87	7.32	13.79	21.29	29.89	41.47	54.19	54.48	7.01	3.55	3.52	0.15	0.40	C25
0.29	0.32	0.41	0.56	0.65	1.06	1.14	0.82	1.36	1.76	0.37	0.23	0.23	0.01	0.03	C30-C31
0.10	0.17	0.25	0.34	0.77	0.93	0.99	2.34	2.47	3.17	0.35	0.18	0.18	0.01	0.02	C32
20.99	37.49	57.82	85.61	122.77	158.17	191.36	234.58	275.08	263.08	54.31	30.28	29.79	1.74	3.48	C33-C34
0.73	0.93	1.37	1.71	2.15	2.57	2.37	2.92	2.80	3.06	0.97	0.62	0.61	0.04	0.07	C37-C38
0.64	1.01	1.33	1.70	2.36	2.85	4.38	5.48	6.55	6.64	1.36	0.94	0.91	0.05	0.09	C40-C41
0.18	0.35	0.42	0.81	1.13	1.44	2.09	2.31	3.01	3.32	0.56	0.33	0.32	0.02	0.04	C43
0.87	1.34	1.94	3.08	4.83	7.78	12.05	17.62	23.80	33.68	3.17	1.66	1.63	0.07	0.17	C44
0.07	0.10	0.14	0.29	0.57	0.58	0.47	0.70	0.49	0.52	0.17	0.10	0.10	0.01	0.01	C45
0.00	0.01	0.03	0.03	0.05	0.01	0.08	0.00	0.00	0.10	0.01	0.01	0.01	0.00	0.00	C46
0.66	0.80	1.05	1.41	1.81	2.22	2.37	3.19	3.66	3.58	1.01	0.72	0.72	0.04	0.07	C47,C49
62.60	96.45	95.52	102.87	111.72	101.47	86.18	84.49	76.30	56.82	51.94	35.04	32.91	2.64	3.58	C50
0.32	0.49	0.63	0.71	1.28	1.65	1.97	2.77	3.01	3.68	0.61	0.35	0.34	0.02	0.04	C51
0.22	0.39	0.46	0.76	0.67	0.93	1.16	1.10	1.28	0.78	0.35	0.21	0.21	0.01	0.02	C52
20.53	29.98	37.01	37.27	32.87	27.26	26.93	23.40	19.97	12.40	17.05	11.78	10.94	0.91	1.18	C53
7.36	15.53	25.88	27.67	22.90	20.87	16.99	13.57	10.25	6.85	10.05	6.43	6.26	0.53	0.72	C54
1.62	2.69	3.57	3.47	3.12	3.25	2.90	3.53	3.38	3.17	1.65	1.07	1.02	0.08	0.11	C55
7.03	12.82	15.63	16.48	17.67	18.99	18.07	17.92	16.14	10.12	8.63	5.93	5.63	0.42	0.61	C56
0.52	0.93	1.33	1.47	1.68	2.10	1.54	1.49	1.24	1.30	0.71	0.45	0.44	0.03	0.05	C57
0.15	0.10	0.09	0.03	0.01	0.00	0.02	0.00	0.00	0.00	0.07	0.08	0.07	0.01	0.01	C58
—	—	—	—	—	—	—	—	—	—	—	—	—	—	—	C60
—	—	—	—	—	—	—	—	—	—	—	—	—	—	—	C61
—	—	—	—	—	—	—	—	—	—	—	—	—	—	—	C62
—	—	—	—	—	—	—	—	—	—	—	—	—	—	—	C63
1.60	3.16	4.67	6.47	8.38	10.69	11.12	12.93	13.09	11.62	3.65	2.19	2.18	0.14	0.25	C64
0.09	0.10	0.30	0.53	0.92	1.81	2.60	4.26	4.53	3.89	0.57	0.29	0.28	0.01	0.03	C65
0.08	0.14	0.31	0.54	1.30	2.00	3.19	4.84	6.09	4.67	0.68	0.34	0.33	0.01	0.04	C66
0.55	0.92	1.84	2.76	5.13	7.65	12.13	18.07	24.05	25.74	2.93	1.49	1.47	0.06	0.16	C67
0.00	0.04	0.10	0.13	0.27	0.42	0.59	0.46	0.95	1.14	0.13	0.06	0.06	0.00	0.01	C68
0.04	0.06	0.10	0.10	0.20	0.20	0.30	0.27	0.58	0.57	0.12	0.09	0.12	0.01	0.01	C69
6.16	9.16	12.91	16.44	20.87	23.47	26.84	29.79	32.40	29.73	9.78	6.41	6.32	0.42	0.67	C70-C72,D32-D33,D42-D43
58.67	64.36	66.17	63.69	46.75	33.38	20.63	11.87	8.69	6.28	37.55	31.83	27.25	2.29	2.56	C73
0.12	0.23	0.31	0.44	0.39	0.71	0.76	0.85	1.11	1.09	0.27	0.17	0.18	0.01	0.02	C74
0.55	0.46	0.65	0.78	0.94	0.97	0.87	0.79	0.74	0.36	0.47	0.36	0.33	0.02	0.03	C75
0.12	0.25	0.34	0.37	0.31	0.51	0.51	0.70	0.70	0.52	0.31	0.29	0.26	0.02	0.02	C81
2.62	3.78	5.41	7.60	10.15	13.26	17.06	18.65	20.50	13.60	4.88	3.04	2.94	0.18	0.33	C82-C86,C96
0.08	0.10	0.11	0.16	0.18	0.35	0.34	0.30	0.29	0.36	0.10	0.07	0.07	0.00	0.01	C88
0.40	1.00	1.79	2.77	4.22	6.24	7.44	7.91	8.19	5.55	1.77	0.99	0.98	0.05	0.12	C90
0.41	0.58	0.88	1.16	1.39	2.03	3.02	2.71	2.64	1.87	1.06	0.90	1.09	0.06	0.08	C91
2.12	2.58	3.54	4.58	5.85	8.13	10.46	12.84	14.41	11.42	3.44	2.35	2.29	0.14	0.23	C92-C94,D45-D47
0.53	0.74	1.16	1.45	1.92	2.88	3.70	5.32	6.88	5.50	1.28	0.89	0.94	0.05	0.10	C95
2.80	4.80	6.40	8.03	10.40	13.55	19.97	24.98	34.71	43.33	6.10	3.59	3.55	0.20	0.37	O & U
227.35	338.68	424.12	505.74	611.70	719.93	841.00	1 011.36	1 163.00	1 113.50	311.77	196.73	187.06	12.52	20.33	C00-C97,D32-D33,D42-D43,D45-D47
226.48	337.34	422.18	502.66	606.87	712.15	828.95	993.74	1 139.20	1 079.83	308.60	195.07	185.43	12.45	20.16	C00-C97,D32-D33,D42-D43,D45-D47 exc. C44

附表 1-7　2019 年全国农村肿瘤登记地区男女合计癌症发病主要指标

部位	Site	病例数 No. cases	构成 Freq./%	年龄组								
				0~	1~4	5~9	10~14	15~19	20~24	25~29	30~34	35~39
唇	Lip	1 219	0.12	0.03	0.02	0.02	0.01	0.01	0.04	0.04	0.06	0.08
舌	Tongue	2 748	0.27	0.03	0.01	0.01	0.02	0.04	0.02	0.09	0.22	0.36
口	Mouth	3 932	0.38	0.06	0.02	0.05	0.07	0.05	0.06	0.06	0.17	0.28
唾液腺	Salivary gland	2 154	0.21	0.00	0.02	0.04	0.06	0.12	0.14	0.28	0.31	0.34
扁桃体	Tonsil	543	0.05	0.00	0.01	0.02	0.01	0.02	0.01	0.03	0.05	0.07
其他口咽	Other oropharynx	941	0.09	0.00	0.01	0.01	0.01	0.02	0.02	0.02	0.03	0.06
鼻咽	Nasopharynx	13 610	1.33	0.06	0.03	0.05	0.17	0.44	0.39	0.88	1.77	2.95
下咽	Hypopharynx	1 555	0.15	0.00	0.00	0.00	0.00	0.01	0.02	0.01	0.02	0.06
咽,部位不明	Pharynx unspecified	837	0.08	0.03	0.01	0.00	0.01	0.01	0.02	0.01	0.02	0.02
食管	Esophagus	68 377	6.69	0.03	0.00	0.00	0.02	0.08	0.11	0.17	0.25	0.49
胃	Stomach	95 488	9.34	0.11	0.04	0.02	0.04	0.32	0.47	1.11	1.96	3.18
小肠	Small intestine	4 253	0.42	0.03	0.01	0.00	0.00	0.04	0.05	0.10	0.15	0.27
结肠	Colon	43 656	4.27	0.00	0.02	0.00	0.05	0.18	0.40	0.93	1.81	2.90
直肠	Rectum	51 413	5.03	0.00	0.01	0.00	0.02	0.13	0.32	0.90	1.51	2.25
肛门	Anus	1 400	0.14	0.00	0.01	0.00	0.00	0.01	0.02	0.02	0.08	0.11
肝脏	Liver	100 453	9.83	0.88	0.39	0.12	0.15	0.39	0.63	2.07	4.51	8.35
胆囊及其他	Gallbladder etc.	14 138	1.38	0.00	0.02	0.01	0.00	0.03	0.05	0.08	0.19	0.40
胰腺	Pancreas	23 149	2.26	0.03	0.01	0.00	0.04	0.05	0.12	0.19	0.39	0.77
鼻、鼻窦及其他	Nose, sinuses etc.	1 621	0.16	0.03	0.02	0.05	0.06	0.04	0.11	0.07	0.12	0.23
喉	Larynx	5 936	0.58	0.03	0.01	0.03	0.00	0.05	0.03	0.06	0.07	0.15
气管、支气管、肺	Trachea, bronchus & lung	228 176	22.32	0.03	0.07	0.04	0.05	0.63	0.86	1.88	3.99	7.96
其他胸腔器官	Other thoracic organs	3 338	0.33	0.17	0.12	0.07	0.10	0.15	0.13	0.26	0.34	0.38
骨	Bone	6 646	0.65	0.20	0.21	0.56	1.12	1.17	0.60	0.60	0.62	0.61
皮肤黑色素瘤	Melanoma of skin	1 743	0.17	0.09	0.05	0.03	0.01	0.06	0.04	0.07	0.12	0.16
皮肤其他	Other skin	9 590	0.94	0.03	0.15	0.10	0.09	0.21	0.23	0.25	0.41	0.56
间皮瘤	Mesothelioma	436	0.04	0.00	0.00	0.00	0.00	0.01	0.00	0.02	0.01	0.03
卡波西肉瘤	Kaposi sarcoma	73	0.01	0.00	0.01	0.00	0.00	0.02	0.01	0.00	0.01	0.03
结缔组织、软组织	Connective & soft tissue	3 324	0.33	0.37	0.35	0.26	0.26	0.31	0.24	0.44	0.49	0.56
乳腺	Breast	63 831	6.35	0.00	0.01	0.00	0.07	0.79	2.39	6.51	14.95	29.79
外阴	Vulva	821	0.08	0.06	0.01	0.01	0.01	0.01	0.06	0.05	0.07	0.20
阴道	Vagina	500	0.05	0.00	0.06	0.00	0.00	0.00	0.01	0.03	0.03	0.08
子宫颈	Cervix uteri	33 381	3.27	0.00	0.00	0.00	0.00	0.18	0.68	3.25	8.32	15.59
子宫体	Corpus uteri	13 952	1.36	0.00	0.00	0.00	0.01	0.09	0.25	0.71	1.47	3.15
子宫,部位不明	Uterus unspecified	3 897	0.38	0.00	0.00	0.00	0.00	0.03	0.11	0.40	0.83	1.39
卵巢	Ovary	12 693	1.24	0.12	0.06	0.11	0.58	1.33	1.98	2.67	2.79	3.41
其他女性生殖器官	Other female genital organs	974	0.10	0.00	0.00	0.01	0.04	0.09	0.10	0.10	0.15	0.24
胎盘	Placenta	133	0.01	0.00	0.00	0.00	0.00	0.00	0.12	0.22	0.17	0.12
阴茎	Penis	1 408	0.14	0.00	0.00	0.00	0.00	0.03	0.02	0.09	0.09	0.15
前列腺	Prostate	19 733	1.93	0.00	0.01	0.01	0.00	0.03	0.02	0.04	0.06	0.08
睾丸	Testis	788	0.08	0.97	0.32	0.05	0.08	0.24	0.37	0.50	0.64	0.59
其他男性生殖器官	Other male genital organs	256	0.03	0.00	0.02	0.01	0.01	0.06	0.01	0.01	0.01	0.02
肾	Kidney	11 321	1.11	0.63	0.57	0.17	0.09	0.12	0.16	0.40	0.78	1.20
肾盂	Renal pelvis	1 367	0.13	0.00	0.02	0.01	0.00	0.02	0.02	0.01	0.01	0.02
输尿管	Ureter	1 496	0.15	0.00	0.00	0.00	0.00	0.01	0.00	0.00	0.03	0.02
膀胱	Bladder	18 644	1.82	0.00	0.05	0.01	0.01	0.07	0.13	0.26	0.40	0.75
其他泌尿器官	Other urinary organs	417	0.04	0.03	0.01	0.00	0.00	0.01	0.01	0.00	0.01	0.04
眼	Eye	611	0.06	0.57	0.56	0.04	0.03	0.01	0.04	0.02	0.05	0.06
脑、神经系统	Brain, nervous system	28 730	2.81	1.96	1.72	1.92	1.84	1.70	1.73	2.31	2.90	3.83
甲状腺	Thyroid	51 167	5.00	0.00	0.01	0.07	0.33	1.34	5.23	12.83	16.88	20.70
肾上腺	Adrenal gland	1 006	0.10	0.26	0.18	0.07	0.01	0.03	0.03	0.09	0.11	0.12
其他内分泌腺	Other endocrine	1 540	0.15	0.00	0.04	0.06	0.12	0.12	0.14	0.19	0.28	0.41
霍奇金淋巴瘤	Hodgkin lymphoma	1 039	0.10	0.03	0.02	0.10	0.13	0.14	0.22	0.16	0.21	0.22
非霍奇金淋巴瘤	Non-Hodgkin lymphoma	14 360	1.40	0.23	0.57	0.45	0.52	0.55	0.64	0.92	1.18	1.72
免疫增生性疾病	Immunoproliferative diseases	194	0.02	0.00	0.01	0.00	0.00	0.00	0.01	0.00	0.00	0.01
多发性骨髓瘤	Multiple myeloma	5 134	0.50	0.06	0.01	0.02	0.04	0.07	0.06	0.05	0.12	0.20
淋巴细胞白血病	Lymphoid leukemia	3 910	0.38	0.77	2.32	1.27	0.97	0.65	0.47	0.45	0.50	0.45
髓系白血病	Myeloid leukemia	10 468	1.02	1.90	0.88	0.66	0.78	1.08	1.07	1.20	1.50	1.57
白血病,未特指	Leukemia unspecified	7 122	0.70	1.96	1.51	1.06	0.98	0.95	0.74	0.84	0.82	0.99
其他或未指明部位	Other and unspecified	19 575	1.91	1.31	1.15	0.76	0.73	0.81	0.78	0.96	1.24	1.78
所有部位合计	All sites	1 022 334	100.00	12.57	11.50	8.32	9.39	13.62	19.56	38.37	61.20	94.43
所有部位除外 C44	All sites except C44	1 012 744	99.06	12.54	11.36	8.22	9.30	13.41	19.33	38.12	60.79	93.87

Appendix Table 1-7　Cancer incidence in rural registration areas of China, both sexes in 2019

Age group										粗率 Crude rate/ 100 000⁻¹	中标率 ASR China/ 100 000⁻¹	世标率 ASR world/ 100 000⁻¹	累积率 Cum. Rate/%		ICD-10
40~44	45~49	50~54	55~59	60~64	65~69	70~74	75~79	80~84	85+				0~64	0~74	
0.12	0.21	0.37	0.41	0.71	1.08	1.35	1.99	1.85	2.23	0.34	0.21	0.20	0.01	0.02	C00
0.56	0.78	1.28	1.39	1.97	2.27	2.31	2.34	2.07	1.63	0.76	0.50	0.49	0.03	0.06	C01-C02
0.45	0.81	1.48	1.76	2.51	3.32	4.58	4.92	4.84	5.21	1.09	0.68	0.67	0.04	0.08	C03-C06
0.46	0.66	0.91	1.07	1.28	1.57	1.50	1.41	1.49	1.57	0.60	0.43	0.41	0.03	0.04	C07-C08
0.06	0.16	0.22	0.34	0.33	0.40	0.42	0.59	0.45	0.49	0.15	0.10	0.10	0.01	0.01	C09
0.11	0.22	0.31	0.52	0.66	0.87	0.99	1.07	1.04	0.87	0.26	0.16	0.16	0.01	0.02	C10
4.35	5.90	7.10	7.58	8.07	7.69	7.67	6.77	6.75	4.86	3.78	2.74	2.55	0.20	0.28	C11
0.08	0.28	0.69	1.01	1.46	1.46	1.70	1.39	1.23	0.76	0.43	0.26	0.26	0.02	0.03	C12-C13
0.05	0.12	0.22	0.41	0.60	0.79	1.10	0.89	1.55	1.33	0.23	0.14	0.14	0.01	0.02	C14
1.70	4.65	12.69	22.68	47.65	75.66	102.55	123.32	127.91	117.99	19.00	10.64	10.69	0.45	1.34	C15
5.94	11.76	22.70	36.65	66.03	97.29	128.21	154.69	161.23	141.83	26.53	15.43	15.33	0.75	1.88	C16
0.50	0.89	1.53	1.95	3.10	4.09	4.61	4.97	4.94	4.64	1.18	0.72	0.72	0.04	0.09	C17
4.75	7.98	12.69	18.59	28.79	39.53	51.82	61.58	67.21	61.22	12.13	7.34	7.18	0.40	0.85	C18
4.85	9.30	15.42	21.76	35.57	49.02	62.79	72.70	76.55	66.65	14.28	8.53	8.42	0.46	1.02	C19-C20
0.14	0.29	0.45	0.55	0.80	1.25	1.42	1.95	2.37	2.66	0.39	0.24	0.23	0.01	0.03	C21
17.15	26.96	39.47	47.81	67.87	84.44	97.14	109.90	117.37	113.18	27.91	17.46	17.08	1.08	1.99	C22
0.82	1.56	3.31	4.63	9.68	13.76	18.71	23.82	27.95	27.04	3.93	2.24	2.23	0.10	0.27	C23-C24
1.53	3.06	5.67	8.73	15.07	22.06	29.53	36.92	44.25	44.50	6.43	3.70	3.68	0.18	0.44	C25
0.30	0.47	0.63	0.73	1.00	1.23	1.46	1.62	1.49	1.41	0.45	0.31	0.30	0.02	0.03	C30-C31
0.34	0.73	1.84	2.96	4.91	6.07	7.86	7.97	6.95	5.43	1.65	0.97	0.98	0.06	0.13	C32
15.50	31.37	61.32	97.26	162.61	233.67	295.64	342.26	348.24	310.42	63.39	37.05	36.92	1.92	4.56	C33-C34
0.61	0.88	1.28	1.77	2.21	2.88	2.71	2.79	2.43	2.09	0.93	0.64	0.62	0.04	0.07	C37-C38
0.95	1.22	1.84	2.23	3.45	4.87	6.26	7.93	8.18	7.79	1.85	1.36	1.34	0.08	0.13	C40-C41
0.30	0.38	0.54	0.67	1.10	1.53	1.72	2.26	2.26	2.25	0.48	0.31	0.31	0.02	0.03	C43
0.89	1.25	2.05	2.88	4.56	6.90	10.78	15.42	23.31	33.23	2.66	1.55	1.54	0.07	0.16	C44
0.04	0.13	0.16	0.24	0.27	0.36	0.53	0.58	0.41	0.35	0.12	0.08	0.07	0.00	0.01	C45
0.02	0.02	0.03	0.01	0.03	0.03	0.05	0.09	0.06	0.14	0.02	0.02	0.01	0.00	0.00	C46
0.66	0.97	1.17	1.37	1.70	2.03	2.35	2.74	2.85	3.29	0.92	0.70	0.68	0.04	0.07	C47,C49
52.10	77.35	77.05	71.22	70.30	61.02	49.69	40.05	32.29	27.10	36.35	26.23	24.28	2.01	2.57	C50
0.23	0.38	0.56	0.68	1.04	1.15	1.94	2.05	2.12	1.88	0.47	0.29	0.28	0.02	0.03	C51
0.30	0.34	0.44	0.48	0.63	0.70	0.94	0.99	0.89	0.54	0.28	0.18	0.18	0.01	0.02	C52
24.50	34.05	41.17	39.65	36.26	32.28	32.30	29.80	22.86	15.53	19.01	13.48	12.48	1.02	1.34	C53
6.83	13.47	21.58	21.53	17.44	15.47	11.87	8.82	7.96	4.98	7.95	5.24	5.07	0.43	0.57	C54
2.54	3.90	4.52	4.09	4.25	4.08	4.37	4.46	5.26	3.50	2.22	1.52	1.42	0.11	0.15	C55
6.55	11.12	14.44	14.30	14.76	15.35	15.30	13.46	10.76	5.34	7.23	5.13	4.86	0.37	0.52	C56
0.54	0.89	1.01	1.15	1.19	1.36	1.30	0.97	0.89	0.49	0.55	0.38	0.36	0.03	0.04	C57
0.14	0.12	0.07	0.02	0.01	0.00	0.00	0.00	0.00	0.04	0.08	0.08	0.07	0.01	0.01	C58
0.38	0.63	1.07	1.13	1.97	2.25	3.18	3.88	5.09	3.57	0.76	0.48	0.47	0.03	0.05	C60
0.14	0.52	1.74	5.30	16.61	36.65	70.48	110.51	133.95	136.38	10.70	6.10	5.99	0.12	0.66	C61
0.49	0.43	0.38	0.40	0.36	0.44	0.75	0.75	0.88	1.17	0.43	0.40	0.38	0.02	0.03	C62
0.05	0.11	0.19	0.21	0.24	0.46	0.58	0.87	0.76	0.55	0.14	0.09	0.09	0.00	0.01	C63
1.94	2.91	4.81	6.44	7.47	9.88	10.06	9.71	9.63	7.47	3.15	2.06	2.04	0.14	0.23	C64
0.10	0.15	0.34	0.65	0.88	1.44	1.75	2.15	2.21	1.95	0.38	0.22	0.22	0.01	0.03	C65
0.06	0.15	0.22	0.48	1.04	1.71	2.12	2.82	2.94	2.09	0.42	0.24	0.23	0.01	0.03	C66
1.11	2.07	3.85	6.54	11.25	16.22	24.17	33.83	40.92	40.72	5.18	2.96	2.93	0.13	0.33	C67
0.03	0.04	0.07	0.18	0.27	0.47	0.55	0.60	0.62	0.71	0.12	0.07	0.07	0.00	0.01	C68
0.06	0.14	0.16	0.15	0.31	0.31	0.49	0.64	0.81	0.62	0.17	0.12	0.16	0.01	0.01	C69
5.65	7.76	10.73	12.87	17.12	20.76	23.51	24.89	25.25	24.98	7.98	5.68	5.59	0.36	0.58	C70-C72,D32-D33,D42-D43
23.36	24.83	26.56	26.48	18.84	14.05	9.74	7.38	5.31	4.29	14.22	12.26	10.63	0.89	1.01	C73
0.19	0.31	0.44	0.46	0.61	0.72	0.71	0.74	0.74	0.90	0.28	0.20	0.20	0.01	0.02	C74
0.43	0.50	0.63	0.79	0.85	0.87	0.91	0.77	0.81	0.62	0.43	0.33	0.31	0.02	0.03	C75
0.20	0.22	0.34	0.34	0.58	0.59	0.70	0.93	0.77	0.68	0.29	0.23	0.22	0.01	0.02	C81
2.07	3.23	4.85	6.28	9.26	12.00	14.99	15.30	14.68	11.76	3.99	2.69	2.63	0.16	0.30	C82-C86,C96
0.02	0.03	0.05	0.06	0.15	0.22	0.23	0.33	0.23	0.14	0.05	0.03	0.03	0.00	0.00	C88
0.35	0.85	1.53	2.36	4.08	5.62	6.11	7.28	5.54	3.94	1.43	0.86	0.86	0.05	0.11	C90
0.49	0.74	0.90	1.03	1.61	2.37	2.75	3.02	2.82	2.01	1.09	0.93	1.05	0.06	0.08	C91
1.89	2.62	3.39	3.85	5.56	7.11	8.73	10.82	9.82	7.60	2.91	2.18	2.13	0.13	0.21	C92-C94,D45-D47
1.13	1.32	1.82	2.04	3.20	4.69	6.36	8.31	7.46	7.09	1.98	1.53	1.58	0.09	0.14	C95
2.54	4.14	6.16	7.54	11.15	15.66	20.11	24.12	27.72	30.05	5.44	3.55	3.53	0.20	0.38	O & U
151.24	235.76	345.83	446.63	650.59	867.72	1 079.35	1 257.39	1 315.47	1 205.23	284.02	180.21	175.48	10.43	20.17	C00-C97,D32-D33, D42-D43,D45-D47
150.35	234.51	343.78	443.76	646.03	860.82	1 068.58	1 241.98	1 292.16	1 172.00	281.36	178.66	173.94	10.37	20.01	C00-C97,D32-D33, D42-D43,D45-D47 exc. C44

附表 1-8　2019 年全国农村肿瘤登记地区男性癌症发病主要指标

	部位 Site	病例数 No. cases	构成 Freq./%	年龄组								
				0~	1~4	5~9	10~14	15~19	20~24	25~29	30~34	35~39
唇	Lip	717	0.13	0.05	0.02	0.03	0.02	0.02	0.03	0.05	0.04	0.05
舌	Tongue	1 914	0.34	0.05	0.01	0.02	0.03	0.05	0.03	0.12	0.28	0.47
口	Mouth	2 604	0.46	0.05	0.02	0.05	0.08	0.05	0.07	0.07	0.21	0.34
唾液腺	Salivary gland	1 203	0.21	0.00	0.03	0.05	0.04	0.09	0.12	0.22	0.28	0.35
扁桃体	Tonsil	392	0.07	0.00	0.01	0.03	0.00	0.01	0.00	0.02	0.04	0.14
其他口咽	Other oropharynx	775	0.14	0.00	0.01	0.02	0.00	0.03	0.02	0.01	0.04	0.08
鼻咽	Nasopharynx	9 675	1.70	0.05	0.05	0.06	0.22	0.66	0.49	1.07	2.32	4.00
下咽	Hypopharynx	1 432	0.25	0.00	0.00	0.00	0.00	0.02	0.02	0.01	0.02	0.08
咽,部位不明	Pharynx unspecified	656	0.12	0.00	0.01	0.01	0.02	0.01	0.02	0.01	0.04	0.02
食管	Esophagus	49 968	8.78	0.05	0.00	0.00	0.03	0.14	0.06	0.17	0.30	0.65
胃	Stomach	66 947	11.77	0.16	0.06	0.03	0.06	0.42	0.44	0.93	1.81	3.16
小肠	Small intestine	2 434	0.43	0.00	0.00	0.00	0.00	0.00	0.06	0.12	0.15	0.34
结肠	Colon	24 872	4.37	0.00	0.02	0.00	0.05	0.25	0.50	1.01	2.02	3.04
直肠	Rectum	31 157	5.48	0.00	0.02	0.01	0.03	0.17	0.36	0.99	1.54	2.32
肛门	Anus	790	0.14	0.00	0.01	0.00	0.00	0.01	0.04	0.02	0.07	0.10
肝脏	Liver	74 813	13.15	1.03	0.41	0.18	0.18	0.52	0.97	3.21	7.21	13.89
胆囊及其他	Gallbladder etc.	6 831	1.20	0.00	0.03	0.01	0.00	0.04	0.02	0.06	0.18	0.34
胰腺	Pancreas	13 382	2.35	0.00	0.01	0.00	0.03	0.04	0.08	0.19	0.39	0.95
鼻、鼻窦及其他	Nose, sinuses etc.	1 013	0.18	0.00	0.02	0.04	0.06	0.04	0.11	0.07	0.11	0.24
喉	Larynx	5 318	0.93	0.05	0.00	0.04	0.01	0.06	0.03	0.05	0.10	0.21
气管、支气管、肺	Trachea, bronchus & lung	149 481	26.27	0.05	0.09	0.05	0.04	0.76	0.84	1.48	3.67	7.38
其他胸腔器官	Other thoracic organs	2 032	0.36	0.22	0.13	0.07	0.16	0.17	0.17	0.30	0.47	0.43
骨	Bone	3 781	0.66	0.16	0.20	0.61	1.21	1.41	0.75	0.71	0.69	0.63
皮肤黑色素瘤	Melanoma of skin	878	0.15	0.05	0.05	0.01	0.01	0.04	0.03	0.04	0.10	0.14
皮肤其他	Other skin	4 741	0.83	0.05	0.13	0.14	0.10	0.22	0.21	0.29	0.42	0.51
间皮瘤	Mesothelioma	239	0.04	0.00	0.00	0.00	0.00	0.00	0.00	0.03	0.01	0.02
卡波西肉瘤	Kaposi sarcoma	50	0.01	0.00	0.00	0.00	0.00	0.03	0.01	0.01	0.01	0.04
结缔组织、软组织	Connective & soft tissue	1 780	0.31	0.32	0.26	0.28	0.31	0.27	0.26	0.45	0.48	0.56
乳腺	Breast	1 117	0.20	0.11	0.01	0.01	0.02	0.02	0.03	0.07	0.13	0.21
外阴	Vulva	—	—	—	—	—	—	—	—	—	—	—
阴道	Vagina	—	—	—	—	—	—	—	—	—	—	—
子宫颈	Cervix uteri	—	—	—	—	—	—	—	—	—	—	—
子宫体	Corpus uteri	—	—	—	—	—	—	—	—	—	—	—
子宫,部位不明	Uterus unspecified	—	—	—	—	—	—	—	—	—	—	—
卵巢	Ovary	—	—	—	—	—	—	—	—	—	—	—
其他女性生殖器官	Other female genital organs	—	—	—	—	—	—	—	—	—	—	—
胎盘	Placenta	—	—	—	—	—	—	—	—	—	—	—
阴茎	Penis	1 408	0.25	0.00	0.00	0.00	0.00	0.00	0.03	0.02	0.09	0.15
前列腺	Prostate	19 733	3.47	0.00	0.01	0.01	0.00	0.03	0.02	0.04	0.06	0.08
睾丸	Testis	788	0.14	0.97	0.32	0.05	0.08	0.24	0.37	0.50	0.64	0.59
其他男性生殖器官	Other male genital organs	256	0.04	0.00	0.02	0.01	0.01	0.06	0.01	0.01	0.01	0.02
肾	Kidney	7 204	1.27	0.49	0.54	0.15	0.09	0.11	0.17	0.46	1.03	1.60
肾盂	Renal pelvis	845	0.15	0.00	0.02	0.01	0.00	0.01	0.03	0.01	0.01	0.01
输尿管	Ureter	843	0.15	0.00	0.00	0.00	0.00	0.01	0.00	0.00	0.03	0.02
膀胱	Bladder	14 958	2.63	0.00	0.07	0.03	0.03	0.10	0.18	0.42	0.58	1.07
其他泌尿器官	Other urinary organs	247	0.04	0.05	0.01	0.00	0.01	0.01	0.00	0.00	0.01	0.05
眼	Eye	334	0.06	0.54	0.55	0.06	0.01	0.01	0.05	0.03	0.08	0.06
脑、神经系统	Brain, nervous system	13 309	2.34	2.11	1.82	2.02	1.95	1.83	1.62	2.41	2.98	3.60
甲状腺	Thyroid	11 772	2.07	0.00	0.02	0.10	0.19	0.51	2.60	6.47	8.89	10.49
肾上腺	Adrenal gland	564	0.10	0.43	0.15	0.08	0.02	0.04	0.03	0.10	0.06	0.14
其他内分泌腺	Other endocrine	725	0.13	0.00	0.07	0.08	0.16	0.11	0.12	0.14	0.28	0.38
霍奇金淋巴瘤	Hodgkin lymphoma	659	0.12	0.00	0.01	0.14	0.15	0.17	0.24	0.19	0.23	0.30
非霍奇金淋巴瘤	Non-Hodgkin lymphoma	8 439	1.48	0.16	0.66	0.55	0.64	0.73	0.72	1.06	1.29	1.87
免疫增生性疾病	Immunoproliferative diseases	115	0.02	0.00	0.01	0.00	0.00	0.01	0.00	0.00	0.00	0.02
多发性骨髓瘤	Multiple myeloma	2 923	0.51	0.11	0.00	0.02	0.00	0.08	0.07	0.07	0.16	0.27
淋巴细胞白血病	Lymphoid leukemia	2 298	0.40	0.76	2.58	1.32	1.07	0.75	0.58	0.52	0.58	0.50
髓系白血病	Myeloid leukemia	5 919	1.04	1.89	0.93	0.76	0.78	1.25	1.12	1.28	1.66	1.77
白血病,未特指	Leukemia unspecified	4 031	0.71	1.73	1.68	1.06	1.01	1.08	0.86	0.93	0.88	1.07
其他或未指明部位	Other and unspecified	10 665	1.87	1.30	1.20	0.85	0.76	0.83	0.78	0.87	1.23	1.62
所有部位合计	All sites	569 027	100.00	13.08	12.30	9.07	9.73	13.51	15.35	27.34	43.91	66.33
所有部位除外 C44	All sites except C44	564 286	99.17	13.03	12.17	8.92	9.63	13.29	15.14	27.05	43.49	65.82

Appendix Table 1-8　Cancer incidence in rural registration areas of China, male in 2019

Age group										粗率 Crude rate/ 100 000⁻¹	中标率 ASR China/ 100 000⁻¹	世标率 ASR world/ 100 000⁻¹	累积率 Cum. Rate/%		ICD-10
40~44	45~49	50~54	55~59	60~64	65~69	70~74	75~79	80~84	85+				0~64	0~74	
0.14	0.20	0.39	0.49	1.00	1.33	1.70	2.57	1.98	3.16	0.39	0.24	0.25	0.01	0.03	C00
0.83	1.09	1.85	2.00	2.82	3.14	3.23	3.14	2.73	1.99	1.04	0.70	0.68	0.05	0.08	C01-C02
0.63	1.14	2.04	2.27	3.49	4.64	6.21	6.45	5.93	7.22	1.41	0.91	0.90	0.05	0.11	C03-C06
0.33	0.63	1.05	1.31	1.44	2.02	1.85	2.00	1.93	1.99	0.65	0.46	0.44	0.03	0.05	C07-C08
0.09	0.23	0.33	0.50	0.55	0.62	0.58	0.85	0.55	0.69	0.21	0.14	0.14	0.01	0.02	C09
0.14	0.36	0.49	0.87	1.18	1.57	1.63	1.82	1.77	1.51	0.42	0.27	0.27	0.02	0.03	C10
6.12	8.32	9.80	11.18	11.70	11.09	11.14	9.77	9.75	6.67	5.25	3.84	3.60	0.28	0.39	C11
0.14	0.49	1.24	1.87	2.76	2.76	3.23	2.62	2.40	1.51	0.78	0.48	0.49	0.03	0.06	C12-C13
0.05	0.21	0.32	0.67	1.05	1.28	1.72	1.52	2.27	2.20	0.36	0.22	0.22	0.01	0.03	C14
2.46	7.72	20.82	37.09	76.06	115.81	150.28	174.68	179.76	159.47	27.10	16.06	16.19	0.73	2.06	C15
6.71	14.27	30.79	52.94	99.09	146.28	190.22	227.34	228.43	196.59	36.31	21.95	21.93	1.05	2.74	C16
0.63	1.00	1.84	2.22	3.55	4.73	5.25	5.71	6.09	6.12	1.32	0.84	0.83	0.05	0.10	C17
5.51	8.84	14.17	21.62	34.68	46.46	61.28	70.80	78.60	72.86	13.49	8.51	8.36	0.46	1.00	C18
5.44	10.44	18.36	26.50	44.79	63.03	78.81	92.47	97.47	82.01	16.90	10.47	10.37	0.55	1.26	C19-C20
0.12	0.29	0.46	0.66	0.96	1.65	1.68	2.18	2.86	3.16	0.43	0.27	0.26	0.01	0.03	C21
28.31	44.38	63.35	76.78	103.27	125.06	134.48	150.32	159.76	148.75	40.58	26.60	25.96	1.71	3.01	C22
0.85	1.52	3.27	4.72	9.65	13.78	19.32	23.62	26.14	27.43	3.71	2.23	2.23	0.10	0.27	C23-C24
1.92	3.76	7.30	10.76	18.42	26.31	34.60	41.71	50.18	52.52	7.26	4.41	4.39	0.22	0.52	C25
0.31	0.52	0.83	0.92	1.40	1.66	1.96	2.21	1.68	1.99	0.55	0.37	0.37	0.02	0.04	C30-C31
0.57	1.23	3.36	5.45	8.94	11.38	14.37	14.44	12.74	10.59	2.88	1.76	1.78	0.10	0.23	C32
15.32	33.83	74.09	124.99	218.89	325.89	418.28	486.51	492.43	447.21	81.08	48.99	49.05	2.41	6.13	C33-C34
0.68	0.94	1.52	2.17	2.76	3.71	3.21	3.42	3.15	3.09	1.10	0.78	0.76	0.05	0.08	C37-C38
1.01	1.20	2.21	2.34	4.03	5.59	7.58	8.94	10.13	10.31	2.05	1.55	1.52	0.08	0.15	C40-C41
0.32	0.38	0.48	0.67	1.15	1.50	1.95	2.65	2.65	2.34	0.48	0.31	0.31	0.02	0.03	C43
0.95	1.29	2.11	2.93	4.82	7.54	11.64	15.86	23.12	31.00	2.57	1.61	1.59	0.07	0.17	C44
0.05	0.09	0.17	0.29	0.28	0.45	0.58	0.67	0.55	0.55	0.13	0.08	0.08	0.00	0.01	C45
0.02	0.03	0.03	0.02	0.05	0.06	0.10	0.13	0.04	0.07	0.03	0.02	0.02	0.00	0.00	C46
0.65	1.00	1.18	1.42	1.77	2.22	2.75	3.65	3.74	3.78	0.97	0.74	0.71	0.04	0.07	C47,C49
0.42	0.77	0.99	1.15	1.34	1.96	2.03	1.85	2.27	1.65	0.61	0.41	0.39	0.03	0.05	C50
—	—	—	—	—	—	—	—	—	—	—	—	—	—	—	C51
—	—	—	—	—	—	—	—	—	—	—	—	—	—	—	C52
—	—	—	—	—	—	—	—	—	—	—	—	—	—	—	C53
—	—	—	—	—	—	—	—	—	—	—	—	—	—	—	C54
—	—	—	—	—	—	—	—	—	—	—	—	—	—	—	C55
—	—	—	—	—	—	—	—	—	—	—	—	—	—	—	C56
—	—	—	—	—	—	—	—	—	—	—	—	—	—	—	C57
—	—	—	—	—	—	—	—	—	—	—	—	—	—	—	C58
0.38	0.63	1.07	1.13	1.97	2.25	3.18	3.88	5.09	3.57	0.76	0.48	0.47	0.03	0.05	C60
0.14	0.52	1.74	5.30	16.61	36.65	70.48	110.51	133.95	136.38	10.70	6.10	5.99	0.12	0.66	C61
0.49	0.43	0.38	0.40	0.36	0.44	0.75	0.75	0.88	1.17	0.43	0.40	0.38	0.02	0.03	C62
0.05	0.11	0.19	0.21	0.24	0.46	0.58	0.87	0.76	0.55	0.14	0.09	0.09	0.00	0.01	C63
2.34	3.58	5.99	8.54	9.66	13.13	12.97	11.98	12.65	10.65	3.91	2.61	2.58	0.17	0.30	C64
0.14	0.23	0.43	0.86	1.24	1.70	2.00	2.57	2.98	2.68	0.46	0.28	0.28	0.02	0.03	C65
0.08	0.18	0.27	0.68	1.29	1.81	2.30	3.06	3.19	3.09	0.46	0.27	0.27	0.01	0.03	C66
1.68	3.25	6.07	10.33	18.60	26.93	39.41	56.59	71.41	78.84	8.11	4.88	4.84	0.21	0.54	C67
0.05	0.05	0.07	0.26	0.20	0.56	0.63	0.80	1.01	1.17	0.13	0.08	0.08	0.00	0.01	C68
0.08	0.15	0.14	0.21	0.35	0.29	0.55	0.64	0.97	1.03	0.18	0.14	0.17	0.01	0.01	C69
5.50	7.05	9.12	11.06	15.71	19.61	22.05	23.21	24.29	24.13	7.22	5.36	5.27	0.33	0.54	C70-C72,D32-D33,D42-D43
10.33	10.01	10.27	11.03	8.48	6.78	5.61	4.39	3.24	2.54	6.38	5.68	4.86	0.40	0.46	C73
0.21	0.31	0.47	0.53	0.65	0.86	0.82	0.77	1.01	1.65	0.31	0.22	0.23	0.01	0.02	C74
0.32	0.38	0.43	0.88	0.83	0.91	1.00	0.72	0.67	1.03	0.39	0.31	0.30	0.02	0.03	C75
0.23	0.23	0.44	0.43	0.82	0.83	0.83	1.21	1.13	0.96	0.36	0.29	0.27	0.02	0.03	C81
2.46	3.85	5.55	7.25	10.73	14.15	18.53	18.43	18.03	16.77	4.58	3.17	3.11	0.19	0.35	C82-C86,C96
0.02	0.02	0.06	0.03	0.17	0.28	0.30	0.46	0.42	0.27	0.06	0.04	0.04	0.00	0.00	C88
0.32	0.97	1.71	2.55	4.40	6.45	7.04	9.18	6.98	6.26	1.59	0.99	0.99	0.05	0.12	C90
0.57	0.80	0.92	1.10	1.95	2.95	3.56	4.09	3.11	3.09	1.25	1.07	1.20	0.06	0.10	C91
2.09	2.70	3.67	4.27	6.14	8.33	10.16	13.57	12.74	9.97	3.21	2.44	2.38	0.14	0.24	C92-C94,D45-D47
1.38	1.51	1.98	2.24	3.58	5.22	7.49	9.87	9.41	9.49	2.19	1.72	1.76	0.10	0.16	C95
2.31	4.08	5.99	8.41	12.59	18.49	24.26	28.12	33.58	35.13	5.78	3.86	3.86	0.21	0.42	O & U
111.88	187.22	321.79	474.51	778.48	1 102.58	1 406.17	1 665.56	1 758.59	1 638.87	308.63	195.70	193.52	10.36	22.90	C00-C97,D32-D33,D42-D43,D45-D47
110.92	185.93	319.67	471.58	773.66	1 095.04	1 394.53	1 649.70	1 735.47	1 607.87	306.06	194.09	191.93	10.29	22.74	C00-C97,D32-D33,D42-D43,D45-D47 exc. C44

附表 1-9　2019 年全国农村肿瘤登记地区女性癌症发病主要指标

部位	Site	病例数 No. cases	构成 Freq./%	0~	1~4	5~9	10~14	15~19	20~24	25~29	30~34	35~39
唇	Lip	502	0.11	0.00	0.01	0.02	0.01	0.00	0.05	0.03	0.07	0.11
舌	Tongue	834	0.18	0.00	0.00	0.01	0.01	0.02	0.01	0.06	0.16	0.24
口	Mouth	1 328	0.29	0.06	0.03	0.05	0.06	0.04	0.06	0.05	0.13	0.22
唾液腺	Salivary gland	951	0.21	0.00	0.01	0.03	0.07	0.15	0.16	0.34	0.35	0.34
扁桃体	Tonsil	151	0.03	0.00	0.00	0.02	0.02	0.03	0.02	0.04	0.05	0.00
其他口咽	Other oropharynx	166	0.04	0.00	0.01	0.00	0.02	0.00	0.02	0.03	0.01	0.05
鼻咽	Nasopharynx	3 935	0.87	0.06	0.01	0.04	0.11	0.18	0.29	0.67	1.18	1.85
下咽	Hypopharynx	123	0.03	0.00	0.00	0.01	0.00	0.00	0.02	0.01	0.02	0.03
咽,部位不明	Pharynx unspecified	181	0.04	0.06	0.00	0.00	0.00	0.01	0.03	0.00	0.01	0.01
食管	Esophagus	18 409	4.06	0.00	0.00	0.00	0.02	0.01	0.17	0.17	0.19	0.32
胃	Stomach	28 541	6.30	0.06	0.03	0.02	0.02	0.21	0.50	1.31	2.11	3.21
小肠	Small intestine	1 819	0.40	0.06	0.01	0.00	0.00	0.08	0.05	0.07	0.14	0.20
结肠	Colon	18 784	4.14	0.00	0.01	0.01	0.04	0.09	0.30	0.84	1.59	2.76
直肠	Rectum	20 256	4.47	0.00	0.00	0.00	0.01	0.08	0.27	0.79	1.48	2.18
肛门	Anus	610	0.13	0.00	0.00	0.00	0.01	0.01	0.00	0.02	0.10	0.11
肝脏	Liver	25 640	5.66	0.72	0.37	0.06	0.11	0.25	0.25	0.83	1.67	2.48
胆囊及其他	Gallbladder etc.	7 307	1.61	0.00	0.00	0.01	0.00	0.02	0.10	0.10	0.21	0.47
胰腺	Pancreas	9 767	2.15	0.00	0.01	0.00	0.05	0.06	0.16	0.20	0.39	0.58
鼻、鼻窦及其他	Nose, sinuses etc.	608	0.13	0.06	0.03	0.06	0.06	0.03	0.11	0.07	0.13	0.22
喉	Larynx	618	0.14	0.00	0.03	0.01	0.00	0.04	0.02	0.06	0.04	0.08
气管、支气管、肺	Trachea, bronchus & lung	78 695	17.36	0.00	0.04	0.03	0.07	0.49	0.89	2.30	4.33	8.58
其他胸腔器官	Other thoracic organs	1 306	0.29	0.12	0.12	0.06	0.03	0.13	0.09	0.22	0.21	0.32
骨	Bone	2 865	0.63	0.24	0.22	0.50	1.00	0.90	0.43	0.48	0.56	0.58
皮肤黑色素瘤	Melanoma of skin	865	0.19	0.12	0.05	0.05	0.01	0.09	0.05	0.09	0.13	0.18
皮肤其他	Other skin	4 849	1.07	0.00	0.17	0.04	0.08	0.19	0.25	0.20	0.40	0.62
间皮瘤	Mesothelioma	197	0.04	0.00	0.00	0.00	0.00	0.01	0.00	0.02	0.01	0.04
卡波西肉瘤	Kaposi sarcoma	23	0.01	0.00	0.01	0.00	0.00	0.00	0.01	0.00	0.00	0.02
结缔组织、软组织	Connective & soft tissue	1 544	0.34	0.42	0.45	0.23	0.21	0.36	0.21	0.44	0.51	0.56
乳腺	Breast	63 831	14.08	0.00	0.01	0.00	0.07	0.79	2.39	6.51	14.95	29.79
外阴	Vulva	821	0.18	0.06	0.01	0.01	0.01	0.01	0.06	0.05	0.07	0.20
阴道	Vagina	500	0.11	0.00	0.06	0.00	0.00	0.00	0.01	0.03	0.03	0.08
子宫颈	Cervix uteri	33 381	7.36	0.00	0.00	0.00	0.00	0.18	0.68	3.25	8.32	15.59
子宫体	Corpus uteri	13 952	3.08	0.00	0.00	0.00	0.01	0.09	0.25	0.71	1.47	3.15
子宫,部位不明	Uterus unspecified	3 897	0.86	0.00	0.00	0.00	0.00	0.03	0.11	0.40	0.83	1.39
卵巢	Ovary	12 693	2.80	0.12	0.06	0.11	0.58	1.33	1.98	2.67	2.79	3.41
其他女性生殖器官	Other female genital organs	974	0.21	0.00	0.00	0.01	0.04	0.09	0.10	0.10	0.15	0.24
胎盘	Placenta	133	0.03	0.00	0.00	0.00	0.00	0.05	0.12	0.22	0.17	0.12
阴茎	Penis	—	—	—	—	—	—	—	—	—	—	—
前列腺	Prostate	—	—	—	—	—	—	—	—	—	—	—
睾丸	Testis	—	—	—	—	—	—	—	—	—	—	—
其他男性生殖器官	Other male genital organs	—	—	—	—	—	—	—	—	—	—	—
肾	Kidney	4 117	0.91	0.78	0.60	0.19	0.08	0.12	0.15	0.34	0.51	0.78
肾盂	Renal pelvis	522	0.12	0.00	0.01	0.01	0.00	0.02	0.00	0.01	0.01	0.03
输尿管	Ureter	653	0.14	0.00	0.00	0.00	0.00	0.00	0.01	0.00	0.02	0.02
膀胱	Bladder	3 686	0.81	0.00	0.03	0.00	0.00	0.03	0.07	0.10	0.21	0.42
其他泌尿器官	Other urinary organs	170	0.04	0.00	0.00	0.00	0.00	0.01	0.02	0.01	0.01	0.03
眼	Eye	277	0.06	0.60	0.56	0.01	0.05	0.00	0.03	0.01	0.02	0.06
脑、神经系统	Brain, nervous system	15 421	3.40	1.80	1.62	1.82	1.71	1.56	1.84	2.20	2.82	4.08
甲状腺	Thyroid	39 395	8.69	0.00	0.00	0.04	0.50	2.30	8.12	19.71	25.28	31.50
肾上腺	Adrenal gland	442	0.10	0.06	0.21	0.06	0.01	0.02	0.03	0.06	0.16	0.09
其他内分泌腺	Other endocrine	815	0.18	0.00	0.01	0.04	0.06	0.13	0.15	0.25	0.27	0.45
霍奇金淋巴瘤	Hodgkin lymphoma	380	0.08	0.06	0.04	0.05	0.10	0.10	0.19	0.12	0.20	0.14
非霍奇金淋巴瘤	Non-Hodgkin lymphoma	5 921	1.31	0.30	0.47	0.33	0.39	0.36	0.56	0.77	1.05	1.55
免疫增生性疾病	Immunoproliferative diseases	79	0.02	0.00	0.01	0.00	0.00	0.00	0.00	0.01	0.00	0.00
多发性骨髓瘤	Multiple myeloma	2 211	0.49	0.00	0.01	0.03	0.04	0.04	0.06	0.03	0.08	0.13
淋巴细胞白血病	Lymphoid leukemia	1 612	0.36	0.78	2.03	1.20	0.85	0.54	0.36	0.37	0.42	0.40
髓系白血病	Myeloid leukemia	4 549	1.00	1.92	0.82	0.55	0.79	0.87	1.02	1.12	1.34	1.36
白血病,未特指	Leukemia unspecified	3 091	0.68	2.22	1.32	1.06	0.95	0.81	0.60	0.73	0.75	0.90
其他或未指明部位	Other and unspecified	8 910	1.97	1.32	1.09	0.66	0.69	0.79	0.78	1.06	1.26	1.95
所有部位合计	All sites	453 307	100.00	11.99	10.62	7.47	9.00	13.75	24.18	50.28	79.38	124.18
所有部位除外 C44	All sites except C44	448 458	98.93	11.99	10.45	7.42	8.91	13.56	23.93	50.08	78.98	123.56

Appendix Table 1-9　Cancer incidence in rural registration areas of China,female in 2019

Age group										粗率 Crude rate/ 100 000⁻¹	中标率 ASR China/ 100 000⁻¹	世标率 ASR world/ 100 000⁻¹	累积率 Cum. Rate/%		ICD-10
40~44	45~49	50~54	55~59	60~64	65~69	70~74	75~79	80~84	85+				0~64	0~74	
0.10	0.22	0.36	0.33	0.41	0.83	1.00	1.46	1.74	1.62	0.29	0.17	0.16	0.01	0.02	C00
0.28	0.47	0.69	0.78	1.09	1.41	1.42	1.60	1.54	1.39	0.48	0.30	0.29	0.02	0.03	C01-C02
0.25	0.48	0.90	1.24	1.49	2.02	3.00	3.51	3.96	3.90	0.76	0.45	0.44	0.03	0.05	C03-C06
0.60	0.69	0.78	0.83	1.11	1.13	1.17	0.87	1.13	1.30	0.54	0.41	0.38	0.03	0.04	C07-C08
0.02	0.08	0.11	0.16	0.11	0.19	0.26	0.35	0.38	0.36	0.09	0.06	0.06	0.00	0.01	C09
0.08	0.07	0.12	0.16	0.14	0.19	0.36	0.38	0.44	0.45	0.09	0.06	0.06	0.00	0.01	C10
2.47	3.39	4.33	3.92	4.34	4.34	4.29	4.03	4.30	3.68	2.24	1.61	1.49	0.11	0.16	C11
0.02	0.05	0.12	0.14	0.14	0.18	0.21	0.26	0.27	0.27	0.07	0.04	0.04	0.00	0.00	C12-C13
0.05	0.04	0.11	0.14	0.13	0.31	0.50	0.31	0.96	0.76	0.10	0.06	0.06	0.00	0.01	C14
0.91	1.46	4.36	8.04	18.51	36.07	56.13	76.21	85.76	90.91	10.48	5.37	5.33	0.17	0.63	C15
5.13	9.15	14.40	20.11	32.11	48.97	67.90	88.05	106.60	106.08	16.26	9.13	8.93	0.44	1.03	C16
0.37	0.78	1.22	1.68	2.64	3.47	3.98	4.29	4.00	3.68	1.04	0.61	0.61	0.04	0.07	C17
3.95	7.09	11.17	15.50	22.75	32.69	42.63	53.11	57.95	53.62	10.70	6.20	6.04	0.33	0.71	C18
4.22	8.11	12.41	16.95	26.10	35.21	47.21	54.57	59.55	56.63	11.54	6.64	6.52	0.36	0.78	C19-C20
0.16	0.29	0.44	0.43	0.64	0.86	1.17	1.74	1.98	2.33	0.35	0.20	0.20	0.01	0.02	C21
5.39	8.87	15.02	18.39	31.56	44.37	60.83	72.82	82.92	89.97	14.60	8.27	8.17	0.43	0.95	C22
0.80	1.61	3.35	4.55	9.70	13.74	18.12	24.00	29.42	26.79	4.16	2.25	2.24	0.10	0.26	C23-C24
1.11	2.32	3.99	6.67	11.63	17.87	24.59	32.53	39.43	39.26	5.56	3.01	2.98	0.14	0.35	C25
0.29	0.42	0.42	0.55	0.59	0.81	0.97	1.08	1.33	1.03	0.35	0.24	0.23	0.01	0.02	C30-C31
0.10	0.22	0.28	0.44	0.78	0.84	1.52	2.03	2.25	2.06	0.35	0.20	0.20	0.01	0.02	C32
15.69	28.81	48.22	69.10	104.87	142.72	176.38	209.95	231.03	221.13	44.82	25.61	25.30	1.42	3.01	C33-C34
0.53	0.82	1.03	1.35	1.65	2.05	2.22	2.22	1.84	1.44	0.74	0.50	0.49	0.03	0.05	C37-C38
0.89	1.23	1.46	2.13	2.86	4.15	4.97	7.00	6.59	6.15	1.63	1.17	1.15	0.07	0.11	C40-C41
0.28	0.38	0.60	0.67	1.05	1.56	1.51	1.91	1.95	2.20	0.49	0.31	0.31	0.02	0.03	C43
0.83	1.20	1.99	2.82	4.29	6.27	9.94	15.02	23.47	34.69	2.76	1.49	1.48	0.07	0.15	C44
0.02	0.17	0.15	0.18	0.26	0.27	0.47	0.50	0.31	0.22	0.11	0.07	0.07	0.00	0.01	C45
0.02	0.01	0.03	0.01	0.02	0.01	0.00	0.05	0.07	0.18	0.01	0.01	0.01	0.00	0.00	C46
0.67	0.95	1.15	1.32	1.62	1.84	1.96	1.91	2.12	2.96	0.88	0.66	0.65	0.04	0.06	C47,C49
52.10	77.35	77.05	71.22	70.30	61.02	49.69	40.05	32.29	27.10	36.35	26.23	24.28	2.01	2.57	C50
0.23	0.38	0.56	0.68	1.04	1.15	1.94	2.05	2.12	1.88	0.47	0.29	0.28	0.02	0.03	C51
0.30	0.34	0.44	0.48	0.63	0.70	0.94	0.99	0.89	0.54	0.28	0.18	0.18	0.01	0.02	C52
24.50	34.05	41.17	39.65	36.26	32.28	32.30	29.80	22.86	15.53	19.01	13.48	12.48	1.02	1.34	C53
6.83	13.47	21.58	21.53	17.44	15.47	11.87	8.82	7.96	4.98	7.95	5.24	5.07	0.43	0.57	C54
2.54	3.90	4.52	4.09	4.25	4.08	4.37	4.46	5.26	3.50	2.22	1.52	1.42	0.11	0.15	C55
6.55	11.12	14.44	14.30	14.76	15.35	15.30	13.46	10.76	5.34	7.23	5.13	4.86	0.37	0.52	C56
0.54	0.89	1.01	1.15	1.19	1.36	1.30	0.97	0.89	0.49	0.55	0.38	0.36	0.03	0.04	C57
0.14	0.12	0.07	0.02	0.01	0.00	0.00	0.02	0.00	0.04	0.08	0.08	0.07	0.01	0.01	C58
—	—	—	—	—	—	—	—	—	—	—	—	—	—	—	C60
—	—	—	—	—	—	—	—	—	—	—	—	—	—	—	C61
—	—	—	—	—	—	—	—	—	—	—	—	—	—	—	C62
—	—	—	—	—	—	—	—	—	—	—	—	—	—	—	C63
1.52	2.21	3.60	4.32	5.21	6.67	7.22	7.64	7.17	5.38	2.34	1.50	1.50	0.10	0.17	C64
0.06	0.08	0.24	0.44	0.50	1.18	1.51	1.77	1.57	1.48	0.30	0.16	0.16	0.01	0.02	C65
0.04	0.12	0.17	0.27	0.79	1.60	1.94	2.59	2.73	1.44	0.37	0.20	0.20	0.01	0.02	C66
0.51	0.85	1.58	2.70	3.71	5.67	9.34	12.94	16.13	15.84	2.10	1.15	1.12	0.05	0.13	C67
0.02	0.03	0.07	0.10	0.33	0.39	0.47	0.42	0.31	0.40	0.10	0.06	0.06	0.00	0.01	C68
0.05	0.14	0.18	0.09	0.27	0.32	0.44	0.64	0.68	0.36	0.16	0.11	0.15	0.01	0.01	C69
5.82	8.50	12.38	14.72	18.56	21.89	24.93	26.43	26.03	25.53	8.78	6.00	5.90	0.39	0.62	C70-C72,D32-D33,D42-D43
37.10	40.21	43.26	42.17	29.46	21.22	13.76	10.11	7.00	5.43	22.44	19.11	16.63	1.40	1.57	C73
0.17	0.30	0.40	0.40	0.56	0.57	0.60	0.71	0.51	0.40	0.25	0.18	0.18	0.01	0.02	C74
0.53	0.63	0.83	0.71	0.86	0.84	0.83	0.83	0.92	0.36	0.46	0.36	0.33	0.02	0.03	C75
0.17	0.22	0.25	0.24	0.32	0.35	0.57	0.68	0.48	0.49	0.22	0.18	0.17	0.01	0.02	C81
1.65	2.59	4.13	5.30	7.76	9.89	11.54	12.42	11.96	8.48	3.37	2.21	2.15	0.13	0.24	C82-C86,C96
0.02	0.03	0.05	0.10	0.12	0.17	0.16	0.21	0.07	0.04	0.04	0.03	0.03	0.00	0.00	C88
0.38	0.71	1.34	2.17	3.75	4.81	5.20	5.54	4.37	2.42	1.26	0.74	0.74	0.04	0.09	C90
0.40	0.67	0.89	0.95	1.26	1.81	1.96	2.05	2.70	1.30	0.92	0.79	0.90	0.05	0.07	C91
1.68	2.53	3.09	3.42	4.97	5.91	7.33	8.30	7.45	6.06	2.59	1.92	1.88	0.12	0.19	C92-C94,D45-D47
0.87	1.12	1.66	1.84	2.82	4.18	5.26	6.88	5.88	5.52	1.76	1.35	1.40	0.08	0.13	C95
2.78	4.20	6.33	6.67	9.67	12.87	16.08	20.46	22.96	26.74	5.07	3.26	3.22	0.19	0.33	O & U
192.72	286.13	370.49	418.33	519.37	636.11	761.57	883.00	955.26	922.15	258.18	166.95	159.57	10.53	17.52	C00-C97,D32-D33, D42-D43,D45-D47
191.89	284.93	368.50	415.51	515.08	629.84	751.63	867.99	931.79	887.47	255.42	165.46	158.09	10.47	17.37	C00-C97,D32-D33, D42-D43, D45-D47 exc. C44

附表 1-10 2019 年全国肿瘤登记地区男女合计癌症死亡主要指标

部位	Site	死亡数 No. deaths	构成 Freq./%	年龄组								
				0~	1~4	5~9	10~14	15~19	20~24	25~29	30~34	35~39
唇	Lip	537	0.05	0.00	0.00	0.00	0.01	0.00	0.00	0.00	0.01	0.00
舌	Tongue	2 715	0.25	0.00	0.00	0.01	0.00	0.00	0.01	0.03	0.07	0.09
口	Mouth	3 761	0.35	0.00	0.01	0.00	0.01	0.01	0.01	0.02	0.02	0.08
唾液腺	Salivary gland	1 241	0.11	0.00	0.00	0.00	0.01	0.02	0.01	0.02	0.02	0.04
扁桃体	Tonsil	458	0.04	0.00	0.00	0.00	0.00	0.01	0.00	0.00	0.00	0.00
其他口咽	Other oropharynx	1 007	0.09	0.00	0.00	0.01	0.00	0.00	0.00	0.00	0.02	0.03
鼻咽	Nasopharynx	12 138	1.12	0.03	0.01	0.00	0.02	0.08	0.07	0.15	0.36	0.68
下咽	Hypopharynx	1 733	0.16	0.02	0.00	0.00	0.00	0.01	0.00	0.00	0.01	0.01
咽,部位不明	Pharynx unspecified	1 302	0.12	0.02	0.00	0.00	0.00	0.01	0.00	0.00	0.01	0.02
食管	Esophagus	84 828	7.80	0.10	0.02	0.00	0.00	0.07	0.02	0.06	0.09	0.16
胃	Stomach	119 847	11.02	0.13	0.06	0.02	0.02	0.13	0.21	0.53	1.05	1.67
小肠	Small intestine	4 605	0.42	0.03	0.00	0.00	0.00	0.00	0.01	0.03	0.05	0.10
结肠	Colon	42 809	3.94	0.00	0.01	0.00	0.01	0.09	0.12	0.29	0.58	0.79
直肠	Rectum	48 477	4.46	0.05	0.02	0.01	0.01	0.09	0.11	0.25	0.52	0.71
肛门	Anus	1 605	0.15	0.00	0.00	0.00	0.00	0.00	0.01	0.01	0.02	0.04
肝脏	Liver	149 617	13.76	0.89	0.16	0.07	0.11	0.35	0.39	1.22	2.92	5.55
胆囊及其他	Gallbladder etc.	19 651	1.81	0.03	0.00	0.00	0.00	0.01	0.00	0.02	0.08	0.17
胰腺	Pancreas	40 421	3.72	0.03	0.02	0.01	0.01	0.02	0.04	0.10	0.21	0.48
鼻、鼻窦及其他	Nose, sinuses etc.	1 413	0.13	0.00	0.01	0.01	0.01	0.02	0.01	0.03	0.04	0.04
喉	Larynx	6 789	0.62	0.03	0.01	0.01	0.00	0.01	0.01	0.01	0.03	0.06
气管、支气管、肺	Trachea, bronchus & lung	303 211	27.88	0.88	0.05	0.03	0.04	0.41	0.25	0.59	1.35	2.58
其他胸腔器官	Other thoracic organs	3 191	0.29	0.06	0.00	0.03	0.05	0.06	0.07	0.08	0.10	0.11
骨	Bone	7 859	0.72	0.05	0.05	0.07	0.28	0.41	0.33	0.23	0.25	0.22
皮肤黑色素瘤	Melanoma of skin	1 792	0.16	0.00	0.00	0.01	0.01	0.01	0.01	0.01	0.05	0.06
皮肤其他	Other skin	5 309	0.49	0.03	0.01	0.02	0.01	0.03	0.04	0.03	0.07	0.07
间皮瘤	Mesothelioma	643	0.06	0.00	0.00	0.00	0.00	0.00	0.00	0.02	0.01	0.01
卡波西肉瘤	Kaposi sarcoma	141	0.01	0.02	0.00	0.01	0.00	0.01	0.01	0.01	0.01	0.02
结缔组织、软组织	Connective & soft tissue	2 198	0.20	0.08	0.13	0.08	0.07	0.09	0.07	0.09	0.13	0.13
乳腺	Breast	28 607	2.70	0.10	0.03	0.01	0.01	0.06	0.10	0.57	1.73	3.50
外阴	Vulva	600	0.06	0.00	0.00	0.00	0.00	0.00	0.00	0.00	0.03	0.04
阴道	Vagina	365	0.03	0.00	0.00	0.00	0.00	0.00	0.00	0.01	0.01	0.02
子宫颈	Cervix uteri	17 198	1.58	0.10	0.01	0.00	0.00	0.04	0.13	0.33	0.98	1.82
子宫体	Corpus uteri	5 873	0.54	0.03	0.01	0.00	0.00	0.02	0.03	0.07	0.19	0.30
子宫,部位不明	Uterus unspecified	2 512	0.23	0.10	0.00	0.00	0.00	0.02	0.02	0.05	0.09	0.16
卵巢	Ovary	11 043	1.02	0.03	0.01	0.01	0.06	0.11	0.21	0.30	0.32	0.64
其他女性生殖器官	Other female genital organs	605	0.06	0.00	0.00	0.00	0.00	0.01	0.01	0.02	0.01	0.03
胎盘	Placenta	28	0.00	0.00	0.00	0.00	0.00	0.01	0.00	0.01	0.03	0.01
阴茎	Penis	878	0.08	0.00	0.00	0.00	0.00	0.00	0.00	0.03	0.03	0.04
前列腺	Prostate	17 004	1.56	0.00	0.02	0.00	0.00	0.00	0.01	0.03	0.02	0.03
睾丸	Testis	351	0.03	0.00	0.01	0.01	0.01	0.05	0.07	0.08	0.10	0.06
其他男性生殖器官	Other male genital organs	196	0.02	0.00	0.00	0.00	0.01	0.01	0.02	0.00	0.02	0.01
肾	Kidney	8 583	0.79	0.10	0.10	0.04	0.03	0.06	0.04	0.10	0.10	0.14
肾盂	Renal pelvis	1 416	0.13	0.00	0.00	0.00	0.00	0.01	0.01	0.00	0.02	0.02
输尿管	Ureter	1 615	0.15	0.00	0.00	0.00	0.00	0.00	0.00	0.00	0.01	0.00
膀胱	Bladder	15 781	1.45	0.02	0.01	0.00	0.00	0.02	0.01	0.01	0.04	0.09
其他泌尿器官	Other urinary organs	358	0.03	0.02	0.00	0.00	0.00	0.00	0.00	0.00	0.00	0.01
眼	Eye	427	0.04	0.08	0.13	0.03	0.01	0.00	0.01	0.00	0.01	0.02
脑、神经系统	Brain, nervous system	27 014	2.48	1.10	0.96	0.98	0.85	0.72	0.65	0.88	1.04	1.45
甲状腺	Thyroid	4 193	0.39	0.00	0.01	0.00	0.01	0.00	0.04	0.08	0.13	0.16
肾上腺	Adrenal gland	1 058	0.10	0.03	0.07	0.07	0.00	0.02	0.02	0.02	0.02	0.04
其他内分泌腺	Other endocrine	703	0.06	0.02	0.02	0.02	0.03	0.04	0.02	0.02	0.03	0.03
霍奇金淋巴瘤	Hodgkin lymphoma	943	0.09	0.00	0.01	0.02	0.01	0.00	0.02	0.02	0.05	0.03
非霍奇金淋巴瘤	Non-Hodgkin lymphoma	15 262	1.40	0.19	0.11	0.12	0.16	0.24	0.28	0.27	0.35	0.54
免疫增生性疾病	Immunoproliferative diseases	132	0.01	0.00	0.00	0.00	0.00	0.00	0.00	0.00	0.00	0.00
多发性骨髓瘤	Multiple myeloma	6 311	0.58	0.00	0.02	0.00	0.04	0.06	0.05	0.04	0.03	0.08
淋巴细胞白血病	Lymphoid leukemia	4 409	0.41	0.40	0.33	0.33	0.35	0.42	0.32	0.28	0.35	0.31
髓系白血病	Myeloid leukemia	10 090	0.93	0.30	0.28	0.14	0.23	0.33	0.32	0.39	0.40	0.59
白血病,未特指	Leukemia unspecified	9 435	0.87	0.86	0.50	0.39	0.49	0.59	0.49	0.45	0.48	0.52
其他或未指明部位	Other and unspecified	24 504	2.25	0.35	0.38	0.21	0.28	0.36	0.28	0.40	0.43	0.66
所有部位合计	All sites	1 087 549	100.00	6.11	3.59	2.80	3.21	5.03	4.66	7.53	13.33	21.91
所有部位除外 C44	All sites except C44	1 082 240	99.51	6.08	3.58	2.78	3.20	5.00	4.63	7.50	13.26	21.84

Appendix Table 1-10　Cancer mortality in　registration areas of China,both sexes in 2019

Age group										粗率 Crude rate/ 100 000⁻¹	中标率 ASR China/ 100 000⁻¹	世标率 ASR world/ 100 000⁻¹	累积率 Cum. Rate/%		ICD-10
40~44	45~49	50~54	55~59	60~64	65~69	70~74	75~79	80~84	85+				0~64	0~74	
0.02	0.03	0.05	0.08	0.13	0.20	0.34	0.58	0.69	1.54	0.09	0.05	0.05	0.00	0.00	C00
0.20	0.29	0.48	0.66	1.06	1.30	1.58	2.13	2.35	2.50	0.43	0.26	0.25	0.01	0.03	C01-C02
0.13	0.26	0.49	0.82	1.20	1.62	2.78	3.52	4.35	5.88	0.60	0.33	0.33	0.02	0.04	C03-C06
0.06	0.13	0.19	0.27	0.43	0.62	0.69	0.77	1.33	1.98	0.20	0.11	0.11	0.01	0.01	C07-C08
0.02	0.05	0.10	0.17	0.18	0.18	0.27	0.36	0.35	0.43	0.07	0.04	0.04	0.00	0.00	C09
0.04	0.08	0.15	0.26	0.36	0.61	0.67	0.80	0.80	0.93	0.16	0.09	0.09	0.00	0.01	C10
1.20	1.98	2.93	3.68	4.68	5.39	6.29	6.61	7.10	5.98	1.93	1.21	1.18	0.08	0.14	C11
0.04	0.15	0.33	0.61	0.85	0.97	1.16	1.06	1.09	0.95	0.28	0.16	0.16	0.01	0.02	C12-C13
0.03	0.08	0.14	0.30	0.47	0.51	1.03	1.38	1.69	1.55	0.21	0.11	0.11	0.01	0.01	C14
0.76	2.53	7.29	13.00	27.48	46.17	70.29	97.82	116.94	121.82	13.50	7.18	7.18	0.26	0.84	C15
2.92	5.97	11.12	18.32	36.66	59.80	92.46	132.77	168.34	179.39	19.07	10.36	10.24	0.39	1.15	C16
0.16	0.32	0.59	0.84	1.52	2.38	3.21	4.38	5.81	5.98	0.73	0.41	0.40	0.02	0.05	C17
1.35	2.31	4.01	6.60	11.69	17.94	27.55	43.00	69.01	92.97	6.81	3.63	3.61	0.14	0.37	C18
1.47	2.95	5.31	7.63	13.85	21.94	33.42	49.11	72.27	89.06	7.71	4.16	4.13	0.16	0.44	C19-C20
0.05	0.13	0.19	0.22	0.50	0.77	1.07	1.46	2.45	2.68	0.26	0.14	0.14	0.01	0.01	C21
11.99	19.74	30.28	37.67	53.92	69.27	85.94	107.02	123.44	134.87	23.81	14.20	13.96	0.82	1.60	C22
0.45	0.86	1.87	3.11	6.29	9.62	14.84	20.40	28.26	33.78	3.13	1.67	1.67	0.06	0.19	C23-C24
0.95	2.41	4.45	7.42	13.81	20.71	29.50	40.81	52.23	56.90	6.43	3.50	3.50	0.15	0.40	C25
0.10	0.12	0.25	0.29	0.53	0.63	0.80	1.11	1.30	1.83	0.22	0.13	0.13	0.01	0.01	C30-C31
0.14	0.32	0.73	1.45	2.38	3.52	5.19	7.03	8.15	8.66	1.08	0.59	0.59	0.03	0.07	C32
6.15	14.51	31.68	54.71	103.75	163.79	231.80	318.86	386.55	396.36	48.25	26.23	26.19	1.08	3.06	C33-C34
0.18	0.33	0.54	0.78	1.13	1.47	1.83	2.46	2.81	2.96	0.51	0.31	0.31	0.02	0.03	C37-C38
0.33	0.58	1.03	1.36	2.27	3.49	5.74	6.76	8.11	9.18	1.25	0.79	0.77	0.04	0.08	C40-C41
0.11	0.18	0.22	0.33	0.47	0.84	1.03	1.59	2.29	3.05	0.29	0.16	0.16	0.01	0.02	C43
0.15	0.25	0.38	0.56	0.89	1.42	2.53	5.00	9.50	22.95	0.84	0.41	0.43	0.01	0.03	C44
0.02	0.04	0.11	0.21	0.27	0.36	0.35	0.51	0.44	0.66	0.10	0.06	0.06	0.00	0.01	C45
0.01	0.02	0.02	0.03	0.05	0.05	0.05	0.08	0.11	0.13	0.02	0.02	0.02	0.00	0.00	C46
0.17	0.23	0.28	0.36	0.65	0.88	1.12	1.56	2.10	2.89	0.35	0.23	0.23	0.01	0.02	C47,C49
6.31	10.45	15.37	17.15	20.04	21.98	21.52	27.15	34.39	48.63	9.24	5.57	5.42	0.38	0.59	C50
0.06	0.06	0.20	0.21	0.29	0.46	0.82	1.05	1.77	1.61	0.19	0.10	0.10	0.00	0.01	C51
0.03	0.10	0.12	0.17	0.22	0.27	0.43	0.69	0.88	0.58	0.12	0.07	0.06	0.00	0.01	C52
3.62	6.80	9.43	10.78	11.11	12.67	16.04	19.76	19.66	18.14	5.55	3.39	3.27	0.23	0.37	C53
0.83	1.43	2.64	3.79	4.48	5.70	6.29	7.07	7.64	7.77	1.90	1.09	1.08	0.07	0.13	C54
0.38	0.64	1.17	1.17	1.61	2.13	2.90	3.57	4.41	4.09	0.81	0.47	0.46	0.03	0.05	C55
1.55	3.57	5.62	6.53	8.60	10.18	12.13	12.37	13.07	9.70	3.57	2.12	2.09	0.14	0.25	C56
0.08	0.09	0.28	0.36	0.44	0.53	0.71	0.81	0.91	1.11	0.20	0.11	0.11	0.01	0.01	C57
0.01	0.01	0.01	0.01	0.01	0.01	0.01	0.00	0.02	0.02	0.01	0.01	0.01	0.00	0.00	C58
0.08	0.16	0.24	0.27	0.51	0.75	1.06	1.51	2.76	4.47	0.28	0.16	0.16	0.01	0.02	C60
0.06	0.21	0.53	1.38	4.25	9.52	22.12	48.76	92.71	162.60	5.33	2.72	2.77	0.03	0.19	C61
0.06	0.10	0.08	0.10	0.14	0.20	0.25	0.43	0.83	1.29	0.11	0.08	0.08	0.00	0.01	C62
0.01	0.03	0.04	0.04	0.09	0.12	0.27	0.52	0.71	0.82	0.06	0.04	0.04	0.00	0.00	C63
0.28	0.57	0.96	1.82	2.63	4.03	5.64	7.88	11.60	13.28	1.37	0.76	0.76	0.03	0.08	C64
0.01	0.06	0.12	0.18	0.41	0.64	0.98	1.46	2.17	3.41	0.23	0.12	0.12	0.00	0.01	C65
0.01	0.04	0.08	0.17	0.40	0.73	1.38	1.82	2.87	3.60	0.26	0.13	0.13	0.00	0.01	C66
0.15	0.35	0.74	1.27	2.75	5.35	9.97	19.09	33.36	53.39	2.51	1.21	1.22	0.03	0.10	C67
0.01	0.01	0.03	0.06	0.09	0.12	0.16	0.36	0.63	1.25	0.06	0.03	0.03	0.00	0.00	C68
0.02	0.03	0.03	0.06	0.08	0.13	0.27	0.37	0.51	0.89	0.07	0.04	0.05	0.00	0.00	C69
1.99	3.16	4.49	5.96	8.52	11.53	15.19	18.36	22.34	24.22	4.30	2.81	2.81	0.16	0.29	C70-C72,D32-D33,D42-D43
0.27	0.41	0.59	0.94	1.35	1.88	2.59	3.40	4.67	5.22	0.67	0.39	0.38	0.02	0.04	C73
0.05	0.08	0.14	0.22	0.37	0.47	0.59	0.85	1.12	1.16	0.17	0.10	0.11	0.01	0.01	C74
0.05	0.06	0.09	0.13	0.23	0.30	0.44	0.43	0.64	0.92	0.11	0.07	0.07	0.00	0.01	C75
0.05	0.07	0.16	0.16	0.32	0.41	0.59	0.75	0.91	1.27	0.15	0.09	0.09	0.00	0.01	C81
0.73	1.17	1.90	2.83	4.90	7.29	10.20	14.67	17.83	16.02	2.43	1.45	1.42	0.07	0.16	C82-C86,C96
0.00	0.01	0.01	0.02	0.05	0.08	0.09	0.17	0.19	0.20	0.02	0.01	0.01	0.00	0.00	C88
0.12	0.35	0.78	1.27	2.29	3.55	5.08	6.08	7.03	5.57	1.00	0.57	0.57	0.03	0.07	C90
0.31	0.42	0.57	0.78	1.05	1.64	2.12	2.87	3.62	4.09	0.70	0.53	0.53	0.03	0.05	C91
0.67	0.93	1.29	1.89	3.12	4.32	6.29	8.17	10.25	9.90	1.61	1.03	1.01	0.05	0.11	C92-C94,D45-D47
0.62	0.83	1.31	1.58	2.44	3.86	5.64	7.47	8.53	8.24	1.50	1.04	1.04	0.05	0.10	C95
1.11	1.81	3.27	4.61	7.15	11.07	15.58	21.72	29.33	39.31	3.90	2.25	2.26	0.10	0.24	O & U
42.12	78.97	139.55	206.73	351.64	526.80	749.50	1 037.78	1 327.42	1 503.21	173.06	97.19	96.51	4.41	10.79	C00-C97,D32-D33, D42-D43,D45-D47
41.97	78.71	139.17	206.17	350.76	525.38	746.97	1 032.78	1 317.92	1 480.26	172.21	96.78	96.08	4.40	10.76	C00-C97,D32-D33, D42-D43, D45-D47 exc. C44

附表 1-11　2019 年全国肿瘤登记地区男性癌症死亡主要指标

部位	Site	死亡数 No. deaths	构成 Freq./%	0~	1~4	5~9	10~14	15~19	20~24	25~29	30~34	35~39
唇	Lip	360	0.05	0.00	0.00	0.00	0.01	0.01	0.00	0.00	0.01	0.00
舌	Tongue	1 940	0.28	0.00	0.01	0.02	0.00	0.00	0.01	0.03	0.10	0.12
口	Mouth	2 601	0.37	0.00	0.01	0.01	0.02	0.01	0.02	0.03	0.04	0.13
唾液腺	Salivary gland	814	0.12	0.00	0.00	0.00	0.00	0.04	0.01	0.03	0.02	0.03
扁桃体	Tonsil	376	0.05	0.00	0.00	0.01	0.00	0.01	0.01	0.00	0.01	0.01
其他口咽	Other oropharynx	875	0.13	0.00	0.00	0.01	0.01	0.00	0.00	0.01	0.02	0.06
鼻咽	Nasopharynx	9 055	1.30	0.06	0.01	0.00	0.03	0.09	0.10	0.18	0.47	1.11
下咽	Hypopharynx	1 627	0.23	0.03	0.01	0.00	0.00	0.01	0.01	0.00	0.01	0.02
咽,部位不明	Pharynx unspecified	1 003	0.14	0.03	0.00	0.01	0.00	0.00	0.00	0.01	0.02	0.02
食管	Esophagus	63 651	9.11	0.18	0.04	0.00	0.00	0.11	0.03	0.10	0.15	0.26
胃	Stomach	83 246	11.92	0.12	0.07	0.01	0.02	0.18	0.20	0.53	0.95	1.63
小肠	Small intestine	2 759	0.39	0.00	0.00	0.00	0.00	0.00	0.00	0.03	0.06	0.12
结肠	Colon	24 232	3.47	0.00	0.02	0.00	0.01	0.12	0.14	0.30	0.71	0.86
直肠	Rectum	30 126	4.31	0.03	0.03	0.01	0.01	0.12	0.14	0.30	0.58	0.76
肛门	Anus	932	0.13	0.00	0.00	0.00	0.00	0.01	0.00	0.01	0.02	0.05
肝脏	Liver	110 868	15.87	1.07	0.18	0.11	0.16	0.45	0.55	1.90	4.92	9.46
胆囊及其他	Gallbladder etc.	9 384	1.34	0.03	0.00	0.00	0.00	0.02	0.00	0.02	0.09	0.17
胰腺	Pancreas	23 184	3.32	0.06	0.01	0.01	0.01	0.03	0.05	0.10	0.26	0.62
鼻、鼻窦及其他	Nose, sinuses etc.	928	0.13	0.00	0.01	0.00	0.01	0.02	0.02	0.04	0.04	0.07
喉	Larynx	6 023	0.86	0.03	0.01	0.01	0.00	0.01	0.02	0.01	0.05	0.10
气管、支气管、肺	Trachea, bronchus & lung	212 974	30.49	1.16	0.05	0.03	0.05	0.58	0.32	0.63	1.74	2.97
其他胸腔器官	Other thoracic organs	2 064	0.30	0.03	0.03	0.04	0.06	0.09	0.10	0.13	0.11	0.13
骨	Bone	4 777	0.68	0.09	0.07	0.07	0.28	0.50	0.44	0.30	0.31	0.29
皮肤黑色素瘤	Melanoma of skin	944	0.14	0.00	0.01	0.00	0.01	0.01	0.01	0.01	0.04	0.03
皮肤其他	Other skin	2 924	0.42	0.03	0.01	0.02	0.01	0.04	0.03	0.04	0.09	0.08
间皮瘤	Mesothelioma	376	0.05	0.00	0.01	0.00	0.00	0.00	0.01	0.01	0.01	0.02
卡波西肉瘤	Kaposi sarcoma	84	0.01	0.00	0.00	0.01	0.01	0.01	0.02	0.01	0.00	0.03
结缔组织、软组织	Connective & soft tissue	1 299	0.19	0.03	0.14	0.10	0.09	0.07	0.07	0.10	0.15	0.15
乳腺	Breast	757	0.11	0.00	0.00	0.00	0.00	0.00	0.01	0.00	0.02	0.04
外阴	Vulva	—	—	—	—	—	—	—	—	—	—	—
阴道	Vagina	—	—	—	—	—	—	—	—	—	—	—
子宫颈	Cervix uteri	—	—	—	—	—	—	—	—	—	—	—
子宫体	Corpus uteri	—	—	—	—	—	—	—	—	—	—	—
子宫,部位不明	Uterus unspecified	—	—	—	—	—	—	—	—	—	—	—
卵巢	Ovary	—	—	—	—	—	—	—	—	—	—	—
其他女性生殖器官	Other female genital organs	—	—	—	—	—	—	—	—	—	—	—
胎盘	Placenta	—	—	—	—	—	—	—	—	—	—	—
阴茎	Penis	878	0.13	0.00	0.00	0.01	0.00	0.00	0.00	0.03	0.03	0.04
前列腺	Prostate	17 004	2.43	0.00	0.02	0.00	0.01	0.04	0.01	0.03	0.02	0.03
睾丸	Testis	351	0.05	0.00	0.01	0.00	0.01	0.05	0.07	0.08	0.10	0.06
其他男性生殖器官	Other male genital organs	196	0.03	0.00	0.00	0.00	0.01	0.01	0.02	0.00	0.02	0.01
肾	Kidney	5 676	0.81	0.06	0.09	0.04	0.02	0.08	0.04	0.11	0.12	0.18
肾盂	Renal pelvis	840	0.12	0.00	0.00	0.00	0.00	0.01	0.00	0.00	0.03	0.03
输尿管	Ureter	867	0.12	0.00	0.00	0.00	0.00	0.01	0.00	0.01	0.01	0.00
膀胱	Bladder	12 424	1.78	0.00	0.01	0.00	0.01	0.03	0.03	0.02	0.08	0.11
其他泌尿器官	Other urinary organs	210	0.03	0.03	0.00	0.01	0.00	0.01	0.00	0.00	0.00	0.01
眼	Eye	238	0.03	0.03	0.15	0.02	0.02	0.01	0.01	0.00	0.00	0.02
脑、神经系统	Brain, nervous system	14 845	2.13	1.13	0.93	1.08	0.94	0.77	0.71	1.05	1.20	1.73
甲状腺	Thyroid	1 579	0.23	0.00	0.01	0.00	0.01	0.01	0.03	0.03	0.10	0.11
肾上腺	Adrenal gland	629	0.09	0.03	0.07	0.07	0.00	0.02	0.01	0.02	0.02	0.04
其他内分泌腺	Other endocrine	414	0.06	0.03	0.03	0.02	0.02	0.06	0.04	0.02	0.03	0.03
霍奇金淋巴瘤	Hodgkin lymphoma	607	0.09	0.00	0.01	0.03	0.01	0.01	0.02	0.03	0.07	0.05
非霍奇金淋巴瘤	Non-Hodgkin lymphoma	9 359	1.34	0.24	0.13	0.16	0.20	0.28	0.36	0.31	0.47	0.64
免疫增生性疾病	Immunoproliferative diseases	96	0.01	0.00	0.00	0.00	0.00	0.00	0.00	0.00	0.00	0.00
多发性骨髓瘤	Multiple myeloma	3 673	0.53	0.00	0.02	0.02	0.04	0.04	0.06	0.05	0.03	0.10
淋巴细胞白血病	Lymphoid leukemia	2 580	0.37	0.30	0.34	0.35	0.35	0.51	0.42	0.34	0.47	0.34
髓系白血病	Myeloid leukemia	5 996	0.86	0.24	0.31	0.16	0.24	0.38	0.34	0.51	0.43	0.67
白血病,未特指	Leukemia unspecified	5 460	0.78	0.79	0.56	0.41	0.48	0.70	0.59	0.52	0.57	0.65
其他或未指明部位	Other and unspecified	14 387	2.06	0.52	0.38	0.22	0.32	0.40	0.29	0.44	0.49	0.75
所有部位合计	All sites	698 492	100.00	6.39	3.77	3.08	3.44	5.92	5.33	8.44	15.30	24.93
所有部位除外 C44	All sites except C44	695 568	99.58	6.36	3.77	3.06	3.44	5.87	5.30	8.40	15.21	24.86

Appendix Table 1-11　Cancer mortality in registration areas of China, male in 2019

Age group										粗率 Crude rate/ 100 000⁻¹	中标率 ASR China/ 100 000⁻¹	世标率 ASR world/ 100 000⁻¹	累积率 Cum. Rate/%		ICD-10
40~44	45~49	50~54	55~59	60~64	65~69	70~74	75~79	80~84	85+				0~64	0~74	
0.03	0.05	0.08	0.10	0.19	0.29	0.53	0.89	0.92	1.93	0.11	0.07	0.07	0.00	0.01	C00
0.30	0.43	0.78	1.08	1.71	1.95	2.25	2.98	2.60	2.97	0.61	0.38	0.37	0.02	0.04	C01-C02
0.20	0.41	0.78	1.34	1.88	2.33	3.84	5.02	5.25	7.79	0.82	0.48	0.48	0.02	0.06	C03-C06
0.06	0.19	0.24	0.41	0.63	0.87	0.88	1.06	1.84	2.61	0.26	0.15	0.15	0.01	0.02	C07-C08
0.03	0.08	0.17	0.30	0.34	0.27	0.46	0.55	0.48	0.57	0.12	0.07	0.07	0.00	0.01	C09
0.06	0.15	0.28	0.48	0.65	1.12	1.12	1.45	1.50	1.64	0.27	0.17	0.16	0.01	0.02	C10
1.91	3.02	4.51	5.65	7.00	8.18	9.72	9.93	10.41	8.40	2.84	1.84	1.79	0.12	0.21	C11
0.07	0.28	0.62	1.17	1.63	1.86	2.22	2.02	2.14	2.04	0.51	0.30	0.31	0.02	0.04	C12-C13
0.04	0.13	0.23	0.53	0.80	0.85	1.63	2.10	2.49	2.50	0.31	0.18	0.18	0.01	0.02	C14
1.28	4.34	12.83	23.17	46.69	75.54	108.45	144.96	168.69	170.25	19.96	11.37	11.40	0.45	1.36	C15
3.15	7.38	15.28	26.36	55.66	90.72	139.35	196.92	242.12	254.37	26.11	14.98	14.88	0.56	1.71	C16
0.20	0.38	0.78	1.13	1.91	2.91	3.84	5.36	7.05	8.51	0.87	0.51	0.50	0.02	0.06	C17
1.45	2.55	4.58	7.97	14.76	21.94	33.51	50.57	80.68	114.62	7.60	4.34	4.33	0.17	0.44	C18
1.63	3.52	6.71	10.09	18.73	29.72	44.61	64.90	91.86	116.94	9.45	5.42	5.40	0.21	0.58	C19-C20
0.05	0.15	0.25	0.27	0.61	1.00	1.29	1.77	2.76	3.29	0.29	0.17	0.17	0.01	0.02	C21
20.33	33.44	49.95	61.77	84.02	104.34	121.07	147.69	164.43	179.79	34.77	21.88	21.47	1.34	2.46	C22
0.51	0.84	1.91	3.33	6.39	9.77	15.17	19.97	27.00	33.36	2.94	1.68	1.68	0.07	0.19	C23-C24
1.24	3.20	5.84	9.66	17.24	25.08	34.13	46.15	57.67	66.82	7.27	4.22	4.22	0.19	0.49	C25
0.11	0.18	0.33	0.40	0.71	0.89	1.14	1.56	1.68	2.40	0.29	0.18	0.18	0.01	0.02	C30-C31
0.25	0.57	1.34	2.77	4.42	6.57	9.57	12.68	15.11	16.62	1.89	1.09	1.09	0.05	0.13	C32
7.59	18.70	44.57	80.35	156.92	248.70	346.71	468.13	550.90	570.12	66.80	38.39	38.43	1.57	4.55	C33-C34
0.21	0.42	0.70	1.09	1.55	2.00	2.42	3.32	3.50	3.97	0.65	0.42	0.41	0.02	0.05	C37-C38
0.40	0.74	1.35	1.66	2.93	4.37	7.21	8.49	9.95	11.80	1.50	0.99	0.97	0.05	0.10	C40-C41
0.09	0.20	0.24	0.27	0.54	0.96	1.16	1.80	2.70	3.86	0.30	0.18	0.17	0.01	0.02	C43
0.15	0.32	0.50	0.66	1.20	1.95	3.39	6.01	11.54	23.95	0.92	0.50	0.52	0.02	0.04	C44
0.02	0.04	0.12	0.25	0.34	0.45	0.37	0.49	0.67	0.97	0.12	0.07	0.07	0.00	0.01	C45
0.01	0.03	0.02	0.04	0.05	0.06	0.07	0.13	0.14	0.14	0.03	0.02	0.02	0.00	0.00	C46
0.15	0.30	0.32	0.47	0.79	1.16	1.31	1.95	2.60	3.86	0.41	0.28	0.28	0.01	0.03	C47, C49
0.06	0.19	0.20	0.40	0.46	0.72	1.02	1.15	1.82	2.75	0.24	0.14	0.14	0.01	0.02	C50
—	—	—	—	—	—	—	—	—	—	—	—	—	—	—	C51
—	—	—	—	—	—	—	—	—	—	—	—	—	—	—	C52
—	—	—	—	—	—	—	—	—	—	—	—	—	—	—	C53
—	—	—	—	—	—	—	—	—	—	—	—	—	—	—	C54
—	—	—	—	—	—	—	—	—	—	—	—	—	—	—	C55
—	—	—	—	—	—	—	—	—	—	—	—	—	—	—	C56
—	—	—	—	—	—	—	—	—	—	—	—	—	—	—	C57
—	—	—	—	—	—	—	—	—	—	—	—	—	—	—	C58
0.08	0.16	0.24	0.27	0.51	0.75	1.06	1.51	2.76	4.47	0.28	0.16	0.16	0.01	0.02	C60
0.06	0.21	0.53	1.38	4.25	9.52	22.12	48.76	92.71	162.60	5.33	2.72	2.77	0.03	0.19	C61
0.06	0.10	0.08	0.10	0.14	0.20	0.25	0.43	0.83	1.29	0.11	0.08	0.08	0.00	0.01	C62
0.01	0.03	0.04	0.04	0.09	0.12	0.27	0.52	0.71	0.82	0.06	0.04	0.04	0.00	0.00	C63
0.35	0.82	1.30	2.62	3.74	5.70	7.91	10.32	15.44	19.63	1.78	1.04	1.05	0.05	0.12	C64
0.01	0.07	0.20	0.27	0.56	0.79	1.18	1.67	2.72	3.86	0.26	0.15	0.15	0.01	0.02	C65
0.01	0.05	0.09	0.21	0.52	0.95	1.54	2.05	2.86	3.83	0.27	0.15	0.15	0.00	0.02	C66
0.19	0.50	1.12	2.11	4.66	8.79	16.23	31.59	59.03	100.10	3.90	2.05	2.09	0.04	0.17	C67
0.01	0.01	0.03	0.07	0.11	0.13	0.20	0.34	0.76	1.97	0.07	0.04	0.04	0.00	0.00	C68
0.03	0.04	0.04	0.09	0.10	0.16	0.33	0.49	0.39	0.93	0.07	0.05	0.06	0.00	0.00	C69
2.40	3.64	5.26	6.86	10.10	13.08	16.60	19.69	23.66	24.63	4.66	3.18	3.16	0.18	0.33	C70-C72,D32-D33,D42-D43
0.21	0.28	0.40	0.77	1.20	1.62	1.99	2.58	3.48	3.86	0.50	0.30	0.30	0.02	0.03	C73
0.08	0.11	0.15	0.30	0.47	0.60	0.70	0.97	1.50	1.57	0.20	0.12	0.13	0.01	0.01	C74
0.06	0.06	0.10	0.17	0.29	0.35	0.49	0.58	0.88	1.29	0.13	0.09	0.09	0.00	0.01	C75
0.05	0.08	0.22	0.24	0.45	0.56	0.71	0.90	1.29	1.89	0.19	0.12	0.12	0.01	0.01	C81
0.90	1.51	2.37	3.74	6.09	9.20	12.89	18.09	23.25	22.27	2.94	1.83	1.80	0.09	0.20	C82-C86, C96
0.00	0.01	0.01	0.02	0.07	0.09	0.13	0.27	0.32	0.39	0.03	0.02	0.02	0.00	0.00	C88
0.15	0.41	0.82	1.42	2.57	4.32	6.35	7.47	9.17	7.65	1.15	0.68	0.68	0.03	0.08	C90
0.30	0.42	0.57	0.80	1.27	2.02	2.74	3.75	4.61	5.43	0.81	0.62	0.62	0.03	0.06	C91
0.76	0.99	1.54	2.20	3.74	5.35	7.74	10.33	13.64	14.59	1.88	1.24	1.22	0.06	0.13	C92-C94, D45-D47
0.72	1.02	1.53	1.84	2.80	4.39	6.74	9.06	10.92	10.98	1.71	1.22	1.21	0.06	0.12	C95
1.28	2.20	3.96	5.80	8.96	14.14	19.29	26.70	35.36	46.30	4.51	2.75	2.75	0.13	0.29	O & U
49.34	94.94	176.15	274.47	483.42	729.41	1 025.90	1 408.01	1 776.80	2 059.20	219.09	129.10	128.62	5.75	14.52	C00-C97,D32-D33, D42-D43,D45-D47
49.18	94.62	175.65	273.81	482.22	727.47	1 022.52	1 402.00	1 765.26	2 035.25	218.17	128.59	128.11	5.73	14.48	C00-C97,D32-D33, D42-D43,D45-D47 exc. C44

附表 1-12　2019 年全国肿瘤登记地区女性癌症死亡主要指标

部位 Site		死亡数 No. deaths	构成 Freq./%	0~	1~4	5~9	10~14	15~19	20~24	25~29	30~34	35~39
唇	Lip	177	0.05	0.00	0.00	0.01	0.00	0.00	0.00	0.00	0.00	0.00
舌	Tongue	775	0.20	0.00	0.00	0.00	0.00	0.01	0.01	0.03	0.04	0.05
口	Mouth	1 160	0.30	0.00	0.01	0.00	0.01	0.01	0.01	0.00	0.00	0.04
唾液腺	Salivary gland	427	0.11	0.00	0.00	0.00	0.01	0.00	0.02	0.02	0.02	0.05
扁桃体	Tonsil	82	0.02	0.00	0.00	0.00	0.00	0.00	0.00	0.00	0.00	0.00
其他口咽	Other oropharynx	132	0.03	0.00	0.00	0.01	0.00	0.01	0.00	0.00	0.02	0.01
鼻咽	Nasopharynx	3 083	0.79	0.00	0.00	0.01	0.01	0.07	0.04	0.11	0.25	0.25
下咽	Hypopharynx	106	0.03	0.00	0.00	0.00	0.00	0.00	0.00	0.00	0.00	0.00
咽，部位不明	Pharynx unspecified	299	0.08	0.00	0.01	0.00	0.00	0.01	0.01	0.00	0.00	0.02
食管	Esophagus	21 177	5.44	0.00	0.00	0.00	0.01	0.03	0.02	0.02	0.03	0.05
胃	Stomach	36 601	9.41	0.13	0.05	0.02	0.03	0.07	0.22	0.53	1.15	1.70
小肠	Small intestine	1 846	0.47	0.07	0.00	0.00	0.00	0.01	0.02	0.04	0.09
结肠	Colon	18 577	4.77	0.00	0.00	0.00	0.02	0.06	0.10	0.28	0.44	0.71
直肠	Rectum	18 351	4.72	0.07	0.01	0.01	0.00	0.05	0.07	0.21	0.46	0.66
肛门	Anus	673	0.17	0.00	0.00	0.00	0.00	0.01	0.00	0.01	0.02	0.03
肝脏	Liver	38 749	9.96	0.70	0.15	0.03	0.06	0.23	0.21	0.51	0.91	1.58
胆囊及其他	Gallbladder etc.	10 267	2.64	0.03	0.00	0.00	0.00	0.01	0.01	0.03	0.07	0.18
胰腺	Pancreas	17 237	4.43	0.00	0.02	0.00	0.00	0.01	0.02	0.10	0.16	0.33
鼻、鼻窦及其他	Nose, sinuses etc.	485	0.12	0.00	0.01	0.01	0.01	0.03	0.01	0.02	0.04	0.02
喉	Larynx	766	0.20	0.03	0.01	0.00	0.00	0.01	0.00	0.01	0.01	0.01
气管、支气管、肺	Trachea, bronchus & lung	90 237	23.19	0.57	0.05	0.04	0.04	0.22	0.17	0.54	0.96	2.18
其他胸腔器官	Other thoracic organs	1 127	0.29	0.10	0.02	0.01	0.00	0.04	0.04	0.03	0.09	0.08
骨	Bone	3 082	0.79	0.00	0.03	0.08	0.29	0.31	0.22	0.16	0.19	0.15
皮肤黑色素瘤	Melanoma of skin	848	0.22	0.00	0.00	0.00	0.01	0.01	0.01	0.01	0.06	0.08
皮肤其他	Other skin	2 385	0.61	0.03	0.02	0.02	0.01	0.03	0.04	0.01	0.05	0.06
间皮瘤	Mesothelioma	267	0.07	0.00	0.00	0.00	0.00	0.00	0.01	0.03	0.01	0.01
卡波西肉瘤	Kaposi sarcoma	57	0.01	0.03	0.01	0.00	0.00	0.01	0.01	0.00	0.01	0.00
结缔组织、软组织	Connective & soft tissue	899	0.23	0.13	0.11	0.06	0.04	0.12	0.07	0.07	0.11	0.11
乳腺	Breast	28 607	7.35	0.10	0.03	0.01	0.01	0.06	0.10	0.57	1.73	3.50
外阴	Vulva	600	0.15	0.00	0.00	0.00	0.00	0.00	0.00	0.00	0.03	0.04
阴道	Vagina	365	0.09	0.00	0.00	0.00	0.00	0.00	0.00	0.01	0.01	0.02
子宫颈	Cervix uteri	17 198	4.42	0.10	0.01	0.00	0.00	0.04	0.13	0.33	0.98	1.82
子宫体	Corpus uteri	5 873	1.51	0.03	0.01	0.00	0.00	0.02	0.03	0.07	0.19	0.30
子宫，部位不明	Uterus unspecified	2 512	0.65	0.10	0.00	0.00	0.00	0.02	0.02	0.05	0.09	0.16
卵巢	Ovary	11 043	2.84	0.03	0.01	0.01	0.06	0.11	0.21	0.30	0.32	0.64
其他女性生殖器官	Other female genital organs	605	0.16	0.00	0.00	0.00	0.00	0.01	0.01	0.02	0.01	0.03
胎盘	Placenta	28	0.01	0.00	0.00	0.00	0.00	0.01	0.00	0.01	0.03	0.01
阴茎	Penis	—	—	—	—	—	—	—	—	—	—	—
前列腺	Prostate	—	—	—	—	—	—	—	—	—	—	—
睾丸	Testis	—	—	—	—	—	—	—	—	—	—	—
其他男性生殖器官	Other male genital organs	—	—	—	—	—	—	—	—	—	—	—
肾	Kidney	2 907	0.75	0.13	0.12	0.04	0.04	0.05	0.03	0.08	0.08	0.09
肾盂	Renal pelvis	576	0.15	0.00	0.00	0.01	0.00	0.00	0.01	0.00	0.00	0.00
输尿管	Ureter	748	0.19	0.00	0.00	0.00	0.01	0.00	0.00	0.00	0.00	0.00
膀胱	Bladder	3 357	0.86	0.03	0.01	0.01	0.00	0.00	0.00	0.00	0.01	0.06
其他泌尿器官	Other urinary organs	148	0.04	0.00	0.00	0.00	0.00	0.00	0.00	0.00	0.00	0.00
眼	Eye	189	0.05	0.13	0.10	0.03	0.00	0.00	0.01	0.00	0.02	0.02
脑、神经系统	Brain, nervous system	12 169	3.13	1.07	1.00	0.87	0.75	0.66	0.58	0.69	0.88	1.17
甲状腺	Thyroid	2 614	0.67	0.00	0.01	0.00	0.01	0.02	0.04	0.13	0.17	0.20
肾上腺	Adrenal gland	429	0.11	0.03	0.07	0.07	0.00	0.01	0.03	0.02	0.02	0.04
其他内分泌腺	Other endocrine	289	0.07	0.00	0.01	0.02	0.05	0.02	0.01	0.03	0.02	0.02
霍奇金淋巴瘤	Hodgkin lymphoma	336	0.09	0.00	0.01	0.00	0.01	0.03	0.02	0.01	0.02	0.02
非霍奇金淋巴瘤	Non-Hodgkin lymphoma	5 903	1.52	0.13	0.09	0.08	0.12	0.20	0.19	0.22	0.23	0.44
免疫增生性疾病	Immunoproliferative diseases	36	0.01	0.00	0.00	0.00	0.00	0.00	0.00	0.00	0.00	0.00
多发性骨髓瘤	Multiple myeloma	2 638	0.68	0.00	0.01	0.01	0.03	0.09	0.00	0.03	0.03	0.05
淋巴细胞白血病	Lymphoid leukemia	1 829	0.47	0.50	0.32	0.31	0.35	0.32	0.22	0.22	0.22	0.27
髓系白血病	Myeloid leukemia	4 094	1.05	0.37	0.24	0.12	0.21	0.28	0.29	0.27	0.36	0.50
白血病，未特指	Leukemia unspecified	3 975	1.02	0.94	0.45	0.38	0.50	0.47	0.38	0.37	0.38	0.39
其他或未指明部位	Other and unspecified	10 117	2.60	0.17	0.38	0.21	0.22	0.31	0.28	0.35	0.36	0.58
所有部位合计	All sites	389 057	100.00	5.81	3.39	2.48	2.94	4.04	3.94	6.58	11.34	18.85
所有部位除外 C44	All sites except C44	386 672	99.39	5.77	3.37	2.46	2.93	4.01	3.90	6.57	11.29	18.78

Appendix Table 1-12　Cancer mortality in registration areas of China, female in 2019

Age group										粗率 Crude rate/ 100 000⁻¹	中标率 ASR China/ 100 000⁻¹	世标率 ASR world/ 100 000⁻¹	累积率 Cum. Rate/%		ICD-10
40~44	45~49	50~54	55~59	60~64	65~69	70~74	75~79	80~84	85+				0~64	0~74	
0.01	0.01	0.02	0.05	0.07	0.12	0.16	0.31	0.50	1.28	0.06	0.03	0.03	0.00	0.00	C00
0.09	0.14	0.17	0.23	0.41	0.67	0.94	1.35	2.15	2.19	0.25	0.14	0.13	0.01	0.01	C01-C02
0.07	0.12	0.19	0.30	0.53	0.94	1.76	2.17	3.62	4.60	0.37	0.18	0.18	0.01	0.02	C03-C06
0.05	0.08	0.13	0.12	0.23	0.38	0.51	0.50	0.91	1.56	0.14	0.08	0.08	0.00	0.01	C07-C08
0.00	0.01	0.02	0.03	0.01	0.09	0.08	0.19	0.24	0.34	0.03	0.01	0.01	0.00	0.00	C09
0.01	0.00	0.02	0.04	0.07	0.12	0.23	0.21	0.24	0.46	0.04	0.02	0.02	0.00	0.00	C10
0.47	0.92	1.32	1.69	2.34	2.67	3.00	3.61	4.41	4.36	1.00	0.60	0.58	0.04	0.07	C11
0.00	0.01	0.03	0.05	0.06	0.11	0.14	0.19	0.24	0.22	0.03	0.02	0.02	0.00	0.00	C12-C13
0.03	0.02	0.04	0.06	0.14	0.19	0.46	0.73	1.05	0.91	0.10	0.05	0.05	0.00	0.00	C14
0.22	0.67	1.64	2.71	8.09	17.68	33.75	55.39	75.01	89.23	6.84	3.20	3.16	0.07	0.32	C15
2.68	4.52	6.87	10.19	17.48	29.80	47.56	75.03	108.54	128.93	11.82	6.04	5.92	0.23	0.61	C16
0.13	0.25	0.39	0.56	1.13	1.87	2.60	3.51	4.80	4.28	0.60	0.32	0.31	0.01	0.04	C17
1.25	2.07	3.43	5.22	8.58	14.07	21.86	36.18	59.55	78.40	6.00	2.97	2.94	0.11	0.29	C18
1.31	2.37	3.88	5.15	8.93	14.39	22.70	34.89	56.39	70.29	5.93	2.98	2.94	0.12	0.30	C19-C20
0.05	0.10	0.11	0.17	0.38	0.55	1.18	2.20	2.26		0.22	0.11	0.11	0.00	0.01	C21
3.43	5.72	10.24	13.31	23.54	35.25	52.30	70.42	90.22	104.63	12.52	6.65	6.58	0.30	0.74	C22
0.39	0.88	1.83	2.89	6.18	9.47	14.52	20.79	29.28	34.07	3.32	1.65	1.65	0.06	0.18	C23-C24
0.65	1.61	3.03	5.15	10.35	16.46	25.07	36.01	47.82	50.22	5.57	2.81	2.80	0.11	0.31	C25
0.08	0.07	0.17	0.18	0.34	0.37	0.47	0.70	0.99	1.44	0.16	0.09	0.09	0.00	0.01	C30-C31
0.03	0.06	0.11	0.13	0.33	0.56	1.01	1.94	2.50	3.30	0.25	0.12	0.12	0.00	0.01	C32
4.68	10.22	18.53	28.79	50.08	81.41	121.78	184.51	253.34	279.40	29.15	14.77	14.65	0.58	1.60	C33-C34
0.15	0.23	0.39	0.46	0.70	0.95	1.26	1.69	2.24	2.29	0.36	0.21	0.21	0.01	0.02	C37-C38
0.25	0.41	0.70	1.06	1.61	2.65	4.34	5.21	6.61	7.41	1.00	0.60	0.58	0.03	0.06	C40-C41
0.13	0.16	0.20	0.38	0.40	0.71	0.91	1.39	1.96	2.50	0.27	0.15	0.15	0.01	0.02	C43
0.14	0.19	0.26	0.45	0.57	0.91	1.71	4.09	7.84	22.28	0.77	0.33	0.35	0.01	0.02	C44
0.02	0.03	0.09	0.16	0.19	0.27	0.32	0.53	0.26	0.46	0.09	0.05	0.05	0.00	0.01	C45
0.01	0.01	0.01	0.02	0.05	0.04	0.03	0.04	0.09	0.12	0.02	0.01	0.01	0.00	0.00	C46
0.18	0.17	0.23	0.24	0.51	0.61	0.94	1.21	1.70	2.24	0.29	0.19	0.19	0.01	0.02	C47,C49
6.31	10.45	15.37	17.15	20.04	21.98	21.52	27.15	34.39	48.63	9.24	5.57	5.42	0.38	0.59	C50
0.06	0.06	0.20	0.21	0.29	0.46	0.82	1.05	1.77	1.61	0.19	0.10	0.10	0.00	0.01	C51
0.03	0.10	0.12	0.17	0.22	0.27	0.43	0.69	0.88	0.58	0.12	0.07	0.06	0.00	0.01	C52
3.62	6.80	9.43	10.78	11.11	12.67	16.04	19.76	19.66	18.14	5.55	3.39	3.27	0.23	0.37	C53
0.83	1.43	2.64	3.79	4.48	5.70	6.29	7.07	7.64	7.77	1.90	1.09	1.08	0.07	0.13	C54
0.38	0.64	1.17	1.17	1.61	2.13	2.90	3.57	4.41	4.09	0.81	0.47	0.46	0.03	0.05	C55
1.55	3.57	5.62	6.53	8.60	10.18	12.13	12.37	13.07	9.70	3.57	2.12	2.09	0.14	0.25	C56
0.08	0.09	0.28	0.36	0.44	0.53	0.71	0.81	0.91	1.11	0.20	0.11	0.11	0.01	0.01	C57
0.01	0.01	0.01	0.01	0.01	0.01	0.01	0.00	0.02	0.02	0.01	0.01	0.01	0.00	0.00	C58
—	—	—	—	—	—	—	—	—	—	—	—	—	—	—	C60
—	—	—	—	—	—	—	—	—	—	—	—	—	—	—	C61
—	—	—	—	—	—	—	—	—	—	—	—	—	—	—	C62
—	—	—	—	—	—	—	—	—	—	—	—	—	—	—	C63
0.20	0.32	0.61	1.01	1.51	2.41	3.47	5.68	8.50	9.00	0.94	0.49	0.49	0.02	0.05	C64
0.00	0.04	0.04	0.09	0.26	0.49	0.80	1.28	1.72	3.10	0.19	0.09	0.09	0.00	0.01	C65
0.01	0.04	0.06	0.14	0.28	0.52	1.22	1.62	2.88	3.44	0.24	0.11	0.11	0.00	0.01	C66
0.12	0.19	0.35	0.41	0.82	2.01	3.97	7.84	12.57	21.95	1.08	0.48	0.48	0.01	0.04	C67
0.01	0.00	0.02	0.04	0.07	0.11	0.12	0.37	0.52	0.77	0.05	0.02	0.02	0.00	0.00	C68
0.02	0.01	0.02	0.03	0.06	0.10	0.22	0.27	0.60	0.87	0.06	0.04	0.04	0.00	0.00	C69
1.57	2.66	3.71	5.04	6.92	10.03	13.84	17.16	21.27	23.94	3.93	2.45	2.45	0.13	0.25	C70-C72,D32-D33,D42-D43
0.33	0.54	0.80	1.10	1.50	2.13	3.16	4.13	5.64	6.14	0.84	0.48	0.46	0.02	0.05	C73
0.03	0.06	0.13	0.14	0.26	0.34	0.50	0.74	0.82	0.89	0.14	0.08	0.09	0.00	0.01	C74
0.04	0.06	0.08	0.09	0.17	0.24	0.40	0.31	0.45	0.67	0.14	0.06	0.06	0.00	0.01	C75
0.05	0.06	0.10	0.08	0.19	0.26	0.49	0.61	0.60	0.84	0.11	0.06	0.06	0.00	0.01	C81
0.56	0.82	1.42	1.91	3.71	5.44	7.63	11.60	13.44	11.81	1.91	1.08	1.06	0.05	0.12	C82-C86,C96
0.00	0.00	0.00	0.02	0.06	0.06	0.05	0.08	0.07	0.07	0.01	0.01	0.01	0.00	0.00	C88
0.09	0.28	0.74	1.12	2.01	2.80	3.87	4.83	5.30	4.16	0.85	0.46	0.46	0.02	0.06	C90
0.31	0.42	0.57	0.76	0.82	1.26	1.53	2.07	2.82	2.29	0.59	0.44	0.45	0.03	0.04	C91
0.58	0.86	1.04	1.59	2.50	3.32	4.90	6.23	7.51	6.74	1.32	0.83	0.82	0.04	0.09	C92-C94,D45-D47
0.52	0.64	1.08	1.32	2.08	3.35	4.58	6.04	6.59	6.40	1.28	0.87	0.87	0.05	0.08	C95
0.93	1.40	2.57	3.40	5.31	8.09	12.03	17.24	24.44	34.60	3.27	1.78	1.78	0.08	0.18	O & U
34.72	62.61	102.25	138.25	218.63	330.21	484.86	704.55	963.20	1 128.99	125.66	67.13	66.33	3.05	7.13	C00-C97,D32-D33,D42-D43,D45-D47
34.58	62.42	101.99	137.80	218.06	329.30	483.15	700.45	955.36	1 106.71	124.89	66.80	65.98	3.04	7.11	C00-C97,D32-D33,D42-D43,D45-D47 exc. C44

附表 1-13　2019 年全国城市肿瘤登记地区男女合计癌症死亡主要指标

部位 Site		死亡数 No. deaths	构成 Freq. /%	年龄组								
				0~	1~4	5~9	10~14	15~19	20~24	25~29	30~34	35~39
唇	Lip	186	0.04	0.00	0.00	0.00	0.01	0.01	0.00	0.01	0.00	0.00
舌	Tongue	1 340	0.28	0.00	0.01	0.01	0.00	0.01	0.01	0.02	0.09	0.09
口	Mouth	1 755	0.37	0.00	0.01	0.00	0.02	0.00	0.01	0.01	0.02	0.09
唾液腺	Salivary gland	592	0.12	0.00	0.00	0.00	0.01	0.02	0.00	0.02	0.03	0.05
扁桃体	Tonsil	219	0.05	0.00	0.00	0.01	0.00	0.01	0.00	0.01	0.01	0.00
其他口咽	Other oropharynx	476	0.10	0.00	0.00	0.00	0.01	0.00	0.00	0.01	0.02	0.03
鼻咽	Nasopharynx	5 048	1.06	0.00	0.00	0.01	0.02	0.10	0.07	0.14	0.30	0.57
下咽	Hypopharynx	910	0.19	0.00	0.00	0.00	0.00	0.01	0.00	0.01	0.01	0.02
咽,部位不明	Pharynx unspecified	550	0.12	0.00	0.00	0.00	0.00	0.02	0.00	0.00	0.00	0.01
食管	Esophagus	30 006	6.29	0.00	0.01	0.00	0.00	0.10	0.01	0.06	0.06	0.14
胃	Stomach	48 089	10.07	0.00	0.01	0.01	0.02	0.20	0.19	0.49	0.93	1.62
小肠	Small intestine	2 378	0.50	0.00	0.00	0.00	0.00	0.00	0.01	0.02	0.03	0.14
结肠	Colon	23 936	5.01	0.00	0.00	0.00	0.01	0.07	0.07	0.30	0.58	0.83
直肠	Rectum	21 944	4.60	0.00	0.01	0.00	0.01	0.09	0.09	0.19	0.47	0.66
肛门	Anus	607	0.13	0.00	0.00	0.00	0.00	0.01	0.01	0.01	0.01	0.03
肝脏	Liver	60 262	12.62	0.22	0.17	0.06	0.09	0.37	0.22	0.96	2.35	4.48
胆囊及其他	Gallbladder etc.	9 466	1.98	0.00	0.00	0.00	0.00	0.00	0.00	0.03	0.07	0.19
胰腺	Pancreas	20 035	4.20	0.00	0.02	0.01	0.01	0.00	0.03	0.12	0.24	0.46
鼻、鼻窦及其他	Nose, sinuses etc.	629	0.13	0.00	0.01	0.01	0.02	0.00	0.01	0.03	0.04	0.03
喉	Larynx	3 069	0.64	0.00	0.01	0.01	0.00	0.00	0.01	0.00	0.02	0.04
气管、支气管、肺	Trachea, bronchus & lung	133 105	27.88	0.11	0.02	0.02	0.05	0.68	0.19	0.46	1.10	2.19
其他胸腔器官	Other thoracic organs	1 614	0.34	0.07	0.02	0.02	0.06	0.09	0.10	0.09	0.10	0.13
骨	Bone	2 909	0.61	0.04	0.06	0.05	0.32	0.35	0.31	0.21	0.18	0.24
皮肤黑色素瘤	Melanoma of skin	900	0.19	0.00	0.01	0.01	0.01	0.02	0.03	0.02	0.05	0.08
皮肤其他	Other skin	2 096	0.44	0.04	0.00	0.01	0.02	0.06	0.05	0.02	0.05	0.04
间皮瘤	Mesothelioma	350	0.07	0.00	0.01	0.00	0.00	0.00	0.02	0.02	0.01	0.01
卡波西肉瘤	Kaposi sarcoma	74	0.02	0.04	0.00	0.01	0.00	0.00	0.01	0.01	0.01	0.03
结缔组织、软组织	Connective & soft tissue	1 118	0.23	0.04	0.18	0.12	0.08	0.16	0.07	0.07	0.17	0.15
乳腺	Breast	14 338	3.08	0.00	0.00	0.01	0.02	0.08	0.07	0.55	1.80	3.51
外阴	Vulva	295	0.06	0.00	0.00	0.00	0.00	0.00	0.00	0.01	0.01	0.03
阴道	Vagina	170	0.04	0.00	0.00	0.00	0.00	0.00	0.00	0.00	0.01	0.04
子宫颈	Cervix uteri	6 822	1.43	0.00	0.00	0.00	0.00	0.05	0.11	0.22	1.03	1.73
子宫体	Corpus uteri	2 642	0.55	0.00	0.00	0.00	0.00	0.00	0.03	0.00	0.07	0.29
子宫,部位不明	Uterus unspecified	899	0.19	0.00	0.00	0.00	0.00	0.00	0.00	0.05	0.06	0.12
卵巢	Ovary	5 599	1.17	0.00	0.02	0.01	0.05	0.12	0.22	0.35	0.45	0.60
其他女性生殖器官	Other female genital organs	320	0.07	0.00	0.00	0.00	0.00	0.03	0.01	0.02	0.00	0.06
胎盘	Placenta	10	0.00	0.00	0.00	0.00	0.00	0.00	0.00	0.00	0.02	0.00
阴茎	Penis	384	0.08	0.00	0.00	0.00	0.01	0.00	0.00	0.01	0.01	0.03
前列腺	Prostate	9 093	1.90	0.00	0.00	0.00	0.00	0.00	0.08	0.03	0.03	0.04
睾丸	Testis	140	0.03	0.00	0.00	0.00	0.00	0.05	0.10	0.10	0.08	0.10
其他男性生殖器官	Other male genital organs	104	0.02	0.00	0.00	0.00	0.00	0.03	0.00	0.01	0.01	0.01
肾	Kidney	4 675	0.98	0.07	0.14	0.01	0.05	0.06	0.04	0.08	0.09	0.12
肾盂	Renal pelvis	828	0.17	0.00	0.00	0.00	0.00	0.00	0.01	0.00	0.02	0.02
输尿管	Ureter	987	0.21	0.00	0.00	0.00	0.01	0.01	0.00	0.00	0.01	0.01
膀胱	Bladder	7 746	1.62	0.04	0.00	0.01	0.00	0.04	0.01	0.01	0.05	0.07
其他泌尿器官	Other urinary organs	198	0.04	0.00	0.00	0.01	0.00	0.00	0.00	0.00	0.00	0.01
眼	Eye	178	0.04	0.11	0.09	0.02	0.01	0.00	0.01	0.00	0.00	0.02
脑、神经系统	Brain, nervous system	11 164	2.34	1.20	1.00	1.06	0.83	0.64	0.58	0.76	0.97	1.25
甲状腺	Thyroid	1 908	0.40	0.00	0.01	0.00	0.01	0.00	0.04	0.07	0.14	0.16
肾上腺	Adrenal gland	555	0.12	0.04	0.09	0.07	0.00	0.02	0.03	0.03	0.01	0.05
其他内分泌腺	Other endocrine	319	0.07	0.00	0.03	0.02	0.01	0.09	0.04	0.02	0.03	0.02
霍奇金淋巴瘤	Hodgkin lymphoma	403	0.08	0.00	0.02	0.02	0.00	0.02	0.04	0.01	0.05	0.04
非霍奇金淋巴瘤	Non-Hodgkin lymphoma	7 518	1.57	0.25	0.08	0.11	0.14	0.21	0.24	0.27	0.40	0.54
免疫增生性疾病	Immunoproliferative diseases	80	0.02	0.00	0.00	0.00	0.00	0.00	0.00	0.00	0.00	0.00
多发性骨髓瘤	Multiple myeloma	3 283	0.69	0.00	0.01	0.03	0.05	0.10	0.06	0.06	0.03	0.08
淋巴细胞白血病	Lymphoid leukemia	2 035	0.43	0.33	0.38	0.35	0.41	0.39	0.35	0.22	0.28	0.34
髓系白血病	Myeloid leukemia	5 188	1.09	0.44	0.33	0.10	0.23	0.42	0.27	0.34	0.41	0.63
白血病,未特指	Leukemia unspecified	3 497	0.73	0.66	0.40	0.26	0.36	0.51	0.36	0.37	0.31	0.34
其他或未指明部位	Other and unspecified	11 990	2.51	0.44	0.42	0.17	0.23	0.40	0.24	0.34	0.43	0.62
所有部位合计	All sites	477 415	100.00	4.11	3.55	2.63	3.10	5.60	4.10	6.57	12.08	20.02
所有部位除外 C44	All sites except C44	475 319	99.56	4.08	3.55	2.62	3.08	5.54	4.06	6.56	12.03	19.97

274

CHINA CANCER REGISTRY ANNUAL REPORT 2022

Appendix Table 1-13　Cancer mortality in urban registration areas of China, both sexes in 2019

40~44	45~49	50~54	55~59	60~64	65~69	70~74	75~79	80~84	85+	粗率 Crude rate/ 100 000⁻¹	中标率 ASR China/ 100 000⁻¹	世标率 ASR world/ 100 000⁻¹	累积率 Cum. Rate/% 0~64	0~74	ICD-10
0.01	0.01	0.04	0.06	0.09	0.12	0.22	0.45	0.75	1.38	0.07	0.03	0.03	0.00	0.00	C00
0.19	0.31	0.55	0.83	1.14	1.40	1.65	2.51	2.89	2.97	0.50	0.29	0.28	0.02	0.03	C01-C02
0.16	0.26	0.50	1.00	1.30	1.67	2.75	3.43	4.76	6.76	0.65	0.35	0.35	0.02	0.04	C03-C06
0.06	0.11	0.21	0.34	0.39	0.64	0.73	0.94	1.46	2.29	0.22	0.12	0.12	0.01	0.01	C07-C08
0.01	0.05	0.13	0.23	0.19	0.20	0.20	0.37	0.41	0.31	0.08	0.05	0.05	0.00	0.01	C09
0.02	0.10	0.19	0.31	0.36	0.61	0.62	0.92	0.96	1.10	0.18	0.10	0.10	0.01	0.01	C10
1.04	1.80	2.86	3.39	4.56	5.39	6.20	6.50	6.70	5.63	1.88	1.15	1.12	0.07	0.13	C11
0.04	0.17	0.41	0.79	1.07	1.07	1.31	1.30	1.14	1.38	0.34	0.19	0.19	0.01	0.02	C12-C13
0.02	0.07	0.15	0.37	0.48	0.44	0.89	1.39	1.50	1.44	0.20	0.11	0.11	0.01	0.01	C14
0.52	2.19	6.53	12.22	23.01	37.13	54.43	75.32	89.95	95.46	11.18	5.79	5.81	0.22	0.68	C15
2.77	5.51	10.00	16.81	32.91	53.43	80.74	120.38	158.18	173.82	17.91	9.40	9.30	0.36	1.03	C16
0.10	0.32	0.65	0.99	1.66	2.84	3.76	5.27	7.40	7.92	0.89	0.47	0.47	0.02	0.05	C17
1.53	2.56	4.44	8.14	14.52	22.33	34.00	55.48	92.37	125.56	8.92	4.50	4.49	0.17	0.45	C18
1.27	2.60	5.20	7.72	14.28	22.70	33.27	49.93	76.79	98.85	8.17	4.21	4.20	0.16	0.44	C19-C20
0.06	0.10	0.17	0.23	0.46	0.58	0.85	1.28	2.07	2.42	0.23	0.12	0.12	0.01	0.01	C21
10.27	17.38	27.34	35.36	48.89	63.39	77.33	100.29	122.39	138.43	22.45	12.90	12.72	0.74	1.44	C22
0.42	0.86	1.92	3.23	6.70	10.19	14.88	22.78	33.85	40.80	3.53	1.79	1.79	0.07	0.19	C23-C24
0.98	2.50	4.77	8.23	15.69	22.85	32.67	46.21	61.48	67.99	7.46	3.91	3.91	0.17	0.44	C25
0.08	0.12	0.21	0.31	0.56	0.63	0.86	1.13	1.48	1.80	0.23	0.13	0.13	0.01	0.01	C30-C31
0.11	0.31	0.73	1.60	2.43	3.63	5.12	6.98	8.52	9.94	1.14	0.60	0.60	0.03	0.07	C32
5.36	13.31	28.95	53.35	101.81	160.16	224.18	324.75	410.94	436.71	49.58	25.89	25.87	1.04	2.96	C33-C34
0.20	0.35	0.60	0.93	1.23	1.64	2.06	3.01	3.67	3.52	0.60	0.36	0.36	0.02	0.04	C37-C38
0.25	0.52	0.86	1.10	1.81	2.87	4.31	5.87	7.81	8.53	1.08	0.67	0.66	0.03	0.07	C40-C41
0.13	0.21	0.25	0.35	0.52	0.98	1.13	1.73	2.53	3.73	0.34	0.19	0.18	0.01	0.02	C43
0.09	0.18	0.38	0.46	0.77	1.13	2.31	4.33	8.59	21.04	0.78	0.36	0.38	0.01	0.03	C44
0.02	0.03	0.10	0.22	0.36	0.51	0.46	0.57	0.52	0.98	0.13	0.07	0.07	0.00	0.01	C45
0.00	0.01	0.01	0.05	0.07	0.04	0.09	0.06	0.18	0.15	0.03	0.02	0.02	0.00	0.00	C46
0.15	0.24	0.35	0.39	0.72	0.98	1.20	2.01	2.69	3.46	0.42	0.27	0.27	0.01	0.03	C47,C49
6.42	11.27	15.93	19.27	22.63	25.19	25.07	32.98	45.66	64.19	10.70	6.19	6.05	0.41	0.66	C50
0.08	0.07	0.22	0.22	0.25	0.52	1.01	1.10	2.06	2.02	0.22	0.11	0.11	0.00	0.01	C51
0.02	0.10	0.12	0.23	0.19	0.34	0.38	0.58	1.15	0.67	0.13	0.07	0.07	0.00	0.01	C52
3.45	6.64	8.55	10.46	9.71	11.00	13.21	16.80	18.08	15.72	5.09	3.09	2.97	0.21	0.33	C53
0.87	1.34	2.30	3.91	4.81	5.96	6.28	7.73	8.11	8.56	1.97	1.10	1.10	0.07	0.13	C54
0.33	0.56	1.09	1.10	1.24	1.65	1.88	2.80	3.87	3.32	0.67	0.38	0.37	0.02	0.04	C55
1.58	3.92	6.08	7.50	9.66	11.87	14.37	14.88	17.21	12.66	4.18	2.42	2.39	0.15	0.28	C56
0.09	0.06	0.35	0.40	0.49	0.73	0.87	0.91	1.15	1.40	0.24	0.13	0.13	0.01	0.02	C57
0.01	0.01	0.01	0.02	0.01	0.01	0.00	0.00	0.04	0.00	0.01	0.01	0.00	0.00	0.00	C58
0.07	0.12	0.24	0.20	0.60	0.68	1.22	1.42	2.86	4.92	0.29	0.15	0.16	0.01	0.02	C60
0.06	0.20	0.57	1.67	4.47	10.98	25.08	57.08	115.28	201.14	6.76	3.22	3.29	0.04	0.22	C61
0.05	0.08	0.06	0.04	0.18	0.12	0.25	0.31	0.82	1.19	0.10	0.08	0.07	0.00	0.01	C62
0.00	0.03	0.05	0.06	0.08	0.18	0.38	0.66	0.76	1.12	0.08	0.04	0.04	0.00	0.00	C63
0.25	0.65	1.08	1.99	3.09	5.10	7.00	10.19	15.76	18.23	1.74	0.92	0.92	0.04	0.10	C64
0.00	0.06	0.12	0.23	0.53	0.85	1.22	1.90	3.05	4.99	0.31	0.15	0.15	0.01	0.02	C65
0.02	0.07	0.09	0.19	0.55	0.97	1.72	2.41	4.31	5.66	0.37	0.18	0.18	0.00	0.02	C66
0.12	0.33	0.66	1.39	2.95	5.59	10.50	20.56	37.38	63.47	2.89	1.31	1.34	0.03	0.11	C67
0.02	0.00	0.02	0.08	0.08	0.09	0.20	0.41	0.89	1.96	0.07	0.03	0.03	0.00	0.00	C68
0.01	0.02	0.03	0.08	0.10	0.11	0.23	0.32	0.62	0.80	0.07	0.04	0.05	0.00	0.00	C69
1.56	2.92	4.14	5.67	7.94	10.61	14.45	18.34	22.92	24.35	4.16	2.64	2.65	0.15	0.27	C70-C72,D32-D33,D42-D43
0.25	0.43	0.61	1.00	1.28	2.01	2.72	3.58	4.94	5.44	0.71	0.41	0.39	0.01	0.04	C73
0.05	0.11	0.18	0.28	0.38	0.54	0.65	1.12	1.53	1.41	0.21	0.12	0.13	0.01	0.01	C74
0.03	0.06	0.11	0.12	0.25	0.31	0.47	0.42	0.64	0.98	0.12	0.08	0.08	0.00	0.01	C75
0.07	0.06	0.14	0.16	0.32	0.38	0.52	0.81	0.64	1.59	0.15	0.09	0.09	0.00	0.01	C81
0.80	1.11	2.12	3.05	5.20	7.83	11.17	17.38	23.08	20.25	2.80	1.59	1.55	0.07	0.17	C82-C86,C96
0.00	0.00	0.01	0.04	0.06	0.06	0.08	0.15	0.23	0.34	0.03	0.02	0.02	0.00	0.00	C88
0.11	0.35	0.91	1.39	2.56	3.87	6.08	7.76	9.27	7.95	1.22	0.67	0.66	0.03	0.08	C90
0.30	0.41	0.56	0.83	1.01	1.82	2.36	3.08	4.62	4.40	0.76	0.55	0.56	0.03	0.05	C91
0.75	0.94	1.36	2.27	3.62	5.26	6.99	10.39	13.64	13.03	1.93	1.18	1.16	0.06	0.12	C92-C94,D45-D47
0.43	0.65	1.03	1.37	1.91	3.29	5.05	6.53	8.86	8.63	1.30	0.85	0.86	0.04	0.08	C95
1.21	1.86	3.50	4.99	7.55	11.54	16.72	24.72	36.06	50.86	4.47	2.45	2.46	0.11	0.25	O & U
38.47	74.53	132.97	206.86	344.89	515.39	722.52	1 045.15	1 408.76	1 649.89	177.82	95.88	95.42	4.28	10.47	C00-C97,D32-D33, D42-D43,D45-D47
38.38	74.35	132.58	206.40	344.13	514.26	720.21	1 040.82	1 400.17	1 628.85	177.04	95.52	95.04	4.27	10.44	C00-C97,D32-D33, D42-D43,D45-D47 exc. C44

部位 Site		死亡数 No. deaths	构成 Freq./%	0~	1~4	5~9	10~14	15~19	20~24	25~29	30~34	35~39
唇	Lip	124	0.04	0.00	0.00	0.00	0.01	0.02	0.00	0.01	0.01	0.00
舌	Tongue	931	0.31	0.00	0.02	0.03	0.00	0.00	0.00	0.03	0.13	0.12
口	Mouth	1 196	0.39	0.00	0.02	0.00	0.03	0.00	0.01	0.01	0.05	0.13
唾液腺	Salivary gland	387	0.13	0.00	0.00	0.00	0.00	0.05	0.00	0.02	0.04	0.04
扁桃体	Tonsil	182	0.06	0.00	0.00	0.01	0.00	0.02	0.00	0.01	0.02	0.00
其他口咽	Other oropharynx	416	0.14	0.00	0.00	0.00	0.01	0.00	0.00	0.02	0.01	0.04
鼻咽	Nasopharynx	3 779	1.25	0.00	0.00	0.00	0.03	0.14	0.10	0.12	0.38	0.92
下咽	Hypopharynx	865	0.29	0.00	0.00	0.00	0.00	0.02	0.00	0.01	0.01	0.04
咽,部位不明	Pharynx unspecified	428	0.14	0.00	0.00	0.00	0.00	0.00	0.00	0.00	0.01	0.01
食管	Esophagus	23 326	7.69	0.00	0.02	0.00	0.00	0.15	0.01	0.10	0.08	0.21
胃	Stomach	33 157	10.93	0.00	0.02	0.00	0.01	0.31	0.15	0.53	0.72	1.47
小肠	Small intestine	1 427	0.47	0.00	0.00	0.00	0.00	0.00	0.01	0.01	0.03	0.17
结肠	Colon	13 502	4.45	0.00	0.00	0.00	0.00	0.06	0.08	0.25	0.72	0.84
直肠	Rectum	13 621	4.49	0.00	0.02	0.01	0.00	0.14	0.09	0.18	0.48	0.68
肛门	Anus	345	0.11	0.00	0.00	0.00	0.00	0.00	0.01	0.00	0.00	0.03
肝脏	Liver	44 457	14.65	0.21	0.20	0.11	0.13	0.44	0.28	1.39	3.97	7.62
胆囊及其他	Gallbladder etc.	4 475	1.47	0.00	0.00	0.00	0.00	0.03	0.00	0.02	0.06	0.17
胰腺	Pancreas	11 308	3.73	0.00	0.03	0.01	0.01	0.03	0.01	0.10	0.30	0.57
鼻、鼻窦及其他	Nose,sinuses etc.	425	0.14	0.00	0.00	0.01	0.00	0.03	0.01	0.04	0.06	0.04
喉	Larynx	2 758	0.91	0.00	0.02	0.01	0.00	0.00	0.01	0.00	0.04	0.09
气管、支气管、肺	Trachea,bronchus & lung	93 230	30.72	0.14	0.02	0.01	0.06	1.01	0.27	0.46	1.41	2.45
其他胸腔器官	Other thoracic organs	1 003	0.33	0.00	0.05	0.03	0.06	0.09	0.10	0.14	0.10	0.14
骨	Bone	1 734	0.57	0.07	0.08	0.05	0.31	0.49	0.39	0.25	0.20	0.33
皮肤黑色素瘤	Melanoma of skin	475	0.16	0.00	0.02	0.00	0.01	0.02	0.03	0.02	0.04	0.05
皮肤其他	Other skin	1 208	0.40	0.07	0.00	0.00	0.01	0.06	0.04	0.03	0.06	0.03
间皮瘤	Mesothelioma	217	0.07	0.00	0.02	0.00	0.00	0.00	0.03	0.02	0.02	0.02
卡波西肉瘤	Kaposi sarcoma	40	0.01	0.00	0.00	0.00	0.00	0.02	0.03	0.01	0.00	0.02
结缔组织、软组织	Connective & soft tissue	670	0.22	0.07	0.20	0.12	0.12	0.11	0.06	0.08	0.19	0.17
乳腺	Breast	384	0.13	0.00	0.00	0.00	0.00	0.00	0.00	0.00	0.04	0.06
外阴	Vulva	—	—	—	—	—	—	—	—	—	—	—
阴道	Vagina	—	—	—	—	—	—	—	—	—	—	—
子宫颈	Cervix uteri	—	—	—	—	—	—	—	—	—	—	—
子宫体	Corpus uteri	—	—	—	—	—	—	—	—	—	—	—
子宫,部位不明	Uterus unspecified	—	—	—	—	—	—	—	—	—	—	—
卵巢	Ovary	—	—	—	—	—	—	—	—	—	—	—
其他女性生殖器官	Other female genital organs	—	—	—	—	—	—	—	—	—	—	—
胎盘	Placenta	—	—	—	—	—	—	—	—	—	—	—
阴茎	Penis	384	0.13	0.00	0.00	0.01	0.00	0.00	0.00	0.01	0.01	0.03
前列腺	Prostate	9 093	3.00	0.00	0.00	0.00	0.00	0.08	0.03	0.03	0.03	0.04
睾丸	Testis	140	0.05	0.00	0.00	0.01	0.00	0.05	0.10	0.10	0.08	0.10
其他男性生殖器官	Other male genital organs	104	0.03	0.00	0.00	0.00	0.00	0.03	0.00	0.01	0.01	0.01
肾	Kidney	3 093	1.02	0.00	0.12	0.03	0.01	0.06	0.05	0.08	0.07	0.19
肾盂	Renal pelvis	477	0.16	0.00	0.00	0.00	0.00	0.03	0.00	0.00	0.03	0.05
输尿管	Ureter	518	0.17	0.00	0.00	0.00	0.00	0.00	0.00	0.00	0.02	0.01
膀胱	Bladder	6 024	1.99	0.00	0.00	0.00	0.00	0.08	0.03	0.01	0.08	0.11
其他泌尿器官	Other urinary organs	111	0.04	0.00	0.00	0.01	0.00	0.00	0.00	0.00	0.00	0.01
眼	Eye	96	0.03	0.00	0.11	0.00	0.01	0.00	0.01	0.00	0.01	0.02
脑、神经系统	Brain,nervous system	6 072	2.00	1.11	0.97	1.14	0.89	0.75	0.63	1.00	1.10	1.45
甲状腺	Thyroid	741	0.24	0.00	0.00	0.00	0.00	0.01	0.02	0.04	0.03	0.10	0.13
肾上腺	Adrenal gland	332	0.11	0.07	0.09	0.09	0.00	0.03	0.01	0.01	0.02	0.04
其他内分泌腺	Other endocrine	199	0.07	0.00	0.05	0.03	0.01	0.14	0.08	0.01	0.04	0.02
霍奇金淋巴瘤	Hodgkin lymphoma	257	0.08	0.00	0.02	0.03	0.00	0.02	0.04	0.01	0.06	0.05
非霍奇金淋巴瘤	Non-Hodgkin lymphoma	4 564	1.50	0.35	0.12	0.13	0.18	0.26	0.31	0.32	0.55	0.72
免疫增生性疾病	Immunoproliferative diseases	55	0.02	0.00	0.02	0.00	0.00	0.00	0.00	0.00	0.00	0.00
多发性骨髓瘤	Multiple myeloma	1 912	0.63	0.00	0.02	0.03	0.06	0.09	0.00	0.08	0.04	0.10
淋巴细胞白血病	Lymphoid leukemia	1 192	0.39	0.21	0.36	0.42	0.43	0.43	0.46	0.26	0.43	0.42
髓系白血病	Myeloid leukemia	3 089	1.02	0.28	0.30	0.15	0.30	0.52	0.30	0.44	0.37	0.77
白血病,未特指	Leukemia unspecified	2 014	0.66	0.63	0.45	0.26	0.34	0.61	0.44	0.37	0.38	0.39
其他或未指明部位	Other and unspecified	6 930	2.28	0.70	0.42	0.08	0.28	0.49	0.24	0.45	0.47	0.66
所有部位合计	All sites	303 467	100.00	3.90	3.72	2.83	3.38	6.87	4.60	7.10	13.08	21.78
所有部位除外 C44	All sites except C44	302 259	99.60	3.83	3.72	2.83	3.37	6.80	4.57	7.06	13.01	21.75

Appendix Table 1-14　Cancer mortality in urban registration areas of China, male in 2019

40~44	45~49	50~54	55~59	60~64	65~69	70~74	75~79	80~84	85+	粗率 Crude rate/ 100 000⁻¹	中标率 ASR China/ 100 000⁻¹	世标率 ASR world/ 100 000⁻¹	累积率 Cum. Rate/% 0~64	0~74	ICD-10
0.02	0.01	0.05	0.08	0.14	0.18	0.34	0.76	1.02	1.79	0.09	0.05	0.05	0.00	0.00	C00
0.29	0.45	0.90	1.33	1.89	2.10	2.37	3.43	3.06	2.76	0.69	0.42	0.41	0.03	0.05	C01-C02
0.22	0.41	0.83	1.69	2.04	2.35	3.79	4.85	5.46	8.57	0.89	0.51	0.51	0.03	0.06	C03-C06
0.07	0.17	0.29	0.56	0.64	0.92	0.88	1.18	1.84	2.98	0.29	0.17	0.17	0.01	0.02	C07-C08
0.02	0.09	0.25	0.43	0.37	0.30	0.34	0.62	0.51	0.37	0.14	0.08	0.08	0.01	0.01	C09
0.04	0.20	0.37	0.59	0.64	1.19	1.08	1.70	1.68	1.79	0.31	0.18	0.18	0.01	0.02	C10
1.67	2.78	4.48	5.14	7.06	8.41	9.60	9.81	10.15	8.19	2.81	1.76	1.72	0.11	0.20	C11
0.09	0.32	0.77	1.51	2.12	2.13	2.55	2.56	2.24	2.98	0.64	0.37	0.38	0.02	0.05	C12-C13
0.03	0.14	0.27	0.69	0.84	0.73	1.46	2.04	2.14	2.16	0.32	0.18	0.18	0.01	0.02	C14
0.89	3.85	11.98	22.58	41.30	63.80	86.47	114.40	135.17	138.34	17.35	9.56	9.64	0.41	1.16	C15
2.80	6.56	13.31	24.23	50.50	81.68	122.07	180.22	229.09	248.75	24.66	13.59	13.52	0.50	1.52	C16
0.10	0.39	0.81	1.35	2.16	3.66	4.48	6.62	8.97	10.88	1.06	0.59	0.59	0.03	0.07	C17
1.60	2.78	5.08	9.98	18.86	27.45	42.43	64.81	109.06	152.65	10.04	5.41	5.43	0.20	0.55	C18
1.38	2.94	6.56	10.44	19.70	31.47	45.20	65.81	96.98	131.04	10.13	5.52	5.55	0.21	0.60	C19-C20
0.04	0.12	0.25	0.30	0.61	0.71	1.08	1.46	2.04	2.91	0.26	0.14	0.14	0.01	0.02	C21
17.82	29.90	46.15	58.91	78.01	96.68	110.64	137.97	159.03	180.58	33.07	20.04	19.75	1.22	2.26	C22
0.51	0.80	1.94	3.69	6.92	10.60	15.05	21.70	32.73	39.48	3.33	1.81	1.82	0.07	0.20	C23-C24
1.27	3.37	6.38	10.78	19.77	28.33	37.59	50.25	65.32	78.82	8.41	4.69	4.71	0.21	0.54	C25
0.11	0.18	0.28	0.43	0.76	1.03	1.28	1.70	1.99	2.01	0.32	0.19	0.19	0.01	0.02	C30-C31
0.20	0.59	1.36	3.13	4.58	6.94	9.83	12.93	15.96	18.55	2.05	1.13	1.14	0.05	0.13	C32
6.33	16.54	40.63	78.70	158.39	249.79	343.09	478.38	571.27	619.75	69.34	38.25	38.37	1.53	4.50	C33-C34
0.22	0.44	0.80	1.35	1.65	2.17	2.59	4.05	4.33	4.32	0.75	0.46	0.45	0.03	0.05	C37-C38
0.28	0.68	1.15	1.40	2.26	3.69	5.16	6.86	9.38	11.62	1.29	0.83	0.82	0.04	0.08	C40-C41
0.10	0.27	0.25	0.32	0.63	1.14	1.22	1.73	3.21	4.84	0.35	0.20	0.20	0.01	0.02	C43
0.10	0.23	0.54	0.55	1.14	1.62	3.18	5.20	11.01	24.66	0.90	0.46	0.48	0.01	0.04	C44
0.03	0.03	0.12	0.29	0.47	0.70	0.45	0.69	0.82	1.42	0.16	0.09	0.10	0.01	0.01	C45
0.00	0.02	0.02	0.06	0.06	0.04	0.11	0.14	0.15	0.30	0.03	0.02	0.02	0.00	0.00	C46
0.16	0.31	0.41	0.57	0.88	1.37	1.53	2.53	3.21	4.77	0.50	0.33	0.33	0.02	0.03	C47,C49
0.10	0.25	0.19	0.46	0.43	0.80	1.13	1.21	2.14	4.10	0.29	0.16	0.16	0.01	0.02	C50
—	—	—	—	—	—	—	—	—	—	—	—	—	—	—	C51
—	—	—	—	—	—	—	—	—	—	—	—	—	—	—	C52
—	—	—	—	—	—	—	—	—	—	—	—	—	—	—	C53
—	—	—	—	—	—	—	—	—	—	—	—	—	—	—	C54
—	—	—	—	—	—	—	—	—	—	—	—	—	—	—	C55
—	—	—	—	—	—	—	—	—	—	—	—	—	—	—	C56
—	—	—	—	—	—	—	—	—	—	—	—	—	—	—	C57
—	—	—	—	—	—	—	—	—	—	—	—	—	—	—	C58
0.07	0.12	0.24	0.20	0.60	0.68	1.22	1.42	2.86	4.92	0.29	0.15	0.16	0.01	0.02	C60
0.06	0.20	0.57	1.67	4.47	10.98	25.08	57.08	115.28	201.14	6.76	3.22	3.29	0.04	0.22	C61
0.05	0.08	0.06	0.04	0.18	0.12	0.25	0.31	0.82	1.19	0.10	0.08	0.07	0.00	0.01	C62
0.00	0.03	0.05	0.06	0.08	0.18	0.38	0.66	0.76	1.12	0.08	0.04	0.04	0.00	0.01	C63
0.38	0.92	1.59	2.99	4.51	7.43	9.92	12.82	20.85	26.30	2.30	1.28	1.29	0.05	0.14	C64
0.00	0.09	0.21	0.37	0.71	1.04	1.37	2.29	3.67	5.44	0.35	0.19	0.19	0.01	0.02	C65
0.01	0.07	0.09	0.20	0.72	1.31	1.85	2.88	4.28	5.89	0.39	0.20	0.21	0.01	0.02	C66
0.20	0.46	0.98	2.32	5.08	9.20	17.19	34.07	64.35	115.77	4.48	2.21	2.27	0.05	0.18	C67
0.02	0.01	0.02	0.09	0.12	0.10	0.20	0.35	1.07	2.91	0.08	0.04	0.04	0.00	0.00	C68
0.01	0.03	0.04	0.11	0.11	0.13	0.32	0.38	0.56	0.89	0.07	0.04	0.05	0.00	0.00	C69
1.72	3.30	4.88	6.79	9.71	12.19	15.66	19.41	24.02	24.58	4.52	2.99	2.99	0.17	0.31	C70-C72,D32-D33,D42-D43
0.15	0.32	0.46	0.86	1.15	1.93	2.03	2.70	3.88	4.32	0.55	0.33	0.32	0.02	0.04	C73
0.10	0.16	0.22	0.38	0.52	0.65	0.83	1.32	1.99	1.56	0.25	0.15	0.16	0.01	0.02	C74
0.02	0.08	0.14	0.16	0.34	0.40	0.54	0.55	0.92	1.27	0.15	0.10	0.10	0.01	0.01	C75
0.07	0.05	0.19	0.26	0.44	0.56	0.61	0.94	1.02	2.31	0.19	0.12	0.12	0.01	0.01	C81
0.92	1.42	2.71	3.91	6.47	9.77	13.86	21.56	30.54	28.68	3.39	2.02	1.97	0.09	0.21	C82-C86,C96
0.01	0.01	0.01	0.03	0.08	0.09	0.20	0.35	0.46	0.60	0.04	0.02	0.02	0.00	0.00	C88
0.16	0.45	1.02	1.58	2.89	4.65	7.46	9.63	12.29	10.80	1.42	0.81	0.81	0.03	0.09	C90
0.29	0.44	0.57	0.86	1.26	2.23	2.91	3.85	6.22	6.63	0.89	0.65	0.65	0.03	0.06	C91
0.75	1.04	1.61	2.65	4.50	6.58	8.81	13.59	17.79	19.00	2.30	1.44	1.42	0.07	0.15	C92-C94,D45-D47
0.56	0.84	1.22	1.54	2.24	3.85	6.22	7.83	11.06	11.40	1.50	1.01	1.01	0.05	0.10	C95
1.45	2.14	4.17	6.45	9.54	14.79	20.82	30.60	42.06	59.67	5.15	2.98	3.00	0.13	0.31	O & U
43.46	87.10	167.47	275.05	480.55	720.86	994.72	1 410.21	1 856.71	2 247.75	225.72	127.26	127.26	5.59	14.16	C00-C97,D32-D33, D42-D43,D45-D47
43.36	86.87	166.93	274.51	479.40	719.24	991.54	1 405.01	1 845.70	2 223.09	224.82	126.80	126.78	5.57	14.12	C00-C97,D32-D33, D42-D43,D45-D47 exc. C44

部位 Site		死亡数 No. deaths	构成 Freq./%	年龄组								
				0~	1~4	5~9	10~14	15~19	20~24	25~29	30~34	35~39
唇	Lip	62	0.04	0.00	0.00	0.00	0.00	0.00	0.00	0.00	0.00	0.00
舌	Tongue	409	0.24	0.00	0.00	0.00	0.00	0.02	0.03	0.00	0.04	0.06
口	Mouth	559	0.32	0.00	0.00	0.00	0.02	0.00	0.01	0.00	0.00	0.05
唾液腺	Salivary gland	205	0.12	0.00	0.00	0.00	0.02	0.00	0.00	0.02	0.03	0.07
扁桃体	Tonsil	37	0.02	0.00	0.00	0.00	0.00	0.00	0.00	0.01	0.00	0.00
其他口咽	Other oropharynx	60	0.03	0.00	0.00	0.00	0.00	0.00	0.00	0.00	0.03	0.02
鼻咽	Nasopharynx	1 269	0.73	0.00	0.00	0.01	0.00	0.07	0.04	0.16	0.23	0.22
下咽	Hypopharynx	45	0.03	0.00	0.00	0.00	0.00	0.00	0.00	0.00	0.01	0.00
咽,部位不明	Pharynx unspecified	122	0.07	0.00	0.00	0.00	0.00	0.03	0.00	0.00	0.00	0.02
食管	Esophagus	6 680	3.84	0.00	0.00	0.00	0.00	0.05	0.01	0.01	0.04	0.07
胃	Stomach	14 932	8.58	0.00	0.00	0.03	0.03	0.08	0.23	0.45	1.14	1.76
小肠	Small intestine	951	0.55	0.00	0.00	0.00	0.00	0.00	0.00	0.02	0.04	0.10
结肠	Colon	10 434	6.00	0.00	0.00	0.00	0.00	0.08	0.07	0.35	0.44	0.83
直肠	Rectum	8 323	4.78	0.00	0.00	0.00	0.00	0.03	0.08	0.21	0.46	0.64
肛门	Anus	262	0.15	0.00	0.00	0.00	0.00	0.02	0.00	0.01	0.02	0.03
肝脏	Liver	15 805	9.09	0.23	0.14	0.01	0.03	0.29	0.15	0.53	0.80	1.44
胆囊及其他	Gallbladder etc.	4 991	2.87	0.00	0.00	0.00	0.00	0.00	0.00	0.03	0.07	0.21
胰腺	Pancreas	8 727	5.02	0.00	0.02	0.00	0.00	0.05	0.14	0.19	0.35
鼻、鼻窦及其他	Nose, sinuses etc.	204	0.12	0.00	0.02	0.00	0.03	0.02	0.00	0.02	0.02	0.02
喉	Larynx	311	0.18	0.00	0.00	0.00	0.00	0.00	0.00	0.00	0.00	0.00
气管、支气管、肺	Trachea, bronchus & lung	39 875	22.92	0.08	0.02	0.03	0.03	0.32	0.11	0.46	0.80	1.94
其他胸腔器官	Other thoracic organs	611	0.35	0.15	0.00	0.01	0.07	0.08	0.09	0.05	0.10	0.12
骨	Bone	1 175	0.68	0.00	0.03	0.04	0.33	0.20	0.23	0.17	0.16	0.15
皮肤黑色素瘤	Melanoma of skin	425	0.24	0.00	0.00	0.00	0.00	0.00	0.03	0.02	0.06	0.11
皮肤其他	Other skin	888	0.51	0.00	0.00	0.03	0.02	0.05	0.05	0.00	0.03	0.06
间皮瘤	Mesothelioma	133	0.08	0.00	0.00	0.00	0.00	0.00	0.01	0.01	0.01	0.00
卡波西肉瘤	Kaposi sarcoma	34	0.02	0.08	0.00	0.01	0.00	0.00	0.00	0.00	0.02	0.04
结缔组织、软组织	Connective & soft tissue	448	0.26	0.00	0.15	0.12	0.03	0.22	0.08	0.05	0.14	0.13
乳腺	Breast	14 338	8.24	0.00	0.00	0.01	0.02	0.08	0.07	0.55	1.80	3.51
外阴	Vulva	295	0.17	0.00	0.00	0.00	0.00	0.00	0.00	0.01	0.01	0.03
阴道	Vagina	170	0.10	0.00	0.00	0.00	0.00	0.00	0.00	0.00	0.01	0.04
子宫颈	Cervix uteri	6 822	3.92	0.00	0.00	0.00	0.00	0.05	0.11	0.22	1.03	1.73
子宫体	Corpus uteri	2 642	1.52	0.00	0.00	0.00	0.00	0.03	0.00	0.07	0.17	0.29
子宫,部位不明	Uterus unspecified	899	0.52	0.00	0.00	0.00	0.00	0.00	0.00	0.05	0.06	0.12
卵巢	Ovary	5 599	3.22	0.00	0.02	0.01	0.05	0.12	0.22	0.35	0.45	0.60
其他女性生殖器官	Other female genital organs	320	0.18	0.00	0.00	0.00	0.00	0.03	0.01	0.02	0.00	0.06
胎盘	Placenta	10	0.01	0.00	0.00	0.00	0.00	0.00	0.00	0.00	0.02	0.00
阴茎	Penis	—	—	—	—	—	—	—	—	—	—	—
前列腺	Prostate	—	—	—	—	—	—	—	—	—	—	—
睾丸	Testis	—	—	—	—	—	—	—	—	—	—	—
其他男性生殖器官	Other male genital organs	—	—	—	—	—	—	—	—	—	—	—
肾	Kidney	1 582	0.91	0.15	0.15	0.00	0.08	0.05	0.03	0.08	0.10	0.06
肾盂	Renal pelvis	351	0.20	0.00	0.00	0.00	0.00	0.00	0.01	0.00	0.01	0.00
输尿管	Ureter	469	0.27	0.00	0.00	0.00	0.02	0.00	0.00	0.00	0.00	0.01
膀胱	Bladder	1 722	0.99	0.08	0.00	0.01	0.00	0.00	0.00	0.00	0.00	0.03
其他泌尿器官	Other urinary organs	87	0.05	0.00	0.00	0.00	0.00	0.00	0.00	0.00	0.00	0.01
眼	Eye	82	0.05	0.23	0.07	0.04	0.00	0.00	0.01	0.00	0.00	0.02
脑、神经系统	Brain, nervous system	5 092	2.93	1.30	1.03	0.97	0.76	0.52	0.53	0.52	0.84	1.05
甲状腺	Thyroid	1 167	0.67	0.00	0.02	0.00	0.00	0.02	0.04	0.12	0.17	0.20
肾上腺	Adrenal gland	223	0.13	0.00	0.09	0.04	0.00	0.02	0.04	0.04	0.01	0.07
其他内分泌腺	Other endocrine	120	0.07	0.00	0.02	0.01	0.00	0.03	0.00	0.03	0.02	0.02
霍奇金淋巴瘤	Hodgkin lymphoma	146	0.08	0.00	0.02	0.01	0.00	0.02	0.04	0.01	0.03	0.03
非霍奇金淋巴瘤	Non-Hodgkin lymphoma	2 954	1.70	0.15	0.03	0.09	0.10	0.15	0.16	0.21	0.25	0.36
免疫增生性疾病	Immunoproliferative diseases	25	0.01	0.00	0.00	0.00	0.00	0.00	0.00	0.00	0.00	0.00
多发性骨髓瘤	Multiple myeloma	1 371	0.79	0.00	0.00	0.00	0.03	0.03	0.10	0.04	0.03	0.07
淋巴细胞白血病	Lymphoid leukemia	843	0.48	0.46	0.41	0.28	0.38	0.35	0.23	0.18	0.14	0.26
髓系白血病	Myeloid leukemia	2 099	1.21	0.61	0.36	0.04	0.17	0.30	0.24	0.24	0.45	0.48
白血病,未特指	Leukemia unspecified	1 483	0.85	0.69	0.34	0.25	0.38	0.41	0.27	0.36	0.25	0.28
其他或未指明部位	Other and unspecified	5 060	2.91	0.15	0.43	0.26	0.18	0.30	0.23	0.23	0.40	0.57
所有部位合计	All sites	173 948	100.00	4.34	3.35	2.41	2.78	4.20	3.58	6.04	11.12	18.31
所有部位除外 C44	All sites except C44	173 060	99.49	4.34	3.35	2.38	2.76	4.15	3.52	6.04	11.09	18.25

Appendix Table 1-15　Cancer mortality in urban registration areas of China,female in 2019

Age group										粗率 Crude rate/ 100 000⁻¹	中标率 ASR China/ 100 000⁻¹	世标率 ASR world/ 100 000⁻¹	累积率 Cum. Rate/%		ICD-10
40~44	45~49	50~54	55~59	60~64	65~69	70~74	75~79	80~84	85+	Crude rate/ 100 000⁻¹	ASR China/ 100 000⁻¹	ASR world/ 100 000⁻¹	0~64	0~74	ICD-10
0.00	0.02	0.03	0.04	0.04	0.07	0.11	0.18	0.54	1.09	0.05	0.02	0.02	0.00	0.00	C00
0.10	0.18	0.20	0.32	0.39	0.73	0.97	1.70	2.76	3.11	0.31	0.16	0.15	0.01	0.02	C01-C02
0.10	0.11	0.17	0.30	0.56	1.02	1.78	2.19	4.20	5.50	0.42	0.20	0.20	0.01	0.02	C03-C06
0.06	0.05	0.13	0.12	0.15	0.38	0.59	0.73	1.15	1.82	0.15	0.08	0.08	0.00	0.01	C07-C08
0.00	0.02	0.02	0.03	0.01	0.10	0.06	0.15	0.33	0.26	0.03	0.01	0.01	0.00	0.00	C09
0.01	0.01	0.01	0.03	0.08	0.06	0.19	0.24	0.37	0.62	0.04	0.02	0.02	0.00	0.00	C10
0.41	0.81	1.22	1.63	2.09	2.51	3.00	3.59	3.91	3.84	0.95	0.56	0.54	0.03	0.06	C11
0.00	0.01	0.04	0.08	0.04	0.07	0.15	0.18	0.25	0.26	0.03	0.02	0.02	0.00	0.00	C12-C13
0.01	0.01	0.03	0.04	0.13	0.17	0.36	0.82	0.99	0.93	0.09	0.05	0.04	0.00	0.00	C14
0.16	0.53	1.02	1.81	4.93	11.80	24.37	41.01	53.44	65.59	4.98	2.26	2.22	0.04	0.22	C15
2.73	4.45	6.64	9.34	15.51	26.60	41.98	67.85	100.92	121.63	11.14	5.56	5.43	0.21	0.55	C16
0.10	0.25	0.49	0.64	1.17	2.06	3.09	4.08	6.13	5.86	0.71	0.36	0.35	0.01	0.04	C17
1.46	2.34	3.79	6.29	10.23	17.46	26.08	47.28	78.89	106.69	7.78	3.67	3.64	0.13	0.35	C18
1.17	2.26	3.82	4.98	8.91	14.37	22.07	35.99	60.48	76.43	6.21	3.00	2.96	0.11	0.30	C19-C20
0.08	0.08	0.08	0.15	0.31	0.45	0.63	1.13	2.10	2.08	0.20	0.10	0.10	0.00	0.01	C21
2.79	4.80	8.33	11.68	20.08	31.78	46.08	67.21	92.81	109.07	11.79	6.00	5.94	0.26	0.64	C22
0.33	0.92	1.89	2.77	6.50	9.80	14.71	23.73	34.75	41.72	3.72	1.77	1.77	0.06	0.19	C23-C24
0.70	1.62	3.14	5.66	11.66	17.63	28.05	42.66	58.38	60.45	6.51	3.18	3.15	0.12	0.35	C25
0.06	0.05	0.14	0.19	0.36	0.25	0.47	0.64	1.07	1.66	0.15	0.08	0.08	0.00	0.01	C30-C31
0.02	0.04	0.10	0.05	0.31	0.49	0.70	1.76	2.51	3.94	0.23	0.10	0.10	0.00	0.01	C32
4.39	10.07	17.15	27.86	45.83	75.01	112.64	189.89	281.47	309.21	29.75	14.43	14.28	0.55	1.48	C33-C34
0.19	0.26	0.40	0.52	0.81	1.13	1.56	2.10	3.13	2.96	0.46	0.27	0.26	0.01	0.03	C37-C38
0.22	0.37	0.57	0.79	1.36	2.09	3.51	4.99	6.55	6.38	0.88	0.52	0.50	0.02	0.05	C40-C41
0.16	0.15	0.25	0.38	0.42	0.83	1.06	1.73	1.98	2.96	0.32	0.17	0.17	0.01	0.02	C43
0.08	0.14	0.23	0.38	0.39	0.66	1.50	3.56	6.63	18.52	0.66	0.27	0.28	0.01	0.02	C44
0.02	0.02	0.09	0.15	0.26	0.34	0.47	0.46	0.29	0.67	0.10	0.05	0.05	0.00	0.01	C45
0.01	0.01	0.01	0.04	0.08	0.03	0.06	0.00	0.21	0.05	0.03	0.02	0.02	0.00	0.00	C46
0.15	0.18	0.29	0.22	0.57	0.62	0.89	1.55	2.26	2.54	0.33	0.22	0.22	0.01	0.02	C47,C49
6.42	11.27	15.93	19.27	22.63	25.19	25.07	32.98	45.66	64.19	10.70	6.19	6.05	0.41	0.66	C50
0.08	0.07	0.22	0.22	0.25	0.52	1.01	1.10	2.06	2.02	0.22	0.11	0.11	0.00	0.01	C51
0.02	0.10	0.12	0.23	0.19	0.34	0.38	0.58	1.15	0.67	0.13	0.07	0.07	0.00	0.01	C52
3.45	6.64	8.55	10.46	9.71	11.00	13.21	16.80	18.08	15.72	5.09	3.09	2.97	0.21	0.33	C53
0.87	1.34	2.30	3.91	4.81	5.96	6.28	7.73	8.11	8.56	1.97	1.10	1.10	0.07	0.13	C54
0.33	0.56	1.09	1.10	1.24	1.65	1.88	2.80	3.87	3.32	0.67	0.38	0.37	0.02	0.04	C55
1.58	3.92	6.08	7.50	9.66	11.87	14.37	14.88	17.21	12.66	4.18	2.42	2.39	0.15	0.28	C56
0.09	0.06	0.35	0.40	0.49	0.73	0.87	0.91	1.15	1.40	0.24	0.13	0.13	0.01	0.02	C57
0.01	0.01	0.01	0.02	0.01	0.01	0.00	0.00	0.04	0.00	0.01	0.01	0.00	0.00	0.00	C58
—	—	—	—	—	—	—	—	—	—	—	—	—		—	C60
—	—	—	—	—	—	—	—	—	—	—	—	—		—	C61
—	—	—	—	—	—	—	—	—	—	—	—	—		—	C62
—	—	—	—	—	—	—	—	—	—	—	—	—		—	C63
0.12	0.37	0.55	0.98	1.69	2.88	4.27	7.88	11.65	12.61	1.18	0.59	0.58	0.02	0.06	C64
0.01	0.04	0.04	0.10	0.36	0.66	1.08	1.55	2.55	4.67	0.26	0.11	0.12	0.00	0.01	C65
0.03	0.06	0.09	0.18	0.38	0.65	1.61	2.01	4.32	5.50	0.35	0.16	0.16	0.00	0.02	C66
0.05	0.20	0.33	0.45	0.84	2.16	4.23	8.70	15.60	27.03	1.28	0.53	0.54	0.01	0.04	C67
0.02	0.00	0.02	0.06	0.05	0.07	0.19	0.46	0.74	1.30	0.06	0.03	0.03	0.00	0.00	C68
0.01	0.01	0.03	0.04	0.10	0.08	0.15	0.27	0.66	0.73	0.06	0.03	0.04	0.00	0.00	C69
1.41	2.53	3.38	4.55	6.20	9.11	13.32	17.40	22.03	24.18	3.80	2.31	2.32	0.12	0.23	C70-C72,D32-D33,D42-D43
0.35	0.53	0.76	1.14	1.40	2.09	3.36	4.35	5.81	6.23	0.87	0.48	0.46	0.02	0.05	C73
0.01	0.06	0.14	0.18	0.25	0.44	0.49	0.94	1.15	1.30	0.17	0.10	0.10	0.00	0.01	C74
0.04	0.04	0.08	0.09	0.17	0.23	0.40	0.30	0.41	0.78	0.09	0.05	0.05	0.00	0.01	C75
0.07	0.06	0.09	0.06	0.20	0.20	0.44	0.70	0.33	1.09	0.11	0.06	0.06	0.00	0.01	C81
0.67	0.81	1.53	2.20	3.95	5.99	8.65	13.72	17.05	14.37	2.20	1.19	1.16	0.05	0.13	C82-C86,C96
0.00	0.00	0.01	0.01	0.04	0.07	0.11	0.12	0.12	0.16	0.02	0.01	0.01	0.00	0.00	C88
0.06	0.24	0.79	1.20	2.24	3.13	4.78	6.12	6.83	5.97	1.02	0.54	0.54	0.02	0.06	C90
0.30	0.38	0.55	0.79	0.76	1.43	1.84	2.40	3.34	2.85	0.63	0.45	0.47	0.03	0.04	C91
0.74	0.83	1.11	1.89	2.75	4.00	5.28	7.58	10.29	8.87	1.57	0.94	0.92	0.05	0.09	C92-C94,D45-D47
0.31	0.46	0.84	1.20	1.58	2.77	3.95	5.39	7.08	6.69	1.11	0.71	0.71	0.04	0.07	C95
0.97	1.57	2.83	3.53	5.58	8.46	12.87	19.56	31.21	44.73	3.78	1.95	1.95	0.09	0.19	O & U
33.53	61.90	98.09	138.28	210.70	320.23	467.20	724.65	1 047.02	1 233.47	129.78	66.85	66.02	2.97	6.91	C00-C97,D32-D33, D42-D43,D45-D47
33.45	61.76	97.86	137.90	210.30	319.56	465.70	721.09	1 040.39	1 214.95	129.11	66.57	65.74	2.97	6.89	C00-C97,D32-D33, D42-D43,D45-D47 exc. C44

部位 Site		死亡数 No. deaths	构成 Freq. /%	年龄组								
				0~	1~4	5~9	10~14	15~19	20~24	25~29	30~34	35~39
唇	Lip	351	0.06	0.00	0.00	0.00	0.00	0.00	0.00	0.00	0.01	0.01
舌	Tongue	1 375	0.23	0.00	0.00	0.00	0.00	0.00	0.01	0.03	0.06	0.09
口	Mouth	2 006	0.33	0.00	0.01	0.00	0.00	0.01	0.01	0.03	0.03	0.07
唾液腺	Salivary gland	649	0.11	0.00	0.00	0.00	0.00	0.02	0.02	0.03	0.01	0.02
扁桃体	Tonsil	239	0.04	0.00	0.00	0.00	0.00	0.01	0.00	0.00	0.00	0.01
其他口咽	Other oropharynx	531	0.09	0.00	0.00	0.01	0.00	0.01	0.00	0.00	0.02	0.04
鼻咽	Nasopharynx	7 090	1.16	0.06	0.01	0.00	0.02	0.07	0.07	0.16	0.41	0.78
下咽	Hypopharynx	823	0.13	0.03	0.01	0.00	0.00	0.00	0.00	0.00	0.00	0.01
咽,部位不明	Pharynx unspecified	752	0.12	0.03	0.01	0.00	0.00	0.00	0.00	0.01	0.01	0.02
食管	Esophagus	54 822	8.99	0.17	0.03	0.00	0.00	0.05	0.03	0.06	0.11	0.17
胃	Stomach	71 758	11.76	0.23	0.10	0.02	0.02	0.09	0.22	0.56	1.14	1.71
小肠	Small intestine	2 227	0.37	0.06	0.00	0.00	0.00	0.00	0.01	0.03	0.06	0.08
结肠	Colon	18 873	3.09	0.00	0.02	0.00	0.02	0.11	0.15	0.29	0.58	0.75
直肠	Rectum	26 533	4.35	0.09	0.03	0.01	0.01	0.09	0.12	0.30	0.56	0.75
肛门	Anus	998	0.16	0.00	0.00	0.00	0.00	0.00	0.00	0.01	0.02	0.05
肝脏	Liver	89 355	14.65	1.42	0.16	0.08	0.13	0.33	0.50	1.41	3.39	6.47
胆囊及其他	Gallbladder etc.	10 185	1.67	0.06	0.00	0.00	0.00	0.01	0.00	0.02	0.09	0.16
胰腺	Pancreas	20 386	3.34	0.06	0.01	0.00	0.00	0.03	0.04	0.08	0.18	0.49
鼻、鼻窦及其他	Nose, sinuses etc.	784	0.13	0.00	0.01	0.01	0.00	0.03	0.01	0.03	0.05	0.05
喉	Larynx	3 720	0.61	0.06	0.01	0.00	0.00	0.01	0.01	0.02	0.04	0.07
气管、支气管、肺	Trachea, bronchus & lung	170 106	27.88	1.48	0.08	0.04	0.04	0.24	0.29	0.68	1.55	2.91
其他胸腔器官	Other thoracic organs	1 577	0.26	0.06	0.02	0.03	0.04	0.05	0.05	0.07	0.10	0.09
骨	Bone	4 950	0.81	0.06	0.04	0.09	0.26	0.45	0.35	0.24	0.30	0.21
皮肤黑色素瘤	Melanoma of skin	892	0.15	0.00	0.00	0.00	0.00	0.01	0.00	0.01	0.05	0.04
皮肤其他	Other skin	3 213	0.53	0.03	0.02	0.03	0.00	0.02	0.03	0.04	0.09	0.09
间皮瘤	Mesothelioma	293	0.05	0.00	0.00	0.00	0.00	0.00	0.02	0.00	0.00	0.02
卡波西肉瘤	Kaposi sarcoma	67	0.01	0.00	0.01	0.00	0.00	0.01	0.01	0.01	0.00	0.02
结缔组织、软组织	Connective & soft tissue	1 080	0.18	0.11	0.08	0.05	0.06	0.05	0.07	0.10	0.11	0.11
乳腺	Breast	14 269	2.40	0.18	0.05	0.00	0.01	0.04	0.12	0.59	1.67	3.48
外阴	Vulva	305	0.05	0.00	0.00	0.00	0.00	0.00	0.00	0.00	0.04	0.04
阴道	Vagina	195	0.03	0.00	0.00	0.00	0.00	0.00	0.00	0.02	0.01	0.01
子宫颈	Cervix uteri	10 376	1.70	0.18	0.03	0.00	0.00	0.03	0.15	0.42	0.93	1.90
子宫体	Corpus uteri	3 231	0.53	0.06	0.01	0.00	0.00	0.01	0.05	0.06	0.22	0.30
子宫,部位不明	Uterus unspecified	1 613	0.26	0.18	0.00	0.00	0.00	0.03	0.03	0.05	0.11	0.20
卵巢	Ovary	5 444	0.89	0.06	0.00	0.00	0.06	0.10	0.20	0.26	0.21	0.68
其他女性生殖器官	Other female genital organs	285	0.05	0.00	0.00	0.00	0.00	0.00	0.00	0.02	0.01	0.00
胎盘	Placenta	18	0.00	0.00	0.00	0.00	0.00	0.00	0.02	0.04	0.03	
阴茎	Penis	494	0.08	0.00	0.00	0.00	0.00	0.00	0.00	0.04	0.05	0.05
前列腺	Prostate	7 911	1.30	0.00	0.03	0.00	0.00	0.01	0.02	0.02	0.02	0.02
睾丸	Testis	211	0.03	0.00	0.02	0.01	0.01	0.05	0.05	0.07	0.11	0.02
其他男性生殖器官	Other male genital organs	92	0.02	0.00	0.00	0.00	0.02	0.01	0.02	0.00	0.02	0.01
肾	Kidney	3 908	0.64	0.11	0.08	0.06	0.02	0.07	0.04	0.10	0.11	0.15
肾盂	Renal pelvis	588	0.10	0.00	0.00	0.00	0.00	0.00	0.00	0.00	0.02	0.01
输尿管	Ureter	628	0.10	0.00	0.00	0.00	0.00	0.00	0.00	0.01	0.00	0.00
膀胱	Bladder	8 035	1.32	0.00	0.02	0.00	0.00	0.00	0.01	0.02	0.04	0.10
其他泌尿器官	Other urinary organs	160	0.03	0.03	0.00	0.00	0.00	0.00	0.00	0.00	0.00	0.00
眼	Eye	249	0.04	0.06	0.15	0.03	0.01	0.00	0.00	0.00	0.01	0.02
脑、神经系统	Brain, nervous system	15 850	2.60	1.02	0.94	0.93	0.87	0.77	0.70	0.96	1.10	1.63
甲状腺	Thyroid	2 285	0.37	0.00	0.01	0.00	0.00	0.02	0.03	0.08	0.13	0.15
肾上腺	Adrenal gland	503	0.08	0.03	0.06	0.07	0.00	0.01	0.01	0.02	0.03	0.03
其他内分泌腺	Other endocrine	384	0.06	0.03	0.01	0.02	0.05	0.01	0.01	0.03	0.03	0.03
霍奇金淋巴瘤	Hodgkin lymphoma	540	0.09	0.00	0.00	0.02	0.02	0.00	0.03	0.05	0.03	
非霍奇金淋巴瘤	Non-Hodgkin lymphoma	7 744	1.27	0.14	0.13	0.13	0.17	0.26	0.31	0.27	0.31	0.54
免疫增生性疾病	Immunoproliferative diseases	52	0.01	0.00	0.00	0.00	0.00	0.00	0.00	0.00	0.00	0.00
多发性骨髓瘤	Multiple myeloma	3 028	0.50	0.00	0.02	0.01	0.03	0.04	0.04	0.03	0.03	0.07
淋巴细胞白血病	Lymphoid leukemia	2 374	0.39	0.45	0.30	0.32	0.31	0.43	0.30	0.33	0.40	0.28
髓系白血病	Myeloid leukemia	4 902	0.80	0.20	0.24	0.17	0.22	0.28	0.35	0.43	0.39	0.55
白血病,未特指	Leukemia unspecified	5 938	0.97	1.02	0.58	0.49	0.57	0.64	0.58	0.51	0.61	0.69
其他或未指明部位	Other and unspecified	12 514	2.05	0.28	0.35	0.25	0.30	0.33	0.32	0.44	0.42	0.70
所有部位合计	All sites	610 134	100.00	7.68	3.62	2.92	3.28	4.68	5.05	8.25	14.33	23.54
所有部位除外 C44	All sites except C44	606 921	99.47	7.65	3.60	2.89	3.27	4.66	5.02	8.21	14.24	23.45

Appendix Table 1-16　Cancer mortality in rural registration areas of China, both sexes in 2019

Age group										粗率 Crude rate/ 100 000⁻¹	中标率 ASR China/ 100 000⁻¹	世标率 ASR world/ 100 000⁻¹	累积率 Cum. Rate/%		ICD-10
40~44	45~49	50~54	55~59	60~64	65~69	70~74	75~79	80~84	85+				0~64	0~74	
0.03	0.04	0.06	0.09	0.16	0.27	0.43	0.68	0.64	1.68	0.10	0.05	0.05	0.00	0.01	C00
0.21	0.27	0.42	0.52	1.00	1.22	1.54	1.83	1.90	2.09	0.38	0.23	0.23	0.01	0.03	C01-C02
0.12	0.26	0.48	0.68	1.13	1.59	2.80	3.58	4.01	5.10	0.56	0.32	0.32	0.01	0.04	C03-C06
0.05	0.15	0.17	0.21	0.46	0.61	0.66	0.64	1.23	1.71	0.18	0.11	0.11	0.01	0.01	C07-C08
0.02	0.04	0.07	0.12	0.16	0.17	0.32	0.34	0.30	0.54	0.07	0.04	0.04	0.00	0.00	C09
0.05	0.05	0.13	0.22	0.36	0.62	0.70	0.70	0.68	0.79	0.15	0.09	0.09	0.00	0.01	C10
1.32	2.12	2.98	3.90	4.77	5.38	6.35	6.69	7.43	6.30	1.97	1.26	1.23	0.08	0.14	C11
0.03	0.13	0.27	0.47	0.67	0.89	1.04	0.87	1.06	0.57	0.23	0.13	0.14	0.01	0.02	C12-C13
0.05	0.08	0.13	0.24	0.46	0.57	1.13	1.36	1.85	1.66	0.21	0.12	0.12	0.01	0.01	C14
0.94	2.77	7.82	13.61	31.10	53.11	82.23	114.89	139.27	145.22	15.23	8.26	8.25	0.28	0.96	C15
3.04	6.31	11.90	19.52	39.70	64.69	101.27	142.17	176.74	184.34	19.94	11.10	10.98	0.42	1.25	C16
0.21	0.31	0.54	0.73	1.41	2.03	2.79	3.71	4.49	4.26	0.62	0.36	0.35	0.02	0.04	C17
1.21	2.13	3.70	5.38	9.39	14.57	22.71	33.53	49.68	64.04	5.24	2.94	2.90	0.12	0.30	C18
1.62	3.21	5.39	7.56	13.51	21.35	33.53	48.48	68.53	80.36	7.37	4.12	4.07	0.17	0.44	C19-C20
0.05	0.15	0.20	0.21	0.53	0.92	1.12	1.60	2.77	2.90	0.28	0.16	0.15	0.01	0.02	C21
13.33	21.47	32.34	39.51	57.99	73.79	92.42	112.14	124.31	131.70	24.82	15.20	14.91	0.89	1.72	C22
0.48	0.86	1.84	3.01	5.95	9.18	14.81	18.59	23.63	27.56	2.83	1.56	1.56	0.06	0.18	C23-C24
0.92	2.35	4.22	6.77	12.28	19.07	27.11	36.71	44.57	47.05	5.66	3.18	3.17	0.14	0.37	C25
0.11	0.13	0.27	0.27	0.50	0.62	0.75	1.09	1.15	1.85	0.22	0.13	0.13	0.01	0.01	C30-C31
0.17	0.32	0.73	1.34	2.34	3.43	5.25	7.06	7.84	7.52	1.03	0.58	0.58	0.03	0.07	C32
6.78	15.39	33.58	55.79	105.32	166.58	237.54	314.39	366.37	360.54	47.26	26.48	26.40	1.11	3.14	C33-C34
0.16	0.30	0.50	0.65	1.05	1.34	1.65	2.04	2.09	2.47	0.44	0.28	0.27	0.02	0.03	C37-C38
0.39	0.62	1.14	1.57	2.65	3.98	6.82	7.44	8.35	9.75	1.38	0.88	0.86	0.04	0.10	C40-C41
0.09	0.16	0.21	0.30	0.44	0.72	0.95	1.48	2.09	2.44	0.25	0.14	0.14	0.01	0.01	C43
0.19	0.31	0.38	0.63	0.98	1.65	2.70	5.51	10.25	24.65	0.89	0.46	0.47	0.01	0.04	C44
0.02	0.04	0.11	0.19	0.18	0.23	0.26	0.47	0.38	0.38	0.08	0.05	0.05	0.00	0.01	C45
0.01	0.02	0.02	0.01	0.03	0.06	0.02	0.10	0.06	0.11	0.02	0.01	0.01	0.00	0.00	C46
0.18	0.23	0.23	0.33	0.59	0.81	1.06	1.22	1.62	2.39	0.30	0.20	0.20	0.01	0.02	C47,C49
6.23	9.84	14.98	15.44	17.91	19.46	18.80	22.63	25.04	35.18	8.13	5.07	4.91	0.35	0.54	C50
0.04	0.06	0.19	0.20	0.32	0.42	0.66	1.01	1.54	1.26	0.17	0.10	0.09	0.00	0.01	C51
0.04	0.10	0.12	0.13	0.24	0.22	0.47	0.78	0.65	0.49	0.11	0.06	0.06	0.00	0.01	C52
3.76	6.92	10.05	11.04	12.26	13.99	18.21	22.07	20.98	20.24	5.91	3.63	3.51	0.24	0.40	C53
0.79	1.50	2.89	3.70	4.21	5.49	6.30	6.55	7.24	7.09	1.84	1.08	1.07	0.07	0.13	C54
0.42	0.69	1.23	1.23	1.91	2.51	3.68	4.17	4.85	4.76	0.92	0.53	0.52	0.03	0.06	C55
1.52	3.31	5.29	5.75	7.73	8.86	10.41	10.42	9.63	7.13	3.10	1.89	1.86	0.13	0.22	C56
0.07	0.11	0.23	0.33	0.40	0.36	0.58	0.73	0.72	0.85	0.16	0.09	0.09	0.01	0.01	C57
0.01	0.01	0.01	0.00	0.01	0.00	0.02	0.00	0.00	0.04	0.01	0.01	0.01	0.00	0.00	C58
0.08	0.19	0.25	0.32	0.44	0.80	0.95	1.57	2.69	4.06	0.27	0.16	0.16	0.01	0.02	C60
0.07	0.21	0.50	1.15	4.08	8.42	19.93	42.59	74.10	127.03	4.29	2.31	2.34	0.03	0.17	C61
0.06	0.11	0.09	0.15	0.11	0.27	0.25	0.51	0.84	1.37	0.11	0.08	0.08	0.00	0.01	C62
0.02	0.03	0.04	0.03	0.09	0.08	0.18	0.41	0.67	0.55	0.05	0.03	0.03	0.00	0.00	C63
0.30	0.52	0.88	1.68	2.25	3.21	4.62	6.12	8.16	8.88	1.09	0.64	0.64	0.03	0.07	C64
0.01	0.05	0.12	0.14	0.31	0.47	0.80	1.13	1.43	2.01	0.16	0.09	0.09	0.00	0.01	C65
0.00	0.03	0.07	0.16	0.28	0.55	1.12	1.38	1.68	1.76	0.17	0.09	0.09	0.00	0.01	C66
0.18	0.36	0.80	1.16	2.58	5.17	9.56	17.98	30.04	44.44	2.23	1.13	1.13	0.03	0.10	C67
0.00	0.01	0.03	0.04	0.09	0.14	0.13	0.32	0.41	0.62	0.04	0.02	0.02	0.00	0.00	C68
0.03	0.04	0.03	0.04	0.06	0.14	0.30	0.41	0.41	0.98	0.07	0.05	0.05	0.00	0.00	C69
2.32	3.33	4.74	6.19	8.99	12.25	15.75	18.37	21.86	24.11	4.40	2.95	2.93	0.17	0.31	C70-C72,D32-D33,D42-D43
0.28	0.39	0.58	0.88	1.41	1.78	2.50	3.26	4.45	5.02	0.63	0.38	0.37	0.02	0.04	C73
0.05	0.07	0.11	0.18	0.35	0.41	0.55	0.65	0.79	0.95	0.14	0.09	0.09	0.00	0.01	C74
0.06	0.06	0.08	0.13	0.21	0.28	0.43	0.44	0.64	0.87	0.11	0.07	0.07	0.00	0.01	C75
0.03	0.08	0.18	0.16	0.32	0.43	0.65	0.70	1.13	0.98	0.15	0.09	0.09	0.00	0.01	C81
0.69	1.21	1.75	2.65	4.66	6.88	9.47	12.62	13.49	12.27	2.15	1.33	1.31	0.07	0.15	C82-C86,C96
0.00	0.01	0.00	0.02	0.04	0.07	0.04	0.12	0.11	0.08	0.01	0.01	0.01	0.00	0.00	C88
0.12	0.35	0.69	1.17	2.08	3.30	4.33	4.81	5.18	3.45	0.84	0.49	0.49	0.02	0.05	C90
0.32	0.43	0.58	0.74	1.08	1.50	1.95	2.71	2.79	2.80	0.66	0.51	0.51	0.03	0.05	C91
0.61	0.92	1.24	1.59	2.72	3.60	5.75	6.49	7.44	7.11	1.36	0.92	0.90	0.05	0.10	C92-C94,D45-D47
0.77	0.97	1.50	1.75	2.88	4.30	6.08	8.19	8.25	7.90	1.65	1.18	1.18	0.06	0.11	C95
1.03	1.77	3.11	4.30	6.82	10.70	14.73	19.44	23.77	29.05	3.48	2.10	2.09	0.10	0.23	O & U
44.98	82.22	144.15	206.63	357.11	535.56	769.81	1 032.19	1 260.12	1 373.01	169.51	98.10	97.21	4.51	11.03	C00-C97,D32-D33, D42-D43,D45-D47
44.79	81.91	143.77	206.00	356.13	533.91	767.11	1 026.68	1 249.87	1 348.36	168.61	97.65	96.74	4.49	11.00	C00-C97,D32-D33, D42-D43,D45-D47 exc. C44

部位 Site		死亡数 No. deaths	构成 Freq. /%	年龄组								
				0~	1~4	5~9	10~14	15~19	20~24	25~29	30~34	35~39
唇	Lip	236	0.06	0.00	0.00	0.00	0.01	0.00	0.00	0.00	0.01	0.01
舌	Tongue	1 009	0.26	0.00	0.00	0.01	0.00	0.00	0.02	0.02	0.08	0.13
口	Mouth	1 405	0.36	0.00	0.00	0.01	0.01	0.01	0.02	0.05	0.04	0.12
唾液腺	Salivary gland	427	0.11	0.00	0.00	0.00	0.00	0.04	0.01	0.03	0.01	0.02
扁桃体	Tonsil	194	0.05	0.00	0.00	0.00	0.00	0.01	0.01	0.00	0.00	0.02
其他口咽	Other oropharynx	459	0.12	0.00	0.00	0.01	0.00	0.00	0.00	0.00	0.03	0.07
鼻咽	Nasopharynx	5 276	1.34	0.11	0.02	0.00	0.03	0.07	0.10	0.22	0.54	1.26
下咽	Hypopharynx	762	0.19	0.05	0.01	0.00	0.00	0.01	0.01	0.00	0.01	0.01
咽,部位不明	Pharynx unspecified	575	0.15	0.05	0.00	0.01	0.00	0.00	0.00	0.01	0.02	0.03
食管	Esophagus	40 325	10.21	0.32	0.06	0.01	0.00	0.08	0.03	0.09	0.20	0.30
胃	Stomach	50 089	12.68	0.22	0.10	0.02	0.02	0.10	0.24	0.52	1.13	1.77
小肠	Small intestine	1 332	0.34	0.00	0.00	0.00	0.00	0.00	0.00	0.04	0.08	0.08
结肠	Colon	10 730	2.72	0.00	0.03	0.00	0.01	0.16	0.17	0.34	0.71	0.88
直肠	Rectum	16 505	4.18	0.05	0.03	0.01	0.02	0.11	0.17	0.38	0.65	0.82
肛门	Anus	587	0.15	0.00	0.00	0.00	0.00	0.01	0.01	0.01	0.03	0.06
肝脏	Liver	66 411	16.81	1.73	0.16	0.11	0.17	0.45	0.72	2.26	5.65	10.96
胆囊及其他	Gallbladder etc.	4 909	1.24	0.05	0.00	0.00	0.01	0.00	0.02	0.11	0.17
胰腺	Pancreas	11 876	3.01	0.11	0.00	0.01	0.01	0.03	0.08	0.09	0.23	0.65
鼻、鼻窦及其他	Nose, sinuses etc.	503	0.13	0.00	0.01	0.00	0.00	0.02	0.02	0.04	0.03	0.09
喉	Larynx	3 265	0.83	0.05	0.00	0.01	0.00	0.01	0.02	0.01	0.06	0.11
气管、支气管、肺	Trachea, bronchus & lung	119 744	30.31	1.95	0.08	0.04	0.04	0.31	0.36	0.76	1.99	3.40
其他胸腔器官	Other thoracic organs	1 061	0.27	0.05	0.01	0.05	0.06	0.08	0.10	0.12	0.12	0.13
骨	Bone	3 043	0.77	0.11	0.06	0.08	0.26	0.51	0.47	0.33	0.39	0.27
皮肤黑色素瘤	Melanoma of skin	469	0.12	0.00	0.00	0.01	0.00	0.00	0.00	0.01	0.05	0.02
皮肤其他	Other skin	1 716	0.43	0.00	0.01	0.04	0.00	0.03	0.03	0.05	0.11	0.12
间皮瘤	Mesothelioma	159	0.04	0.00	0.00	0.00	0.00	0.00	0.01	0.00	0.02
卡波西肉瘤	Kaposi sarcoma	44	0.01	0.00	0.00	0.01	0.01	0.01	0.01	0.01	0.01	0.03
结缔组织、软组织	Connective & soft tissue	629	0.16	0.00	0.09	0.08	0.07	0.05	0.08	0.12	0.12	0.13
乳腺	Breast	373	0.09	0.00	0.00	0.00	0.00	0.00	0.01	0.00	0.00	0.02
外阴	Vulva	—	—	—	—	—	—	—	—	—	—	—
阴道	Vagina	—	—	—	—	—	—	—	—	—	—	—
子宫颈	Cervix uteri	—	—	—	—	—	—	—	—	—	—	—
子宫体	Corpus uteri	—	—	—	—	—	—	—	—	—	—	—
子宫,部位不明	Uterus unspecified	—	—	—	—	—	—	—	—	—	—	—
卵巢	Ovary	—	—	—	—	—	—	—	—	—	—	—
其他女性生殖器官	Other female genital organs	—	—	—	—	—	—	—	—	—	—	—
胎盘	Placenta	—	—	—	—	—	—	—	—	—	—	—
阴茎	Penis	494	0.13	0.00	0.00	0.00	0.00	0.00	0.00	0.04	0.05	0.05
前列腺	Prostate	7 911	2.00	0.00	0.03	0.00	0.01	0.02	0.00	0.02	0.02	0.02
睾丸	Testis	211	0.05	0.00	0.02	0.01	0.00	0.05	0.05	0.07	0.11	0.02
其他男性生殖器官	Other male genital organs	92	0.02	0.00	0.00	0.00	0.02	0.01	0.02	0.00	0.02	0.01
肾	Kidney	2 583	0.65	0.11	0.07	0.04	0.02	0.08	0.03	0.13	0.15	0.17
肾盂	Renal pelvis	363	0.09	0.00	0.00	0.00	0.00	0.00	0.00	0.00	0.04	0.02
输尿管	Ureter	349	0.09	0.00	0.00	0.00	0.00	0.00	0.00	0.01	0.00	0.00
膀胱	Bladder	6 400	1.62	0.00	0.02	0.00	0.01	0.00	0.03	0.02	0.08	0.11
其他泌尿器官	Other urinary organs	99	0.03	0.05	0.00	0.00	0.00	0.01	0.00	0.00	0.01	0.01
眼	Eye	142	0.04	0.05	0.18	0.04	0.02	0.01	0.00	0.01	0.00	0.02
脑、神经系统	Brain, nervous system	8 773	2.22	1.14	0.90	1.05	0.97	0.78	0.77	1.08	1.27	1.96
甲状腺	Thyroid	838	0.21	0.00	0.00	0.01	0.00	0.01	0.02	0.02	0.09	0.10
肾上腺	Adrenal gland	297	0.08	0.00	0.06	0.06	0.00	0.01	0.00	0.02	0.01	0.04
其他内分泌腺	Other endocrine	215	0.05	0.05	0.01	0.02	0.02	0.01	0.00	0.02	0.02	0.05
霍奇金淋巴瘤	Hodgkin lymphoma	350	0.09	0.00	0.00	0.04	0.02	0.01	0.01	0.04	0.07	0.06
非霍奇金淋巴瘤	Non-Hodgkin lymphoma	4 795	1.21	0.16	0.13	0.18	0.21	0.29	0.40	0.31	0.41	0.57
免疫增生性疾病	Immunoproliferative diseases	41	0.01	0.00	0.00	0.00	0.00	0.00	0.00	0.00	0.00	0.00
多发性骨髓瘤	Multiple myeloma	1 761	0.45	0.00	0.02	0.02	0.04	0.00	0.04	0.03	0.03	0.10
淋巴细胞白血病	Lymphoid leukemia	1 388	0.35	0.38	0.33	0.30	0.30	0.56	0.38	0.40	0.50	0.27
髓系白血病	Myeloid leukemia	2 907	0.74	0.22	0.32	0.17	0.21	0.29	0.38	0.56	0.48	0.59
白血病,未特指	Leukemia unspecified	3 446	0.87	0.92	0.63	0.50	0.57	0.75	0.70	0.62	0.72	0.87
其他或未指明部位	Other and unspecified	7 457	1.89	0.38	0.36	0.31	0.35	0.34	0.31	0.43	0.51	0.81
所有部位合计	All sites	395 025	100.00	8.32	3.81	3.25	3.48	5.33	5.83	9.41	17.00	27.52
所有部位除外 C44	All sites except C44	393 309	99.57	8.32	3.80	3.22	3.48	5.30	5.80	9.35	16.89	27.40

Appendix Table 1-17　Cancer mortality in rural registration areas of China, male in 2019

Age group										粗率 Crude rate/ 100 000⁻¹	中标率 ASR China/ 100 000⁻¹	世标率 ASR world/ 100 000⁻¹	累积率 Cum. Rate/%		ICD-10
40~44	45~49	50~54	55~59	60~64	65~69	70~74	75~79	80~84	85+				0~64	0~74	
0.05	0.08	0.10	0.12	0.22	0.37	0.67	0.98	0.84	2.06	0.13	0.08	0.08	0.00	0.01	C00
0.32	0.41	0.69	0.88	1.56	1.84	2.16	2.65	2.23	3.16	0.55	0.35	0.34	0.02	0.04	C01-C02
0.18	0.40	0.75	1.06	1.74	2.32	3.88	5.14	5.09	7.08	0.76	0.46	0.46	0.02	0.05	C03-C06
0.06	0.20	0.21	0.30	0.62	0.83	0.88	0.98	1.85	2.27	0.23	0.14	0.14	0.01	0.02	C07-C08
0.05	0.07	0.12	0.20	0.32	0.26	0.55	0.49	0.46	0.76	0.11	0.07	0.07	0.00	0.01	C09
0.08	0.11	0.22	0.39	0.66	1.08	1.15	1.26	1.34	1.51	0.25	0.15	0.15	0.01	0.02	C10
2.10	3.19	4.53	6.05	6.95	8.01	9.81	10.02	10.63	8.59	2.86	1.90	1.84	0.13	0.21	C11
0.06	0.25	0.51	0.90	1.24	1.66	1.98	1.62	2.06	1.17	0.41	0.25	0.26	0.02	0.03	C12-C13
0.05	0.13	0.20	0.40	0.77	0.94	1.75	2.13	2.77	2.82	0.31	0.19	0.19	0.01	0.02	C14
1.57	4.68	13.42	23.64	50.98	84.38	124.70	167.62	196.32	199.69	21.87	12.75	12.77	0.48	1.52	C15
3.42	7.98	16.65	28.04	59.77	97.53	152.13	209.30	252.85	259.56	27.17	16.04	15.91	0.60	1.85	C16
0.27	0.37	0.75	0.96	1.70	2.34	3.36	4.42	5.46	6.32	0.72	0.44	0.44	0.02	0.05	C17
1.34	2.38	4.23	6.38	11.50	17.78	26.91	40.02	57.29	79.53	5.82	3.49	3.46	0.14	0.36	C18
1.81	3.95	6.82	9.81	17.95	28.40	44.18	64.23	87.63	103.93	8.95	5.33	5.28	0.21	0.58	C19-C20
0.06	0.17	0.26	0.24	0.61	1.22	1.45	2.00	3.36	3.64	0.32	0.19	0.19	0.01	0.02	C21
22.25	35.98	52.58	64.04	88.80	110.12	128.78	154.90	168.88	179.06	36.02	23.26	22.76	1.42	2.62	C22
0.52	0.87	1.88	3.04	5.97	9.14	15.25	18.68	22.28	27.70	2.66	1.57	1.57	0.06	0.18	C23-C24
1.22	3.07	5.46	8.77	15.22	22.64	31.57	43.10	51.36	55.75	6.44	3.85	3.84	0.17	0.45	C25
0.11	0.18	0.36	0.38	0.67	0.78	1.03	1.46	1.43	2.75	0.27	0.17	0.17	0.01	0.02	C30-C31
0.29	0.55	1.33	2.48	4.29	6.28	9.37	12.49	14.42	14.85	1.77	1.05	1.05	0.05	0.12	C32
8.54	20.26	47.31	81.66	155.74	247.87	349.39	460.52	534.12	524.34	64.95	38.45	38.41	1.60	4.59	C33-C34
0.20	0.40	0.63	0.89	1.46	1.87	2.30	2.78	2.82	3.64	0.58	0.38	0.38	0.02	0.04	C37-C38
0.50	0.79	1.49	1.87	3.45	4.88	8.73	9.69	10.42	11.96	1.65	1.10	1.08	0.05	0.12	C40-C41
0.08	0.15	0.24	0.23	0.48	0.83	1.12	1.85	2.27	2.96	0.25	0.15	0.15	0.01	0.02	C43
0.20	0.39	0.47	0.75	1.24	2.20	3.55	6.60	11.98	23.30	0.93	0.54	0.54	0.02	0.05	C44
0.02	0.05	0.12	0.21	0.24	0.26	0.32	0.33	0.55	0.55	0.09	0.05	0.05	0.00	0.01	C45
0.02	0.03	0.03	0.02	0.04	0.08	0.03	0.13	0.13	0.00	0.02	0.02	0.02	0.00	0.00	C46
0.15	0.30	0.27	0.39	0.72	1.01	1.15	1.52	2.10	3.02	0.34	0.24	0.24	0.01	0.02	C47,C49
0.04	0.15	0.21	0.35	0.49	0.65	0.93	1.11	1.56	1.51	0.20	0.12	0.12	0.01	0.01	C50
—	—	—	—	—	—	—	—	—	—	—	—	—	—	—	C51
—	—	—	—	—	—	—	—	—	—	—	—	—	—	—	C52
—	—	—	—	—	—	—	—	—	—	—	—	—	—	—	C53
—	—	—	—	—	—	—	—	—	—	—	—	—	—	—	C54
—	—	—	—	—	—	—	—	—	—	—	—	—	—	—	C55
—	—	—	—	—	—	—	—	—	—	—	—	—	—	—	C56
—	—	—	—	—	—	—	—	—	—	—	—	—	—	—	C57
—	—	—	—	—	—	—	—	—	—	—	—	—	—	—	C58
0.08	0.19	0.25	0.32	0.44	0.80	0.95	1.57	2.69	4.06	0.27	0.16	0.16	0.01	0.02	C60
0.07	0.21	0.50	1.15	4.08	8.42	19.93	42.59	74.10	127.03	4.29	2.31	2.34	0.03	0.17	C61
0.06	0.11	0.09	0.15	0.11	0.27	0.25	0.51	0.84	1.37	0.11	0.08	0.08	0.00	0.01	C62
0.02	0.03	0.04	0.03	0.09	0.08	0.18	0.41	0.67	0.55	0.05	0.03	0.03	0.00	0.00	C63
0.33	0.75	1.10	2.32	3.12	4.40	6.43	8.46	10.97	13.47	1.40	0.86	0.86	0.04	0.10	C64
0.02	0.06	0.20	0.20	0.45	0.59	1.03	1.21	1.93	2.41	0.20	0.12	0.12	0.00	0.01	C65
0.01	0.04	0.09	0.21	0.35	0.68	1.32	1.44	1.68	1.92	0.19	0.11	0.11	0.00	0.01	C66
0.18	0.52	1.22	1.94	4.33	8.48	15.52	29.76	54.64	85.65	3.47	1.92	1.94	0.04	0.16	C67
0.01	0.02	0.05	0.06	0.10	0.16	0.20	0.33	0.50	1.10	0.05	0.03	0.03	0.00	0.00	C68
0.04	0.05	0.05	0.07	0.09	0.18	0.33	0.57	0.25	0.96	0.08	0.05	0.06	0.00	0.01	C69
2.91	3.89	5.52	6.92	10.42	13.76	17.30	19.89	23.37	24.68	4.76	3.33	3.29	0.19	0.35	C70-C72,D32-D33,D42-D43
0.26	0.25	0.35	0.70	1.23	1.39	1.96	2.49	3.15	3.44	0.45	0.29	0.28	0.02	0.03	C73
0.07	0.08	0.10	0.25	0.43	0.56	0.60	0.72	1.09	1.58	0.16	0.10	0.11	0.01	0.01	C74
0.08	0.04	0.08	0.17	0.26	0.31	0.45	0.59	0.84	1.31	0.12	0.08	0.08	0.00	0.01	C75
0.03	0.09	0.24	0.22	0.46	0.56	0.78	0.87	1.51	1.51	0.19	0.12	0.12	0.01	0.01	C81
0.88	1.58	2.14	3.61	5.79	8.78	12.17	15.52	17.23	16.36	2.60	1.68	1.65	0.08	0.19	C82-C86,C96
0.00	0.01	0.01	0.02	0.07	0.09	0.08	0.21	0.21	0.21	0.02	0.01	0.01	0.00	0.00	C88
0.14	0.38	0.69	1.29	2.33	4.08	5.53	5.86	6.60	4.74	0.96	0.58	0.58	0.03	0.07	C90
0.32	0.41	0.58	0.76	1.27	1.86	2.61	3.68	3.28	4.33	0.75	0.60	0.59	0.03	0.05	C91
0.77	0.95	1.49	1.84	3.14	4.42	6.94	7.92	10.21	10.52	1.58	1.09	1.07	0.06	0.11	C92-C94,D45-D47
0.84	1.15	1.75	2.07	3.25	4.79	7.13	9.97	10.80	10.59	1.87	1.38	1.37	0.07	0.13	C95
1.15	2.24	3.81	5.30	8.51	13.64	18.17	23.80	29.84	33.96	4.04	2.56	2.55	0.12	0.28	O & U
53.81	100.59	182.17	274.00	485.71	735.86	1 048.95	1 406.37	1 710.93	1 885.23	214.26	130.31	129.43	5.86	14.79	C00-C97,D32-D33, D42-D43,D45-D47
53.61	100.20	181.70	273.25	484.47	733.67	1 045.40	1 399.77	1 698.95	1 861.93	213.33	129.78	128.89	5.85	14.74	C00-C97,D32-D33, D42-D43, D45-D47 exc. C44

部位 Site		死亡数 No. deaths	构成 Freq. /%	年龄组								
				0~	1~4	5~9	10~14	15~19	20~24	25~29	30~34	35~39
唇	Lip	115	0.05	0.00	0.00	0.01	0.00	0.00	0.00	0.00	0.01	0.01
舌	Tongue	366	0.17	0.00	0.00	0.00	0.00	0.00	0.00	0.05	0.04	0.04
口	Mouth	601	0.28	0.00	0.01	0.00	0.00	0.01	0.00	0.00	0.01	0.03
唾液腺	Salivary gland	222	0.10	0.00	0.00	0.00	0.01	0.00	0.03	0.02	0.01	0.03
扁桃体	Tonsil	45	0.02	0.00	0.00	0.00	0.00	0.00	0.00	0.00	0.00	0.00
其他口咽	Other oropharynx	72	0.03	0.00	0.00	0.01	0.00	0.01	0.00	0.00	0.01	0.00
鼻咽	Nasopharynx	1 814	0.84	0.00	0.00	0.00	0.01	0.06	0.04	0.08	0.26	0.28
下咽	Hypopharynx	61	0.03	0.00	0.00	0.00	0.00	0.00	0.00	0.00	0.00	0.01
咽,部位不明	Pharynx unspecified	177	0.08	0.00	0.01	0.00	0.00	0.00	0.01	0.00	0.00	0.02
食管	Esophagus	14 497	6.74	0.00	0.00	0.00	0.01	0.01	0.03	0.03	0.02	0.03
胃	Stomach	21 669	10.07	0.24	0.09	0.02	0.02	0.06	0.21	0.59	1.15	1.65
小肠	Small intestine	895	0.42	0.12	0.00	0.00	0.00	0.00	0.02	0.02	0.04	0.08
结肠	Colon	8 143	3.79	0.00	0.00	0.00	0.03	0.04	0.12	0.23	0.45	0.61
直肠	Rectum	10 028	4.66	0.12	0.03	0.01	0.00	0.06	0.07	0.21	0.47	0.68
肛门	Anus	411	0.19	0.00	0.00	0.00	0.00	0.00	0.00	0.01	0.01	0.03
肝脏	Liver	22 944	10.67	1.08	0.15	0.04	0.07	0.19	0.26	0.49	1.00	1.71
胆囊及其他	Gallbladder etc.	5 276	2.45	0.06	0.00	0.00	0.01	0.01	0.02	0.07	0.15	
胰腺	Pancreas	8 510	3.96	0.00	0.03	0.00	0.00	0.02	0.00	0.07	0.13	0.32
鼻、鼻窦及其他	Nose, sinuses etc.	281	0.13	0.00	0.00	0.01	0.00	0.03	0.01	0.02	0.07	0.02
喉	Larynx	455	0.21	0.06	0.01	0.00	0.00	0.01	0.00	0.02	0.01	0.03
气管、支气管、肺	Trachea, bronchus & lung	50 362	23.41	0.96	0.08	0.04	0.04	0.15	0.21	0.60	1.09	2.39
其他胸腔器官	Other thoracic organs	516	0.24	0.06	0.04	0.01	0.00	0.01	0.00	0.02	0.08	0.04
骨	Bone	1 907	0.89	0.00	0.03	0.10	0.26	0.38	0.22	0.15	0.21	0.15
皮肤黑色素瘤	Melanoma of skin	423	0.20	0.00	0.00	0.00	0.01	0.00	0.00	0.01	0.06	0.06
皮肤其他	Other skin	1 497	0.70	0.06	0.04	0.02	0.01	0.01	0.03	0.02	0.07	0.07
间皮瘤	Mesothelioma	134	0.06	0.00	0.00	0.00	0.00	0.00	0.01	0.04	0.01	0.01
卡波西肉瘤	Kaposi sarcoma	23	0.01	0.00	0.01	0.00	0.00	0.00	0.01	0.01	0.00	0.01
结缔组织、软组织	Connective & soft tissue	451	0.21	0.24	0.08	0.02	0.04	0.05	0.07	0.09	0.09	0.08
乳腺	Breast	14 269	6.63	0.18	0.05	0.01	0.01	0.04	0.12	0.59	1.67	3.48
外阴	Vulva	305	0.14	0.00	0.00	0.00	0.00	0.00	0.00	0.00	0.04	0.04
阴道	Vagina	195	0.09	0.00	0.00	0.00	0.00	0.00	0.00	0.02	0.01	0.01
子宫颈	Cervix uteri	10 376	4.82	0.18	0.03	0.01	0.00	0.03	0.15	0.42	0.93	1.90
子宫体	Corpus uteri	3 231	1.50	0.06	0.01	0.00	0.00	0.00	0.05	0.06	0.22	0.30
子宫,部位不明	Uterus unspecified	1 613	0.75	0.18	0.00	0.00	0.00	0.03	0.03	0.05	0.11	0.20
卵巢	Ovary	5 444	2.53	0.06	0.00	0.00	0.06	0.10	0.20	0.26	0.21	0.68
其他女性生殖器官	Other female genital organs	285	0.13	0.00	0.00	0.00	0.00	0.00	0.00	0.02	0.01	0.00
胎盘	Placenta	18	0.01	0.00	0.00	0.00	0.00	0.01	0.00	0.02	0.04	0.03
阴茎	Penis	—	—	—	—	—	—	—	—	—	—	—
前列腺	Prostate	—	—	—	—	—	—	—	—	—	—	—
睾丸	Testis	—	—	—	—	—	—	—	—	—	—	—
其他男性生殖器官	Other male genital organs	—	—	—	—	—	—	—	—	—	—	—
肾	Kidney	1 325	0.62	0.12	0.09	0.07	0.02	0.04	0.04	0.07	0.07	0.12
肾盂	Renal pelvis	225	0.10	0.00	0.00	0.01	0.00	0.00	0.01	0.01	0.00	0.00
输尿管	Ureter	279	0.13	0.00	0.00	0.00	0.00	0.00	0.00	0.00	0.00	0.00
膀胱	Bladder	1 635	0.76	0.00	0.01	0.00	0.00	0.00	0.00	0.01	0.00	0.09
其他泌尿器官	Other urinary organs	61	0.03	0.00	0.00	0.00	0.00	0.00	0.00	0.00	0.00	0.00
眼	Eye	107	0.05	0.06	0.12	0.02	0.00	0.00	0.01	0.00	0.03	0.02
脑、神经系统	Brain, nervous system	7 077	3.29	0.90	0.99	0.80	0.75	0.75	0.62	0.83	0.92	1.28
甲状腺	Thyroid	1 447	0.67	0.00	0.00	0.00	0.01	0.02	0.05	0.15	0.17	0.20
肾上腺	Adrenal gland	206	0.10	0.06	0.06	0.08	0.00	0.01	0.02	0.01	0.04	0.03
其他内分泌腺	Other endocrine	169	0.08	0.00	0.01	0.03	0.08	0.01	0.00	0.03	0.03	0.02
霍奇金淋巴瘤	Hodgkin lymphoma	190	0.09	0.00	0.00	0.00	0.02	0.03	0.00	0.01	0.02	0.01
非霍奇金淋巴瘤	Non-Hodgkin lymphoma	2 949	1.37	0.12	0.13	0.07	0.13	0.23	0.21	0.23	0.21	0.50
免疫增生性疾病	Immunoproliferative diseases	11	0.01	0.00	0.00	0.00	0.00	0.00	0.00	0.00	0.00	0.00
多发性骨髓瘤	Multiple myeloma	1 267	0.59	0.00	0.03	0.00	0.00	0.03	0.08	0.03	0.02	0.04
淋巴细胞白血病	Lymphoid leukemia	986	0.46	0.54	0.26	0.34	0.33	0.29	0.21	0.25	0.28	0.28
髓系白血病	Myeloid leukemia	1 995	0.93	0.18	0.15	0.17	0.24	0.27	0.33	0.29	0.29	0.51
白血病,未特指	Leukemia unspecified	2 492	1.16	1.14	0.53	0.47	0.57	0.51	0.45	0.39	0.49	0.49
其他或未指明部位	Other and unspecified	5 057	2.35	0.18	0.35	0.17	0.25	0.31	0.32	0.44	0.33	0.58
所有部位合计	All sites	215 109	100.00	6.96	3.41	2.53	3.04	3.93	4.20	6.99	11.53	19.32
所有部位除外 C44	All sites except C44	213 612	99.30	6.90	3.38	2.51	3.03	3.92	4.17	6.97	11.46	19.26

Appendix Table 1-18　Cancer mortality in rural registration areas of China, female in 2019

40~44	45~49	50~54	55~59	60~64	65~69	70~74	75~79	80~84	85+	粗率 Crude rate/ 100 000⁻¹	中标率 ASR China/ 100 000⁻¹	世标率 ASR world/ 100 000⁻¹	累积率 Cum. Rate/% 0~64	0~74	ICD-10
0.02	0.00	0.02	0.06	0.10	0.17	0.19	0.40	0.48	1.44	0.07	0.03	0.03	0.00	0.00	C00
0.09	0.12	0.15	0.16	0.42	0.62	0.92	1.08	1.64	1.39	0.21	0.12	0.11	0.01	0.01	C01-C02
0.05	0.12	0.21	0.29	0.50	0.87	1.75	2.15	3.14	3.81	0.34	0.17	0.17	0.01	0.02	C03-C06
0.04	0.10	0.12	0.11	0.29	0.39	0.45	0.33	0.72	1.35	0.13	0.07	0.07	0.00	0.01	C07-C08
0.00	0.01	0.02	0.03	0.01	0.08	0.10	0.21	0.17	0.40	0.03	0.01	0.01	0.00	0.00	C09
0.02	0.00	0.03	0.05	0.06	0.17	0.26	0.19	0.14	0.31	0.04	0.02	0.02	0.00	0.00	C10
0.51	1.00	1.40	1.73	2.54	2.79	3.00	3.63	4.82	4.80	1.03	0.62	0.61	0.04	0.07	C11
0.01	0.02	0.03	0.03	0.09	0.13	0.13	0.19	0.24	0.18	0.03	0.02	0.02	0.00	0.00	C12-C13
0.04	0.03	0.05	0.08	0.15	0.20	0.53	0.66	1.09	0.90	0.10	0.05	0.05	0.00	0.01	C14
0.28	0.78	2.08	3.44	10.70	22.27	40.93	66.53	92.90	109.67	8.26	3.95	3.91	0.09	0.40	C15
2.63	4.57	7.02	10.87	19.10	32.31	51.83	80.60	114.87	135.24	12.34	6.42	6.30	0.24	0.66	C16
0.15	0.25	0.33	0.49	1.11	1.72	2.23	3.06	3.69	2.92	0.51	0.28	0.28	0.01	0.03	C17
1.07	1.87	3.17	4.36	7.23	11.41	18.62	27.58	43.49	53.94	4.64	2.41	2.37	0.10	0.25	C18
1.42	2.45	3.93	5.29	8.95	14.40	23.19	34.04	52.99	64.97	5.71	2.97	2.93	0.12	0.31	C19-C20
0.03	0.12	0.14	0.19	0.44	0.63	1.02	1.23	2.29	2.42	0.23	0.12	0.12	0.00	0.01	C21
3.94	6.40	11.58	14.62	26.39	37.96	57.07	72.91	88.08	100.78	13.07	7.15	7.09	0.34	0.81	C22
0.43	0.85	1.79	2.99	5.92	9.21	14.38	18.51	24.74	27.46	3.00	1.55	1.55	0.06	0.18	C23-C24
0.60	1.61	2.95	4.74	9.27	15.54	22.78	30.86	39.05	41.37	4.85	2.52	2.51	0.10	0.29	C25
0.10	0.08	0.18	0.16	0.33	0.46	0.47	0.75	0.92	1.26	0.16	0.10	0.09	0.01	0.01	C30-C31
0.04	0.08	0.11	0.18	0.34	0.62	1.25	2.07	2.49	2.74	0.26	0.13	0.13	0.00	0.01	C32
4.92	10.33	19.50	29.54	53.59	86.42	128.78	180.34	230.01	253.61	28.68	15.03	14.93	0.61	1.69	C33-C34
0.11	0.21	0.38	0.42	0.62	0.82	1.02	1.37	1.50	1.71	0.29	0.17	0.17	0.01	0.02	C37-C38
0.28	0.44	0.79	1.27	1.83	3.08	4.97	5.37	6.66	8.30	1.09	0.66	0.65	0.03	0.07	C40-C41
0.10	0.16	0.17	0.38	0.39	0.62	0.79	1.13	1.95	2.11	0.24	0.14	0.13	0.01	0.01	C43
0.18	0.22	0.28	0.51	0.72	1.10	1.88	4.50	8.85	25.53	0.85	0.37	0.40	0.01	0.03	C44
0.02	0.04	0.09	0.17	0.13	0.21	0.21	0.59	0.24	0.27	0.08	0.05	0.04	0.00	0.00	C45
0.01	0.01	0.01	0.01	0.03	0.04	0.00	0.07	0.00	0.18	0.01	0.01	0.01	0.00	0.00	C46
0.21	0.16	0.19	0.26	0.45	0.61	0.97	0.94	1.23	1.97	0.26	0.17	0.17	0.01	0.02	C47,C49
6.23	9.84	14.98	15.44	17.91	19.46	18.80	22.63	25.04	35.18	8.13	5.07	4.91	0.35	0.54	C50
0.04	0.06	0.19	0.20	0.32	0.42	0.66	1.01	1.54	1.26	0.17	0.10	0.09	0.00	0.01	C51
0.04	0.10	0.12	0.13	0.24	0.22	0.47	0.78	0.65	0.49	0.11	0.06	0.06	0.00	0.01	C52
3.76	6.92	10.05	11.04	12.26	13.99	18.21	22.07	20.98	20.24	5.91	3.63	3.51	0.24	0.40	C53
0.79	1.50	2.89	3.70	4.21	5.49	6.30	6.55	7.24	7.09	1.84	1.08	1.07	0.07	0.13	C54
0.42	0.69	1.23	1.23	1.91	2.51	3.68	4.17	4.85	4.76	0.92	0.53	0.52	0.03	0.06	C55
1.52	3.31	5.29	5.75	7.73	8.86	10.41	10.42	9.63	7.13	3.10	1.89	1.86	0.13	0.22	C56
0.07	0.11	0.23	0.33	0.40	0.36	0.58	0.73	0.72	0.85	0.16	0.09	0.09	0.01	0.01	C57
0.01	0.01	0.01	0.00	0.01	0.00	0.02	0.00	0.00	0.04	0.01	0.01	0.01	—	—	C58
—	—	—	—	—	—	—	—	—	—	—	—	—	—	—	C60
—	—	—	—	—	—	—	—	—	—	—	—	—	—	—	C61
—	—	—	—	—	—	—	—	—	—	—	—	—	—	—	C62
—	—	—	—	—	—	—	—	—	—	—	—	—	—	—	C63
0.26	0.29	0.65	1.03	1.36	2.04	2.87	3.98	5.88	5.88	0.75	0.42	0.42	0.02	0.05	C64
0.00	0.05	0.04	0.08	0.18	0.35	0.58	1.06	1.02	1.75	0.13	0.06	0.06	0.00	0.01	C65
0.00	0.02	0.05	0.10	0.20	0.42	0.92	1.32	1.67	1.66	0.16	0.08	0.08	0.00	0.01	C66
0.18	0.18	0.36	0.38	0.80	1.90	3.77	7.17	10.04	17.54	0.93	0.44	0.44	0.01	0.04	C67
0.00	0.01	0.01	0.03	0.09	0.13	0.06	0.31	0.34	0.31	0.03	0.02	0.02	0.00	0.00	C68
0.02	0.02	0.01	0.02	0.03	0.11	0.28	0.26	0.55	0.99	0.06	0.04	0.04	0.00	0.00	C69
1.69	2.75	3.93	5.44	7.52	10.76	14.25	16.97	20.64	23.74	4.03	2.56	2.56	0.14	0.27	C70-C72,D32-D33,D42-D43
0.30	0.54	0.82	1.07	1.58	2.17	3.01	3.96	5.50	6.06	0.82	0.48	0.46	0.02	0.05	C73
0.04	0.05	0.12	0.11	0.27	0.27	0.50	0.59	0.55	0.54	0.12	0.07	0.08	0.00	0.01	C74
0.03	0.08	0.09	0.10	0.17	0.25	0.40	0.31	0.48	0.58	0.11	0.07	0.07	0.00	0.01	C75
0.03	0.06	0.11	0.10	0.19	0.31	0.52	0.54	0.82	0.63	0.11	0.07	0.07	0.00	0.01	C81
0.48	0.83	1.35	1.68	3.50	5.00	6.85	9.95	10.45	9.60	1.68	0.99	0.97	0.05	0.11	C82-C86,C96
0.00	0.00	0.00	0.02	0.01	0.06	0.00	0.05	0.03	0.00	0.01	0.00	0.00	0.00	0.00	C88
0.11	0.32	0.70	1.05	1.83	2.54	3.17	3.84	4.03	2.60	0.72	0.41	0.41	0.02	0.05	C90
0.32	0.45	0.59	0.73	0.87	1.14	1.30	1.17	2.39	1.79	0.56	0.43	0.44	0.03	0.04	C91
0.45	0.89	0.99	1.34	2.29	2.79	4.60	5.19	5.19	4.89	1.14	0.75	0.73	0.04	0.08	C92-C94,D45-D47
0.69	0.78	1.25	1.42	2.49	3.81	5.07	6.55	6.18	6.15	1.42	0.99	1.00	0.05	0.10	C95
0.90	1.28	2.39	3.29	5.10	7.80	11.38	15.44	18.83	25.85	2.88	1.65	1.65	0.08	0.17	O & U
35.68	63.14	105.17	138.23	225.17	338.03	498.39	688.97	893.66	1 038.64	122.52	67.30	66.51	3.12	7.30	C00-C97,D32-D33, D42-D43,D45-D47
35.49	62.92	104.89	137.72	224.45	336.92	496.51	684.46	884.81	1 013.11	121.66	66.92	66.11	3.10	7.27	C00-C97,D32-D33, D42-D43, D45-D47 exc. C44

附录 2　2019 年全国东中西部肿瘤登记地区癌症发病与死亡结果

附表 2-1　2019 年全国东部肿瘤登记地区癌症发病主要指标

Appendix Table 2-1　Cancer incidence in Eastern registration areas of China, 2019

部位 Site		男性 Male 病例数 No. cases	构成 Freq./%	粗率 Crude rate/ $100\,000^{-1}$	世标率 ASR world/ $100\,000^{-1}$	累积率 Cum. Rate/% 0~64	0~74	女性 Female 病例数 No. cases	构成 Freq./%	粗率 Crude rate/ $100\,000^{-1}$	世标率 ASR world/ $100\,000^{-1}$	累积率 Cum. Rate/% 0~64	0~74	ICD-10
唇	Lip	285	0.06	0.22	0.12	0.01	0.01	226	0.05	0.18	0.09	0.00	0.01	C00
舌	Tongue	1 526	0.31	1.20	0.72	0.05	0.09	941	0.22	0.75	0.41	0.03	0.05	C01-C02
口	Mouth	1 927	0.39	1.51	0.87	0.05	0.10	1 140	0.26	0.90	0.46	0.02	0.05	C03-C06
唾液腺	Salivary gland	1 042	0.21	0.82	0.51	0.03	0.06	772	0.18	0.61	0.41	0.03	0.04	C07-C08
扁桃体	Tonsil	392	0.08	0.31	0.19	0.01	0.02	136	0.03	0.11	0.06	0.00	0.01	C09
其他口咽	Other oropharynx	625	0.13	0.49	0.29	0.02	0.03	108	0.02	0.09	0.05	0.00	0.00	C10
鼻咽	Nasopharynx	7 010	1.43	5.50	3.63	0.28	0.39	2 660	0.61	2.11	1.38	0.11	0.14	C11
下咽	Hypopharynx	1 650	0.34	1.29	0.74	0.05	0.10	114	0.03	0.09	0.05	0.00	0.01	C12-C13
咽,部位不明	Pharynx unspecified	439	0.09	0.34	0.19	0.01	0.02	97	0.02	0.08	0.04	0.00	0.00	C14
食管	Esophagus	31 974	6.54	25.08	13.42	0.65	1.70	11 268	2.58	8.93	3.91	0.11	0.45	C15
胃	Stomach	54 894	11.23	43.06	23.26	1.10	2.91	23 807	5.45	18.86	9.41	0.47	1.09	C16
小肠	Small intestine	2 258	0.46	1.77	0.99	0.06	0.12	1 625	0.37	1.29	0.66	0.04	0.08	C17
结肠	Colon	30 839	6.31	24.19	13.30	0.70	1.59	23 096	5.29	18.30	9.14	0.47	1.06	C18
直肠	Rectum	27 745	5.68	21.77	12.11	0.68	1.49	16 966	3.89	13.44	6.88	0.39	0.82	C19-C20
肛门	Anus	437	0.09	0.34	0.19	0.01	0.02	356	0.08	0.28	0.14	0.01	0.02	C21
肝脏	Liver	47 896	9.80	37.57	22.03	1.47	2.56	16 614	3.81	13.16	6.52	0.32	0.75	C22
胆囊及其他	Gallbladder etc.	6 623	1.36	5.20	2.75	0.12	0.33	6 700	1.53	5.31	2.47	0.11	0.28	C23-C24
胰腺	Pancreas	13 150	2.69	10.32	5.53	0.27	0.66	10 268	2.35	8.14	3.80	0.16	0.44	C25
鼻、鼻窦及其他	Nose, sinuses etc.	766	0.16	0.60	0.36	0.02	0.04	404	0.09	0.32	0.19	0.01	0.01	C30-C31
喉	Larynx	4 937	1.01	3.87	2.16	0.13	0.28	369	0.08	0.29	0.14	0.01	0.01	C32
气管、支气管、肺	Trachea, bronchus & lung	121 428	24.84	95.26	51.64	2.51	6.47	80 169	18.37	63.53	33.45	2.01	3.96	C33-C34
其他胸腔器官	Other thoracic organs	1 803	0.37	1.41	0.93	0.06	0.10	1 226	0.28	0.97	0.59	0.04	0.07	C37-C38
骨	Bone	2 220	0.45	1.74	1.24	0.07	0.12	1 713	0.39	1.36	0.88	0.05	0.08	C40-C41
皮肤黑色素瘤	Melanoma of skin	867	0.18	0.68	0.39	0.02	0.04	836	0.19	0.66	0.37	0.02	0.04	C43
皮肤其他	Other skin	4 570	0.93	3.59	1.94	0.08	0.20	4 765	1.09	3.78	1.77	0.07	0.18	C44
间皮瘤	Mesothelioma	313	0.06	0.25	0.14	0.01	0.02	259	0.06	0.21	0.11	0.01	0.01	C45
卡波西肉瘤	Kaposi sarcoma	45	0.01	0.04	0.02	0.00	0.00	27	0.01	0.02	0.01	0.00	0.00	C46
结缔组织、软组织	Connective & soft tissue	1 693	0.35	1.33	0.92	0.06	0.09	1 348	0.31	1.07	0.73	0.05	0.07	C47, C49
乳腺	Breast	624	0.13	0.49	0.28	0.02	0.03	71 099	16.29	56.34	35.25	2.84	3.82	C50
外阴	Vulva	—	—	—	—	—	—	787	0.18	0.62	0.33	0.02	0.04	C51
阴道	Vagina	—	—	—	—	—	—	383	0.09	0.30	0.18	0.01	0.02	C52
子宫颈	Cervix uteri	—	—	—	—	—	—	20 363	4.66	16.14	10.20	0.85	1.09	C53
子宫体	Corpus uteri	—	—	—	—	—	—	13 991	3.21	11.09	6.73	0.57	0.77	C54
子宫,部位不明	Uterus unspecified	—	—	—	—	—	—	2 028	0.46	1.61	0.95	0.07	0.10	C55
卵巢	Ovary	—	—	—	—	—	—	11 039	2.53	8.75	5.54	0.41	0.60	C56
其他女性生殖器官	Other female genital organs	—	—	—	—	—	—	931	0.21	0.74	0.44	0.03	0.05	C57
胎盘	Placenta	—	—	—	—	—	—	93	0.02	0.07	0.06	0.00	0.01	C58
阴茎	Penis	1 089	0.22	0.85	0.46	0.02	0.05	—	—	—	—	—	—	C60
前列腺	Prostate	24 833	5.08	19.48	9.65	0.22	1.12							C61
睾丸	Testis	704	0.14	0.55	0.50	0.03	0.04							C62
其他男性生殖器官	Other male genital organs	336	0.07	0.26	0.15	0.01	0.02							C63
肾	Kidney	10 158	2.08	7.97	4.85	0.33	0.57	5 050	1.16	4.00	2.34	0.16	0.27	C64
肾盂	Renal pelvis	1 083	0.22	0.85	0.46	0.02	0.06	757	0.17	0.60	0.28	0.01	0.03	C65
输尿管	Ureter	1 182	0.24	0.93	0.49	0.02	0.06	912	0.21	0.72	0.33	0.01	0.04	C66
膀胱	Bladder	15 510	3.17	12.17	6.45	0.28	0.74	3 871	0.89	3.07	1.44	0.06	0.16	C67
其他泌尿器官	Other urinary organs	237	0.05	0.19	0.10	0.00	0.01	164	0.04	0.13	0.06	0.00	0.01	C68
眼	Eye	198	0.04	0.16	0.15	0.01	0.01	157	0.04	0.12	0.14	0.01	0.01	C69
脑、神经系统	Brain, nervous system	10 753	2.20	8.44	5.75	0.37	0.59	14 243	3.26	11.29	7.00	0.47	0.75	C70-C72, D32-D33, D42-D43
甲状腺	Thyroid	19 586	4.01	15.36	11.64	0.95	1.06	56 674	12.98	44.91	32.94	2.76	3.08	C73
肾上腺	Adrenal gland	468	0.10	0.37	0.26	0.02	0.03	353	0.08	0.28	0.20	0.01	0.02	C74
其他内分泌腺	Other endocrine	684	0.14	0.54	0.39	0.03	0.04	717	0.16	0.57	0.39	0.03	0.04	C75
霍奇金淋巴瘤	Hodgkin lymphoma	468	0.10	0.37	0.29	0.02	0.03	354	0.08	0.28	0.24	0.02	0.02	C81
非霍奇金淋巴瘤	Non-Hodgkin lymphoma	8 963	1.83	7.03	4.34	0.25	0.48	6 798	1.56	5.39	3.10	0.19	0.35	C82-C86, C96
免疫增生性疾病	Immunoproliferative diseases	231	0.05	0.18	0.10	0.00	0.01	123	0.03	0.10	0.05	0.00	0.01	C88
多发性骨髓瘤	Multiple myeloma	3 080	0.63	2.42	1.33	0.07	0.16	2 352	0.54	1.86	0.98	0.06	0.12	C90
淋巴细胞白血病	Lymphoid leukemia	2 350	0.48	1.84	1.77	0.09	0.13	1 614	0.37	1.28	1.30	0.07	0.10	C91
髓系白血病	Myeloid leukemia	7 057	1.44	5.54	3.70	0.21	0.38	5 310	1.22	4.21	2.76	0.17	0.28	C92-C94, D45-D47
白血病,未特指	Leukemia unspecified	2 127	0.44	1.67	1.14	0.06	0.11	1 637	0.38	1.30	0.88	0.05	0.08	C95
其他或未指明部位	Other and unspecified	7 700	1.58	6.04	3.53	0.18	0.38	6 715	1.54	5.32	2.90	0.16	0.30	O & U
所有部位合计	All sites	488 775	100.00	383.43	218.36	11.76	25.68	436 525	100.00	345.90	201.15	13.58	21.91	C00-C97, D32-D33, D42-D43, D45-D47
所有部位除外 C44	All sites except C44	484 205	99.07	379.84	216.42	11.68	25.47	431 760	98.91	342.12	199.37	13.51	21.72	C00-C97, D32-D33, D42-D43, D45-D47 exc. C44

Appendix 2   Cancer incidence and mortality in Eastern, Central and Western registration areas of China, 2019

附表 2-2　2019 年全国东部城市肿瘤登记地区癌症发病主要指标

Appendix Table 2-2　Cancer incidence in Eastern urban registration areas of China, 2019

部位 Site		男性 Male						女性 Female						ICD-10
		病例数 No. cases	构成 Freq./%	粗率 Crude rate/ $100\,000^{-1}$	世标率 ASR world/ $100\,000^{-1}$	累积率 Cum. Rate/% 0~64	0~74	病例数 No. cases	构成 Freq./%	粗率 Crude rate/ $100\,000^{-1}$	世标率 ASR world/ $100\,000^{-1}$	累积率 Cum. Rate/% 0~64	0~74	
唇	Lip	117	0.05	0.18	0.10	0.00	0.01	101	0.04	0.15	0.08	0.00	0.01	C00
舌	Tongue	929	0.36	1.44	0.86	0.06	0.10	572	0.24	0.87	0.46	0.03	0.05	C01-C02
口	Mouth	1 110	0.43	1.72	0.97	0.06	0.11	628	0.26	0.96	0.48	0.02	0.06	C03-C06
唾液腺	Salivary gland	582	0.22	0.90	0.56	0.04	0.06	423	0.18	0.65	0.43	0.03	0.04	C07-C08
扁桃体	Tonsil	221	0.09	0.34	0.21	0.02	0.02	85	0.04	0.13	0.07	0.01	0.01	C09
其他口咽	Other oropharynx	373	0.14	0.58	0.33	0.02	0.04	62	0.03	0.09	0.05	0.00	0.01	C10
鼻咽	Nasopharynx	3 894	1.50	6.03	3.95	0.31	0.42	1 480	0.61	2.26	1.51	0.12	0.15	C11
下咽	Hypopharynx	973	0.38	1.51	0.85	0.06	0.11	64	0.03	0.10	0.05	0.00	0.01	C12-C13
咽, 部位不明	Pharynx unspecified	247	0.10	0.38	0.21	0.01	0.02	53	0.02	0.08	0.04	0.00	0.00	C14
食管	Esophagus	13 313	5.14	20.61	10.91	0.58	1.38	3 710	1.54	5.67	2.43	0.07	0.28	C15
胃	Stomach	26 303	10.16	40.72	21.54	1.05	2.69	11 698	4.85	17.88	8.87	0.46	1.02	C16
小肠	Small intestine	1 231	0.48	1.91	1.03	0.06	0.12	908	0.38	1.39	0.70	0.04	0.08	C17
结肠	Colon	18 715	7.23	28.97	15.48	0.80	1.84	14 032	5.81	21.45	10.50	0.54	1.21	C18
直肠	Rectum	15 644	6.04	24.22	13.21	0.75	1.62	9 370	3.88	14.32	7.26	0.41	0.86	C19-C20
肛门	Anus	206	0.08	0.32	0.17	0.01	0.02	162	0.07	0.25	0.13	0.01	0.02	C21
肝脏	Liver	23 995	9.27	37.15	21.38	1.44	2.49	8 164	3.38	12.48	6.05	0.30	0.68	C22
胆囊及其他	Gallbladder etc.	3 385	1.31	5.24	2.69	0.12	0.32	3 511	1.45	5.37	2.42	0.10	0.27	C23-C24
胰腺	Pancreas	6 974	2.69	10.80	5.65	0.28	0.67	5 530	2.29	8.45	3.86	0.16	0.44	C25
鼻、鼻窦及其他	Nose, sinuses etc.	402	0.16	0.62	0.37	0.02	0.04	231	0.10	0.35	0.21	0.01	0.02	C30-C31
喉	Larynx	2 782	1.07	4.31	2.36	0.15	0.31	208	0.09	0.32	0.15	0.01	0.02	C32
气管、支气管、肺	Trachea, bronchus & lung	62 973	24.32	97.49	51.86	2.61	6.45	43 941	18.21	67.17	35.14	2.16	4.11	C33-C34
其他胸腔器官	Other thoracic organs	1 040	0.40	1.61	1.04	0.07	0.11	700	0.29	1.07	0.65	0.04	0.07	C37-C38
骨	Bone	1 053	0.41	1.63	1.14	0.06	0.11	811	0.34	1.24	0.79	0.05	0.08	C40-C41
皮肤黑色素瘤	Melanoma of skin	470	0.18	0.73	0.40	0.02	0.04	429	0.18	0.66	0.35	0.02	0.04	C43
皮肤其他	Other skin	2 483	0.96	3.84	2.05	0.09	0.21	2 602	1.08	3.98	1.89	0.08	0.20	C44
间皮瘤	Mesothelioma	202	0.08	0.31	0.17	0.01	0.02	155	0.06	0.24	0.13	0.01	0.02	C45
卡波西肉瘤	Kaposi sarcoma	31	0.01	0.05	0.04	0.00	0.00	13	0.01	0.02	0.01	0.00	0.00	C46
结缔组织、软组织	Connective & soft tissue	970	0.37	1.50	1.03	0.06	0.10	753	0.31	1.15	0.78	0.05	0.07	C47, C49
乳腺	Breast	325	0.13	0.50	0.28	0.02	0.03	42 162	17.47	64.45	39.63	3.18	4.32	C50
外阴	Vulva	—	—	—	—	—	—	477	0.20	0.73	0.38	0.02	0.04	C51
阴道	Vagina	—	—	—	—	—	—	226	0.09	0.35	0.20	0.01	0.02	C52
子宫颈	Cervix uteri	—	—	—	—	—	—	10 440	4.33	15.96	10.06	0.85	1.08	C53
子宫体	Corpus uteri	—	—	—	—	—	—	8 051	3.34	12.31	7.46	0.63	0.85	C54
子宫, 部位不明	Uterus unspecified	—	—	—	—	—	—	1 041	0.43	1.59	0.93	0.07	0.10	C55
卵巢	Ovary	—	—	—	—	—	—	6 181	2.56	9.45	5.96	0.44	0.64	C56
其他女性生殖器官	Other female genital organs	—	—	—	—	—	—	519	0.22	0.79	0.46	0.03	0.05	C57
胎盘	Placenta	—	—	—	—	—	—	42	0.02	0.06	0.06	0.00	0.00	C58
阴茎	Penis	552	0.21	0.85	0.45	0.03	0.05	—	—	—	—	—	—	C60
前列腺	Prostate	14 539	5.62	22.51	10.89	0.26	1.27	—	—	—	—	—	—	C61
睾丸	Testis	391	0.15	0.61	0.54	0.04	0.04	—	—	—	—	—	—	C62
其他男性生殖器官	Other male genital organs	199	0.08	0.31	0.17	0.01	0.02	—	—	—	—	—	—	C63
肾	Kidney	6 239	2.41	9.66	5.74	0.40	0.68	3 049	1.26	4.66	2.67	0.18	0.31	C64
肾盂	Renal pelvis	660	0.25	1.02	0.54	0.03	0.06	470	0.19	0.72	0.33	0.01	0.04	C65
输尿管	Ureter	742	0.29	1.15	0.59	0.03	0.07	577	0.24	0.88	0.39	0.01	0.04	C66
膀胱	Bladder	8 753	3.38	13.55	6.99	0.31	0.80	2 278	0.94	3.48	1.59	0.07	0.17	C67
其他泌尿器官	Other urinary organs	133	0.05	0.21	0.10	0.00	0.01	105	0.04	0.16	0.07	0.00	0.01	C68
眼	Eye	102	0.04	0.16	0.17	0.01	0.01	76	0.03	0.12	0.14	0.01	0.01	C69
脑、神经系统	Brain, nervous system	5 700	2.20	8.82	5.95	0.39	0.60	7 728	3.20	11.81	7.31	0.50	0.78	C70-C72, D32-D33, D42-D43
甲状腺	Thyroid	12 159	4.70	18.82	14.21	1.16	1.29	33 354	13.82	50.99	37.29	3.12	3.46	C73
肾上腺	Adrenal gland	244	0.09	0.38	0.27	0.02	0.03	177	0.07	0.27	0.19	0.01	0.02	C74
其他内分泌腺	Other endocrine	312	0.12	0.48	0.36	0.02	0.04	313	0.13	0.48	0.33	0.02	0.03	C75
霍奇金淋巴瘤	Hodgkin lymphoma	265	0.10	0.41	0.33	0.02	0.03	215	0.09	0.33	0.30	0.02	0.02	C81
非霍奇金淋巴瘤	Non-Hodgkin lymphoma	4 974	1.92	7.70	4.70	0.28	0.51	3 899	1.62	5.96	3.43	0.21	0.39	C82-C86, C96
免疫增生性疾病	Immunoproliferative diseases	140	0.05	0.22	0.12	0.01	0.02	65	0.03	0.10	0.05	0.00	0.01	C88
多发性骨髓瘤	Multiple myeloma	1 649	0.64	2.55	1.37	0.07	0.17	1 317	0.55	2.01	1.04	0.06	0.13	C90
淋巴细胞白血病	Lymphoid leukemia	1 217	0.47	1.88	1.81	0.10	0.13	830	0.34	1.27	1.32	0.07	0.10	C91
髓系白血病	Myeloid leukemia	3 909	1.51	6.05	3.91	0.22	0.40	2 940	1.22	4.49	2.85	0.17	0.29	C92-C94, D45-D47
白血病, 未特指	Leukemia unspecified	947	0.37	1.47	0.99	0.05	0.09	724	0.30	1.11	0.73	0.04	0.07	C95
其他或未指明部位	Other and unspecified	4 135	1.60	6.40	3.63	0.19	0.39	3 705	1.54	5.66	3.04	0.17	0.36	O & U
所有部位合计	All sites	258 904	100.00	400.80	224.66	12.43	26.18	241 357	100.00	368.95	213.70	14.66	23.10	C00-C97, D32-D33, D42-D43, D45-D47
所有部位除外 C44	All sites except C44	256 421	99.04	396.96	222.61	12.34	25.96	238 755	98.92	364.97	211.81	14.58	22.90	C00-C97, D32-D33, D42-D43, D45-D47 exc. C44

部位 Site		男性 Male						女性 Female						ICD-10
		病例数 No. cases	构成 Freq./%	粗率 Crude rate/ 100 000^{-1}	世标率 ASR world/ 100 000^{-1}	累积率 Cum. Rate/%		病例数 No. cases	构成 Freq./%	粗率 Crude rate/ 100 000^{-1}	世标率 ASR world/ 100 000^{-1}	累积率 Cum. Rate/%		
						0~64	0~74					0~64	0~74	
唇	Lip	168	0.07	0.27	0.15	0.01	0.02	125	0.06	0.21	0.10	0.00	0.01	C00
舌	Tongue	597	0.26	0.95	0.58	0.04	0.07	369	0.19	0.61	0.35	0.02	0.04	C01-C02
口	Mouth	817	0.36	1.30	0.76	0.05	0.09	512	0.26	0.84	0.45	0.03	0.05	C03-C06
唾液腺	Salivary gland	460	0.20	0.73	0.47	0.03	0.05	349	0.18	0.57	0.39	0.03	0.04	C07-C08
扁桃体	Tonsil	171	0.07	0.27	0.16	0.01	0.02	51	0.03	0.08	0.05	0.00	0.01	C09
其他口咽	Other oropharynx	252	0.11	0.40	0.24	0.02	0.03	46	0.02	0.08	0.04	0.00	0.00	C10
鼻咽	Nasopharynx	3 116	1.36	4.96	3.30	0.25	0.36	1 180	0.60	1.94	1.25	0.09	0.13	C11
下咽	Hypopharynx	677	0.29	1.08	0.63	0.04	0.08	50	0.03	0.08	0.04	0.00	0.00	C12-C13
咽,部位不明	Pharynx unspecified	192	0.08	0.31	0.17	0.01	0.02	44	0.02	0.07	0.04	0.00	0.00	C14
食管	Esophagus	18 661	8.12	29.68	16.13	0.72	2.04	7 558	3.87	12.43	5.54	0.15	0.65	C15
胃	Stomach	28 591	12.44	45.47	25.08	1.15	3.15	12 109	6.20	19.92	10.00	0.48	1.17	C16
小肠	Small intestine	1 027	0.45	1.63	0.95	0.06	0.12	717	0.37	1.18	0.62	0.03	0.08	C17
结肠	Colon	12 124	5.27	19.28	10.94	0.58	1.33	9 064	4.64	14.91	7.65	0.39	0.90	C18
直肠	Rectum	12 101	5.26	19.25	10.92	0.60	1.34	7 596	3.89	12.50	6.47	0.36	0.77	C19-C20
肛门	Anus	231	0.10	0.37	0.21	0.01	0.02	194	0.10	0.32	0.16	0.01	0.02	C21
肝脏	Liver	23 901	10.40	38.01	22.72	1.50	2.64	8 450	4.33	13.90	7.03	0.35	0.83	C22
胆囊及其他	Gallbladder etc.	3 238	1.41	5.15	2.81	0.12	0.34	3 189	1.63	5.25	2.51	0.11	0.29	C23-C24
胰腺	Pancreas	6 176	2.69	9.82	5.41	0.26	0.65	4 738	2.43	7.80	3.73	0.16	0.43	C25
鼻、鼻窦及其他	Nose, sinuses etc.	364	0.16	0.58	0.36	0.02	0.04	173	0.09	0.28	0.16	0.01	0.02	C30-C31
喉	Larynx	2 155	0.94	3.43	1.95	0.11	0.25	161	0.08	0.26	0.13	0.01	0.01	C32
气管、支气管、肺	Trachea, bronchus & lung	58 455	25.43	92.97	51.40	2.41	6.49	36 228	18.56	59.60	31.62	1.84	3.81	C33-C34
其他胸腔器官	Other thoracic organs	763	0.33	1.21	0.81	0.05	0.09	526	0.27	0.87	0.53	0.03	0.06	C37-C38
骨	Bone	1 167	0.51	1.86	1.33	0.07	0.13	902	0.46	1.48	0.98	0.05	0.09	C40-C41
皮肤黑色素瘤	Melanoma of skin	397	0.17	0.63	0.38	0.02	0.04	407	0.21	0.67	0.38	0.02	0.04	C43
皮肤其他	Other skin	2 087	0.91	3.32	1.83	0.07	0.19	2 163	1.11	3.56	1.65	0.06	0.16	C44
间皮瘤	Mesothelioma	111	0.05	0.18	0.10	0.01	0.01	104	0.05	0.17	0.10	0.01	0.01	C45
卡波西肉瘤	Kaposi sarcoma	14	0.01	0.02	0.01	0.00	0.00	14	0.01	0.02	0.01	0.00	0.00	C46
结缔组织、软组织	Connective & soft tissue	723	0.31	1.15	0.81	0.05	0.08	590	0.30	0.98	0.69	0.04	0.07	C47, C49
乳腺	Breast	299	0.13	0.48	0.28	0.02	0.03	28 937	14.83	47.61	30.42	2.48	3.28	C50
外阴	Vulva	—	—	—	—	—	—	310	0.16	0.51	0.28	0.02	0.03	C51
阴道	Vagina	—	—	—	—	—	—	157	0.08	0.26	0.16	0.01	0.02	C52
子宫颈	Cervix uteri	—	—	—	—	—	—	9 923	5.08	16.33	10.36	0.85	1.10	C53
子宫体	Corpus uteri	—	—	—	—	—	—	5 940	3.04	9.77	5.94	0.51	0.68	C54
子宫,部位不明	Uterus unspecified	—	—	—	—	—	—	987	0.51	1.62	0.98	0.07	0.11	C55
卵巢	Ovary	—	—	—	—	—	—	4 858	2.49	7.99	5.09	0.38	0.56	C56
其他女性生殖器官	Other female genital organs	—	—	—	—	—	—	412	0.21	0.68	0.41	0.03	0.05	C57
胎盘	Placenta	—	—	—	—	—	—	51	0.03	0.08	0.07	0.01	0.01	C58
阴茎	Penis	537	0.23	0.85	0.47	0.02	0.06	—	—	—	—	—	—	C60
前列腺	Prostate	10 294	4.48	16.37	8.31	0.18	0.96	—	—	—	—	—	—	C61
睾丸	Testis	313	0.14	0.50	0.46	0.03	0.04	—	—	—	—	—	—	C62
其他男性生殖器官	Other male genital organs	137	0.06	0.22	0.13	0.01	0.01	—	—	—	—	—	—	C63
肾	Kidney	3 919	1.70	6.23	3.90	0.26	0.46	2 001	1.03	3.29	1.98	0.13	0.22	C64
肾盂	Renal pelvis	423	0.18	0.67	0.37	0.02	0.05	287	0.15	0.47	0.24	0.01	0.03	C65
输尿管	Ureter	440	0.19	0.70	0.38	0.02	0.05	315	0.17	0.55	0.27	0.01	0.04	C66
膀胱	Bladder	6 757	2.94	10.75	5.85	0.25	0.67	1 593	0.82	2.62	1.27	0.06	0.15	C67
其他泌尿器官	Other urinary organs	104	0.05	0.17	0.09	0.00	0.01	59	0.03	0.10	0.05	0.00	0.01	C68
眼	Eye	96	0.04	0.15	0.13	0.01	0.01	81	0.04	0.13	0.13	0.01	0.01	C69
脑、神经系统	Brain, nervous system	5 053	2.20	8.04	5.54	0.35	0.58	6 515	3.34	10.72	6.66	0.44	0.72	C70-C72, D32-D33, D42-D43
甲状腺	Thyroid	7 427	3.23	11.81	8.94	0.73	0.83	23 320	11.95	38.37	28.16	2.37	2.66	C73
肾上腺	Adrenal gland	224	0.10	0.36	0.25	0.02	0.03	176	0.09	0.29	0.21	0.01	0.02	C74
其他内分泌腺	Other endocrine	372	0.16	0.59	0.42	0.03	0.05	404	0.21	0.66	0.45	0.03	0.05	C75
霍奇金淋巴瘤	Hodgkin lymphoma	203	0.09	0.32	0.25	0.02	0.02	139	0.07	0.23	0.18	0.01	0.02	C81
非霍奇金淋巴瘤	Non-Hodgkin lymphoma	3 989	1.74	6.34	3.97	0.23	0.45	2 899	1.49	4.77	2.74	0.16	0.31	C82-C86, C96
免疫增生性疾病	Immunoproliferative diseases	91	0.04	0.14	0.08	0.00	0.01	58	0.03	0.10	0.06	0.00	0.01	C88
多发性骨髓瘤	Multiple myeloma	1 431	0.62	2.28	1.29	0.06	0.16	1 035	0.53	1.70	0.91	0.05	0.12	C90
淋巴细胞白血病	Lymphoid leukemia	1 133	0.49	1.80	1.73	0.09	0.14	784	0.40	1.29	1.27	0.07	0.10	C91
髓系白血病	Myeloid leukemia	3 148	1.37	5.01	3.48	0.20	0.35	2 370	1.21	3.90	2.66	0.16	0.27	C92-C94, D45-D47
白血病,未特指	Leukemia unspecified	1 180	0.51	1.88	1.31	0.07	0.12	913	0.47	1.50	1.05	0.06	0.10	C95
其他或未指明部位	Other and unspecified	3 565	1.55	5.67	3.40	0.17	0.38	3 010	1.54	4.95	2.74	0.15	0.29	O & U
所有部位合计	All sites	229 871	100.00	365.58	211.65	11.06	25.15	195 168	100.00	321.09	187.41	12.41	20.60	C00-C97, D32-D33, D42-D43, D45-D47
所有部位除外 C44	All sites except C44	227 784	99.09	362.26	209.82	10.99	24.96	193 005	98.89	317.53	185.76	12.35	20.44	C00-C97, D32-D33, D42-D43, D45-D47 exc. C44

部位 Site		男性 Male						女性 Female						ICD-10
		病例数 No. cases	构成 Freq. /%	粗率 Crude rate/ 100 000⁻¹	世标率 ASR world/ 100 000⁻¹	累积率 Cum. Rate/%		病例数 No. cases	构成 Freq. /%	粗率 Crude rate/ 100 000⁻¹	世标率 ASR world/ 100 000⁻¹	累积率 Cum. Rate/%		
						0~64	0~74					0~64	0~74	
唇	Lip	198	0.09	0.26	0.17	0.01	0.02	119	0.06	0.16	0.09	0.00	0.01	C00
舌	Tongue	1 177	0.51	1.54	1.06	0.08	0.12	371	0.19	0.50	0.31	0.02	0.04	C01-C02
口	Mouth	1 223	0.53	1.60	1.08	0.08	0.12	526	0.27	0.71	0.42	0.02	0.05	C03-C06
唾液腺	Salivary gland	523	0.23	0.68	0.48	0.03	0.05	402	0.21	0.54	0.37	0.03	0.04	C07-C08
扁桃体	Tonsil	186	0.08	0.24	0.17	0.01	0.02	73	0.04	0.10	0.07	0.00	0.01	C09
其他口咽	Other oropharynx	276	0.12	0.36	0.24	0.02	0.03	63	0.03	0.09	0.05	0.00	0.01	C10
鼻咽	Nasopharynx	3 431	1.49	4.48	3.11	0.24	0.35	1 456	0.75	1.97	1.32	0.10	0.14	C11
下咽	Hypopharynx	588	0.25	0.77	0.50	0.03	0.06	55	0.03	0.07	0.05	0.00	0.01	C12-C13
咽,部位不明	Pharynx unspecified	262	0.11	0.34	0.22	0.01	0.03	80	0.04	0.11	0.06	0.00	0.01	C14
食管	Esophagus	18 026	7.82	23.55	14.83	0.64	1.87	7 751	3.99	10.50	5.77	0.19	0.68	C15
胃	Stomach	28 027	12.15	36.62	23.32	1.10	2.92	12 303	6.34	16.67	9.71	0.49	1.11	C16
小肠	Small intestine	1 041	0.45	1.36	0.89	0.05	0.10	855	0.44	1.16	0.71	0.04	0.08	C17
结肠	Colon	10 585	4.59	13.83	8.94	0.49	1.05	8 212	4.23	11.13	6.53	0.35	0.76	C18
直肠	Rectum	11 701	5.07	15.29	9.86	0.53	1.20	8 004	4.12	10.84	6.46	0.37	0.77	C19-C20
肛门	Anus	273	0.12	0.36	0.23	0.01	0.03	233	0.12	0.32	0.18	0.01	0.02	C21
肝脏	Liver	28 471	12.35	37.20	24.55	1.54	2.88	10 899	5.61	14.77	8.64	0.43	1.00	C22
胆囊及其他	Gallbladder etc.	2 676	1.16	3.50	2.23	0.10	0.27	3 182	1.64	4.31	2.45	0.11	0.29	C23-C24
胰腺	Pancreas	4 874	2.11	6.37	4.05	0.21	0.48	3 806	1.96	5.16	2.96	0.14	0.35	C25
鼻、鼻窦及其他	Nose, sinuses etc.	385	0.17	0.50	0.35	0.02	0.04	260	0.13	0.35	0.24	0.01	0.02	C30-C31
喉	Larynx	2 448	1.06	3.20	2.07	0.12	0.26	334	0.17	0.45	0.27	0.01	0.03	C32
气管、支气管、肺	Trachea, bronchus & lung	63 004	27.32	82.31	52.17	2.45	6.47	29 033	14.95	39.34	22.95	1.21	2.70	C33-C34
其他胸腔器官	Other thoracic organs	925	0.40	1.21	0.85	0.06	0.09	599	0.31	0.81	0.55	0.04	0.06	C37-C38
骨	Bone	1 486	0.64	1.94	1.52	0.08	0.15	1 228	0.63	1.66	1.24	0.07	0.12	C40-C41
皮肤黑色素瘤	Melanoma of skin	361	0.16	0.47	0.31	0.02	0.04	352	0.18	0.48	0.31	0.02	0.03	C43
皮肤其他	Other skin	1 788	0.78	2.34	1.52	0.07	0.16	1 611	0.83	2.18	1.24	0.05	0.13	C44
间皮瘤	Mesothelioma	94	0.04	0.12	0.08	0.00	0.01	64	0.03	0.09	0.05	0.00	0.01	C45
卡波西肉瘤	Kaposi sarcoma	19	0.01	0.02	0.02	0.00	0.00	2	0.00	0.00	0.00	0.00	0.00	C46
结缔组织、软组织	Connective & soft tissue	694	0.30	0.91	0.69	0.04	0.07	623	0.32	0.84	0.62	0.04	0.06	C47,C49
乳腺	Breast	508	0.22	0.66	0.45	0.03	0.05	30 670	15.80	41.55	28.06	2.30	2.98	C50
外阴	Vulva	—	—	—	—	—	—	307	0.16	0.42	0.25	0.02	0.03	C51
阴道	Vagina	—	—	—	—	—	—	239	0.12	0.32	0.20	0.01	0.02	C52
子宫颈	Cervix uteri	—	—	—	—	—	—	16 051	8.27	21.75	14.45	1.18	1.58	C53
子宫体	Corpus uteri	—	—	—	—	—	—	6 299	3.24	8.53	5.57	0.47	0.62	C54
子宫,部位不明	Uterus unspecified	—	—	—	—	—	—	1 447	0.75	1.96	1.28	0.10	0.14	C55
卵巢	Ovary	—	—	—	—	—	—	5 438	2.80	7.37	5.04	0.38	0.55	C56
其他女性生殖器官	Other female genital organs	—	—	—	—	—	—	380	0.20	0.51	0.35	0.03	0.04	C57
胎盘	Placenta	—	—	—	—	—	—	45	0.02	0.06	0.05	0.00	0.00	C58
阴茎	Penis	520	0.23	0.68	0.44	0.02	0.05	—	—	—	—	—	—	C60
前列腺	Prostate	7 334	3.18	9.58	5.68	0.11	0.59	—	—	—	—	—	—	C61
睾丸	Testis	297	0.13	0.39	0.34	0.02	0.03	—	—	—	—	—	—	C62
其他男性生殖器官	Other male genital organs	114	0.05	0.15	0.11	0.01	0.01	—	—	—	—	—	—	C63
肾	Kidney	3 336	1.45	4.36	2.95	0.19	0.34	1 978	1.02	2.68	1.75	0.11	0.20	C64
肾盂	Renal pelvis	389	0.17	0.51	0.33	0.02	0.04	221	0.11	0.30	0.17	0.01	0.02	C65
输尿管	Ureter	403	0.17	0.53	0.33	0.01	0.04	289	0.15	0.39	0.22	0.01	0.03	C66
膀胱	Bladder	6 036	2.62	7.89	4.96	0.22	0.56	1 543	0.79	2.09	1.18	0.05	0.13	C67
其他泌尿器官	Other urinary organs	113	0.05	0.15	0.10	0.00	0.01	70	0.04	0.09	0.05	0.00	0.01	C68
眼	Eye	135	0.06	0.18	0.19	0.01	0.01	101	0.05	0.14	0.13	0.01	0.01	C69
脑、神经系统	Brain, nervous system	5 661	2.45	7.40	5.59	0.35	0.57	6 318	3.25	8.56	5.93	0.38	0.62	C70-C72, D32-D33,D42-D43
甲状腺	Thyroid	5 361	2.32	7.00	5.34	0.44	0.50	18 039	9.29	24.44	17.86	1.51	1.70	C73
肾上腺	Adrenal gland	300	0.13	0.39	0.29	0.02	0.03	218	0.11	0.30	0.21	0.01	0.02	C74
其他内分泌腺	Other endocrine	233	0.10	0.30	0.24	0.02	0.03	278	0.14	0.38	0.27	0.02	0.03	C75
霍奇金淋巴瘤	Hodgkin lymphoma	288	0.12	0.38	0.29	0.02	0.03	198	0.10	0.27	0.21	0.01	0.02	C81
非霍奇金淋巴瘤	Non-Hodgkin lymphoma	3 623	1.57	4.73	3.37	0.20	0.37	2 710	1.40	3.67	2.42	0.15	0.26	C82-C86,C96
免疫增生性疾病	Immunoproliferative diseases	35	0.02	0.05	0.03	0.00	0.00	18	0.01	0.02	0.02	0.00	0.00	C88
多发性骨髓瘤	Multiple myeloma	1 273	0.55	1.66	1.10	0.06	0.13	931	0.48	1.26	0.78	0.04	0.10	C90
淋巴细胞白血病	Lymphoid leukemia	948	0.41	1.24	1.19	0.06	0.10	619	0.32	0.84	0.86	0.05	0.06	C91
髓系白血病	Myeloid leukemia	2 267	0.98	2.96	2.24	0.13	0.22	1 676	0.86	2.27	1.66	0.10	0.16	C92-C94, D45-D47
白血病,未特指	Leukemia unspecified	1 835	0.80	2.40	1.98	0.11	0.18	1 350	0.70	1.83	1.50	0.08	0.14	C95
其他或未指明部位	Other and unspecified	4 874	2.11	6.37	4.43	0.23	0.48	4 224	2.18	5.72	3.76	0.21	0.39	O & U
所有部位合计	All sites	230 625	100.00	301.30	197.43	10.35	23.28	194 153	100.00	263.05	167.86	11.05	18.38	C00-C97, D32-D33, D42-D43, D45-D47
所有部位除外 C44	All sites except C44	228 837	99.22	298.96	195.90	10.28	23.12	192 542	99.17	260.87	166.63	11.00	18.26	C00-C97, D32-D33, D42-D43, D45-D47 exc. C44

附表 2-5 2019 年全国中部城市肿瘤登记地区癌症发病主要指标
Appendix Table 2-5 Cancer incidence in Central urban registration areas of China,2019

部位 Site		男性 Male						女性 Female						ICD-10
		病例数 No. cases	构成 Freq./%	粗率 Crude rate/ 100 000⁻¹	世标率 ASR world/ 100 000⁻¹	累积率 Cum. Rate/% 0~64	0~74	病例数 No. cases	构成 Freq./%	粗率 Crude rate/ 100 000⁻¹	世标率 ASR world/ 100 000⁻¹	累积率 Cum. Rate/% 0~64	0~74	
唇	Lip	72	0.08	0.28	0.18	0.01	0.02	48	0.06	0.19	0.10	0.00	0.01	C00
舌	Tongue	496	0.58	1.90	1.25	0.09	0.14	181	0.24	0.70	0.42	0.03	0.05	C01-C02
口	Mouth	531	0.62	2.03	1.32	0.09	0.15	213	0.28	0.83	0.46	0.02	0.05	C03-C06
唾液腺	Salivary gland	184	0.21	0.70	0.48	0.03	0.05	135	0.18	0.52	0.34	0.03	0.03	C07-C08
扁桃体	Tonsil	100	0.12	0.38	0.25	0.02	0.03	29	0.04	0.11	0.07	0.01	0.01	C09
其他口咽	Other oropharynx	110	0.13	0.42	0.27	0.02	0.03	18	0.02	0.07	0.04	0.00	0.01	C10
鼻咽	Nasopharynx	1 027	1.20	3.93	2.64	0.20	0.30	462	0.61	1.79	1.17	0.09	0.13	C11
下咽	Hypopharynx	288	0.34	1.10	0.70	0.05	0.09	15	0.02	0.06	0.04	0.00	0.00	C12-C13
咽,部位不明	Pharynx unspecified	80	0.09	0.31	0.20	0.01	0.02	18	0.02	0.07	0.04	0.00	0.00	C14
食管	Esophagus	5 116	5.97	19.59	11.98	0.56	1.50	1 768	2.33	6.86	3.58	0.10	0.41	C15
胃	Stomach	8 147	9.50	31.20	19.20	0.90	2.39	3 814	5.02	14.80	8.40	0.41	0.96	C16
小肠	Small intestine	408	0.48	1.56	0.98	0.06	0.12	322	0.42	1.25	0.72	0.03	0.08	C17
结肠	Colon	4 997	5.83	19.14	11.81	0.60	1.39	3 869	5.09	15.01	8.44	0.42	0.96	C18
直肠	Rectum	4 643	5.41	17.78	11.10	0.60	1.37	2 964	3.90	11.50	6.63	0.36	0.78	C19-C20
肛门	Anus	80	0.09	0.31	0.19	0.01	0.02	66	0.09	0.26	0.13	0.01	0.01	C21
肝脏	Liver	9 343	10.90	35.78	22.82	1.44	2.64	3 546	4.67	13.76	7.80	0.38	0.87	C22
胆囊及其他	Gallbladder etc.	1 078	1.26	4.13	2.53	0.12	0.30	1 309	1.72	5.08	2.76	0.11	0.32	C23-C24
胰腺	Pancreas	2 041	2.38	7.82	4.80	0.24	0.57	1 545	2.03	6.00	3.30	0.14	0.39	C25
鼻,鼻窦及其他	Nose,sinuses etc.	139	0.16	0.53	0.35	0.02	0.04	90	0.12	0.35	0.22	0.01	0.02	C30-31
喉	Larynx	1 053	1.23	4.03	2.55	0.16	0.32	104	0.14	0.40	0.22	0.01	0.02	C32
气管、支气管、肺	Trachea,bronchus & lung	23 476	27.38	89.91	55.14	2.60	6.81	11 645	15.33	45.19	25.86	1.38	3.00	C33-C34
其他胸腔器官	Other thoracic organs	351	0.41	1.34	0.94	0.06	0.10	245	0.32	0.95	0.61	0.04	0.06	C37-C38
骨	Bone	434	0.51	1.66	1.23	0.07	0.12	364	0.48	1.41	0.96	0.05	0.10	C40-C41
皮肤黑色素瘤	Melanoma of skin	130	0.15	0.50	0.33	0.02	0.04	150	0.20	0.58	0.35	0.02	0.04	C43
皮肤其他	Other skin	698	0.81	2.67	1.67	0.08	0.18	568	0.75	2.20	1.21	0.05	0.12	C44
间皮瘤	Mesothelioma	43	0.05	0.16	0.10	0.01	0.01	34	0.04	0.13	0.08	0.00	0.01	C45
卡波西肉瘤	Kaposi sarcoma	10	0.01	0.04	0.02	0.00	0.00	1	0.00	0.00	0.00	0.00	0.00	C46
结缔组织、软组织	Connective & soft tissue	298	0.35	1.14	0.81	0.05	0.08	237	0.31	0.92	0.66	0.04	0.07	C47,C49
乳腺	Breast	172	0.20	0.66	0.42	0.03	0.05	131 88	17.36	51.18	33.24	2.67	3.62	C50
外阴	Vulva	—	—	—	—	—	—	122	0.16	0.47	0.28	0.02	0.03	C51
阴道	Vagina	—	—	—	—	—	—	83	0.11	0.32	0.19	0.01	0.02	C52
子宫颈	Cervix uteri	—	—	—	—	—	—	5 075	6.68	19.69	12.78	1.05	1.40	C53
子宫体	Corpus uteri	—	—	—	—	—	—	2 395	3.15	9.29	5.91	0.49	0.68	C54
子宫,部位不明	Uterus unspecified	—	—	—	—	—	—	336	0.44	1.30	0.83	0.07	0.09	C55
卵巢	Ovary	—	—	—	—	—	—	2 083	2.74	8.08	5.39	0.40	0.59	C56
其他女性生殖器官	Other female genital organs	—	—	—	—	—	—	166	0.22	0.64	0.41	0.03	0.05	C57
胎盘	Placenta	—	—	—	—	—	—	19	0.03	0.07	0.07	0.01	0.01	C58
阴茎	Penis	180	0.21	0.69	0.42	0.02	0.05	—	—	—	—	—	—	C60
前列腺	Prostate	3 642	4.25	13.95	7.86	0.14	0.79	—	—	—	—	—	—	C61
睾丸	Testis	107	0.12	0.41	0.33	0.02	0.03	—	—	—	—	—	—	C62
其他男性生殖器官	Other male genital organs	59	0.07	0.23	0.15	0.01	0.02	—	—	—	—	—	—	C63
肾	Kidney	1 601	1.87	6.13	4.03	0.25	0.48	859	1.13	3.33	2.08	0.13	0.24	C64
肾盂	Renal pelvis	184	0.21	0.70	0.43	0.02	0.05	126	0.17	0.49	0.26	0.01	0.03	C65
输尿管	Ureter	197	0.23	0.75	0.45	0.02	0.05	147	0.19	0.57	0.31	0.01	0.04	C66
膀胱	Bladder	2 674	3.12	10.24	6.14	0.27	0.68	692	0.91	2.69	1.47	0.06	0.16	C67
其他泌尿器官	Other urinary organs	49	0.06	0.19	0.11	0.01	0.01	25	0.03	0.10	0.05	0.00	0.01	C68
眼	Eye	39	0.05	0.15	0.15	0.01	0.01	30	0.04	0.12	0.11	0.00	0.00	C69
脑、神经系统	Brain,nervous system	1 845	2.15	7.07	5.19	0.32	0.52	2 223	2.93	8.63	5.75	0.35	0.60	C70-C72, D32-D33,D42-D43
甲状腺	Thyroid	3 105	3.62	11.89	8.83	0.73	0.82	9 528	12.54	36.98	26.46	2.25	2.52	C73
肾上腺	Adrenal gland	117	0.14	0.45	0.30	0.02	0.03	79	0.10	0.31	0.20	0.01	0.02	C74
其他内分泌腺	Other endocrine	122	0.14	0.47	0.36	0.02	0.04	138	0.18	0.54	0.38	0.03	0.04	C75
霍奇金淋巴瘤	Hodgkin lymphoma	107	0.12	0.41	0.33	0.02	0.03	74	0.10	0.29	0.25	0.02	0.02	C81
非霍奇金淋巴瘤	Non-Hodgkin lymphoma	1 597	1.86	6.12	4.14	0.24	0.46	1 280	1.68	4.97	3.08	0.18	0.34	C82-C86,C96
免疫增生性疾病	Immunoproliferative diseases	22	0.03	0.08	0.05	0.00	0.01	10	0.01	0.04	0.02	0.00	0.00	C88
多发性骨髓瘤	Multiple myeloma	579	0.68	2.22	1.41	0.07	0.16	418	0.55	1.62	0.98	0.05	0.12	C90
淋巴细胞白血病	Lymphoid leukemia	417	0.49	1.60	1.59	0.08	0.13	251	0.33	0.97	1.07	0.06	0.08	C91
髓系白血病	Myeloid leukemia	1 035	1.21	3.96	2.81	0.15	0.28	746	0.98	2.90	1.99	0.11	0.20	C92-C94, D45-D47
白血病,未特指	Leukemia unspecified	537	0.63	2.06	1.60	0.08	0.15	397	0.52	1.54	1.16	0.06	0.11	C95
其他或未指明部位	Other and unspecified	1 990	2.32	7.62	5.04	0.25	0.55	1 726	2.27	6.70	4.17	0.23	0.44	O & U
所有部位合计	All sites	85 750	100.00	328.42	207.98	10.90	24.25	75 976	100.00	294.84	183.51	12.07	19.97	C00-C97, D32-D33, D42-D43, D45-D47
所有部位除外 C44	All sites except C44	85 052	99.19	325.75	206.31	10.82	24.07	75 408	99.25	292.64	182.30	12.02	19.84	C00-C97,D32-D33,D42-D43, D45-D47 exc. C44

附表 2-6　2019 年全国中部农村肿瘤登记地区癌症发病主要指标

Appendix Table 2-6　Cancer incidence in Central rural registration areas of China,2019

| 部位 Site | | 男性 Male | | | | | | 女性 Female | | | | | | ICD-10 |
| | | 病例数 No. cases | 构成 Freq./% | 粗率 Crude rate/ 100 000⁻¹ | 世标率 ASR world/ 100 000⁻¹ | 累积率 Cum. Rate/% | | 病例数 No. cases | 构成 Freq./% | 粗率 Crude rate/ 100 000⁻¹ | 世标率 ASR world/ 100 000⁻¹ | 累积率 Cum. Rate/% | | |
						0~64	0~74					0~64	0~74	
唇	Lip	126	0.09	0.25	0.17	0.01	0.02	71	0.06	0.15	0.09	0.00	0.01	C00
舌	Tongue	681	0.47	1.35	0.95	0.07	0.11	190	0.16	0.40	0.25	0.02	0.03	C01-C02
口	Mouth	692	0.48	1.37	0.94	0.07	0.11	313	0.26	0.65	0.40	0.02	0.04	C03-C06
唾液腺	Salivary gland	339	0.23	0.67	0.48	0.03	0.05	267	0.23	0.56	0.39	0.03	0.04	C07-C08
扁桃体	Tonsil	86	0.06	0.17	0.12	0.01	0.01	44	0.04	0.09	0.06	0.00	0.01	C09
其他口咽	Other oropharynx	166	0.11	0.33	0.22	0.01	0.03	45	0.04	0.09	0.06	0.00	0.01	C10
鼻咽	Nasopharynx	2 404	1.66	4.77	3.36	0.26	0.37	994	0.84	2.07	1.40	0.11	0.15	C11
下咽	Hypopharynx	300	0.21	0.59	0.39	0.02	0.05	40	0.03	0.08	0.05	0.00	0.01	C12-C13
咽,部位不明	Pharynx unspecified	182	0.13	0.36	0.24	0.01	0.03	62	0.05	0.13	0.08	0.00	0.01	C14
食管	Esophagus	12 910	8.91	25.60	16.37	0.69	2.07	5 983	5.06	12.45	6.97	0.25	0.84	C15
胃	Stomach	19 880	13.72	39.42	25.52	1.21	3.20	8 489	7.18	17.67	10.43	0.53	1.20	C16
小肠	Small intestine	633	0.44	1.26	0.83	0.05	0.10	533	0.45	1.11	0.71	0.05	0.08	C17
结肠	Colon	5 588	3.86	11.08	7.36	0.42	0.87	4 343	3.67	9.04	5.48	0.31	0.65	C18
直肠	Rectum	7 058	4.87	13.99	9.19	0.50	1.11	5 040	4.26	10.49	6.36	0.37	0.76	C19-C20
肛门	Anus	193	0.13	0.38	0.26	0.01	0.03	167	0.14	0.35	0.21	0.01	0.02	C21
肝脏	Liver	19 128	13.20	37.93	25.46	1.60	3.00	7 353	6.22	15.31	9.10	0.47	1.07	C22
胆囊及其他	Gallbladder etc.	1 598	1.10	3.17	2.06	0.10	0.25	1 873	1.58	3.90	2.27	0.11	0.27	C23-C24
胰腺	Pancreas	2 833	1.96	5.62	3.65	0.19	0.44	2 261	1.91	4.71	2.77	0.14	0.33	C25
鼻,鼻窦及其他	Nose,sinuses etc.	246	0.17	0.49	0.34	0.02	0.04	170	0.14	0.35	0.25	0.02	0.02	C30-C31
喉	Larynx	1 395	0.96	2.77	1.81	0.10	0.23	230	0.19	0.48	0.30	0.02	0.03	C32
气管,支气管,肺	Trachea,bronchus & lung	39 528	27.28	78.37	50.55	2.37	6.30	17 388	14.71	36.20	21.34	1.12	2.53	C33-C34
其他胸腔器官	Other thoracic organs	574	0.40	1.14	0.80	0.05	0.09	354	0.30	0.74	0.51	0.03	0.05	C37-C38
骨	Bone	1 052	0.73	2.09	1.65	0.09	0.16	864	0.73	1.80	1.38	0.08	0.13	C40-C41
皮肤黑色素瘤	Melanoma of skin	231	0.16	0.46	0.30	0.02	0.03	202	0.17	0.42	0.28	0.02	0.03	C43
皮肤其他	Other skin	1 090	0.75	2.16	1.44	0.06	0.15	1 043	0.88	2.17	1.25	0.06	0.13	C44
间皮瘤	Mesothelioma	51	0.04	0.10	0.07	0.00	0.01	30	0.03	0.06	0.04	0.00	0.00	C45
卡波西肉瘤	Kaposi sarcoma	9	0.01	0.02	0.01	0.00	0.00	1	0.00	0.00	0.00	0.00	0.00	C46
结缔组织,软组织	Connective & soft tissue	396	0.27	0.79	0.62	0.04	0.06	386	0.33	0.80	0.60	0.04	0.06	C47,C49
乳腺	Breast	336	0.23	0.67	0.46	0.03	0.05	17 482	14.79	36.39	25.20	2.10	2.64	C50
外阴	Vulva	—	—	—	—	—	—	185	0.16	0.39	0.24	0.01	0.03	C51
阴道	Vagina	—	—	—	—	—	—	156	0.13	0.32	0.21	0.01	0.02	C52
子宫颈	Cervix uteri	—	—	—	—	—	—	10 976	9.29	22.85	15.37	1.25	1.67	C53
子宫体	Corpus uteri	—	—	—	—	—	—	3 904	3.30	8.13	5.38	0.46	0.59	C54
子宫,部位不明	Uterus unspecified	—	—	—	—	—	—	1 111	0.94	2.31	1.53	0.12	0.16	C55
卵巢	Ovary	—	—	—	—	—	—	3 355	2.84	6.98	4.84	0.37	0.52	C56
其他女性生殖器官	Other female genital organs	—	—	—	—	—	—	214	0.18	0.45	0.31	0.02	0.03	C57
胎盘	Placenta	—	—	—	—	—	—	26	0.02	0.05	0.05	0.00	0.00	C58
阴茎	Penis	340	0.23	0.67	0.44	0.03	0.05	—	—	—	—	—	—	C60
前列腺	Prostate	3 692	2.55	7.32	4.46	0.09	0.49	—	—	—	—	—	—	C61
睾丸	Testis	190	0.13	0.38	0.34	0.02	0.03	—	—	—	—	—	—	C62
其他男性生殖器官	Other male genital organs	55	0.04	0.11	0.08	0.00	0.01	—	—	—	—	—	—	C63
肾	Kidney	1 735	1.20	3.44	2.37	0.16	0.27	1 119	0.95	2.33	1.56	0.10	0.18	C64
肾盂	Renal pelvis	205	0.14	0.41	0.28	0.02	0.03	95	0.08	0.20	0.12	0.01	0.02	C65
输尿管	Ureter	206	0.14	0.41	0.27	0.01	0.03	142	0.12	0.30	0.17	0.01	0.02	C66
膀胱	Bladder	3 362	2.32	6.67	4.30	0.20	0.50	851	0.72	1.77	1.02	0.05	0.11	C67
其他泌尿器官	Other urinary organs	64	0.04	0.13	0.09	0.00	0.01	45	0.04	0.09	0.06	0.00	0.01	C68
眼	Eye	96	0.07	0.19	0.21	0.01	0.01	71	0.06	0.15	0.15	0.01	0.01	C69
脑、神经系统	Brain,nervous system	3 816	2.63	7.57	5.79	0.36	0.60	4 095	3.47	8.52	6.03	0.39	0.63	C70-C72, D32-D33,D42-D43
甲状腺	Thyroid	2 256	1.56	4.47	3.43	0.28	0.33	8 511	7.20	17.72	13.04	1.09	1.25	C73
肾上腺	Adrenal gland	183	0.13	0.36	0.28	0.02	0.03	139	0.12	0.29	0.21	0.02	0.02	C74
其他内分泌腺	Other endocrine	111	0.08	0.22	0.18	0.01	0.02	140	0.12	0.29	0.21	0.01	0.02	C75
霍奇金淋巴瘤	Hodgkin lymphoma	181	0.12	0.36	0.27	0.02	0.03	124	0.10	0.26	0.20	0.01	0.02	C81
非霍奇金淋巴瘤	Non-Hodgkin lymphoma	2 026	1.40	4.02	2.94	0.18	0.33	1 430	1.21	2.98	2.05	0.13	0.23	C82-C86,C96
免疫增生性疾病	Immunoproliferative diseases	13	0.01	0.03	0.02	0.00	0.00	8	0.01	0.02	0.01	0.00	0.00	C88
多发性骨髓瘤	Multiple myeloma	694	0.48	1.38	0.92	0.05	0.12	513	0.43	1.07	0.67	0.04	0.09	C90
淋巴细胞白血病	Lymphoid leukemia	531	0.37	1.05	0.99	0.05	0.08	368	0.31	0.77	0.75	0.04	0.06	C91
髓系白血病	Myeloid leukemia	1 232	0.85	2.44	1.92	0.12	0.19	930	0.79	1.94	1.48	0.09	0.14	C92-C94, D45-D47
白血病,未特指	Leukemia unspecified	1 298	0.90	2.57	2.18	0.12	0.20	953	0.81	1.98	1.68	0.10	0.15	C95
其他或未指明部位	Other and unspecified	2 884	1.99	5.72	4.08	0.22	0.44	2 498	2.11	5.20	3.52	0.21	0.36	O & U
所有部位合计	All sites	144 875	100.00	287.25	191.48	10.04	22.76	118 177	100.00	246.00	159.09	10.48	17.51	C00-C97, D32-D33, D42-D43, D45-D47
所有部位除外 C44	All sites except C44	143 785	99.25	285.09	190.03	9.98	22.60	117 134	99.12	243.83	157.84	10.42	17.38	C00-C97,D32-D33,D42-D43, D45-D47 exc. C44

附表 2-7　2019 年全国西部肿瘤登记地区癌症发病主要指标

Appendix Table 2-7　Cancer incidence in Western registration areas of China,2019

部位 Site		男性 Male						女性 Female						ICD-10
		病例数 No. cases	构成 Freq./%	粗率 Crude rate/ $100\,000^{-1}$	世标率 ASR world/ $100\,000^{-1}$	累积率 Cum. Rate/%		病例数 No. cases	构成 Freq./%	粗率 Crude rate/ $100\,000^{-1}$	世标率 ASR world/ $100\,000^{-1}$	累积率 Cum. Rate/%		
						0~64	0~74					0~64	0~74	
唇	Lip	544	0.17	0.48	0.31	0.02	0.04	390	0.16	0.36	0.22	0.01	0.02	C00
舌	Tongue	1 057	0.33	0.92	0.60	0.04	0.07	521	0.22	0.48	0.30	0.02	0.03	C01-C02
口	Mouth	1 707	0.53	1.49	0.95	0.05	0.11	829	0.35	0.76	0.47	0.03	0.05	C03-C06
唾液腺	Salivary gland	686	0.21	0.60	0.41	0.03	0.05	563	0.24	0.52	0.35	0.03	0.04	C07-C08
扁桃体	Tonsil	228	0.07	0.20	0.13	0.01	0.01	95	0.04	0.09	0.06	0.00	0.01	C09
其他口咽	Other oropharynx	564	0.17	0.49	0.32	0.02	0.04	111	0.05	0.10	0.07	0.00	0.01	C10
鼻咽	Nasopharynx	6 377	1.97	5.58	3.84	0.30	0.42	2 706	1.13	2.48	1.68	0.13	0.18	C11
下咽	Hypopharynx	809	0.25	0.71	0.46	0.03	0.06	61	0.03	0.06	0.03	0.00	0.00	C12-C13
咽,部位不明	Pharynx unspecified	483	0.15	0.42	0.27	0.01	0.03	122	0.05	0.11	0.06	0.00	0.01	C14
食管	Esophagus	28 461	8.78	24.90	15.49	0.73	1.99	7 539	3.15	6.91	3.75	0.13	0.45	C15
胃	Stomach	30 256	9.33	26.47	16.59	0.85	2.04	13 027	5.45	11.94	6.86	0.35	0.77	C16
小肠	Small intestine	1 346	0.42	1.18	0.75	0.04	0.09	1 035	0.43	0.95	0.57	0.03	0.07	C17
结肠	Colon	13 630	4.20	11.92	7.55	0.40	0.88	10 429	4.36	9.56	5.60	0.31	0.71	C18
直肠	Rectum	19 862	6.13	17.38	10.91	0.56	1.31	12 619	5.28	11.57	6.74	0.36	0.79	C19-C20
肛门	Anus	568	0.18	0.50	0.31	0.01	0.03	405	0.17	0.37	0.22	0.01	0.02	C21
肝脏	Liver	49 871	15.38	43.63	28.50	1.91	3.28	15 649	6.54	14.35	8.40	0.45	0.96	C22
胆囊及其他	Gallbladder etc.	3 586	1.11	3.14	1.95	0.09	0.23	4 091	1.71	3.75	2.11	0.10	0.25	C23-C24
胰腺	Pancreas	7 477	2.31	6.54	4.10	0.21	0.49	5 032	2.10	4.61	2.60	0.12	0.30	C25
鼻、鼻窦及其他	Nose, sinuses etc.	651	0.20	0.57	0.39	0.03	0.04	433	0.18	0.40	0.27	0.02	0.03	C30-C31
喉	Larynx	3 141	0.97	2.75	1.74	0.10	0.22	387	0.16	0.35	0.21	0.01	0.02	C32
气管、支气管、肺	Trachea, bronchus & lung	86 260	26.61	75.46	47.30	2.45	5.84	42 130	17.62	38.62	22.46	1.23	2.63	C33-C34
其他胸腔器官	Other thoracic organs	1 198	0.37	1.05	0.73	0.05	0.08	778	0.33	0.71	0.47	0.03	0.05	C37-C38
骨	Bone	2 394	0.74	2.09	1.51	0.08	0.15	1 740	0.73	1.60	1.11	0.07	0.11	C40-C41
皮肤黑色素瘤	Melanoma of skin	426	0.13	0.37	0.25	0.01	0.03	424	0.18	0.39	0.25	0.01	0.03	C43
皮肤其他	Other skin	2 686	0.83	2.35	1.51	0.07	0.16	2 708	1.13	2.48	1.43	0.07	0.14	C44
间皮瘤	Mesothelioma	127	0.04	0.11	0.07	0.00	0.01	105	0.04	0.10	0.06	0.00	0.01	C45
卡波西肉瘤	Kaposi sarcoma	38	0.01	0.03	0.02	0.00	0.00	14	0.01	0.01	0.01	0.00	0.00	C46
结缔组织、软组织	Connective & soft tissue	1 122	0.35	0.98	0.72	0.04	0.07	925	0.39	0.85	0.65	0.04	0.06	C47,C49
乳腺	Breast	768	0.24	0.67	0.44	0.03	0.05	31 482	13.17	28.86	19.30	1.61	2.02	C50
外阴	Vulva	—	—	—	—	—	—	542	0.23	0.50	0.31	0.02	0.03	C51
阴道	Vagina	—	—	—	—	—	—	339	0.14	0.31	0.20	0.01	0.02	C52
子宫颈	Cervix uteri	—	—	—	—	—	—	19 737	8.25	18.09	11.99	0.97	1.29	C53
子宫体	Corpus uteri	—	—	—	—	—	—	7 081	2.96	6.49	4.20	0.35	0.47	C54
子宫,部位不明	Uterus unspecified	—	—	—	—	—	—	2 629	1.10	2.41	1.57	0.12	0.17	C55
卵巢	Ovary	—	—	—	—	—	—	7 739	3.24	7.09	4.87	0.38	0.52	C56
其他女性生殖器官	Other female genital organs	—	—	—	—	—	—	613	0.26	0.56	0.37	0.03	0.04	C57
胎盘	Placenta	—	—	—	—	—	—	93	0.04	0.09	0.08	0.01	0.01	C58
阴茎	Penis	832	0.26	0.73	0.47	0.03	0.05	—	—	—	—	—	—	C60
前列腺	Prostate	11 166	3.44	9.77	5.61	0.10	0.56	—	—	—	—	—	—	C61
睾丸	Testis	450	0.14	0.39	0.34	0.02	0.02	—	—	—	—	—	—	C62
其他男性生殖器官	Other male genital organs	117	0.04	0.10	0.07	0.00	0.01	—	—	—	—	—	—	C63
肾	Kidney	3 172	0.98	2.78	1.85	0.12	0.21	1 959	0.82	1.80	1.15	0.07	0.13	C64
肾盂	Renal pelvis	440	0.14	0.38	0.24	0.01	0.03	306	0.13	0.28	0.15	0.01	0.02	C65
输尿管	Ureter	411	0.13	0.36	0.22	0.01	0.03	362	0.15	0.33	0.18	0.01	0.02	C66
膀胱	Bladder	8 403	2.59	7.35	4.49	0.18	0.48	2 190	0.92	2.01	1.11	0.05	0.12	C67
其他泌尿器官	Other urinary organs	140	0.04	0.12	0.08	0.00	0.01	105	0.04	0.10	0.06	0.00	0.01	C68
眼	Eye	211	0.07	0.18	0.17	0.01	0.01	176	0.07	0.16	0.14	0.01	0.01	C69
脑、神经系统	Brain, nervous system	7 136	2.20	6.24	4.60	0.29	0.47	7 940	3.32	7.28	5.04	0.33	0.52	C70-C72, D32-D33,D42-D43
甲状腺	Thyroid	4 435	1.37	3.88	2.93	0.23	0.27	14 857	6.21	13.62	10.17	0.84	0.94	C73
肾上腺	Adrenal gland	273	0.08	0.24	0.17	0.01	0.02	228	0.10	0.21	0.15	0.01	0.01	C74
其他内分泌腺	Other endocrine	402	0.12	0.35	0.27	0.02	0.02	453	0.19	0.42	0.30	0.02	0.02	C75
霍奇金淋巴瘤	Hodgkin lymphoma	441	0.14	0.39	0.30	0.02	0.03	249	0.10	0.23	0.17	0.01	0.02	C81
非霍奇金淋巴瘤	Non-Hodgkin lymphoma	4 247	1.31	3.72	2.55	0.15	0.28	2 936	1.23	2.69	1.79	0.12	0.20	C82-C86,C96
免疫增生性疾病	Immunoproliferative diseases	98	0.03	0.09	0.06	0.00	0.01	75	0.03	0.07	0.05	0.00	0.01	C88
多发性骨髓瘤	Multiple myeloma	1 564	0.48	1.37	0.88	0.05	0.10	1 284	0.54	1.18	0.71	0.04	0.09	C90
淋巴细胞白血病	Lymphoid leukemia	1 119	0.35	0.98	0.95	0.05	0.08	796	0.33	0.73	0.70	0.04	0.06	C91
髓系白血病	Myeloid leukemia	2 697	0.83	2.36	1.79	0.11	0.17	2 164	0.91	1.98	1.47	0.09	0.14	C92-C94, D45-D47
白血病,未特指	Leukemia unspecified	2 346	0.72	2.05	1.72	0.09	0.15	1 815	0.76	1.66	1.36	0.08	0.12	C95
其他或未指明部位	Other and unspecified	7 757	2.39	6.79	4.59	0.25	0.50	6 097	2.55	5.59	3.65	0.22	0.38	O & U
所有部位合计	All sites	324 180	100.00	283.61	182.45	9.98	21.35	239 115	100.00	219.21	138.23	9.00	15.08	C00-C97, D32-D33, D42-D43, D45-D47
所有部位除外 C44	All sites except C44	321 494	99.17	281.26	180.94	9.90	21.20	236 407	98.87	216.72	136.80	8.93	14.94	C00-C97,D32-D33,D42-D43, D45-D47 exc. C44

附表 2-8 2019 年全国西部城市肿瘤登记地区癌症发病主要指标
Appendix Table 2-8 Cancer incidence in Western urban registration areas of China, 2019

部位 Site		男性 Male						女性 Female						ICD-10
		病例数 No. cases	构成 Freq./%	粗率 Crude rate/100 000⁻¹	世标率 ASR world/100 000⁻¹	累积率 Cum. Rate/% 0~64	0~74	病例数 No. cases	构成 Freq./%	粗率 Crude rate/100 000⁻¹	世标率 ASR world/100 000⁻¹	累积率 Cum. Rate/% 0~64	0~74	
唇	Lip	121	0.09	0.28	0.18	0.01	0.02	84	0.08	0.20	0.12	0.01	0.01	C00
舌	Tongue	421	0.32	0.97	0.62	0.04	0.07	246	0.25	0.58	0.36	0.02	0.04	C01-C02
口	Mouth	612	0.47	1.42	0.89	0.04	0.10	326	0.33	0.77	0.48	0.03	0.06	C03-C06
唾液腺	Salivary gland	282	0.22	0.65	0.44	0.03	0.05	228	0.23	0.54	0.35	0.02	0.04	C07-C08
扁桃体	Tonsil	93	0.07	0.22	0.14	0.01	0.02	39	0.04	0.09	0.06	0.00	0.01	C09
其他口咽	Other oropharynx	207	0.16	0.48	0.31	0.02	0.04	36	0.04	0.09	0.05	0.00	0.01	C10
鼻咽	Nasopharynx	2 220	1.71	5.13	3.48	0.27	0.38	944	0.95	2.23	1.50	0.11	0.16	C11
下咽	Hypopharynx	352	0.27	0.81	0.52	0.03	0.07	28	0.03	0.07	0.04	0.00	0.00	C12-C13
咽，部位不明	Pharynx unspecified	201	0.16	0.46	0.29	0.02	0.04	47	0.05	0.11	0.06	0.00	0.01	C14
食管	Esophagus	10 012	7.73	23.15	14.39	0.68	1.84	2 651	2.68	6.26	3.43	0.11	0.40	C15
胃	Stomach	11 703	9.03	27.06	16.91	0.86	2.07	5 064	5.12	11.96	6.94	0.36	0.78	C16
小肠	Small intestine	572	0.44	1.32	0.84	0.04	0.10	466	0.47	1.10	0.63	0.04	0.07	C17
结肠	Colon	6 465	4.99	14.95	9.33	0.47	1.08	5 046	5.10	11.92	6.89	0.35	0.79	C18
直肠	Rectum	7 849	6.06	18.15	11.31	0.57	1.35	4 990	5.04	11.79	6.85	0.35	0.80	C19-C20
肛门	Anus	202	0.16	0.47	0.29	0.01	0.03	156	0.16	0.37	0.21	0.01	0.02	C21
肝脏	Liver	18 028	13.91	41.68	26.94	1.77	3.10	5 793	5.85	13.69	8.00	0.40	0.91	C22
胆囊及其他	Gallbladder etc.	1 589	1.23	3.67	2.26	0.10	0.26	1 843	1.86	4.35	2.44	0.11	0.27	C23-C24
胰腺	Pancreas	3 098	2.39	7.16	4.46	0.22	0.53	2 262	2.29	5.34	3.00	0.14	0.34	C25
鼻、鼻窦及其他	Nose, sinuses etc.	248	0.19	0.57	0.39	0.03	0.04	168	0.17	0.40	0.26	0.01	0.03	C30-C31
喉	Larynx	1 373	1.06	3.17	1.99	0.11	0.25	159	0.16	0.38	0.21	0.01	0.02	C32
气管、支气管、肺	Trachea, bronchus & lung	34 700	26.78	80.23	49.96	2.50	6.15	17 033	17.21	40.24	23.44	1.26	2.73	C33-C34
其他胸腔器官	Other thoracic organs	503	0.39	1.16	0.80	0.05	0.09	352	0.36	0.83	0.54	0.03	0.06	C37-C38
骨	Bone	831	0.64	1.92	1.34	0.08	0.14	641	0.65	1.51	1.06	0.06	0.10	C40-C41
皮肤黑色素瘤	Melanoma of skin	176	0.14	0.41	0.27	0.01	0.03	167	0.17	0.39	0.24	0.01	0.03	C43
皮肤其他	Other skin	1 120	0.86	2.59	1.63	0.07	0.16	1 064	1.08	2.51	1.42	0.06	0.14	C44
间皮瘤	Mesothelioma	50	0.04	0.12	0.08	0.00	0.01	42	0.04	0.10	0.06	0.00	0.01	C45
卡波西肉瘤	Kaposi sarcoma	11	0.01	0.03	0.02	0.00	0.00	6	0.01	0.01	0.01	0.00	0.00	C46
结缔组织、软组织	Connective & soft tissue	461	0.36	1.07	0.78	0.05	0.08	362	0.37	0.86	0.65	0.04	0.06	C47, C49
乳腺	Breast	286	0.22	0.66	0.43	0.02	0.05	14 043	14.19	33.18	21.78	1.76	2.32	C50
外阴	Vulva	—	—	—	—	—	—	215	0.22	0.51	0.31	0.02	0.03	C51
阴道	Vagina	—	—	—	—	—	—	152	0.15	0.36	0.23	0.01	0.03	C52
子宫颈	Cervix uteri	—	—	—	—	—	—	7 227	7.30	17.07	11.22	0.91	1.21	C53
子宫体	Corpus uteri	—	—	—	—	—	—	2 973	3.00	7.02	4.52	0.38	0.51	C54
子宫，部位不明	Uterus unspecified	—	—	—	—	—	—	817	0.83	1.93	1.25	0.10	0.13	C55
卵巢	Ovary	—	—	—	—	—	—	3 251	3.29	7.68	5.21	0.39	0.55	C56
其他女性生殖器官	Other female genital organs	—	—	—	—	—	—	265	0.27	0.63	0.41	0.03	0.04	C57
胎盘	Placenta	—	—	—	—	—	—	37	0.04	0.09	0.08	0.01	0.01	C58
阴茎	Penis	301	0.23	0.70	0.44	0.03	0.05	—	—	—	—	—	—	C60
前列腺	Prostate	5 414	4.18	12.52	7.13	0.13	0.70	—	—	—	—	—	—	C61
睾丸	Testis	165	0.13	0.38	0.33	0.02	0.03	—	—	—	—	—	—	C62
其他男性生殖器官	Other male genital organs	53	0.04	0.12	0.09	0.00	0.01	—	—	—	—	—	—	C63
肾	Kidney	1 622	1.25	3.75	2.46	0.15	0.29	962	0.97	2.27	1.42	0.08	0.16	C64
肾盂	Renal pelvis	223	0.17	0.52	0.32	0.01	0.04	166	0.17	0.39	0.21	0.01	0.02	C65
输尿管	Ureter	214	0.17	0.49	0.30	0.01	0.03	185	0.19	0.44	0.24	0.01	0.03	C66
膀胱	Bladder	3 560	2.75	8.23	4.96	0.19	0.54	948	0.96	2.24	1.25	0.05	0.14	C67
其他泌尿器官	Other urinary organs	61	0.05	0.14	0.09	0.00	0.01	39	0.04	0.09	0.05	0.00	0.01	C68
眼	Eye	68	0.05	0.16	0.15	0.01	0.01	51	0.05	0.12	0.09	0.01	0.01	C69
脑、神经系统	Brain, nervous system	2 683	2.07	6.20	4.53	0.28	0.47	3 122	3.15	7.38	5.04	0.32	0.52	C70-C72, D32-D33, D42-D43
甲状腺	Thyroid	2 344	1.81	5.42	4.01	0.32	0.38	7 288	7.36	17.22	12.54	1.03	1.18	C73
肾上腺	Adrenal gland	116	0.09	0.27	0.19	0.01	0.02	101	0.10	0.24	0.17	0.01	0.01	C74
其他内分泌腺	Other endocrine	159	0.12	0.37	0.29	0.02	0.03	182	0.18	0.43	0.31	0.02	0.03	C75
霍奇金淋巴瘤	Hodgkin lymphoma	166	0.13	0.38	0.30	0.02	0.03	130	0.13	0.31	0.22	0.01	0.02	C81
非霍奇金淋巴瘤	Non-Hodgkin lymphoma	1 819	1.40	4.21	2.84	0.16	0.32	1 343	1.36	3.17	2.07	0.13	0.23	C82-C86, C96
免疫增生性疾病	Immunoproliferative diseases	87	0.07	0.20	0.14	0.01	0.02	62	0.06	0.15	0.11	0.01	0.01	C88
多发性骨髓瘤	Multiple myeloma	766	0.59	1.77	1.12	0.06	0.13	621	0.63	1.47	0.88	0.05	0.11	C90
淋巴细胞白血病	Lymphoid leukemia	485	0.37	1.12	1.08	0.06	0.09	336	0.34	0.79	0.75	0.04	0.06	C91
髓系白血病	Myeloid leukemia	1 158	0.89	2.68	1.98	0.12	0.20	915	0.92	2.16	1.56	0.10	0.15	C92-C94, D45-D47
白血病，未特指	Leukemia unspecified	790	0.61	1.83	1.49	0.08	0.14	589	0.60	1.39	1.13	0.06	0.15	C95
其他或未指明部位	Other and unspecified	3 540	2.73	8.19	5.35	0.28	0.58	2 694	2.72	6.36	4.00	0.23	0.42	O & U
所有部位合计	All sites	129 580	100.00	299.62	190.84	10.10	22.23	98 957	100.00	233.80	146.38	9.36	15.97	C00-C97, D32-D33, D42-D43, D45-D47
所有部位除外 C44	All sites except C44	128 460	99.14	297.03	189.22	10.03	22.06	97 893	98.92	231.28	144.96	9.29	15.82	C00-C97, D32-D33, D42-D43, D45-D47 exc. C44

部位 Site		男性 Male						女性 Female						ICD-10
		病例数 No. cases	构成 Freq./%	粗率 Crude rate/ 100 000⁻¹	世标率 ASR world/ 100 000⁻¹	累积率 Cum. Rate/%		病例数 No. cases	构成 Freq./%	粗率 Crude rate/ 100 000⁻¹	世标率 ASR world/ 100 000⁻¹	累积率 Cum. Rate/%		
						0~64	0~74					0~64	0~74	
唇	Lip	423	0.22	0.60	0.39	0.02	0.04	306	0.22	0.46	0.28	0.02	0.03	C00
舌	Tongue	636	0.33	0.90	0.59	0.04	0.07	275	0.20	0.41	0.26	0.02	0.03	C01-C02
口	Mouth	1 095	0.56	1.54	0.99	0.05	0.12	503	0.36	0.75	0.46	0.03	0.05	C03-C06
唾液腺	Salivary gland	404	0.21	0.57	0.40	0.03	0.04	335	0.24	0.50	0.35	0.03	0.04	C07-C08
扁桃体	Tonsil	135	0.07	0.19	0.13	0.01	0.01	56	0.04	0.08	0.06	0.00	0.00	C09
其他口咽	Other oropharynx	357	0.18	0.50	0.33	0.02	0.04	75	0.05	0.11	0.07	0.00	0.01	C10
鼻咽	Nasopharynx	4 157	2.14	5.85	4.06	0.32	0.44	1 762	1.26	2.64	1.79	0.14	0.19	C11
下咽	Hypopharynx	457	0.23	0.64	0.42	0.03	0.05	33	0.02	0.05	0.03	0.00	0.00	C12-C13
咽,部位不明	Pharynx unspecified	282	0.14	0.40	0.25	0.01	0.03	75	0.05	0.11	0.06	0.00	0.01	C14
食管	Esophagus	18 449	9.48	25.96	16.16	0.76	2.08	4 888	3.49	7.32	3.95	0.14	0.48	C15
胃	Stomach	18 553	9.53	26.11	16.40	0.85	2.02	7 963	5.68	11.93	6.80	0.34	0.76	C16
小肠	Small intestine	774	0.40	1.09	0.70	0.04	0.08	569	0.41	0.85	0.52	0.03	0.06	C17
结肠	Colon	7 165	3.68	10.08	6.46	0.36	0.76	5 383	3.84	8.06	4.79	0.28	0.56	C18
直肠	Rectum	12 013	6.17	16.91	10.66	0.55	1.29	7 629	5.44	11.43	6.68	0.36	0.79	C19-C20
肛门	Anus	366	0.19	0.52	0.32	0.02	0.04	249	0.18	0.37	0.22	0.01	0.02	C21
肝脏	Liver	31 843	16.36	44.81	29.47	2.00	3.39	9 856	7.03	14.76	8.67	0.47	1.00	C22
胆囊及其他	Gallbladder etc.	1 997	1.03	2.81	1.75	0.09	0.21	2 248	1.60	3.37	1.91	0.09	0.23	C23-C24
胰腺	Pancreas	4 379	2.25	6.16	3.88	0.20	0.46	2 770	1.98	4.15	2.34	0.11	0.28	C25
鼻,鼻窦及其他	Nose,sinuses etc.	403	0.21	0.57	0.38	0.03	0.04	265	0.19	0.40	0.27	0.02	0.03	C30-C31
喉	Larynx	1 768	0.91	2.49	1.58	0.09	0.20	228	0.16	0.34	0.21	0.01	0.02	C32
气管、支气管、肺	Trachea,bronchus & lung	51 560	26.50	72.56	45.68	2.42	5.66	25 097	17.91	37.60	21.84	1.20	2.56	C33-C34
其他胸腔器官	Other thoracic organs	695	0.36	0.98	0.69	0.04	0.08	426	0.30	0.64	0.42	0.03	0.05	C37-C38
骨	Bone	1 563	0.80	2.20	1.61	0.09	0.16	1 099	0.78	1.65	1.14	0.07	0.12	C40-C41
皮肤黑色素瘤	Melanoma of skin	250	0.13	0.35	0.23	0.01	0.03	257	0.18	0.38	0.25	0.02	0.03	C43
皮肤其他	Other skin	1 566	0.80	2.20	1.44	0.07	0.15	1 644	1.17	2.46	1.43	0.07	0.14	C44
间皮瘤	Mesothelioma	77	0.04	0.11	0.07	0.00	0.01	63	0.04	0.09	0.06	0.00	0.01	C45
卡波西肉瘤	Kaposi sarcoma	27	0.01	0.04	0.03	0.00	0.00	8	0.01	0.01	0.01	0.00	0.00	C46
结缔组织、软组织	Connective & soft tissue	661	0.34	0.93	0.69	0.04	0.07	563	0.40	0.84	0.65	0.04	0.06	C47,C49
乳腺	Breast	482	0.25	0.68	0.45	0.03	0.05	17 439	12.44	26.12	17.76	1.51	1.83	C50
外阴	Vulva	—	—	—	—	—	—	327	0.23	0.49	0.31	0.02	0.03	C51
阴道	Vagina	—	—	—	—	—	—	187	0.13	0.28	0.18	0.01	0.02	C52
子宫颈	Cervix uteri	—	—	—	—	—	—	12 510	8.93	18.74	12.50	1.01	1.35	C53
子宫体	Corpus uteri	—	—	—	—	—	—	4 108	2.93	6.15	3.99	0.34	0.44	C54
子宫,部位不明	Uterus unspecified	—	—	—	—	—	—	1 812	1.29	2.71	1.77	0.14	0.19	C55
卵巢	Ovary	—	—	—	—	—	—	4 488	3.20	6.72	4.66	0.37	0.49	C56
其他女性生殖器官	Other female genital organs	—	—	—	—	—	—	348	0.25	0.52	0.35	0.03	0.04	C57
胎盘	Placenta	—	—	—	—	—	—	56	0.04	0.08	0.08	0.01	0.01	C58
阴茎	Penis	531	0.27	0.75	0.48	0.03	0.05	—	—	—	—	—	—	C60
前列腺	Prostate	5 752	2.96	8.09	4.67	0.08	0.48	—	—	—	—	—	—	C61
睾丸	Testis	285	0.15	0.40	0.34	0.02	0.03	—	—	—	—	—	—	C62
其他男性生殖器官	Other male genital organs	64	0.03	0.09	0.06	0.00	0.01	—	—	—	—	—	—	C63
肾	Kidney	1 550	0.80	2.18	1.48	0.10	0.17	997	0.71	1.49	0.98	0.06	0.10	C64
肾盂	Renal pelvis	217	0.11	0.31	0.19	0.01	0.02	140	0.10	0.21	0.12	0.01	0.01	C65
输尿管	Ureter	197	0.10	0.28	0.17	0.01	0.02	177	0.13	0.27	0.15	0.01	0.02	C66
膀胱	Bladder	4 843	2.49	6.82	4.19	0.18	0.45	1 242	0.89	1.86	1.03	0.05	0.11	C67
其他泌尿器官	Other urinary organs	79	0.04	0.11	0.07	0.00	0.01	66	0.05	0.10	0.06	0.00	0.01	C68
眼	Eye	143	0.07	0.20	0.17	0.01	0.01	125	0.09	0.19	0.16	0.01	0.01	C69
脑、神经系统	Brain,nervous system	4 453	2.29	6.27	4.65	0.30	0.47	4 818	3.44	7.22	5.05	0.34	0.53	C70-C72, D32-D33,D42-D43
甲状腺	Thyroid	2 091	1.07	2.94	2.24	0.18	0.21	7 569	5.40	11.34	8.61	0.71	0.79	C73
肾上腺	Adrenal gland	157	0.08	0.22	0.16	0.01	0.02	127	0.09	0.19	0.13	0.01	0.01	C74
其他内分泌腺	Other endocrine	243	0.12	0.34	0.26	0.02	0.03	271	0.19	0.41	0.29	0.02	0.03	C75
霍奇金淋巴瘤	Hodgkin lymphoma	275	0.14	0.39	0.30	0.02	0.03	119	0.08	0.18	0.14	0.01	0.01	C81
非霍奇金淋巴瘤	Non-Hodgkin lymphoma	2 428	1.25	3.42	2.37	0.15	0.26	1 593	1.14	2.39	1.62	0.11	0.18	C82-C86,C96
免疫增生性疾病	Immunoproliferative diseases	11	0.01	0.02	0.01	0.00	0.00	13	0.01	0.02	0.01	0.00	0.00	C88
多发性骨髓瘤	Multiple myeloma	798	0.41	1.12	0.73	0.04	0.09	663	0.47	0.99	0.60	0.04	0.08	C90
淋巴细胞白血病	Lymphoid leukemia	634	0.33	0.89	0.87	0.05	0.07	460	0.33	0.69	0.66	0.04	0.05	C91
髓系白血病	Myeloid leukemia	1 539	0.79	2.17	1.67	0.11	0.16	1 249	0.89	1.87	1.42	0.09	0.14	C92-C94, D45-D47
白血病,未特指	Leukemia unspecified	1 556	0.80	2.19	1.86	0.10	0.17	1 226	0.87	1.84	1.50	0.09	0.13	C95
其他或未指明部位	Other and unspecified	4 217	2.17	5.93	4.11	0.24	0.45	3 403	2.43	5.10	3.43	0.21	0.36	O & U
所有部位合计	All sites	194 600	100.00	273.87	177.28	9.89	20.83	140 158	100.00	209.96	133.11	8.76	14.53	C00-C97, D32-D33, D42-D43, D45-D47
所有部位除外 C44	All sites except C44	193 034	99.20	271.66	175.84	9.82	20.68	138 514	98.83	207.49	131.68	8.69	14.39	C00-C97,D32-D33, D42-D43, D45-D47 exc. C44

部位 Site		男性 Male						女性 Female						ICD-10
		死亡数 No. deaths	构成 Freq./%	粗率 Crude rate/ 100 000⁻¹	世标率 ASR world/ 100 000⁻¹	累积率 Cum. Rate/%		死亡数 No. deaths	构成 Freq./%	粗率 Crude rate/ 100 000⁻¹	世标率 ASR world/ 100 000⁻¹	累积率 Cum. Rate/%		
						0~64	0~74					0~64	0~74	
唇	Lip	109	0.04	0.09	0.04	0.00	0.00	60	0.03	0.05	0.02	0.00	0.00	C00
舌	Tongue	776	0.25	0.61	0.35	0.02	0.04	391	0.22	0.31	0.14	0.01	0.02	C01-C02
口	Mouth	967	0.32	0.76	0.41	0.02	0.05	518	0.29	0.41	0.18	0.01	0.02	C03-C06
唾液腺	Salivary gland	377	0.12	0.30	0.16	0.01	0.02	199	0.11	0.16	0.08	0.00	0.01	C07-C08
扁桃体	Tonsil	157	0.05	0.12	0.07	0.01	0.01	40	0.02	0.03	0.01	0.00	0.00	C09
其他口咽	Other oropharynx	350	0.11	0.27	0.15	0.01	0.02	52	0.03	0.04	0.02	0.00	0.00	C10
鼻咽	Nasopharynx	3 845	1.26	3.02	1.78	0.12	0.21	1 272	0.71	1.01	0.55	0.03	0.06	C11
下咽	Hypopharynx	840	0.28	0.66	0.37	0.02	0.05	42	0.02	0.03	0.02	0.00	0.00	C12-C13
咽,部位不明	Pharynx unspecified	334	0.11	0.26	0.14	0.01	0.02	93	0.05	0.07	0.04	0.00	0.00	C14
食管	Esophagus	26 325	8.62	20.65	10.63	0.42	1.25	9 401	5.28	7.45	2.98	0.05	0.29	C15
胃	Stomach	38 749	12.69	30.40	15.56	0.55	1.76	17 253	9.68	13.67	6.11	0.23	0.63	C16
小肠	Small intestine	1 323	0.43	1.04	0.55	0.02	0.06	881	0.49	0.70	0.32	0.01	0.04	C17
结肠	Colon	13 253	4.34	10.40	5.30	0.20	0.54	10 339	5.80	8.19	3.51	0.13	0.33	C18
直肠	Rectum	12 625	4.13	9.90	5.09	0.20	0.54	7 699	4.32	6.10	2.67	0.10	0.27	C19-C20
肛门	Anus	289	0.09	0.23	0.12	0.01	0.01	218	0.12	0.17	0.08	0.00	0.01	C21
肝脏	Liver	41 675	13.65	32.69	18.65	1.16	2.16	14 986	8.41	11.87	5.55	0.24	0.62	C22
胆囊及其他	Gallbladder etc.	4 897	1.60	3.84	1.97	0.07	0.22	5 065	2.84	4.01	1.76	0.06	0.19	C23-C24
胰腺	Pancreas	12 057	3.95	9.46	4.98	0.22	0.58	9 395	5.27	7.44	3.32	0.12	0.37	C25
鼻、鼻窦及其他	Nose, sinuses etc.	364	0.12	0.29	0.16	0.01	0.02	184	0.10	0.15	0.07	0.00	0.01	C30-C31
喉	Larynx	2 578	0.84	2.02	1.05	0.05	0.12	299	0.17	0.24	0.10	0.00	0.01	C32
气管、支气管、肺	Trachea, bronchus & lung	90 576	29.67	71.05	36.70	1.40	4.31	41 670	23.38	33.02	14.74	0.56	1.59	C33-C34
其他胸腔器官	Other thoracic organs	936	0.31	0.73	0.44	0.03	0.05	529	0.30	0.42	0.22	0.01	0.02	C37-C38
骨	Bone	1 770	0.58	1.39	0.84	0.04	0.09	1 218	0.68	0.97	0.52	0.02	0.05	C40-C41
皮肤黑色素瘤	Melanoma of skin	512	0.17	0.40	0.21	0.01	0.02	467	0.26	0.37	0.18	0.01	0.02	C43
皮肤其他	Other skin	1 150	0.38	0.90	0.44	0.01	0.03	1 078	0.60	0.85	0.30	0.01	0.02	C44
间皮瘤	Mesothelioma	208	0.07	0.16	0.09	0.00	0.01	148	0.08	0.12	0.06	0.00	0.01	C45
卡波西肉瘤	Kaposi sarcoma	40	0.01	0.03	0.02	0.00	0.00	29	0.02	0.02	0.02	0.00	0.00	C46
结缔组织、软组织	Connective & soft tissue	603	0.20	0.47	0.30	0.02	0.03	431	0.24	0.34	0.21	0.01	0.02	C47,C49
乳腺	Breast	275	0.09	0.22	0.11	0.01	0.01	14 184	7.96	11.24	6.00	0.40	0.66	C50
外阴	Vulva	—	—	—	—	—	—	296	0.17	0.23	0.11	0.00	0.01	C51
阴道	Vagina	—	—	—	—	—	—	154	0.09	0.12	0.06	0.00	0.01	C52
子宫颈	Cervix uteri	—	—	—	—	—	—	5 813	3.26	4.61	2.55	0.18	0.28	C53
子宫体	Corpus uteri	—	—	—	—	—	—	2 473	1.39	1.96	1.03	0.06	0.12	C54
子宫,部位不明	Uterus unspecified	—	—	—	—	—	—	997	0.56	0.79	0.40	0.02	0.05	C55
卵巢	Ovary	—	—	—	—	—	—	5 260	2.95	4.17	2.26	0.14	0.27	C56
其他女性生殖器官	Other female genital organs	—	—	—	—	—	—	296	0.17	0.23	0.12	0.01	0.01	C57
胎盘	Placenta	—	—	—	—	—	—	12	0.01	0.01	0.01	0.00	0.00	C58
阴茎	Penis	374	0.12	0.29	0.15	0.01	0.01	—	—	—	—	—	—	C60
前列腺	Prostate	8 684	2.84	6.81	3.08	0.03	0.20	—	—	—	—	—	—	C61
睾丸	Testis	148	0.05	0.12	0.08	0.00	0.01	—	—	—	—	—	—	C62
其他男性生殖器官	Other male genital organs	100	0.03	0.08	0.04	0.00	0.00	—	—	—	—	—	—	C63
肾	Kidney	3 141	1.03	2.46	1.31	0.06	0.14	1 482	0.83	1.17	0.55	0.02	0.06	C64
肾盂	Renal pelvis	441	0.14	0.35	0.18	0.01	0.02	327	0.18	0.26	0.10	0.00	0.01	C65
输尿管	Ureter	522	0.17	0.41	0.21	0.01	0.02	427	0.24	0.34	0.14	0.00	0.01	C66
膀胱	Bladder	6 179	2.02	4.85	2.27	0.04	0.18	1 716	0.96	1.36	0.51	0.01	0.04	C67
其他泌尿器官	Other urinary organs	114	0.04	0.09	0.04	0.00	0.00	79	0.04	0.06	0.02	0.00	0.00	C68
眼	Eye	81	0.03	0.06	0.05	0.00	0.00	76	0.04	0.06	0.04	0.00	0.00	C69
脑、神经系统	Brain, nervous system	6 162	2.02	4.83	3.04	0.17	0.32	5 316	2.98	4.21	2.39	0.13	0.24	C70-C72, D32-D33,D42-D43
甲状腺	Thyroid	734	0.24	0.58	0.32	0.01	0.04	1 135	0.64	0.90	0.44	0.02	0.05	C73
肾上腺	Adrenal gland	304	0.10	0.24	0.15	0.01	0.01	187	0.10	0.15	0.09	0.00	0.01	C74
其他内分泌腺	Other endocrine	197	0.06	0.15	0.09	0.00	0.01	147	0.08	0.12	0.07	0.00	0.01	C75
霍奇金淋巴瘤	Hodgkin lymphoma	250	0.08	0.20	0.11	0.00	0.01	150	0.08	0.12	0.06	0.00	0.01	C81
非霍奇金淋巴瘤	Non-Hodgkin lymphoma	4 791	1.57	3.76	2.09	0.09	0.23	3 162	1.77	2.51	1.25	0.06	0.14	C82-C86,C96
免疫增生性疾病	Immunoproliferative diseases	70	0.02	0.05	0.03	0.00	0.00	22	0.01	0.02	0.01	0.00	0.00	C88
多发性骨髓瘤	Multiple myeloma	1 889	0.62	1.48	0.78	0.03	0.10	1 394	0.78	1.10	0.55	0.03	0.07	C90
淋巴细胞白血病	Lymphoid leukemia	1 266	0.41	0.99	0.71	0.04	0.06	868	0.49	0.69	0.50	0.03	0.04	C91
髓系白血病	Myeloid leukemia	3 459	1.13	2.71	1.56	0.07	0.16	2 276	1.28	1.80	1.01	0.05	0.11	C92-C94, D45-D47
白血病,未特指	Leukemia unspecified	2 221	0.73	1.74	1.12	0.05	0.11	1 589	0.89	1.26	0.74	0.04	0.08	C95
其他或未指明部位	Other and unspecified	6 239	2.04	4.89	2.65	0.12	0.29	4 418	2.48	3.50	1.64	0.07	0.17	O & U
所有部位合计	All sites	305 326	100.00	239.52	126.74	5.38	14.17	178 213	100.00	141.21	66.41	2.93	7.04	C00-C97, D32-D33, D42-D43, D45-D47
所有部位除外 C44	All sites except C44	304 176	99.62	238.62	126.30	5.37	14.13	177 135	99.40	140.36	66.11	2.93	7.02	C00-C97,D32-D33, D42-D43, D45-D47 exc. C44

附表 2-11　2019 年全国东部城市肿瘤登记地区癌症死亡主要指标

Appendix Table 2-11　Cancer mortality in Eastern urban registration areas of China, 2019

部位 Site		男性 Male						女性 Female						ICD-10
		死亡数 No. deaths	构成 Freq./%	粗率 Crude rate/ 100 000⁻¹	世标率 ASR world/ 100 000⁻¹	累积率 Cum. Rate/%		死亡数 No. deaths	构成 Freq./%	粗率 Crude rate/ 100 000⁻¹	世标率 ASR world/ 100 000⁻¹	累积率 Cum. Rate/%		
						0~64	0~74					0~64	0~74	
唇	Lip	44	0.03	0.07	0.03	0.00	0.00	23	0.02	0.04	0.01	0.00	0.00	C00
舌	Tongue	448	0.29	0.69	0.40	0.03	0.05	234	0.25	0.36	0.16	0.01	0.02	C01-C02
口	Mouth	550	0.36	0.85	0.45	0.03	0.05	281	0.30	0.43	0.18	0.01	0.02	C03-C06
唾液腺	Salivary gland	213	0.14	0.33	0.18	0.01	0.02	105	0.11	0.16	0.08	0.00	0.01	C07-C08
扁桃体	Tonsil	88	0.06	0.14	0.08	0.01	0.01	20	0.02	0.03	0.01	0.00	0.00	C09
其他口咽	Other oropharynx	218	0.14	0.34	0.18	0.01	0.02	35	0.04	0.05	0.02	0.00	0.00	C10
鼻咽	Nasopharynx	2 013	1.31	3.12	1.81	0.12	0.22	670	0.73	1.02	0.55	0.04	0.07	C11
下咽	Hypopharynx	498	0.32	0.77	0.42	0.03	0.05	24	0.03	0.04	0.02	0.00	0.00	C12-C13
咽,部位不明	Pharynx unspecified	170	0.11	0.26	0.14	0.01	0.02	45	0.05	0.07	0.03	0.00	0.00	C14
食管	Esophagus	10 878	7.09	16.84	8.58	0.38	1.02	3 193	3.46	4.88	1.91	0.03	0.18	C15
胃	Stomach	17 997	11.72	27.86	13.91	0.50	1.55	8 247	8.93	12.61	5.58	0.22	0.56	C16
小肠	Small intestine	776	0.51	1.20	0.61	0.03	0.07	498	0.54	0.76	0.34	0.01	0.04	C17
结肠	Colon	7 989	5.20	12.37	6.07	0.22	0.61	6 326	6.85	9.67	4.02	0.14	0.37	C18
直肠	Rectum	6 786	4.42	10.51	5.22	0.20	0.56	4 147	4.49	6.34	2.73	0.11	0.27	C19-C20
肛门	Anus	134	0.09	0.21	0.11	0.01	0.01	107	0.12	0.16	0.07	0.00	0.01	C21
肝脏	Liver	20 228	13.18	31.31	17.43	1.08	2.01	7 276	7.88	11.12	5.03	0.21	0.54	C22
胆囊及其他	Gallbladder etc.	2 548	1.66	3.94	1.95	0.07	0.21	2 663	2.88	4.07	1.73	0.06	0.18	C23-C24
胰腺	Pancreas	6 508	4.24	10.07	5.17	0.23	0.60	5 130	5.55	7.84	3.41	0.12	0.38	C25
鼻、鼻窦及其他	Nose, sinuses etc.	191	0.12	0.30	0.16	0.01	0.02	104	0.11	0.16	0.07	0.00	0.01	C30-C31
喉	Larynx	1 368	0.89	2.12	1.08	0.05	0.12	154	0.17	0.24	0.09	0.00	0.01	C32
气管、支气管、肺	Trachea, bronchus & lung	45 353	29.54	70.21	35.35	1.36	4.11	21 427	23.20	32.75	14.13	0.53	1.45	C33-C34
其他胸腔器官	Other thoracic organs	536	0.35	0.83	0.49	0.03	0.05	327	0.35	0.50	0.26	0.01	0.03	C37-C38
骨	Bone	782	0.51	1.21	0.73	0.03	0.07	541	0.59	0.83	0.46	0.02	0.04	C40-C41
皮肤黑色素瘤	Melanoma of skin	263	0.17	0.41	0.21	0.01	0.02	245	0.27	0.37	0.18	0.01	0.02	C43
皮肤其他	Other skin	554	0.36	0.86	0.40	0.01	0.03	437	0.47	0.67	0.24	0.01	0.01	C44
间皮瘤	Mesothelioma	127	0.08	0.20	0.10	0.01	0.01	78	0.08	0.12	0.06	0.00	0.01	C45
卡波西肉瘤	Kaposi sarcoma	24	0.02	0.04	0.03	0.00	0.00	14	0.02	0.02	0.02	0.00	0.00	C46
结缔组织、软组织	Connective & soft tissue	354	0.23	0.55	0.35	0.02	0.03	234	0.25	0.36	0.23	0.01	0.02	C47, C49
乳腺	Breast	187	0.12	0.29	0.15	0.01	0.02	8 183	8.86	12.51	6.52	0.42	0.71	C50
外阴	Vulva	—	—	—	—	—	—	177	0.19	0.27	0.12	0.00	0.01	C51
阴道	Vagina	—	—	—	—	—	—	81	0.09	0.12	0.06	0.00	0.01	C52
子宫颈	Cervix uteri	—	—	—	—	—	—	2 900	3.14	4.43	2.46	0.18	0.27	C53
子宫体	Corpus uteri	—	—	—	—	—	—	1 375	1.49	2.10	1.09	0.07	0.13	C54
子宫,部位不明	Uterus unspecified	—	—	—	—	—	—	450	0.49	0.69	0.35	0.02	0.04	C55
卵巢	Ovary	—	—	—	—	—	—	3 022	3.27	4.62	2.47	0.16	0.29	C56
其他女性生殖器官	Other female genital organs	—	—	—	—	—	—	180	0.19	0.28	0.15	0.01	0.02	C57
胎盘	Placenta	—	—	—	—	—	—	5	0.01	0.01	0.00	0.00	0.00	C58
阴茎	Penis	181	0.12	0.28	0.14	0.01	0.01	—	—	—	—	—	—	C60
前列腺	Prostate	4 925	3.21	7.62	3.29	0.03	0.21	—	—	—	—	—	—	C61
睾丸	Testis	72	0.05	0.11	0.07	0.00	0.01	—	—	—	—	—	—	C62
其他男性生殖器官	Other male genital organs	62	0.04	0.10	0.05	0.00	0.01	—	—	—	—	—	—	C63
肾	Kidney	1 907	1.24	2.95	1.52	0.06	0.17	902	0.98	1.38	0.61	0.02	0.06	C64
肾盂	Renal pelvis	273	0.18	0.42	0.21	0.01	0.02	203	0.22	0.31	0.12	0.00	0.01	C65
输尿管	Ureter	321	0.21	0.50	0.24	0.01	0.02	284	0.31	0.43	0.17	0.00	0.02	C66
膀胱	Bladder	3 393	2.21	5.25	2.36	0.05	0.18	987	1.07	1.51	0.55	0.01	0.04	C67
其他泌尿器官	Other urinary organs	70	0.05	0.11	0.05	0.00	0.00	53	0.06	0.08	0.03	0.00	0.00	C68
眼	Eye	37	0.02	0.06	0.04	0.00	0.00	40	0.04	0.06	0.04	0.00	0.00	C69
脑、神经系统	Brain, nervous system	3 019	1.97	4.67	2.92	0.17	0.30	2 643	2.86	4.04	2.29	0.12	0.23	C70-C72, D32-D33, D42-D43
甲状腺	Thyroid	410	0.27	0.63	0.34	0.02	0.04	623	0.67	0.95	0.46	0.02	0.05	C73
肾上腺	Adrenal gland	164	0.11	0.25	0.16	0.01	0.02	104	0.11	0.16	0.10	0.01	0.01	C74
其他内分泌腺	Other endocrine	90	0.06	0.14	0.09	0.00	0.01	63	0.07	0.10	0.05	0.00	0.01	C75
霍奇金淋巴瘤	Hodgkin lymphoma	122	0.08	0.19	0.11	0.00	0.01	75	0.08	0.11	0.07	0.00	0.01	C81
非霍奇金淋巴瘤	Non-Hodgkin lymphoma	2 545	1.66	3.94	2.12	0.10	0.22	1 708	1.85	2.61	1.26	0.06	0.14	C82-C86, C96
免疫增生性疾病	Immunoproliferative diseases	37	0.02	0.06	0.03	0.00	0.00	18	0.02	0.03	0.01	0.00	0.00	C88
多发性骨髓瘤	Multiple myeloma	1 017	0.66	1.57	0.80	0.03	0.09	756	0.82	1.16	0.55	0.03	0.06	C90
淋巴细胞白血病	Lymphoid leukemia	602	0.39	0.93	0.64	0.03	0.06	400	0.43	0.61	0.43	0.02	0.04	C91
髓系白血病	Myeloid leukemia	1 936	1.26	3.00	1.65	0.08	0.17	1 249	1.35	1.91	1.04	0.05	0.11	C92-C94, D45-D47
白血病,未特指	Leukemia unspecified	972	0.63	1.50	0.94	0.04	0.09	714	0.77	1.09	0.60	0.03	0.06	C95
其他或未指明部位	Other and unspecified	3 535	2.30	5.47	2.87	0.13	0.30	2 586	2.80	3.95	1.79	0.07	0.18	O & U
所有部位合计	All sites	153 515	100.00	237.65	122.40	5.28	13.53	92 366	100.00	141.19	65.01	2.89	6.74	C00-C97, D32-D33, D42-D43, D45-D47
所有部位除外 C44	All sites except C44	152 961	99.64	236.80	122.00	5.27	13.50	91 929	99.53	140.53	64.77	2.89	6.72	C00-C97, D32-D33, D42-D43, D45-D47 exc. C44

部位 Site		男性 Male						女性 Female						ICD-10
		死亡数 No. deaths	构成 Freq./%	粗率 Crude rate/ $100\,000^{-1}$	世标率 ASR world/ $100\,000^{-1}$	累积率 Cum. Rate/%		死亡数 No. deaths	构成 Freq./%	粗率 Crude rate/ $100\,000^{-1}$	世标率 ASR world/ $100\,000^{-1}$	累积率 Cum. Rate/%		
						0~64	0~74					0~64	0~74	
唇	Lip	65	0.04	0.10	0.05	0.00	0.00	37	0.04	0.06	0.02	0.00	0.00	C00
舌	Tongue	328	0.22	0.52	0.30	0.02	0.04	157	0.18	0.26	0.13	0.01	0.01	C01-C02
口	Mouth	417	0.27	0.66	0.37	0.02	0.04	237	0.28	0.39	0.18	0.01	0.02	C03-C06
唾液腺	Salivary gland	164	0.11	0.26	0.15	0.01	0.01	94	0.11	0.15	0.08	0.00	0.01	C07-C08
扁桃体	Tonsil	69	0.05	0.11	0.06	0.00	0.01	20	0.02	0.03	0.02	0.00	0.00	C09
其他口咽	Other oropharynx	132	0.09	0.21	0.12	0.01	0.02	17	0.02	0.03	0.01	0.00	0.00	C10
鼻咽	Nasopharynx	1 832	1.21	2.91	1.75	0.12	0.20	602	0.70	0.99	0.54	0.03	0.06	C11
下咽	Hypopharynx	342	0.23	0.54	0.31	0.02	0.04	18	0.02	0.03	0.01	0.00	0.00	C12-C13
咽,部位不明	Pharynx unspecified	164	0.11	0.26	0.14	0.01	0.02	48	0.06	0.08	0.04	0.00	0.00	C14
食管	Esophagus	15 447	10.18	24.57	12.87	0.46	1.50	6 208	7.23	10.21	4.17	0.08	0.41	C15
胃	Stomach	20 752	13.67	33.00	17.33	0.59	1.98	9 006	10.49	14.82	6.71	0.24	0.69	C16
小肠	Small intestine	547	0.36	0.87	0.47	0.02	0.05	385	0.45	0.63	0.31	0.01	0.04	C17
结肠	Colon	5 264	3.47	8.37	4.45	0.16	0.46	4 013	4.67	6.60	2.94	0.11	0.29	C18
直肠	Rectum	5 839	3.85	9.29	4.93	0.19	0.52	3 552	4.14	5.84	2.60	0.10	0.26	C19-C20
肛门	Anus	155	0.10	0.25	0.13	0.01	0.02	111	0.13	0.18	0.08	0.00	0.01	C21
肝脏	Liver	21 447	14.13	34.11	19.96	1.24	2.31	7 710	8.98	12.68	6.12	0.28	0.70	C22
胆囊及其他	Gallbladder etc.	2 349	1.55	3.74	1.98	0.07	0.23	2 402	2.80	3.95	1.79	0.07	0.20	C23-C24
胰腺	Pancreas	5 549	3.66	8.82	4.76	0.20	0.55	4 265	4.97	7.02	3.21	0.11	0.36	C25
鼻、鼻窦及其他	Nose,sinuses etc.	173	0.11	0.28	0.16	0.01	0.02	80	0.09	0.13	0.07	0.00	0.01	C30-C31
喉	Larynx	1 210	0.80	1.92	1.03	0.04	0.12	145	0.17	0.24	0.11	0.00	0.01	C32
气管、支气管、肺	Trachea,bronchus & lung	45 223	29.79	71.92	38.14	1.43	4.53	20 243	23.58	33.30	15.40	0.60	1.74	C33-C34
其他胸腔器官	Other thoracic organs	400	0.26	0.64	0.39	0.02	0.04	202	0.24	0.33	0.17	0.01	0.02	C37-C38
骨	Bone	988	0.65	1.57	0.96	0.05	0.10	677	0.79	1.11	0.59	0.03	0.06	C40-C41
皮肤黑色素瘤	Melanoma of skin	249	0.16	0.40	0.21	0.01	0.02	222	0.26	0.37	0.18	0.01	0.02	C43
皮肤其他	Other skin	596	0.39	0.95	0.48	0.01	0.04	641	0.75	1.05	0.38	0.01	0.02	C44
间皮瘤	Mesothelioma	81	0.05	0.13	0.07	0.00	0.01	70	0.08	0.12	0.06	0.00	0.01	C45
卡波西肉瘤	Kaposi sarcoma	16	0.01	0.03	0.02	0.00	0.00	15	0.02	0.02	0.02	0.00	0.00	C46
结缔组织、软组织	Connective & soft tissue	249	0.16	0.40	0.25	0.01	0.03	197	0.23	0.32	0.20	0.01	0.02	C47,C49
乳腺	Breast	88	0.06	0.14	0.07	0.00	0.01	6 001	6.99	9.87	5.43	0.37	0.60	C50
外阴	Vulva	—	—	—	—	—	—	119	0.14	0.20	0.09	0.00	0.01	C51
阴道	Vagina	—	—	—	—	—	—	73	0.09	0.12	0.06	0.00	0.01	C52
子宫颈	Cervix uteri	—	—	—	—	—	—	2 913	3.39	4.79	2.64	0.18	0.29	C53
子宫体	Corpus uteri	—	—	—	—	—	—	1 098	1.28	1.81	0.95	0.06	0.12	C54
子宫,部位不明	Uterus unspecified	—	—	—	—	—	—	547	0.64	0.90	0.45	0.02	0.05	C55
卵巢	Ovary	—	—	—	—	—	—	2 238	2.61	3.68	2.03	0.13	0.24	C56
其他女性生殖器官	Other female genital organs	—	—	—	—	—	—	116	0.14	0.19	0.10	0.01	0.01	C57
胎盘	Placenta	—	—	—	—	—	—	7	0.01	0.01	0.01	0.00	0.00	C58
阴茎	Penis	193	0.13	0.31	0.16	0.01	0.01	—	—	—	—	—	—	C60
前列腺	Prostate	3 759	2.48	5.98	2.85	0.03	0.19	—	—	—	—	—	—	C61
睾丸	Testis	76	0.05	0.12	0.08	0.00	0.01	—	—	—	—	—	—	C62
其他男性生殖器官	Other male genital organs	38	0.03	0.06	0.04	0.00	0.00	—	—	—	—	—	—	C63
肾	Kidney	1 234	0.81	1.96	1.08	0.05	0.12	580	0.68	0.95	0.48	0.02	0.05	C64
肾盂	Renal pelvis	168	0.11	0.27	0.14	0.01	0.02	124	0.14	0.20	0.09	0.00	0.01	C65
输尿管	Ureter	201	0.13	0.32	0.17	0.00	0.02	143	0.17	0.24	0.10	0.00	0.01	C66
膀胱	Bladder	2 786	1.84	4.43	2.17	0.04	0.17	729	0.85	1.20	0.48	0.01	0.04	C67
其他泌尿器官	Other urinary organs	44	0.03	0.07	0.04	0.00	0.00	26	0.03	0.04	0.02	0.00	0.00	C68
眼	Eye	44	0.03	0.07	0.06	0.00	0.00	36	0.04	0.06	0.04	0.00	0.00	C69
脑、神经系统	Brain,nervous system	3 143	2.07	5.00	3.18	0.18	0.34	2 673	3.11	4.40	2.51	0.13	0.26	C70-C72, D32-D33,D42-D43
甲状腺	Thyroid	324	0.21	0.52	0.29	0.01	0.03	512	0.60	0.84	0.41	0.02	0.04	C73
肾上腺	Adrenal gland	140	0.09	0.22	0.15	0.01	0.01	83	0.10	0.14	0.09	0.00	0.01	C74
其他内分泌腺	Other endocrine	107	0.07	0.17	0.10	0.00	0.01	84	0.10	0.14	0.08	0.00	0.00	C75
霍奇金淋巴瘤	Hodgkin lymphoma	128	0.08	0.20	0.11	0.01	0.01	75	0.09	0.12	0.06	0.00	0.01	C81
非霍奇金淋巴瘤	Non-Hodgkin lymphoma	2 246	1.48	3.57	2.05	0.09	0.23	1 454	1.69	2.39	1.23	0.06	0.13	C82-C86,C96
免疫增生性疾病	Immunoproliferative diseases	33	0.02	0.05	0.03	0.00	0.00	4	0.00	0.01	0.00	0.00	0.00	C88
多发性骨髓瘤	Multiple myeloma	872	0.57	1.39	0.76	0.03	0.10	638	0.74	1.05	0.54	0.03	0.07	C90
淋巴细胞白血病	Lymphoid leukemia	664	0.44	1.06	0.78	0.04	0.07	468	0.55	0.77	0.57	0.03	0.05	C91
髓系白血病	Myeloid leukemia	1 523	1.00	2.42	1.46	0.07	0.16	1 027	1.20	1.69	0.98	0.05	0.11	C92-C94,D45-D47
白血病,未特指	Leukemia unspecified	1 249	0.82	1.99	1.31	0.07	0.13	875	1.02	1.44	0.89	0.05	0.09	C95
其他或未指明部位	Other and unspecified	2 704	1.78	4.30	2.40	0.10	0.28	1 832	2.13	3.01	1.48	0.06	0.15	O & U
所有部位合计	All sites	151 811	100.00	241.44	131.34	5.49	14.84	85 847	100.00	141.24	67.95	2.98	7.37	C00-C97, D32-D33, D42-D43, D45-D47
所有部位除外 C44	All sites except C44	151 215	99.61	240.49	130.86	5.48	14.80	85 206	99.25	140.18	67.57	2.97	7.35	C00-C97,D32-D33,D42-D43, D45-D47 exc. C44

附表 2-13 2019 年全国中部肿瘤登记地区癌症死亡主要指标
Appendix Table 2-13 Cancer mortality in Central registration areas of China, 2019

部位 Site		男性 Male						女性 Female						ICD-10
		死亡数 No. deaths	构成 Freq./%	粗率 Crude rate/ 100 000⁻¹	世标率 ASR world/ 100 000⁻¹	累积率 Cum. Rate/% 0~64	0~74	死亡数 No. deaths	构成 Freq./%	粗率 Crude rate/ 100 000⁻¹	世标率 ASR world/ 100 000⁻¹	累积率 Cum. Rate/% 0~64	0~74	
唇	Lip	66	0.04	0.09	0.05	0.00	0.01	35	0.04	0.05	0.02	0.00	0.00	C00
舌	Tongue	455	0.29	0.59	0.40	0.03	0.04	138	0.16	0.19	0.10	0.00	0.01	C01-C02
口	Mouth	594	0.38	0.78	0.50	0.03	0.05	230	0.26	0.31	0.17	0.01	0.02	C03-C06
唾液腺	Salivary gland	184	0.12	0.24	0.16	0.01	0.02	96	0.11	0.13	0.08	0.00	0.01	C07-C08
扁桃体	Tonsil	104	0.07	0.14	0.09	0.01	0.01	17	0.02	0.02	0.01	0.00	0.00	C09
其他口咽	Other oropharynx	174	0.11	0.23	0.15	0.01	0.02	33	0.04	0.04	0.03	0.00	0.00	C10
鼻咽	Nasopharynx	1 657	1.06	2.16	1.44	0.09	0.17	606	0.68	0.82	0.50	0.03	0.06	C11
下咽	Hypopharynx	324	0.21	0.42	0.27	0.02	0.04	32	0.04	0.04	0.02	0.00	0.00	C12-C13
咽,部位不明	Pharynx unspecified	201	0.13	0.26	0.16	0.01	0.02	60	0.07	0.08	0.05	0.00	0.00	C14
食管	Esophagus	13 989	8.93	18.28	11.25	0.39	1.32	5 767	6.50	7.81	4.00	0.09	0.42	C15
胃	Stomach	20 573	13.13	26.88	16.62	0.60	1.93	9 005	10.15	12.20	6.65	0.26	0.70	C16
小肠	Small intestine	700	0.45	0.91	0.58	0.03	0.07	417	0.47	0.56	0.33	0.01	0.04	C17
结肠	Colon	4 866	3.10	6.36	3.98	0.17	0.42	3 743	4.22	5.07	2.77	0.11	0.29	C18
直肠	Rectum	5 953	3.80	7.78	4.82	0.20	0.52	3 734	4.21	5.06	2.76	0.12	0.29	C19-C20
肛门	Anus	198	0.13	0.26	0.16	0.01	0.02	163	0.18	0.22	0.12	0.00	0.01	C21
肝脏	Liver	24 581	15.68	32.11	20.89	1.23	2.42	9 577	10.80	12.98	7.37	0.33	0.84	C22
胆囊及其他	Gallbladder etc.	2 004	1.28	2.62	1.64	0.07	0.19	2 321	2.62	3.14	1.72	0.07	0.20	C23-C24
胰腺	Pancreas	4 513	2.88	5.90	3.70	0.17	0.43	3 266	3.68	4.42	2.46	0.10	0.29	C25
鼻、鼻窦及其他	Nose, sinuses etc.	212	0.14	0.28	0.19	0.01	0.02	110	0.12	0.15	0.09	0.01	0.01	C30-C31
喉	Larynx	1 405	0.90	1.84	1.14	0.05	0.14	205	0.23	0.28	0.14	0.00	0.01	C32
气管、支气管、肺	Trachea, bronchus & lung	49 965	31.88	65.28	40.59	1.60	4.82	19 246	21.70	26.08	14.28	0.57	1.57	C33-C34
其他胸腔器官	Other thoracic organs	481	0.31	0.63	0.42	0.02	0.05	220	0.25	0.30	0.19	0.01	0.02	C37-C38
骨	Bone	1 119	0.71	1.46	1.02	0.05	0.12	690	0.78	0.93	0.58	0.03	0.07	C40-C41
皮肤黑色素瘤	Melanoma of skin	205	0.13	0.27	0.17	0.01	0.02	164	0.18	0.22	0.13	0.01	0.01	C43
皮肤其他	Other skin	715	0.46	0.93	0.56	0.02	0.04	505	0.57	0.68	0.35	0.01	0.02	C44
间皮瘤	Mesothelioma	74	0.05	0.10	0.06	0.00	0.01	43	0.05	0.06	0.04	0.00	0.00	C45
卡波西肉瘤	Kaposi sarcoma	10	0.01	0.01	0.01	0.00	0.00	13	0.01	0.02	0.01	0.00	0.00	C46
结缔组织、软组织	Connective & soft tissue	259	0.17	0.34	0.25	0.01	0.03	197	0.22	0.27	0.18	0.01	0.02	C47, C49
乳腺	Breast	186	0.12	0.24	0.15	0.01	0.02	6 721	7.58	9.11	5.66	0.40	0.63	C50
外阴	Vulva	—	—	—	—	—	—	130	0.15	0.18	0.09	0.00	0.01	C51
阴道	Vagina	—	—	—	—	—	—	77	0.09	0.10	0.06	0.00	0.01	C52
子宫颈	Cervix uteri	—	—	—	—	—	—	4 768	5.37	6.46	3.96	0.26	0.46	C53
子宫体	Corpus uteri	—	—	—	—	—	—	1 418	1.60	1.92	1.16	0.07	0.14	C54
子宫,部位不明	Uterus unspecified	—	—	—	—	—	—	472	0.53	0.64	0.37	0.02	0.04	C55
卵巢	Ovary	—	—	—	—	—	—	2 504	2.82	3.39	2.10	0.14	0.25	C56
其他女性生殖器官	Other female genital organs	—	—	—	—	—	—	125	0.14	0.17	0.10	0.01	0.01	C57
胎盘	Placenta	—	—	—	—	—	—	8	0.01	0.01	0.01	0.00	0.00	C58
阴茎	Penis	221	0.14	0.29	0.18	0.01	0.02	—	—	—	—	—	—	C60
前列腺	Prostate	3 293	2.10	4.30	2.49	0.03	0.18	—	—	—	—	—	—	C61
睾丸	Testis	82	0.05	0.11	0.08	0.00	0.01	—	—	—	—	—	—	C62
其他男性生殖器官	Other male genital organs	47	0.03	0.06	0.04	0.00	0.00	—	—	—	—	—	—	C63
肾	Kidney	1 220	0.78	1.59	1.02	0.05	0.12	667	0.75	0.90	0.52	0.02	0.06	C64
肾盂	Renal pelvis	178	0.11	0.23	0.14	0.01	0.01	102	0.11	0.14	0.08	0.00	0.01	C65
输尿管	Ureter	176	0.11	0.23	0.14	0.00	0.02	145	0.16	0.20	0.10	0.00	0.01	C66
膀胱	Bladder	2 479	1.58	3.24	1.93	0.04	0.17	646	0.73	0.88	0.43	0.01	0.04	C67
其他泌尿器官	Other urinary organs	45	0.03	0.06	0.04	0.00	0.00	32	0.04	0.04	0.02	0.00	0.00	C68
眼	Eye	53	0.03	0.07	0.05	0.00	0.01	36	0.04	0.05	0.03	0.00	0.00	C69
脑、神经系统	Brain, nervous system	3 602	2.30	4.71	3.35	0.19	0.35	2 996	3.38	4.06	2.70	0.14	0.28	C70-C72, D32-D33, D42-D43
甲状腺	Thyroid	357	0.23	0.47	0.30	0.02	0.03	726	0.82	0.98	0.58	0.03	0.06	C73
肾上腺	Adrenal gland	156	0.10	0.20	0.14	0.01	0.01	108	0.12	0.15	0.10	0.01	0.01	C74
其他内分泌腺	Other endocrine	79	0.05	0.10	0.07	0.00	0.01	49	0.06	0.07	0.05	0.00	0.00	C75
霍奇金淋巴瘤	Hodgkin lymphoma	132	0.08	0.17	0.12	0.01	0.01	79	0.09	0.11	0.06	0.00	0.01	C81
非霍奇金淋巴瘤	Non-Hodgkin lymphoma	1 947	1.24	2.54	1.68	0.08	0.19	1 255	1.41	1.70	1.01	0.05	0.11	C82-C86, C96
免疫增生性疾病	Immunoproliferative diseases	14	0.01	0.02	0.01	0.00	0.00	6	0.01	0.01	0.00	0.00	0.00	C88
多发性骨髓瘤	Multiple myeloma	854	0.54	1.12	0.71	0.03	0.09	584	0.66	0.79	0.45	0.02	0.05	C90
淋巴细胞白血病	Lymphoid leukemia	549	0.35	0.72	0.57	0.03	0.05	382	0.43	0.52	0.41	0.02	0.04	C91
髓系白血病	Myeloid leukemia	1 115	0.71	1.46	1.03	0.05	0.11	767	0.86	1.04	0.69	0.04	0.07	C92-C94, D45-D47
白血病,未特指	Leukemia unspecified	1 345	0.86	1.76	1.30	0.07	0.13	1 001	1.13	1.36	1.00	0.05	0.10	C95
其他或未指明部位	Other and unspecified	3 016	1.92	3.94	2.63	0.12	0.28	2 272	2.56	3.08	1.81	0.08	0.19	O & U
所有部位合计	All sites	156 727	100.00	204.75	129.46	5.59	14.74	88 709	100.00	120.19	68.73	3.19	7.50	C00-C97, D32-D33, D42-D43, D45-D47
所有部位除外 C44	All sites except C44	156 012	99.54	203.82	128.90	5.57	14.70	88 204	99.43	119.50	68.38	3.18	7.47	C00-C97, D32-D33, D42-D43, D45-D47 exc. C44

附表 2-14　2019 年全国中部城市肿瘤登记地区癌症死亡主要指标

Appendix Table 2-14　Cancer mortality in Central urban registration areas of China,2019

部位 Site		男性 Male						女性 Female						ICD-10
		死亡数 No. deaths	构成 Freq./%	粗率 Crude rate/100 000⁻¹	世标率 ASR world/100 000⁻¹	累积率 Cum. Rate/%		死亡数 No. deaths	构成 Freq./%	粗率 Crude rate/100 000⁻¹	世标率 ASR world/100 000⁻¹	累积率 Cum. Rate/%		
						0~64	0~74					0~64	0~74	
唇	Lip	37	0.07	0.14	0.08	0.00	0.01	20	0.06	0.08	0.04	0.00	0.00	C00
舌	Tongue	208	0.37	0.80	0.51	0.03	0.06	71	0.22	0.28	0.14	0.01	0.01	C01-C02
口	Mouth	257	0.46	0.98	0.61	0.04	0.06	103	0.32	0.40	0.21	0.01	0.02	C03-C06
唾液腺	Salivary gland	74	0.13	0.28	0.18	0.01	0.02	42	0.13	0.16	0.09	0.00	0.01	C07-C08
扁桃体	Tonsil	46	0.08	0.18	0.12	0.01	0.01	6	0.02	0.02	0.01	0.00	0.00	C09
其他口咽	Other oropharynx	64	0.11	0.25	0.16	0.01	0.02	13	0.04	0.05	0.03	0.00	0.00	C10
鼻咽	Nasopharynx	512	0.91	1.96	1.25	0.08	0.15	163	0.50	0.63	0.37	0.02	0.04	C11
下咽	Hypopharynx	156	0.28	0.60	0.38	0.02	0.05	8	0.02	0.03	0.02	0.00	0.00	C12-C13
咽,部位不明	Pharynx unspecified	82	0.15	0.31	0.19	0.01	0.02	18	0.06	0.07	0.04	0.00	0.00	C14
食管	Esophagus	4 128	7.34	15.81	9.46	0.37	1.12	1 408	4.35	5.46	2.67	0.05	0.26	C15
胃	Stomach	6 072	10.79	23.26	13.72	0.48	1.53	2 790	8.62	10.83	5.70	0.22	0.57	C16
小肠	Small intestine	319	0.57	1.22	0.74	0.03	0.09	180	0.56	0.70	0.39	0.02	0.04	C17
结肠	Colon	2 379	4.23	9.11	5.36	0.20	0.56	1 768	5.46	6.86	3.59	0.13	0.36	C18
直肠	Rectum	2 317	4.12	8.87	5.24	0.21	0.55	1 400	4.33	5.43	2.83	0.11	0.28	C19-C20
肛门	Anus	49	0.09	0.19	0.12	0.01	0.01	49	0.15	0.19	0.09	0.00	0.01	C21
肝脏	Liver	8 064	14.34	30.89	19.35	1.15	2.21	3 115	9.63	12.09	6.59	0.28	0.72	C22
胆囊及其他	Gallbladder etc.	837	1.49	3.21	1.91	0.07	0.21	969	2.99	3.76	1.96	0.07	0.21	C23-C24
胰腺	Pancreas	1 888	3.36	7.23	4.39	0.20	0.51	1 466	4.53	5.69	3.04	0.12	0.34	C25
鼻、鼻窦及其他	Nose, sinuses etc.	87	0.15	0.33	0.22	0.01	0.03	32	0.10	0.12	0.07	0.00	0.01	C30-C31
喉	Larynx	533	0.95	2.04	1.24	0.06	0.15	78	0.24	0.30	0.15	0.00	0.01	C32
气管、支气管、肺	Trachea, bronchus & lung	18 376	32.67	70.38	42.00	1.60	4.92	7 196	22.24	27.93	14.62	0.56	1.51	C33-C34
其他胸腔器官	Other thoracic organs	190	0.34	0.73	0.46	0.03	0.05	109	0.34	0.42	0.27	0.02	0.03	C37-C38
骨	Bone	302	0.54	1.16	0.80	0.04	0.08	216	0.67	0.84	0.51	0.02	0.06	C40-C41
皮肤黑色素瘤	Melanoma of skin	94	0.17	0.36	0.22	0.01	0.02	72	0.22	0.28	0.16	0.01	0.02	C43
皮肤其他	Other skin	262	0.47	1.00	0.55	0.01	0.04	159	0.49	0.62	0.29	0.01	0.02	C44
间皮瘤	Mesothelioma	43	0.08	0.16	0.10	0.00	0.01	27	0.08	0.10	0.06	0.00	0.01	C45
卡波西肉瘤	Kaposi sarcoma	4	0.01	0.02	0.01	0.00	0.00	10	0.03	0.04	0.03	0.00	0.00	C46
结缔组织、软组织	Connective & soft tissue	132	0.23	0.51	0.36	0.02	0.03	97	0.30	0.38	0.25	0.01	0.02	C47,C49
乳腺	Breast	64	0.11	0.25	0.15	0.01	0.02	2 754	8.51	10.69	6.40	0.43	0.71	C50
外阴	Vulva	—	—	—	—	—	—	53	0.16	0.21	0.11	0.01	0.01	C51
阴道	Vagina	—	—	—	—	—	—	24	0.07	0.09	0.05	0.00	0.01	C52
子宫颈	Cervix uteri	—	—	—	—	—	—	1 533	4.74	5.95	3.59	0.25	0.41	C53
子宫体	Corpus uteri	—	—	—	—	—	—	488	1.51	1.89	1.10	0.06	0.13	C54
子宫,部位不明	Uterus unspecified	—	—	—	—	—	—	122	0.38	0.47	0.27	0.01	0.03	C55
卵巢	Ovary	—	—	—	—	—	—	1 038	3.21	4.03	2.42	0.16	0.28	C56
其他女性生殖器官	Other female genital organs	—	—	—	—	—	—	55	0.17	0.21	0.12	0.01	0.01	C57
胎盘	Placenta	—	—	—	—	—	—	3	0.01	0.01	0.01	0.00	0.00	C58
阴茎	Penis	85	0.15	0.33	0.19	0.01	0.02	—	—	—	—	—	—	C60
前列腺	Prostate	1 650	2.93	6.32	3.36	0.03	0.22	—	—	—	—	—	—	C61
睾丸	Testis	25	0.04	0.10	0.07	0.00	0.00	—	—	—	—	—	—	C62
其他男性生殖器官	Other male genital organs	23	0.04	0.09	0.05	0.00	0.00	—	—	—	—	—	—	C63
肾	Kidney	540	0.96	2.07	1.26	0.05	0.15	294	0.91	1.14	0.62	0.02	0.06	C64
肾盂	Renal pelvis	94	0.17	0.36	0.21	0.01	0.02	66	0.20	0.26	0.13	0.00	0.01	C65
输尿管	Ureter	102	0.18	0.39	0.22	0.00	0.02	82	0.25	0.32	0.15	0.00	0.01	C66
膀胱	Bladder	1 043	1.85	3.99	2.24	0.04	0.18	295	0.91	1.14	0.53	0.01	0.04	C67
其他泌尿器官	Other urinary organs	19	0.03	0.07	0.04	0.00	0.00	16	0.05	0.06	0.03	0.00	0.00	C68
眼	Eye	21	0.04	0.08	0.06	0.00	0.01	13	0.04	0.05	0.03	0.00	0.00	C69
脑、神经系统	Brain, nervous system	1 175	2.09	4.50	3.07	0.18	0.32	976	3.02	3.79	2.43	0.12	0.25	C70-C72, D32-D33,D42-D43
甲状腺	Thyroid	129	0.23	0.49	0.30	0.02	0.03	228	0.70	0.88	0.50	0.03	0.05	C73
肾上腺	Adrenal gland	84	0.15	0.32	0.20	0.01	0.02	46	0.14	0.18	0.11	0.00	0.01	C74
其他内分泌腺	Other endocrine	51	0.09	0.20	0.14	0.01	0.02	22	0.07	0.09	0.05	0.00	0.01	C75
霍奇金淋巴瘤	Hodgkin lymphoma	41	0.07	0.16	0.10	0.01	0.01	23	0.07	0.09	0.05	0.00	0.00	C81
非霍奇金淋巴瘤	Non-Hodgkin lymphoma	820	1.46	3.14	1.92	0.09	0.20	548	1.69	2.13	1.18	0.05	0.13	C82-C86,C96
免疫增生性疾病	Immunoproliferative diseases	9	0.02	0.03	0.02	0.00	0.00	4	0.01	0.02	0.01	0.00	0.00	C88
多发性骨髓瘤	Multiple myeloma	406	0.72	1.55	0.97	0.04	0.11	259	0.80	1.01	0.56	0.02	0.06	C90
淋巴细胞白血病	Lymphoid leukemia	228	0.41	0.87	0.68	0.03	0.06	174	0.54	0.68	0.52	0.03	0.05	C91
髓系白血病	Myeloid leukemia	467	0.83	1.79	1.19	0.06	0.12	343	1.06	1.33	0.83	0.04	0.09	C92-C94, D45-D47
白血病,未特指	Leukemia unspecified	409	0.73	1.57	1.08	0.05	0.11	306	0.95	1.19	0.84	0.04	0.08	C95
其他或未指明部位	Other and unspecified	1 252	2.23	4.80	3.08	0.13	0.32	1 007	3.11	3.91	2.18	0.09	0.20	O & U
所有部位合计	All sites	56 249	100.00	215.43	130.31	5.50	14.49	32 357	100.00	125.57	69.05	3.06	7.24	C00-C97, D32-D33, D42-D43, D45-D47
所有部位除外 C44	All sites except C44	55 987	99.53	214.43	129.76	5.48	14.46	32 198	99.51	124.95	68.75	3.06	7.22	C00-C97,D32-D33,D42-D43,D45-D47 exc. C44

部位 Site		男性 Male						女性 Female						ICD-10
		死亡数 No. deaths	构成 Freq./%	粗率 Crude rate/ 100 000⁻¹	世标率 ASR world/ 100 000⁻¹	累积率 Cum. Rate/% 0~64	0~74	死亡数 No. deaths	构成 Freq./%	粗率 Crude rate/ 100 000⁻¹	世标率 ASR world/ 100 000⁻¹	累积率 Cum. Rate/% 0~64	0~74	
唇	Lip	29	0.03	0.06	0.03	0.00	0.00	15	0.03	0.03	0.02	0.00	0.00	C00
舌	Tongue	247	0.25	0.49	0.34	0.02	0.04	67	0.12	0.14	0.08	0.00	0.01	C01-C02
口	Mouth	337	0.34	0.67	0.44	0.02	0.05	127	0.23	0.26	0.14	0.00	0.02	C03-C06
唾液腺	Salivary gland	110	0.11	0.22	0.15	0.01	0.02	54	0.10	0.11	0.07	0.00	0.01	C07-C08
扁桃体	Tonsil	58	0.06	0.12	0.08	0.00	0.01	11	0.02	0.02	0.01	0.00	0.00	C09
其他口咽	Other oropharynx	110	0.11	0.22	0.14	0.01	0.02	20	0.04	0.04	0.03	0.00	0.00	C10
鼻咽	Nasopharynx	1 145	1.14	2.27	1.54	0.10	0.18	443	0.79	0.92	0.57	0.04	0.07	C11
下咽	Hypopharynx	168	0.17	0.33	0.22	0.01	0.03	24	0.04	0.05	0.03	0.00	0.00	C12-C13
咽,部位不明	Pharynx unspecified	119	0.12	0.24	0.15	0.01	0.02	42	0.07	0.09	0.05	0.00	0.01	C14
食管	Esophagus	9 861	9.81	19.55	12.23	0.40	1.42	4 359	7.74	9.07	4.73	0.11	0.50	C15
胃	Stomach	14 501	14.43	28.75	18.17	0.66	2.14	6 215	11.03	12.94	7.18	0.28	0.77	C16
小肠	Small intestine	381	0.38	0.76	0.49	0.03	0.06	237	0.42	0.49	0.29	0.01	0.03	C17
结肠	Colon	2 487	2.48	4.93	3.19	0.15	0.35	1 975	3.50	4.11	2.31	0.10	0.25	C18
直肠	Rectum	3 636	3.62	7.21	4.58	0.19	0.50	2 334	4.14	4.86	2.72	0.12	0.29	C19-C20
肛门	Anus	149	0.15	0.30	0.19	0.01	0.02	114	0.20	0.24	0.13	0.01	0.02	C21
肝脏	Liver	16 517	16.44	32.75	21.71	1.28	2.53	6 462	11.47	13.45	7.80	0.36	0.91	C22
胆囊及其他	Gallbladder etc.	1 167	1.16	2.31	1.49	0.06	0.18	1 352	2.40	2.81	1.58	0.06	0.19	C23-C24
胰腺	Pancreas	2 625	2.61	5.20	3.33	0.15	0.38	1 800	3.19	3.75	2.13	0.09	0.26	C25
鼻,鼻窦及其他	Nose, sinuses etc.	125	0.12	0.25	0.17	0.01	0.02	78	0.14	0.16	0.10	0.01	0.01	C30-C31
喉	Larynx	872	0.87	1.73	1.09	0.05	0.13	127	0.23	0.26	0.14	0.00	0.01	C32
气管、支气管、肺	Trachea, bronchus & lung	31 589	31.44	62.63	39.77	1.60	4.78	12 050	21.38	25.08	14.08	0.58	1.60	C33-C34
其他胸腔器官	Other thoracic organs	291	0.29	0.58	0.39	0.02	0.04	111	0.20	0.23	0.14	0.01	0.02	C37-C38
骨	Bone	817	0.81	1.62	1.14	0.05	0.14	474	0.84	0.99	0.63	0.03	0.07	C40-C41
皮肤黑色素瘤	Melanoma of skin	111	0.11	0.22	0.14	0.01	0.02	92	0.16	0.19	0.12	0.01	0.01	C43
皮肤其他	Other skin	453	0.45	0.90	0.56	0.02	0.05	346	0.61	0.72	0.38	0.01	0.03	C44
间皮瘤	Mesothelioma	31	0.03	0.06	0.04	0.00	0.00	16	0.03	0.03	0.02	0.00	0.00	C45
卡波西肉瘤	Kaposi sarcoma	6	0.01	0.01	0.01	0.00	0.00	3	0.01	0.01	0.01	0.00	0.00	C46
结缔组织、软组织	Connective & soft tissue	127	0.13	0.25	0.19	0.01	0.02	100	0.18	0.21	0.15	0.01	0.02	C47, C49
乳腺	Breast	122	0.12	0.24	0.16	0.01	0.02	3 967	7.04	8.26	5.25	0.38	0.59	C50
外阴	Vulva	—	—	—	—	—	—	77	0.14	0.16	0.08	0.00	0.01	C51
阴道	Vagina	—	—	—	—	—	—	53	0.09	0.11	0.07	0.00	0.01	C52
子宫颈	Cervix uteri	—	—	—	—	—	—	3 235	5.74	6.73	4.17	0.27	0.48	C53
子宫体	Corpus uteri	—	—	—	—	—	—	930	1.65	1.94	1.19	0.08	0.14	C54
子宫,部位不明	Uterus unspecified	—	—	—	—	—	—	350	0.62	0.73	0.43	0.02	0.05	C55
卵巢	Ovary	—	—	—	—	—	—	1 466	2.60	3.05	1.93	0.13	0.23	C56
其他女性生殖器官	Other female genital organs	—	—	—	—	—	—	70	0.12	0.15	0.09	0.01	0.01	C57
胎盘	Placenta	—	—	—	—	—	—	5	0.01	0.01	0.01	0.00	0.00	C58
阴茎	Penis	136	0.14	0.27	0.17	0.01	0.02	—	—	—	—	—	—	C60
前列腺	Prostate	1 643	1.64	3.26	1.96	0.03	0.15	—	—	—	—	—	—	C61
睾丸	Testis	57	0.06	0.11	0.08	0.00	0.01	—	—	—	—	—	—	C62
其他男性生殖器官	Other male genital organs	24	0.02	0.05	0.03	0.00	0.00	—	—	—	—	—	—	C63
肾	Kidney	680	0.68	1.35	0.89	0.04	0.10	373	0.66	0.78	0.47	0.02	0.05	C64
肾盂	Renal pelvis	84	0.08	0.17	0.10	0.00	0.01	36	0.06	0.07	0.04	0.00	0.01	C65
输尿管	Ureter	74	0.07	0.15	0.10	0.00	0.01	63	0.11	0.13	0.07	0.00	0.01	C66
膀胱	Bladder	1 436	1.43	2.85	1.74	0.04	0.16	351	0.62	0.73	0.38	0.01	0.03	C67
其他泌尿器官	Other urinary organs	26	0.03	0.05	0.04	0.00	0.00	16	0.03	0.03	0.02	0.00	0.00	C68
眼	Eye	32	0.03	0.06	0.05	0.00	0.01	23	0.04	0.05	0.04	0.00	0.00	C69
脑、神经系统	Brain, nervous system	2 427	2.42	4.81	3.49	0.20	0.37	2 020	3.58	4.20	2.84	0.16	0.30	C70-C72, D32-D33,D42-D43
甲状腺	Thyroid	228	0.23	0.45	0.30	0.02	0.03	498	0.88	1.04	0.62	0.03	0.07	C73
肾上腺	Adrenal gland	72	0.07	0.14	0.10	0.01	0.01	62	0.11	0.13	0.09	0.01	0.01	C74
其他内分泌腺	Other endocrine	28	0.03	0.06	0.04	0.00	0.00	27	0.05	0.06	0.04	0.00	0.00	C75
霍奇金淋巴瘤	Hodgkin lymphoma	91	0.09	0.18	0.13	0.01	0.01	56	0.10	0.12	0.07	0.00	0.01	C81
非霍奇金淋巴瘤	Non-Hodgkin lymphoma	1 127	1.12	2.23	1.54	0.08	0.18	707	1.25	1.47	0.92	0.05	0.10	C82-C86, C96
免疫增生性疾病	Immunoproliferative diseases	5	0.00	0.01	0.01	0.00	0.00	2	0.00	0.00	0.00	0.00	0.00	C88
多发性骨髓瘤	Multiple myeloma	448	0.45	0.89	0.58	0.03	0.07	325	0.58	0.68	0.40	0.02	0.05	C90
淋巴细胞白血病	Lymphoid leukemia	321	0.32	0.64	0.52	0.03	0.05	208	0.37	0.43	0.35	0.02	0.03	C91
髓系白血病	Myeloid leukemia	648	0.64	1.28	0.94	0.05	0.10	424	0.75	0.88	0.61	0.03	0.06	C92-C94, D45-D47
白血病,未特指	Leukemia unspecified	936	0.93	1.86	1.41	0.08	0.14	695	1.23	1.45	1.09	0.06	0.11	C95
其他或未指明部位	Other and unspecified	1 764	1.76	3.50	2.38	0.11	0.25	1 265	2.24	2.63	1.61	0.07	0.18	O & U
所有部位合计	All sites	100 478	100.00	199.22	128.72	5.64	14.87	56 352	100.00	117.30	68.50	3.25	7.64	C00-C97, D32-D33, D42-D43, D45-D47
所有部位除外 C44	All sites except C44	100 025	99.55	198.33	128.15	5.62	14.82	56 006	99.39	116.58	68.12	3.24	7.61	C00-C97,D32-D33, D42-D43, D45-D47 exc. C44

附表 2-16　2019 年全国西部肿瘤登记地区癌症死亡主要指标

Appendix Table 2-16　Cancer mortality in Western registration areas of China,2019

部位 Site		男性 Male						女性 Female						ICD-10
		死亡数 No. deaths	构成 Freq./%	粗率 Crude rate/ 100 000⁻¹	世标率 ASR world/ 100 000⁻¹	累积率 Cum. Rate/%		死亡数 No. deaths	构成 Freq./%	粗率 Crude rate/ 100 000⁻¹	世标率 ASR world/ 100 000⁻¹	累积率 Cum. Rate/%		
						0~64	0~74					0~64	0~74	
唇	Lip	185	0.08	0.16	0.10	0.00	0.01	82	0.07	0.08	0.04	0.00	0.00	C00
舌	Tongue	705	0.30	0.62	0.39	0.02	0.05	246	0.20	0.23	0.13	0.01	0.01	C01-C02
口	Mouth	1 039	0.44	0.91	0.56	0.02	0.07	411	0.34	0.38	0.20	0.01	0.02	C03-C06
唾液腺	Salivary gland	253	0.11	0.22	0.14	0.01	0.02	130	0.11	0.12	0.07	0.00	0.01	C07-C08
扁桃体	Tonsil	115	0.05	0.10	0.07	0.00	0.01	25	0.02	0.02	0.01	0.00	0.00	C09
其他口咽	Other oropharynx	351	0.15	0.31	0.19	0.01	0.02	47	0.04	0.04	0.03	0.00	0.00	C10
鼻咽	Nasopharynx	3 549	1.51	3.10	2.04	0.14	0.23	1 203	0.99	1.10	0.68	0.04	0.07	C11
下咽	Hypopharynx	463	0.20	0.41	0.26	0.02	0.03	32	0.03	0.03	0.02	0.00	0.00	C12-C13
咽,部位不明	Pharynx unspecified	467	0.20	0.41	0.25	0.01	0.03	146	0.12	0.13	0.07	0.00	0.01	C14
食管	Esophagus	23 345	9.90	20.42	12.53	0.52	1.55	6 002	4.93	5.50	2.84	0.07	0.30	C15
胃	Stomach	23 784	10.09	20.81	12.77	0.54	1.49	10 288	8.46	9.43	5.15	0.21	0.54	C16
小肠	Small intestine	731	0.31	0.64	0.39	0.02	0.04	542	0.45	0.50	0.28	0.01	0.03	C17
结肠	Colon	6 083	2.58	5.32	3.25	0.13	0.34	4 468	3.67	4.10	2.23	0.09	0.24	C18
直肠	Rectum	11 501	4.88	10.06	6.14	0.24	0.68	6 897	5.67	6.32	3.42	0.14	0.36	C19-C20
肛门	Anus	444	0.19	0.39	0.24	0.01	0.03	292	0.24	0.27	0.15	0.01	0.02	C21
肝脏	Liver	44 508	18.88	38.94	25.24	1.62	2.87	14 132	11.62	12.96	7.38	0.35	0.83	C22
胆囊及其他	Gallbladder etc.	2 468	1.05	2.16	1.33	0.06	0.15	2 848	2.34	2.61	1.42	0.06	0.16	C23-C24
胰腺	Pancreas	6 575	2.79	5.75	3.56	0.17	0.41	4 535	3.73	4.16	2.28	0.10	0.26	C25
鼻、鼻窦及其他	Nose,sinuses etc.	350	0.15	0.31	0.19	0.01	0.02	191	0.16	0.18	0.11	0.01	0.01	C30-C31
喉	Larynx	2 035	0.86	1.78	1.10	0.05	0.13	262	0.22	0.24	0.13	0.00	0.01	C32
气管、支气管、肺	Trachea,bronchus & lung	72 239	30.65	63.20	39.08	1.77	4.67	29 230	24.03	26.80	14.72	0.61	1.63	C33-C34
其他胸腔器官	Other thoracic organs	646	0.27	0.57	0.38	0.02	0.04	375	0.31	0.34	0.21	0.01	0.02	C37-C38
骨	Bone	1 884	0.80	1.65	1.10	0.06	0.12	1 172	0.96	1.07	0.67	0.03	0.07	C40-C41
皮肤黑色素瘤	Melanoma of skin	225	0.10	0.20	0.12	0.01	0.01	213	0.18	0.20	0.11	0.01	0.01	C43
皮肤其他	Other skin	1 056	0.45	0.92	0.58	0.02	0.05	801	0.66	0.73	0.39	0.01	0.03	C44
间皮瘤	Mesothelioma	93	0.04	0.08	0.06	0.00	0.01	76	0.06	0.07	0.04	0.00	0.00	C45
卡波西肉瘤	Kaposi sarcoma	34	0.01	0.03	0.02	0.00	0.00	15	0.01	0.01	0.01	0.00	0.00	C46
结缔组织、软组织	Connective & soft tissue	434	0.18	0.38	0.27	0.01	0.02	268	0.22	0.25	0.17	0.01	0.02	C47,C49
乳腺	Breast	296	0.13	0.26	0.16	0.01	0.02	7 673	6.31	7.03	4.45	0.34	0.49	C50
外阴	Vulva	—	—	—	—	—	—	174	0.14	0.16	0.09	0.01	0.01	C51
阴道	Vagina	—	—	—	—	—	—	132	0.11	0.12	0.07	0.00	0.01	C52
子宫颈	Cervix uteri	—	—	—	—	—	—	6 604	5.43	6.05	3.74	0.26	0.43	C53
子宫体	Corpus uteri	—	—	—	—	—	—	1 976	1.62	1.81	1.10	0.07	0.13	C54
子宫,部位不明	Uterus unspecified	—	—	—	—	—	—	1 046	0.86	0.96	0.58	0.04	0.07	C55
卵巢	Ovary	—	—	—	—	—	—	3 267	2.69	3.00	1.86	0.13	0.22	C56
其他女性生殖器官	Other female genital organs	—	—	—	—	—	—	184	0.15	0.17	0.10	0.01	0.01	C57
胎盘	Placenta	—	—	—	—	—	—	8	0.01	0.01	0.01	0.00	0.00	C58
阴茎	Penis	283	0.12	0.25	0.16	0.01	0.02	—	—	—	—	—	—	C60
前列腺	Prostate	4 980	2.11	4.36	2.48	0.03	0.19	—	—	—	—	—	—	C61
睾丸	Testis	121	0.05	0.11	0.08	0.00	0.01	—	—	—	—	—	—	C62
其他男性生殖器官	Other male genital organs	49	0.02	0.04	0.03	0.00	0.00	—	—	—	—	—	—	C63
肾	Kidney	1 298	0.55	1.14	0.72	0.04	0.08	750	0.62	0.69	0.40	0.02	0.04	C64
肾盂	Renal pelvis	220	0.09	0.19	0.12	0.00	0.01	146	0.12	0.13	0.07	0.00	0.01	C65
输尿管	Ureter	169	0.07	0.15	0.09	0.00	0.01	177	0.15	0.16	0.08	0.00	0.01	C66
膀胱	Bladder	3 741	1.59	3.27	1.91	0.04	0.16	990	0.81	0.91	0.46	0.01	0.04	C67
其他泌尿器官	Other urinary organs	50	0.02	0.04	0.03	0.00	0.00	37	0.03	0.03	0.02	0.00	0.00	C68
眼	Eye	104	0.04	0.09	0.07	0.00	0.01	76	0.06	0.07	0.05	0.00	0.00	C69
脑、神经系统	Brain,nervous system	5 065	2.15	4.43	3.18	0.19	0.33	3 845	3.16	3.52	2.36	0.13	0.24	C70-C72, D32-D33,D42-D43
甲状腺	Thyroid	489	0.21	0.43	0.28	0.02	0.03	748	0.61	0.69	0.41	0.02	0.04	C73
肾上腺	Adrenal gland	168	0.07	0.15	0.10	0.01	0.01	134	0.11	0.12	0.08	0.00	0.01	C74
其他内分泌腺	Other endocrine	137	0.06	0.12	0.09	0.00	0.01	92	0.08	0.08	0.06	0.00	0.01	C75
霍奇金淋巴瘤	Hodgkin lymphoma	224	0.10	0.20	0.13	0.01	0.01	106	0.09	0.10	0.06	0.00	0.01	C81
非霍奇金淋巴瘤	Non-Hodgkin lymphoma	2 618	1.11	2.29	1.50	0.08	0.16	1 476	1.21	1.35	0.83	0.04	0.09	C82-C86,C96
免疫增生性疾病	Immunoproliferative diseases	12	0.01	0.01	0.01	0.00	0.00	8	0.01	0.01	0.00	0.00	0.00	C88
多发性骨髓瘤	Multiple myeloma	921	0.39	0.81	0.51	0.02	0.06	651	0.54	0.60	0.36	0.02	0.05	C90
淋巴细胞白血病	Lymphoid leukemia	763	0.32	0.67	0.54	0.03	0.05	575	0.47	0.53	0.42	0.02	0.04	C91
髓系白血病	Myeloid leukemia	1 416	0.60	1.24	0.90	0.05	0.09	1 042	0.86	0.96	0.65	0.04	0.07	C92-C94, D45-D47
白血病,未特指	Leukemia unspecified	1 894	0.80	1.66	1.26	0.07	0.12	1 383	1.14	1.27	0.94	0.05	0.09	C95
其他或未指明部位	Other and unspecified	5 114	2.17	4.47	2.92	0.15	0.31	3 413	2.81	3.13	1.92	0.10	0.20	O & U
所有部位合计	All sites	235 694	100.00	206.20	129.59	6.27	14.81	121 642	100.00	111.51	64.12	3.11	7.00	C00-C97, D32-D33, D42-D43, D45-D47
所有部位除外 C44	All sites except C44	234 638	99.55	205.27	129.02	6.25	14.76	120 841	99.34	110.78	63.73	3.10	6.97	C00-C97,D32-D33,D42-D43, D45-D47 exc. C44

附表 2-17 2019 年全国西部城市肿瘤登记地区癌症死亡主要指标
Appendix Table 2-17 Cancer mortality in Western urban registration areas of China,2019

部位 Site		男性 Male 死亡数 No. deaths	构成 Freq./%	粗率 Crude rate/100 000⁻¹	世标率 ASR world/100 000⁻¹	累积率 Cum. Rate/% 0~64	0~74	女性 Female 死亡数 No. deaths	构成 Freq./%	粗率 Crude rate/100 000⁻¹	世标率 ASR world/100 000⁻¹	累积率 Cum. Rate/% 0~64	0~74	ICD-10
唇	Lip	43	0.05	0.10	0.06	0.00	0.01	19	0.04	0.04	0.02	0.00	0.00	C00
舌	Tongue	270	0.29	0.62	0.39	0.02	0.04	104	0.21	0.25	0.14	0.01	0.02	C01-C02
口	Mouth	388	0.42	0.90	0.55	0.02	0.07	174	0.36	0.41	0.22	0.01	0.02	C03-C06
唾液腺	Salivary gland	100	0.11	0.23	0.15	0.01	0.02	56	0.12	0.13	0.07	0.00	0.01	C07-C08
扁桃体	Tonsil	48	0.05	0.11	0.07	0.00	0.01	11	0.02	0.03	0.01	0.00	0.00	C09
其他口咽	Other oropharynx	134	0.14	0.31	0.19	0.01	0.02	12	0.02	0.03	0.02	0.00	0.00	C10
鼻咽	Nasopharynx	1 250	1.35	2.89	1.87	0.13	0.22	434	0.89	1.03	0.63	0.04	0.07	C11
下咽	Hypopharynx	211	0.23	0.49	0.31	0.02	0.04	13	0.03	0.03	0.02	0.00	0.00	C12-C13
咽,部位不明	Pharynx unspecified	175	0.19	0.40	0.24	0.01	0.03	59	0.12	0.14	0.07	0.00	0.01	C14
食管	Esophagus	8 271	8.92	19.12	11.65	0.47	1.43	2 060	4.24	4.87	2.52	0.06	0.27	C15
胃	Stomach	8 888	9.59	20.55	12.50	0.51	1.45	3 825	7.87	9.04	4.96	0.20	0.53	C16
小肠	Small intestine	327	0.35	0.76	0.45	0.02	0.05	267	0.55	0.63	0.35	0.01	0.04	C17
结肠	Colon	3 099	3.34	7.17	4.29	0.16	0.44	2 308	4.75	5.45	2.92	0.11	0.29	C18
直肠	Rectum	4 468	4.82	10.33	6.24	0.23	0.68	2 748	5.65	6.49	3.49	0.13	0.34	C19-C20
肛门	Anus	161	0.17	0.37	0.23	0.01	0.02	106	0.22	0.25	0.14	0.01	0.01	C21
肝脏	Liver	16 021	17.28	37.04	23.72	1.49	2.70	5 350	11.01	12.64	7.12	0.31	0.79	C22
胆囊及其他	Gallbladder etc.	1 073	1.16	2.48	1.50	0.06	0.16	1 323	2.72	3.13	1.68	0.06	0.18	C23-C24
胰腺	Pancreas	2 868	3.09	6.63	4.07	0.18	0.47	2 087	4.29	4.93	2.69	0.11	0.29	C25
鼻、鼻窦及其他	Nose,sinuses etc.	145	0.16	0.34	0.21	0.01	0.02	68	0.14	0.16	0.10	0.01	0.01	C30-C31
喉	Larynx	852	0.92	1.97	1.20	0.05	0.14	79	0.16	0.19	0.10	0.00	0.01	C32
气管、支气管、肺	Trachea,bronchus & lung	29 249	31.55	67.63	41.41	1.78	4.92	11 132	22.90	26.30	14.29	0.56	1.52	C33-C34
其他胸腔器官	Other thoracic organs	276	0.30	0.64	0.41	0.02	0.05	172	0.35	0.41	0.25	0.01	0.02	C37-C38
骨	Bone	645	0.70	1.49	0.99	0.05	0.10	416	0.86	0.98	0.60	0.03	0.06	C40-C41
皮肤黑色素瘤	Melanoma of skin	116	0.13	0.27	0.17	0.01	0.02	104	0.21	0.25	0.15	0.01	0.02	C43
皮肤其他	Other skin	388	0.42	0.90	0.56	0.02	0.05	290	0.60	0.69	0.36	0.01	0.03	C44
间皮瘤	Mesothelioma	46	0.05	0.11	0.08	0.00	0.01	28	0.06	0.07	0.04	0.00	0.00	C45
卡波西肉瘤	Kaposi sarcoma	12	0.01	0.03	0.02	0.00	0.00	10	0.02	0.02	0.02	0.00	0.00	C46
结缔组织、软组织	Connective & soft tissue	181	0.20	0.42	0.29	0.01	0.03	114	0.23	0.27	0.18	0.01	0.02	C47,C49
乳腺	Breast	133	0.14	0.31	0.19	0.01	0.02	3 361	6.92	7.94	4.95	0.36	0.55	C50
外阴	Vulva	—	—	—	—	—	—	65	0.13	0.15	0.09	0.00	0.01	C51
阴道	Vagina	—	—	—	—	—	—	62	0.13	0.15	0.08	0.00	0.01	C52
子宫颈	Cervix uteri	—	—	—	—	—	—	2 363	4.86	5.58	3.45	0.24	0.39	C53
子宫体	Corpus uteri	—	—	—	—	—	—	772	1.59	1.82	1.11	0.07	0.13	C54
子宫,部位不明	Uterus unspecified	—	—	—	—	—	—	324	0.67	0.77	0.46	0.03	0.05	C55
卵巢	Ovary	—	—	—	—	—	—	1 523	3.13	3.60	2.23	0.14	0.27	C56
其他女性生殖器官	Other female genital organs	—	—	—	—	—	—	85	0.17	0.20	0.12	0.01	0.01	C57
胎盘	Placenta	—	—	—	—	—	—	2	0.00	0.00	0.00	0.00	0.00	C58
阴茎	Penis	118	0.13	0.27	0.17	0.01	0.02	—	—	—	—	—	—	C60
前列腺	Prostate	2 469	2.66	5.71	3.18	0.04	0.22	—	—	—	—	—	—	C61
睾丸	Testis	43	0.05	0.10	0.08	0.01	0.01	—	—	—	—	—	—	C62
其他男性生殖器官	Other male genital organs	19	0.02	0.04	0.03	0.00	0.00	—	—	—	—	—	—	C63
肾	Kidney	629	0.68	1.45	0.90	0.04	0.10	378	0.78	0.89	0.51	0.02	0.05	C64
肾盂	Renal pelvis	109	0.12	0.25	0.16	0.01	0.02	80	0.16	0.19	0.11	0.00	0.01	C65
输尿管	Ureter	95	0.10	0.22	0.13	0.00	0.01	103	0.21	0.24	0.13	0.00	0.01	C66
膀胱	Bladder	1 563	1.69	3.61	2.09	0.05	0.17	435	0.90	1.03	0.51	0.01	0.04	C67
其他泌尿器官	Other urinary organs	21	0.02	0.05	0.03	0.00	0.00	18	0.04	0.04	0.02	0.00	0.00	C68
眼	Eye	38	0.04	0.09	0.06	0.00	0.01	28	0.06	0.07	0.05	0.00	0.00	C69
脑、神经系统	Brain,nervous system	1 859	2.01	4.30	3.06	0.18	0.32	1 456	3.00	3.44	2.30	0.12	0.24	C70-C72,D32-D33,D42-D43
甲状腺	Thyroid	200	0.22	0.46	0.30	0.02	0.03	310	0.64	0.73	0.44	0.02	0.05	C73
肾上腺	Adrenal gland	83	0.09	0.19	0.13	0.01	0.01	73	0.15	0.17	0.10	0.00	0.01	C74
其他内分泌腺	Other endocrine	57	0.06	0.13	0.10	0.00	0.01	34	0.07	0.08	0.06	0.00	0.01	C75
霍奇金淋巴瘤	Hodgkin lymphoma	93	0.10	0.22	0.15	0.01	0.01	47	0.10	0.11	0.07	0.00	0.01	C81
非霍奇金淋巴瘤	Non-Hodgkin lymphoma	1 191	1.28	2.75	1.76	0.09	0.19	688	1.42	1.63	0.97	0.05	0.11	C82-C86,C96
免疫增生性疾病	Immunoproliferative diseases	9	0.01	0.02	0.01	0.00	0.00	3	0.01	0.01	0.00	0.00	0.00	C88
多发性骨髓瘤	Multiple myeloma	480	0.52	1.11	0.69	0.03	0.08	347	0.71	0.82	0.48	0.02	0.06	C90
淋巴细胞白血病	Lymphoid leukemia	360	0.39	0.83	0.66	0.03	0.06	265	0.55	0.63	0.49	0.03	0.04	C91
髓系白血病	Myeloid leukemia	680	0.73	1.57	1.13	0.06	0.11	498	1.02	1.18	0.77	0.04	0.08	C92-C94,D45-D47
白血病,未特指	Leukemia unspecified	629	0.68	1.45	1.08	0.05	0.11	461	0.95	1.09	0.79	0.04	0.07	C95
其他或未指明部位	Other and unspecified	2 124	2.29	4.91	3.12	0.15	0.33	1 453	2.99	3.43	2.08	0.10	0.29	O & U
所有部位合计	All sites	92 707	100.00	214.36	133.02	6.11	15.03	48 603	100.00	114.83	65.53	3.04	7.00	C00-C97,D32-D33,D42-D43,D45-D47
所有部位除外 C44	All sites except C44	92 319	99.58	213.46	132.46	6.09	14.99	48 313	99.40	114.14	65.17	3.03	6.97	C00-C97,D32-D33,D42-D43,D45-D47 exc. C44

附表 2-18　2019 年全国西部农村肿瘤登记地区癌症死亡主要指标

Appendix Table 2-18　Cancer mortality in Western rural registration areas of China,2019

部位 Site		男性 Male						女性 Female						ICD-10
		死亡数 No. deaths	构成 Freq. /%	粗率 Crude rate/ 100 000⁻¹	世标率 ASR world/ 100 000⁻¹	累积率 Cum. Rate/%		死亡数 No. deaths	构成 Freq. /%	粗率 Crude rate/ 100 000⁻¹	世标率 ASR world/ 100 000⁻¹	累积率 Cum. Rate/%		
						0~64	0~74					0~64	0~74	
唇	Lip	142	0.10	0.20	0.13	0.01	0.01	63	0.09	0.09	0.05	0.00	0.00	C00
舌	Tongue	435	0.30	0.61	0.39	0.02	0.05	142	0.19	0.21	0.13	0.01	0.01	C01-C02
口	Mouth	651	0.46	0.92	0.57	0.02	0.07	237	0.32	0.36	0.19	0.01	0.02	C03-C06
唾液腺	Salivary gland	153	0.11	0.22	0.14	0.01	0.02	74	0.10	0.11	0.06	0.00	0.01	C07-C08
扁桃体	Tonsil	67	0.05	0.09	0.06	0.00	0.01	14	0.02	0.02	0.01	0.00	0.00	C09
其他口咽	Other oropharynx	217	0.15	0.31	0.19	0.01	0.02	35	0.05	0.05	0.03	0.00	0.00	C10
鼻咽	Nasopharynx	2 299	1.61	3.24	2.14	0.15	0.25	769	1.05	1.15	0.70	0.05	0.08	C11
下咽	Hypopharynx	252	0.18	0.35	0.23	0.02	0.03	19	0.03	0.03	0.02	0.00	0.00	C12-C13
咽,部位不明	Pharynx unspecified	292	0.20	0.41	0.26	0.01	0.03	87	0.12	0.13	0.07	0.00	0.01	C14
食管	Esophagus	15 074	10.54	21.21	13.06	0.54	1.62	3 942	5.40	5.91	3.04	0.08	0.33	C15
胃	Stomach	14 896	10.42	20.96	12.93	0.56	1.52	6 463	8.85	9.68	5.26	0.21	0.55	C16
小肠	Small intestine	404	0.28	0.57	0.36	0.02	0.04	275	0.38	0.41	0.24	0.01	0.03	C17
结肠	Colon	2 984	2.09	4.20	2.61	0.11	0.28	2 160	2.96	3.24	1.79	0.06	0.20	C18
直肠	Rectum	7 033	4.92	9.90	6.07	0.24	0.68	4 149	5.68	6.22	3.39	0.14	0.37	C19-C20
肛门	Anus	283	0.20	0.40	0.24	0.01	0.03	186	0.25	0.28	0.15	0.01	0.02	C21
肝脏	Liver	28 487	19.92	40.09	26.18	1.70	2.98	8 782	12.02	13.16	7.54	0.37	0.85	C22
胆囊及其他	Gallbladder etc.	1 395	0.98	1.96	1.22	0.06	0.14	1 525	2.09	2.28	1.26	0.05	0.15	C23-C24
胰腺	Pancreas	3 707	2.59	5.22	3.25	0.16	0.38	2 448	3.35	3.67	2.03	0.09	0.24	C25
鼻、鼻窦及其他	Nose, sinuses etc.	205	0.14	0.29	0.18	0.01	0.02	123	0.17	0.18	0.11	0.01	0.01	C30-C31
喉	Larynx	1 183	0.83	1.66	1.04	0.05	0.13	183	0.25	0.27	0.15	0.01	0.02	C32
气管、支气管、肺	Trachea, bronchus & lung	42 990	30.07	60.50	37.64	1.77	4.52	18 098	24.78	27.11	15.00	0.65	1.70	C33-C34
其他胸腔器官	Other thoracic organs	370	0.26	0.52	0.36	0.02	0.04	203	0.28	0.30	0.19	0.01	0.02	C37-C38
骨	Bone	1 239	0.87	1.74	1.17	0.06	0.13	756	1.04	1.13	0.71	0.03	0.08	C40-C41
皮肤黑色素瘤	Melanoma of skin	109	0.08	0.15	0.09	0.00	0.01	109	0.15	0.16	0.09	0.00	0.01	C43
皮肤其他	Other skin	668	0.47	0.94	0.59	0.02	0.06	511	0.70	0.77	0.41	0.01	0.03	C44
间皮瘤	Mesothelioma	47	0.03	0.07	0.04	0.00	0.00	48	0.07	0.07	0.04	0.00	0.00	C45
卡波西肉瘤	Kaposi sarcoma	22	0.02	0.03	0.02	0.00	0.00	5	0.01	0.01	0.00	0.00	0.00	C46
结缔组织、软组织	Connective & soft tissue	253	0.18	0.36	0.25	0.01	0.02	154	0.21	0.23	0.16	0.01	0.02	C47,C49
乳腺	Breast	163	0.11	0.23	0.14	0.01	0.02	4 312	5.90	6.46	4.13	0.32	0.45	C50
外阴	Vulva	—	—	—	—	—	—	109	0.15	0.16	0.09	0.01	0.01	C51
阴道	Vagina	—	—	—	—	—	—	70	0.10	0.10	0.06	0.00	0.01	C52
子宫颈	Cervix uteri	—	—	—	—	—	—	4 241	5.81	6.35	3.92	0.27	0.45	C53
子宫体	Corpus uteri	—	—	—	—	—	—	1 204	1.65	1.80	1.10	0.07	0.13	C54
子宫,部位不明	Uterus unspecified	—	—	—	—	—	—	722	0.99	1.08	0.66	0.04	0.08	C55
卵巢	Ovary	—	—	—	—	—	—	1 744	2.39	2.61	1.64	0.12	0.19	C56
其他女性生殖器官	Other female genital organs	—	—	—	—	—	—	99	0.14	0.15	0.09	0.01	0.01	C57
胎盘	Placenta	—	—	—	—	—	—	6	0.01	0.01	0.01	0.00	0.00	C58
阴茎	Penis	165	0.12	0.23	0.15	0.01	0.01	—	—	—	—	—	—	C60
前列腺	Prostate	2 511	1.76	3.53	2.04	0.03	0.16	—	—	—	—	—	—	C61
睾丸	Testis	78	0.05	0.11	0.08	0.00	0.01	—	—	—	—	—	—	C62
其他男性生殖器官	Other male genital organs	30	0.02	0.04	0.03	0.00	0.00	—	—	—	—	—	—	C63
肾	Kidney	669	0.47	0.94	0.61	0.03	0.07	372	0.51	0.56	0.33	0.01	0.03	C64
肾盂	Renal pelvis	111	0.08	0.16	0.10	0.00	0.01	66	0.09	0.10	0.06	0.00	0.01	C65
输尿管	Ureter	74	0.05	0.10	0.06	0.00	0.01	74	0.10	0.11	0.06	0.00	0.01	C66
膀胱	Bladder	2 178	1.52	3.07	1.80	0.04	0.16	555	0.76	0.83	0.42	0.01	0.04	C67
其他泌尿器官	Other urinary organs	29	0.02	0.04	0.02	0.00	0.00	19	0.03	0.03	0.01	0.00	0.00	C68
眼	Eye	66	0.05	0.09	0.08	0.00	0.00	48	0.07	0.07	0.05	0.00	0.00	C69
脑、神经系统	Brain, nervous system	3 206	2.24	4.51	3.25	0.20	0.34	2 389	3.27	3.58	2.40	0.14	0.25	C70-C72, D32-D33,D42-D43
甲状腺	Thyroid	289	0.20	0.41	0.26	0.02	0.03	438	0.60	0.66	0.39	0.02	0.04	C73
肾上腺	Adrenal gland	85	0.06	0.12	0.08	0.00	0.01	61	0.08	0.09	0.06	0.00	0.01	C74
其他内分泌腺	Other endocrine	80	0.06	0.11	0.08	0.01	0.01	58	0.08	0.09	0.06	0.00	0.01	C75
霍奇金淋巴瘤	Hodgkin lymphoma	131	0.09	0.18	0.12	0.01	0.01	59	0.08	0.09	0.05	0.00	0.01	C81
非霍奇金淋巴瘤	Non-Hodgkin lymphoma	1 427	1.00	2.01	1.34	0.07	0.15	788	1.08	1.18	0.74	0.04	0.08	C82-C86,C96
免疫增生性疾病	Immunoproliferative diseases	3	0.00	0.00	0.00	0.00	0.00	5	0.01	0.01	0.00	0.00	0.00	C88
多发性骨髓瘤	Multiple myeloma	441	0.31	0.62	0.40	0.02	0.05	304	0.42	0.46	0.28	0.02	0.04	C90
淋巴细胞白血病	Lymphoid leukemia	403	0.28	0.57	0.47	0.03	0.04	310	0.42	0.46	0.38	0.02	0.03	C91
髓系白血病	Myeloid leukemia	736	0.51	1.04	0.76	0.04	0.08	544	0.74	0.81	0.57	0.04	0.06	C92-C94, D45-D47
白血病,未特指	Leukemia unspecified	1 265	0.88	1.78	1.38	0.08	0.13	922	1.26	1.38	1.03	0.06	0.10	C95
其他或未指明部位	Other and unspecified	2 990	2.09	4.21	2.80	0.15	0.30	1 960	2.68	2.94	1.82	0.10	0.19	O & U
所有部位合计	All sites	142 987	100.00	201.23	127.45	6.37	14.69	73 039	100.00	109.41	63.26	3.15	7.00	C00-C97, D32-D33, D42-D43, D45-D47
所有部位除外 C44	All sites except C44	142 319	99.53	200.29	126.86	6.34	14.63	72 528	99.30	108.65	62.85	3.14	6.96	C00-C97,D32-D33,D42-D43, D45-D47 exc. C44

鸣　谢

　　《2022中国肿瘤登记年报》编委会对各肿瘤登记处的相关工作人员在本年报出版过程中给予的大力协助,尤其在整理、补充、审核登记资料,以及建档、建库等方面所做出的贡献表示感谢。衷心感谢编写组成员在年报撰写工作付出的辛苦努力。

Acknowledgement

　　The editorial committee of 2022 Chinese Cancer Registry Annual Report would like to express their gratitude to all staffs of cancer registries who have made a great contribution for the report, especially on data reduction, supplements, auditing, and cancer registration database management. Sincere thanks go to all members of the contributors for their great efforts.

肿瘤登记处名单 List of Cancer Registries and Registrars

省(自治区、直辖市) Province (autonomous region, municipality)	肿瘤登记处 Cancer Registry	登记处所在单位 Affiliation	主要工作人员 Staff
北京市	北京市	北京大学肿瘤医院暨北京市肿瘤防治研究所	季加孚　王　宁　刘　硕　李慧超　杨　雷 张　希　李晴雨　李浩鑫
天津市	天津市	天津市疾病预防控制中心	江国虹　王德征　沈成凤　王　冲　寻鲁宁 张　爽　张　辉　郑文龙
	天津市和平区	天津市和平区疾病预防控制中心	杨继平　高　杰
	天津市河东区	天津市河东区疾病预防控制中心	吕丽娜　马　娜　陈　楠　都星月
	天津市河西区	天津市河西区疾病预防控制中心	王　森　段雪旭　张艳艳
	天津市南开区	天津市南开区疾病预防控制中心	王　辉　王　娟　郭晓慧　韩　娜
	天津市河北区	天津市河北区疾病预防控制中心	贾　鑫
	天津市红桥区	天津市红桥区疾病预防控制中心	许海燕
	天津市东丽区	天津市东丽区疾病预防控制中心	苏　玉　刘　贺
	天津市西青区	天津市西青区疾病预防控制中心	窦　斐
	天津市津南区	天津市津南区疾病预防控制中心	李志红　张洪达　王　冲
	天津市北辰区	天津市北辰区疾病预防控制中心	金　莉
	天津市武清区	天津市武清区疾病预防控制中心	肖永刚　吴立波　王　震
	天津市宝坻区	天津市宝坻区疾病预防控制中心	谭孝琼　杨　洋　胡艳杰
	天津市滨海新区	天津市滨海新区疾病预防控制中心	柳艳萍　张炳旭　刘军秋　刘　佳
	天津市宁河区	天津市宁河区疾病预防控制中心	马　建　李金凤　马友田
	天津市静海区	天津市静海区疾病预防控制中心	魏新健　马娟娟
	天津市蓟州区	天津市蓟州区疾病预防控制中心	董金凤　杨　杨　吴佐军
河北省	河北省	河北医科大学第四医院	单保恩　贺宇彤　李道娟　刘言玉　梁　迪 靳　晶　师　金　瞿　峰
	石家庄市	石家庄市疾病预防控制中心	马新颜　梁震宇　高　从　段宇帆
	石家庄市长安区	石家庄市长安区疾病预防控制中心	范志磊　张雪滢　胡晓蒙

省（自治区、直辖市）Province（autonomous region，municipality）	肿瘤登记处 Cancer Registry	登记处所在单位 Affiliation	主要工作人员 Staff
	石家庄市桥西区	石家庄市桥西区疾病预防控制中心	张新娟　尚丽乔　曹朴芳
	石家庄市新华区	石家庄市新华区疾病预防控制中心	于素君　焦玉霞　王艳媛
	石家庄市井陉矿区	石家庄市井陉矿区疾病预防控制中心	辛　玲　魏晓瑞
	石家庄市裕华区	石家庄市裕华区疾病预防控制中心	刘红梅　甘知昊　齐璐莹
	石家庄市藁城区	石家庄市藁城区疾病预防控制中心	田密格　甘利宠　杨亚丛　张　鹏　李欣欣
	石家庄市鹿泉区	石家庄市鹿泉区疾病预防控制中心	贾爱华　任军辉　梁子乔　梁杰坤　张冰冻
	石家庄市栾城区	石家庄市栾城区疾病预防控制中心	赵金永　张　艺　王　媛　崔聿萧
	井陉县	井陉县疾病预防控制中心	刘会林　杜国平　张贤
	正定县	正定县疾病预防控制中心	张玉伟　赵晓静　王　灼　康艳岭
	高邑县	高邑县疾病预防控制中心	张晓娜　邢丽妍
	深泽县	深泽县疾病预防控制中心	刘　毅　张　红　赵　博
	赞皇县	赞皇县疾病预防控制中心	王树革　李　丽　郝月红　吕晓红
	赵县	赵县疾病预防控制中心	高明　程志辉　张肖肖
	辛集市	辛集市疾病预防控制中心	李　娜　万真真　耿　兵
	新乐市	新乐市疾病预防控制中心	董立新　董　旭　田　倩
	迁西县	迁西县疾病预防控制中心	赵金鸽　陈晓东　闫晓宇　田晓宇　冯峻楠　张艳洁　王伟光　赵　珊
	迁安市	迁安市疾病预防控制中心	刘　芳　谌华卿　邵舰伟
	秦皇岛市	秦皇岛市第四医院	熊润红　杨　晋　窦雅琳
	秦皇岛市海港区	秦皇岛市海港医院	姬秀颖　何文静
	秦皇岛市山海关区	秦皇岛市山海关人民医院	王　强　吕文博
	秦皇岛市北戴河区	秦皇岛市北戴河医院	滕　磊　郭珊珊
	秦皇岛市抚宁区	秦皇岛市抚宁区人民医院	任丽云　贾德建楠
	邯郸市邯山区	邯郸市邯山区疾病预防控制中心	张瑞欣　李金娥
	邯郸市峰峰矿区	邯郸市峰峰矿区疾病预防控制中心	黄春广　侯　怡
	大名县	大名县疾病预防控制中心	李　杨　刘肖单　张　赛　李欣欣　孙建冰　杨永花　李占龙

省(自治区、直辖市) Province (autonomous region, municipality)	肿瘤登记处 Cancer Registry	登记处所在单位 Affiliation	主要工作人员 Staff
	涉县	涉县肿瘤防治所	李永伟 温登瑰 李奋君 杨云娥 贾瑞强 张 喻
	磁县	磁县肿瘤防治研究所	宋国慧 陈超 龚妍玮 张 金 高志光 孟凡书
	武安市	武安市疾病预防控制中心	张宙 郭秀杰 卢 昱
	邢台市	邢台市人民医院	刘登湘 王军辉 贾丹丹 张亚琛 刘淑娴
	邢台市襄都区	邢台市襄都区医院	牛丽霞 白 静 赵立鹏
	邢台市信都区	团结路街道办事处社区卫生服务中心	马增瑜 王艳霞
	邢台市高新技术产业开发区	邢台经济开发区医院	田延琼 韩 蕾
	临城县	临城县人民医院	和丽娜 王 童
	内丘县	内丘县疾病预防控制中心	龙云 石胜民 智 玉 房晓芳
	邢台市任泽区	邢台市任泽区人民医院	赵雅芳 吉国强 孟 飞
	保定市	保定市疾病预防控制中心	张雁 赵凤芹 侯 烨 王紫炜 刘玉荣
	保定市竞秀区	保定市竞秀区疾病预防控制中心	张卫君 刘云帆
	保定市莲池区	保定市莲池区疾病预防控制中心	和丽娜 石兴宇
	望都县	望都县疾病预防控制中心	谷朝华 李 曼 程叶文
	安国市	安国市疾病预防控制中心	刘振博 李 辉 魏泽永 董浩楠 陈 邦 王 晟
	张家口市宣化区	张家口市宣化区疾病预防控制中心	支 雯 左存锐 李少英
	张北县	张北县疾病预防控制中心	刘 会 刘东雍
	承德市双桥区	承德市双桥区疾病预防控制中心	管丽娟 李广鲲 王明慧 平 萍 彭媛媛 刘 杰 于秀娟
	丰宁满族自治县	丰宁满族自治县医院	梁树军 颜学文 付杨健娇
	沧州市	沧州市肿瘤防治办公室	朱庆荣 郭艳汝 袁 媛 姬骁亮
	沧州市新华区	沧州市新华区疾病预防控制中心	李文娟 仝建玲
	沧州市运河区	沧州市运河区疾病预防控制中心	付素红 杨秀敏
	海兴县	海兴县疾病预防控制中心	武华倩 王淑丹 张 策
	盐山县	盐山县疾病预防控制中心	巩吉良 陈清彦 边梅芳
	衡水市桃城区	衡水第二人民医院	彭 晔 宋海林 李 燕 李 雪 赵子太
	衡水市冀州区	衡水市冀州区疾病预防控制中心	魏 丹 郭志超 贾向勇 王英林
	枣强县	枣强县人民医院	焦艳莉 杨凤秀
	景县	景县人民医院	梁晓婷 张 蕾 黄爱芹

省(自治区、直辖市) Province (autonomous region, municipality)	肿瘤登记处 Cancer Registry	登记处所在单位 Affiliation	主要工作人员 Staff
	辛集市	辛集市疾病预防控制中心	李 娜　万真真　耿 兵
山西省	山西省	中国医学科学院肿瘤医院山西医院/山西省肿瘤医院	邢念增　张永贞　曹 凌　王俊田　崔王飞
	太原市小店区	太原市小店区疾病预防控制中心	王琳琳
	太原市杏花岭区	太原市杏花岭区疾病预防控制中心	张 英　倪 芳　薛秀丽　朱祥　李 昕
	太原市万柏林区	太原市万柏林区疾病预防控制中心	杜小英
	阳泉市	阳泉市肿瘤防治研究所肿瘤医院	吕利成　郝素花　冯俊青　蒋书琼　萨其拉
	平定县	平定县疾病预防控制中心	贾源瑶　康 平　武金平　李春霞
	盂 县	盂县疾病预防控制中心	韩瑞贞
	襄垣县	襄垣县疾病预防控制中心	李志霞　张 钰
	平顺县	平顺县疾病预防控制中心	贾艳芳
	沁源县	沁源县疾病预防控制中心	张海虹
	阳城县	阳城县肿瘤医院	王新正　元芳梅　李阳　卫 娟
	陵川县	陵川县疾病预防控制中心	秦艺菲
	晋中市榆次区	晋中市榆次区疾病预防控制中心	郑永萍　郭秀峰　董小平　智 伟　李巧凤 闫梦娇　郭 磊
	晋中市太谷区	晋中市太谷区疾病预防控制中心	白建梅　韩 敏
	昔阳县	昔阳县疾病预防控制中心	王晓霞
	寿阳县	寿阳县疾病预防控制中心	张慧玲　郝佐文　霍志强　杨晓静　胡旭强 王俊红　姜艳红
	稷山县	稷山县疾病预防控制中心	谭万霞　赵夏娟
	新绛县	新绛县疾病预防控制中心	郭亚丽　权丽珍　苏 凯
	绛县	绛县疾病预防控制中心	高丽莉　曹 玉
	垣曲县	垣曲县疾病预防控制中心	张红霞　武茹燕　张高辉
	芮城县	芮城县疾病预防控制中心	张成军
	忻州市忻府区	忻州市忻府区疾病预防控制中心	王淑然
	定襄县	定襄县疾病预防控制中心	刘秉华
	原平市	原平市疾病预防控制中心	赵治田　李素琴
	襄汾县	襄汾县疾病预防控制中心	赵雄杰
	洪洞县	洪洞县疾病预防控制中心	侯晓艳　焦燕燕　崔亚丽
	交城县	交城县疾病预防控制中心	冯旭敏

省(自治区、直辖市) Province (autonomous region, municipality)	肿瘤登记处 Cancer Registry	登记处所在单位 Affiliation	主要工作人员 Staff
	临县	临县疾病预防控制中心	刘秀娥 高旭亮
	孝义市	孝义市疾病预防控制中心	冀德恩 张学慧 黄丽
	汾阳市	汾阳市疾病预防控制中心	高生丽 姚若花 黄艳英 殷红钰
内蒙古自治区	内蒙古自治区	内蒙古自治区综合疾病预防控制中心	席云峰 乔丽颖
	呼和浩特市	呼和浩特市疾病预防控制中心	李娜
	武川县	武川县疾病预防控制中心	梁蒙 蔡利萍
	乌海市	乌海市疾病预防控制中心	周娟 王晓敏 冯瑞 赵晶晶 董玉芬 李海云
	赤峰市	赤峰市疾病预防控制中心	张竞丹 刘占学 迟艳玲
	赤峰市红山区	赤峰市红山区疾病预防控制中心	何丽 刘剑飞 安建国 刘岩
	赤峰市元宝山区	赤峰市元宝山区疾病预防控制中心	韩小玉 孟晓东
	赤峰市松山区	赤峰市松山区疾病预防控制中心	王梦元 徐鑫 夏丽红
	巴林左旗	巴林左旗疾病预防控制中心	凌海杰 王文蕊
	敖汉旗	敖汉旗疾病预防控制中心	崔海华 于蕾 刘继莹
	通辽市	通辽市疾病预防控制中心	李智慧 赵丽 倪晓娜
	通辽市科尔沁区	通辽市科尔沁区疾病预防控制中心	周婷婷 高晶 李娜 唐丽梅
	科尔沁左翼中旗	科尔沁左翼中旗疾病预防控制中心	刘艳玲
	科尔沁左翼后旗	科左后旗疾病预防控制中心	李文慧
	开鲁县	开鲁县疾病预防控制中心	吴艳伟 王婉莹 刁玉飞
	库伦旗	库伦旗疾病预防控制中心	于鑫刚 王朝民
	奈曼旗	奈曼旗疾病预防控制中心	倪志华 李丽媛 张永红
	扎鲁特旗	扎鲁特旗疾病预防控制中心	婷婷 王晓琪 姜磊磊
	霍林郭勒市	霍林郭勒市疾病预防控制中心	刘娇 丁丽杰
	呼伦贝尔市	呼伦贝尔市疾病预防控制中心	蔡静明 王勇 柳聪慧
	呼伦贝尔市海拉尔区	呼伦贝尔市海拉尔区疾病预防控制中心	孔程程 孙溯苑
	呼伦贝尔市扎赉诺尔区	呼伦贝尔市呼伦贝尔市扎赉诺尔区疾病预防控制中心	贾丽敏 过亮
	阿荣旗	阿荣旗疾病预防控制中心	郭天骅 高智 高晨雨
	莫力达瓦达斡尔族自治旗	莫力达瓦达斡尔族自治旗疾病预防控制中心	赵占峰

省(自治区、直辖市) Province (autonomous region, municipality)	肿瘤登记处 Cancer Registry	登记处所在单位 Affiliation	主要工作人员 Staff
	鄂伦春自治旗	鄂伦春自治旗疾病预防控制中心	关 伟
	鄂温克族自治旗	鄂温克族自治旗疾病预防控制中心	张艺杰
	陈巴尔虎旗	陈巴尔虎旗疾病预防控制中心	永 梅 图 雅
	新巴尔虎左旗	新巴尔虎左旗疾病预防控制中心	韩明霞
	新巴尔虎右旗	新巴尔虎右旗疾病预防控制中心	塔 娜
	满洲里市	满洲里市疾病预防控制中心	李 颖 迎 春 王 娜
	牙克石市	牙克石市疾病预防控制中心	苏 燕 夏 宇 李覆男
	扎兰屯市	扎兰屯市疾病预防控制中心	李 静 陈 丽 李英杰
	根河市	根河市疾病预防控制中心	钟彦丰 孙林茹
	巴彦淖尔市	巴彦淖尔市疾病预防控制中心	韩爱英 邓海凤
	巴彦淖尔市临河区	巴彦淖尔市临河区疾病预防控制中心	张彩霞 高飞雪 王 芳
	五原县	五原县疾病预防控制中心	彭 娜 王小丽
	杭锦后旗	杭锦后旗疾病预防控制中心	王如博 董悦霞
	锡林郭勒盟	锡林郭勒盟疾病预防控制中心	王树丽 武慧芳
	锡林浩特市	锡林浩特市疾病预防控制中心	李智鹏 马 莉
	苏尼特左旗	苏尼特左旗疾病预防控制中心	乌日勒嘎 苏世齐
	苏尼特右旗	苏尼特右旗疾病预防控制中心	郭凤兰 娜布其
	东乌珠穆沁旗	东乌珠穆沁旗疾病预防控制中心	梅兰花 海 英 高楠楠
	太仆寺旗	太仆寺旗疾病预防控制中心	任红梅 郭振利 康赫赫
辽宁省	辽宁省	辽宁省疾病预防控制中心	穆慧娟
	沈阳市	沈阳市疾病预防控制中心	白 杉 刘 岩 许秀莹 刘权兴 刘新雨
	康平县	康平县疾病预防控制中心	彭红伟 白宇南
	法库县	法库县疾病预防控制中心	曹海洋 白鹤楠 马云丽
	新民市	新民市疾病预防控制中心	刘 丽 梁 浩
	大连市	大连市疾病预防控制中心	王晓锋 梅 丹 林 红 张新慧
	大连市金州区	大连市金州区疾病预防控制中心	李 萌 于世洪 胡秀冰 李 瑶 管修明
	庄河市	庄河市疾病预防控制中心	姜金宏 王丽娜
	鞍山市	鞍山市疾病预防控制中心	徐绍和 王丽娟 尹 晔 张微微 王肖琳 林立强 李绯璇 刘美玲 陈康境 张 颖 袁 媛 洪圣茹
	岫岩满族自治县	岫岩满族自治县疾病预防控制中心	张倩钰

省(自治区、直辖市) Province (autonomous region, municipality)	肿瘤登记处 Cancer Registry	登记处所在单位 Affiliation	主要工作人员 Staff				
	抚顺市	抚顺市疾病预防控制中心	徐 芳	许 威	邓小强	孙雯雯	孙野骞
			付淇予	杨 敏	龙 渊	钱诗雨	孟 桃
			尚莹莹	邓 可	杜 阳	孙继发	徐 哲
	本溪市	本溪市疾病预防控制中心	陈永刚	罗 娜	安晓霞	李海娜	付 艳
			刘 莹	韩 策	赵 楠		
	丹东市	丹东市疾病预防控制中心	邹晓琳	王诗云	孙继绪	秦 玲	盛禹萌
	东港市	东港市疾病预防控制中心	张武武	吕 辉	田玉敏	程笛珈	杨玉倩
			万莉蕾	赵银凤	郭向秋		
	锦州市	锦州市疾病预防控制中心	邵 颖	杨励励	于 雷		
	营口市	营口市疾病预防控制中心	刘 洋	白明宇	陈丽莉	赵 博	黄 颖
			梁 宏	李 颖	周 萍		
	阜新市	阜新市疾病预防控制中心	代晓泽	李鹏莹	徐 飒		
	彰武县	彰武县疾病预防控制中心	王静艳	王 楠			
	辽阳县	辽阳县疾病预防控制中心	何秀玲	李修竹	李迎秋	王武通	高晓楠
	盘锦市	盘锦市疾病预防控制中心	智 鑫	佟丽娟	马家开	杜巧红	邱园园
			刘 飞	王 磊	弓 拓	刘 红	郭文锦
	盘锦市大洼区	盘锦市大洼区疾病预防控制中心	吕建峰	陆 阳	岳 玲	杨 欢	曹凤娥
			李凤芹	许亚杰	张 勇	李浩然	
	建平县	建平县疾病预防控制中心	李宗芬	吕广艳	杨晓光	马佳杰	熊丽杰
吉林省	吉林省	吉林省疾病预防控制中心	郭 伟	朱颖俐	卢欣荣		
	长春市朝阳区	长春市朝阳区疾病预防控制中心	董玉军	李晓霞	王秋实	张天梅	赵红艳
			赵美子	李颂滨			
	德惠市	德惠市疾病预防控制中心	程志芳	凌命新			
	吉林市	吉林市疾病预防控制中心	孙岩海	刘 晔	王丽宇		
	永吉县	永吉县疾病预防控制中心	王晓妍	何晓峰			
	蛟河市	蛟河市疾病预防控制中心	张黎黎	张黎黎			
	桦甸市	桦甸市疾病预防控制中心	王晓丽	李忠诚	王春颖		
	舒兰市	舒兰市疾病预防控制中心	刘巾杰	雷 明	朱 莹	刘萍萍	
	磐石市	磐石市疾病预防控制中心	王艳萍	步 颖			
	四平市铁西区	四平市疾病预防控制中心	谭 丽	魏莉延	曹思淼	刘洪伟	张春雨
	四平市铁东区	四平市疾病预防控制中心	魏莉延	谭 丽	张春雨	刘洪伟	曹思淼
	梨树县	梨树县疾病预防控制中心	王 丹	徐 丹	张玉洁		
	伊通满族自治县	伊通满族自治县疾病预防控制中心	李 成	张 强	王大为	王 佟	

省（自治区、直辖市）Province（autonomous region，municipality）	肿瘤登记处 Cancer Registry	登记处所在单位 Affiliation	主要工作人员 Staff				
	双辽市	双辽市疾病预防控制中心	周颖丽	任立新	陈 华	李冬梅	
	辽源市龙山区	辽源市龙山区卫生健康局	初玉娜				
	东辽县	东辽县疾病预防控制中心	石 鹤				
	通化市	通化市疾病预防控制中心	何 柳	张 琳	魏 霞		
	通化县	通化县疾病预防控制中心	荆 铭	张俊丽	高艳华	孙静玲	
	梅河口市	梅河口市疾病预防控制中心	王 彬	王 越	宋立娟	朱瑞平	
	集安市	集安市疾病预防控制中心	杨 军	张晓虹	金 鑫	姚婷	
	白山市浑江区	白山市疾病预防控制中心	杨宇晨	徐春艳	张非愚		
	抚松县	抚松县疾病预防控制中心	陈祥梅	穆德营			
	松原市宁江区	松原市宁江区疾病预防控制中心	王春梅	郭 迪			
	前郭尔罗斯蒙古族自治县	前郭尔罗斯蒙古族自治县疾病预防控制中心	李静波	吴敬周	李贵麟	李智峰	
	乾安县	乾安县疾病预防控制中心	王艳秋	齐天坤	徐小超	杜华超	
	通榆县	通榆县疾病预防控制中心	李红妍	邓 楠	李 晶		
	大安市	大安市疾病预防控制中心	王 威	李晓秋	刘艳平		
	延吉市	延吉市疾病预防控制中心	方学哲	任 洋	郑春姬		
	图们市	图们市疾病预防控制中心	王嘉玉	郑玉凤			
	敦化市	敦化市疾病预防控制中心	朱晓梅	李秀英	马桂君		
	珲春市	珲春市疾病预防控制中心	李美子	任爱芳			
	龙井市	龙井市疾病预防控制中心	罗艳丽	金秀颖			
	和龙市	和龙市疾病预防控制中心	朱艳艳	徐桐欣	尹佳惠	张 旭	
	汪清县	汪清县疾病预防控制中心	李美娜	刘 宇			
	安图县	安图县疾病预防控制中心	朴顺姬	方立强			
黑龙江省	黑龙江省	黑龙江省癌症中心	宋冰冰 赵 敏	孙惠昕	张茂祥	王婉莹	贾海晗
	哈尔滨市道里区	哈尔滨市道里区疾病预防控制中心	刘旭东 李卓然	王 欣	康 娟	杨媛媛	吴 晗
	哈尔滨市南岗区	哈尔滨市南岗区疾病预防控制中心	于 波	王威娜	王 驰	吴镇原	单晓丽
	哈尔滨市香坊区	哈尔滨市香坊区疾病预防控制中心	宫旭志	李逸足			
	尚志市	尚志市疾病预防控制中心	姜 欣				
	五常市	五常市疾病预防控制中心	周 锐	田伟成			

省（自治区、直辖市）Province (autonomous region, municipality)	肿瘤登记处 Cancer Registry	登记处所在单位 Affiliation	主要工作人员 Staff
	勃利县	勃利县疾病预防控制中心	田鹏　胡月　蒙金　白特　张子明
	牡丹江市东安区	牡丹江市东安区疾病预防控制中心	常蓉　郭净炜
	牡丹江市阳明区	牡丹江市阳明区疾病预防控制中心	姚琳
	牡丹江市爱民区	牡丹江市爱民区疾病预防控制中心	郝庆华
	牡丹江市西安区	牡丹江市西安区疾病预防控制中心	邱红
	海林市	海林市疾病预防控制中心	余斌　周阳　龙江　杨珏琼　牛春英
上海市	上海市	上海市疾病预防控制中心	付晨　施燕　顾凯　吴春晓　庞怡　王春芳　施亮　向詠梅　龚杨明　窦剑明　吴梦吟　章晓聪
	上海市黄浦区	上海市黄浦区疾病预防控制中心	王烨菁　高淑娜　何丽华　杜娟　纪云芳　王一
	上海市徐汇区	上海市徐汇区疾病预防控制中心	钮登　顾海雁　朱菁　徐芊　钱孝琳　徐荆庶　汪逸超
	上海市长宁区	上海市长宁区疾病预防控制中心	庄建林　姜玉　张云　庄尹竹
	上海市静安区	上海市静安区疾病预防控制中心	周洲　方嘉列　杨晓明　王妍敏　高文君　尹晓烈　张敏　褚晓婷
	上海市普陀区	上海市普陀区疾病预防控制中心	沈莉　沈渊　石飞娅　杨丽娟　王若静　桑灏　朱晔　夏妍
	上海市虹口区	上海市虹口区基本预防控制中心	陈道湧　叶景虹　邹弘　赵静　龙家茹　计维　龚盼
	上海市杨浦区	上海市杨浦区疾病预防控制中心	韩雪　赵佳　陈灵颖　周隽隽　李辉　张正征　陈静
	上海市闵行区	上海市闵行区疾病预防控制中心	刘小华　许慧琳　李俊　程颖玲　俞丹丹　李为希　周洁　石安霞　马小玉
	上海市宝山区	上海市宝山区疾病预防控制中心	孟杨　茅俭英　刘世友　李叶　沈方力　蔡卫华　汪金辰　周慧宁
	上海市嘉定区	上海市嘉定区疾病预防控制中心	彭谦　于宏杰　张一英　向芳　黄芳　王亚伟　徐一凡
	上海市浦东新区	上海市浦东新区疾病预防控制中心	林涛　杨琛　张莉　顾梅蓉　乔羽　林上群　段雨彤　王莹莹　吴铮　胡佳　黄华　张美玉　瞿纯洁　朱海明　沈建国　陈亦晨
	上海市金山区	上海市金山区疾病预防控制中心	高霞　朱晓云　林菲　王倩　杨彩霞　夏文霞　张南南

省(自治区、直辖市) Province (autonomous region, municipality)	肿瘤登记处 Cancer Registry	登记处所在单位 Affiliation	主要工作人员 Staff
	上海市松江区	上海市松江区疾病预防控制中心	姜永根 杨 鹏 何静怡 吴毅凌 苏旭燕 陆慧萍
	上海市青浦区	上海市青浦区疾病预防控制中心	王 森 吴 雅 陆 叶 汪月琴 韩荣荣 方利萍
	上海市奉贤区	上海市奉贤区疾病预防控制中心	陈 英 汤海英 张 琳 唐怡菁 邓泽南 徐海峰 黄 芳
	上海市崇明区	上海市崇明区疾病预防控制中心	唐 明 徐 燕 黄玉华 汤佳秀 史爱玉
江苏省	江苏省	江苏省疾病预防控制中心(江苏省公共卫生研究院)	朱宝立 韩仁强 周金意 缪伟刚 俞 浩 罗鹏飞 陶 然
	南京市	南京市疾病预防控制中心	周海茸 洪 忻 王巍巍
	南京市六合区	南京市六合区疾病预防控制中心	杨 爽 尤万喜 王宏晶
	南京市溧水区	南京市溧水区疾病预防控制中心	郑欢欢 傅爱华 李菁玲 郑 继
	南京市高淳区	南京市高淳区疾病预防控制中心	张丁丁 吕惠青 周绿兵
	无锡市	无锡市疾病预防控制中心	杨志杰 钱 云 董昀球 陈 海 刘雅琦
	无锡市锡山区	无锡市锡山区疾病预防控制中心	顾 月 徐红艳
	无锡市惠山区	无锡市惠山区疾病预防控制中心	茹 炯 陈顺平 曹 军
	无锡市滨湖区	无锡市滨湖区疾病预防控制中心	杜 明 刘俊华
	无锡市梁溪区	无锡市梁溪区疾病预防控制中心	王 琳 包海明 徐凌云
	无锡市新吴区	无锡市新吴区疾病预防控制中心	陆绍琦 李 纯 时进进
	江阴市	江阴市疾病预防控制中心	李 莹 刘 娟 章 剑 张燕茹 王敏洁
	宜兴市	宜兴市疾病预防控制中心	任露露 胡 静 乔健健 闵艺璇
	无锡经济开发区	无锡经济开发区疾病预防控制中心	王礼华 王 景 邹志红
	徐州市	徐州市疾病预防控制中心	娄培安 董宗美 张 盼 乔 程 李 婷 陈培培 张 宁 刘 德
	徐州市鼓楼区	徐州市鼓楼区疾病预防控制中心	刘娅娴 蒋晓露
	徐州市云龙区	徐州市云龙区疾病预防控制中心	渠漫漫 宋兆粉
	徐州市贾汪区	徐州市贾汪区疾病预防控制中心	宗 华 李金宇 张 璐 刘禹杉
	徐州市泉山区	徐州市泉山区疾病预防控制中心	赵梦晨 王艳梅 吴海宏 李 念
	邳州市	邳州市疾病预防控制中心	张 明 李军政 娄从民
	常州市	常州市疾病预防控制中心	骆文书 徐文超 姚杏娟 周孟孟
	常州市天宁区	常州市天宁区疾病预防控制中心	颉艳霞 施鸿飞
	常州市钟楼区	常州市钟楼区疾病预防控制中心	吴振霞 崔艳丽

省(自治区、直辖市) Province (autonomous region, municipality)	肿瘤登记处 Cancer Registry	登记处所在单位 Affiliation	主要工作人员 Staff
	常州市新北区	常州市新北区疾病预防控制中心	何　怡　郑蜀贞　张　友
	常州市武进区	常州市武进区疾病预防控制中心	宗　菁　强德仁　孔晓玲　石素逸
	溧阳市	溧阳市疾病预防控制中心	刘建平　浦芸菲　石一辰　金　玲
	常州市金坛区	常州市金坛区疾病预防控制中心	方惠玲　周　鑫　程　鑫　王　姣
	常州经济开发区	常州经开区公共卫生管理服务中心	陈　玉　张端强
	苏州市	苏州市疾病预防控制中心	陆　艳　王临池　崔俊鹏　黄春妍
	苏州市虎丘区	苏州市虎丘区疾病预防控制中心	王从菊
	苏州市吴中区	苏州市吴中区疾病预防控制中心	周　游　顾建芬　马菊萍
	苏州市相城区	苏州市相城区疾病预防控制中心	张　群　毛　赟
	苏州市姑苏区	苏州市姑苏区疾病预防控制中心	张　秋　孔芳芳　吴新凡　徐　焱
	苏州市吴江区	苏州市吴江区疾病预防控制中心	沈建新　张荣艳　彭晓楚　杨　梅　顾思义
	苏州工业园区	苏州工业园区疾病防治中心	翟　静　刘　佳　景　阳　陆梦兰
	常熟市	常熟市疾病预防控制中心	陈冰霞　顾淑君　顾亦斌　陈俐枫　叶映丹 董晨章　朱一宁
	张家港市	张家港市疾病预防控制中心	杜国明　邱　晶　秦敏晔　王洵之　谢　辉
	昆山市	昆山市疾病预防控制中心	张　婷　金亦徐　秦　威　陆吕霖　仝　岚 周　杰　贺方荣
	太仓市	太仓市疾病预防控制中心	张建安　高玲琳　颜小銮　陆鸿滋
	南通市	南通市疾病预防控制中心	徐　红　韩颖颖　潘少聪　王　秦
	南通市通州区	南通市通州区疾病预防控制中心	韩建周　凡丽芸
	南通市崇川区	南通市崇川区疾病预防控制中心	郑会燕　刘海峰
	海安市	海安市疾病预防控制中心	钱　赟　吉　光　张玉成　童海燕
	如东县	如东县疾病预防控制中心	季佳慧　张爱红　吴双玲
	启东市	启东市人民医院	朱　健　陈永胜　王　军　张永辉　丁璐璐 徐源佑　陈建国
	如皋市	如皋市疾病预防控制中心	王书兰　徐培培　许利军　王　磊　吴　琼
	南通市海门区	南通市海门区疾病预防控制中心	杨艳蕾　唐锦高　倪倬健　梁晓健　陈燕熙
	连云港市	连云港市疾病预防控制中心	董建梅　张春道　李伟伟　柴莉莉　秦绪成 马昭君
	连云港市连云区	连云港市连云区疾病预防控制中心	李绪磊　刘　敏　张　琦
	连云港市海州区	连云港市海州区疾病预防控制中心	李炎炎　李佳雨　邓鑫鑫
	连云港市赣榆区	连云港市赣榆区疾病预防控制中心	张晓峰　金　凤　顾绍生

省(自治区、直辖市) Province (autonomous region, municipality)	肿瘤登记处 Cancer Registry	登记处所在单位 Affiliation	主要工作人员 Staff				
	东海县	东海县疾病预防控制中心	马 进 丁东艳	胡书铭	吉园园	彭琪琪	陈世杰
	灌云县	灌云县疾病预防控制中心	马士化	宋 靖	严春华		
	灌南县	灌南县疾病预防控制中心	崔玲波	孟忆宁	陈学琴	丁梦秋	
	连云港经济技术开发区	连云港经济技术开发区疾病预防控制中心	李存禄	宋家胜			
	淮安市	淮安市疾病预防控制中心	沈 欢 梅冬蒙	潘恩春	孙中明	文进博	缪丹丹
	淮安市淮安区	淮安市淮安区疾病预防控制中心	苏 明	王 昕	冯昊琼	孙博文	刘可可
	淮安市淮阴区	淮安市淮阴区疾病预防控制中心	罗国良	袁 瑛	刘 丹	徐 静	李 敏
	淮安市清江浦区	淮安市清江浦区疾病预防控制中心	刘 超	曹慷慷	万福萍		
	涟水县	涟水县疾病预防控制中心	浦继尹	孟宪炜	孝宇新	包雨晴	
	淮安市洪泽区	淮安市洪泽区疾病预防控制中心	陈思红 王 芳	王庶安	曹巧力	袁翠莲	张举巧
	盱眙县	盱眙县疾病预防控制中心	王 裕	吉慧敏	姜其家		
	金湖县	金湖县疾病预防控制中心	何士林	雷茵子			
	盐城市	盐城市疾病预防控制中心	刘付东	吴玲玲	陈建旭	杨子莫	
	盐城市亭湖区	盐城市亭湖区疾病预防控制中心	严莉丽	王 静			
	盐城市盐都区	盐城市盐都区疾病预防控制中心	何 飞	耿 佳			
	响水县	响水县疾病预防控制中心	陈玥华	王 超			
	滨海县	滨海县疾病预防控制中心	蔡 伟	胡 裕			
	阜宁县	阜宁县疾病预防控制中心	杨尚波	张 瑜			
	射阳县	射阳县疾病预防控制中心	戴曙光	陈银宝	戴春云	王颖莹	万能能
	建湖县	建湖县疾病预防控制中心	王 剑	肖 丽	孙动员		
	东台市	东台市疾病预防控制中心	赵建华	史春兰	丁海健		
	盐城市大丰区	盐城市大丰区疾病预防控制中心	顾晓平	顾 昕	曾立明	刘 铭	
	扬州市	扬州市疾病预防控制中心	解 晔	赵 培	王琦玮		
	扬州市广陵区	扬州市广陵区疾病预防控制中心	陈雪筠	居梦天	于 薇		
	扬州市邗江区	扬州市邗江区疾病预防控制中心	孔娴娴	薛安庆	陈俐娜		
	宝应县	宝应县疾病预防控制中心	任 涛 高胜静	朱立文	丁爱红	潘艳玉	王元霞
	仪征市	仪征市疾病预防控制中心	许 琴	魏 婕			
	扬州市江都区	扬州市江都区疾病预防控制中心	王锦云	朱 俊	周冰洁	赵宏达	

省(自治区、直辖市) Province (autonomous region, municipality)	肿瘤登记处 Cancer Registry	登记处所在单位 Affiliation	主要工作人员 Staff				
	镇江市	镇江市疾病预防控制中心	朱月兰	徐 璐	王宏宇	何佳佳	
	丹阳市	丹阳市疾病预防控制中心	陈丽黎	应洪琰	胡佳慧	王佳烨	
	扬中市	扬中市肿瘤防治研究所	华召来 宋统球	周 琴 朱进华	施爱武 戴 春	冯 祥	郭艳霞
	泰州市	泰州市疾病预防控制中心	张德坤 黄 鑫	赵小兰 杜京航	卢海燕	杨家骥	杨玉雪
	泰兴市	泰兴市疾病预防控制中心	刘静琦 蒋 慧	黄素勤	徐 兴	丁华萍	封军莉
	宿迁市	宿迁市疾病预防控制中心	于 蕾	邱玉保	张新楠	井海陵	
	宿迁市宿城区	宿迁市宿城区疾病预防控制中心	陈 英	漆苏洋	张恋恋		
	沭阳县	沭阳县疾病预防控制中心	张晶晶				
	泗阳县	泗阳县疾病预防控制中心	符地宝	姜素清			
	泗洪县	泗洪县疾病预防控制中心	韩嘉仪				
浙江省	浙江省	浙江省肿瘤防治办公室	程向东 龚巍巍	裘燕飞 李辉章	杜灵彬 陈天辉	俞 敏 陈瑶瑶	钟节鸣 周慧娟
	杭州市	杭州市疾病预防控制中心	徐 珏 任艳军	姜彩霞 张 艳	李 标	程宗雪	秦 康
	宁波市鄞州区	宁波市鄞州区疾病预防控制中心	孙晗莹 李小勇	赵 磊	陈 奇	林鸿波	沈 鹏
	慈溪市	慈溪市疾病预防控制中心	吴逸平 罗央努 李 妍	马 旭 黄 文 张 映	罗 丹 王利君 徐 洲	刘 琼 胡 吉	黄振宇 岑 鑫
	温州市鹿城区	温州市鹿城区疾病预防控制中心	谢海斌 周承洁	陈 捷 毛振兴	张沛绮	孙力涵	罗亚莹
	乐清市	乐清市疾病预防控制中心	蒋曙初 胡瑶莹	黄秀丹 林怡珊	虞朋余	孔剑芳	潘寅曙
	嘉兴市	嘉兴市(南湖区)疾病预防控制中心	李雪琴 金 鎏	陈中文 王林红	顾伟玲 周夏芳	谢 亮 金泽彬	陈文燕
	嘉善县	嘉善县肿瘤防治所	沈飞琼 张小红	费兴林	杨金华	李其龙	吕洁萍
	海宁市	海宁市中医院	朱云峰	祝丽娟	杨 靖	陆恩宁	
	湖州市南浔区	湖州市南浔区疾病预防控制中心	杨丽萍 杨晓伟	沈红伟 顾 恒	李 笛 吴小利	詹 伟 陈晓亚	王 毅
	长兴县	长兴县疾病预防控制中心	施长苗 顾建萍	秦家胜 叶 萍	陈 蓉	臧宇凡	陈 芸
	诸暨市	诸暨市疾病预防控制中心	谢锦荣	何 亮	张奇阳	孙迪霞	张光欣
	绍兴市上虞区	绍兴市上虞区疾病预防控制中心	方海平 龚月江	范建强 王少华	丁萍飞	杨晓静	赵之青

省(自治区、直辖市) Province (autonomous region, municipality)	肿瘤登记处 Cancer Registry	登记处所在单位 Affiliation	主要工作人员 Staff				
	金华市婺城区	金华市婺城区疾病预防控制中心	金红艳 韩郸轲	王洪歆 董燕群	陈 佩	陈静英	陆文雯
	永康市	永康市疾病预防控制中心	潘中伟 胡春生	胡云卿 徐玲巧	吴忠顶 陈 璐	胡 浩 沈锦绣	朱洪挺 周美儿
	衢州市柯城区	衢州市柯城区疾病预防控制中心	周文武 王小敏 余肖燕	史玉坤 黄文思	谢海燕 姜晓风	周 萍 陈 莺	徐幼平 程献梅
	开化县	开化县疾病预防控制中心	严传富 万红建	汪德兵 叶 青	项彩英 王贵平	吴芝兰 余 虹	应武群
	舟山市定海区	舟山市定海区疾病预防控制中心	张 彩 蒋志明	李本和	翁永夫	耿晓冬	赵展峰
	岱山县	岱山县疾病预防控制中心	李琼燕 朱夏燕	虞吉寅 鲍玮臻	张彤杰 徐 妮	何存弘	赵剑刚
	仙居县	仙居县疾病预防控制中心	张秀芬 王宇多	应江伟 黄镜泽	李笑琴 周东华	周立新 王敏华	王丽君 吴佳霞
	温岭市	温岭市疾病预防控制中心	范炜钢 陈彩虹	吴丹红 赵秀贞	王玲娜	李 黎	舒 展
	丽水市莲都区	丽水市莲都区疾病预防控制中心	刘海波 何笔通	卢小丽 郑桂爱	徐伟钗 陈晓苗	许 铭	柳伟峰
	龙泉市	龙泉市疾病预防控制中心	钟伟文 叶水菊	梅盛华 尹丽梅	万春松 谢泽久	刘卫红 张美锦	潘伟文 吴国庆
安徽省	安徽省	安徽省疾病预防控制中心	刘志荣	王华东	戴 丹		
	合肥市	合肥市疾病预防控制中心	张小鹏 袁胜祥	李佳佳 何 燕	孙 锋 汪志远	唐 伦 朱晓培	陈晓园 尹晓冬
	长丰县	长丰县疾病预防控制中心	吴海燕	陈 春	孙多壮	周艳辉	
	肥东县	肥东县疾病预防控制中心	陈海涛	徐 旭	张全寿	谈其干	
	肥西县	肥西县疾病预防控制中心	魏九丹	马郭兴	刘玲玲	吴颢璇	解光文
	庐江县	庐江县疾病预防控制中心	左登敏	郑诗佳	吴 骅		
	巢湖市	巢湖市疾病预防控制中心	王义江	刘 涛			
	芜湖市	芜湖市疾病预防控制中心	朱君君 赵丽华	陈佳瑶 王秀丽	盛 娟 吴瑞萍	鲍慧芬 冯花平	丁卫群
	芜湖市繁昌区	芜湖市繁昌区疾病预防控制中心	程 锋	李玉莉			
	南陵县	南陵县疾病预防控制中心	朱景红	陈琪琪	贾运萍		
	蚌埠市	蚌埠市疾病预防控制中心	竟广群 袁 梅	周静静	周国华	陈 艳	尚晓静
	五河县	五河县疾病预防控制中心	田 军 郭永妹	许美菱	郭茂蕴	纪 琼	夏立环

省(自治区、直辖市) Province (autonomous region, municipality)	肿瘤登记处 Cancer Registry	登记处所在单位 Affiliation	主要工作人员 Staff
	淮南市潘集区	淮南市潘集区卫生防疫和食品药品安全服务中心	姚　媛　张　珂
	凤台县	凤台县疾病预防控制中心	秦克波　郭　克　李　涛　缪众众
	马鞍山市	马鞍山市疾病预防控制中心	王　春　吴丹丹　张　燕　秦其荣　娄金海
	当涂县	当涂县疾病预防控制中心	徐　薇　卜维霞　李代平
	濉溪县	濉溪县疾病预防控制中心	赵雪飞　杨　珂　周鹏程　朱　英　蔡秋晨
	铜陵市	铜陵市疾病预防控制中心	吴　刚　刘　睿　何春玲
	铜陵市义安区	铜陵市义安区疾病预防控制中心	张　标　丁　媛　高红霞　杨为务
	安庆市迎江区	安庆市迎江区疾病预防控制中心	蔡　林　朱晓庆
	安庆市大观区	安庆市大观区疾病预防控制中心	刘维正　韦冬玲
	安庆市宜秀区	安庆市宜秀区疾病预防控制中心	鲍克彪　王鹏飞
	怀宁县	怀宁县疾病预防控制中心	刘少鑫　王小爱
	太湖县	太湖县疾病预防控制中心	阮四君　刘会川　王杰梅
	望江县	望江县疾病预防控制中心	周春林　储姣姣
	岳西县	岳西县疾病预防控制中心	范莉莉　储琼瑛
	桐城市	桐城市疾病预防控制中心	王俊武　陈兴国
	潜山市	潜山市疾病预防控制中心	陈娇娇　黄春芳　叶丹丹
	定远县	定远县疾病预防控制中心	俞庆国　张世涛　曹娇娇　杜欣欣
	天长市	天长市疾病预防控制中心	胡　彪　赵培甫　张　浩　任桂云　曹　水　王莲东
	阜阳市颍州区	颍州区疾病预防控制中心	张海峰　郭　青　刘俊辉　王明玉
	阜阳市颍东区	颍东区疾病预防控制中心	马朝阳　孙　涛　陈　雷　徐晓晴　张静静
	阜阳市颍泉区	颍泉区疾病预防控制中心	刘　军　张存红　韩士顶　尹雷雷
	太和县	太和县疾病预防控制中心	王允田　张西才　张怡楠　李诗童
	阜南县	阜南县疾病预防控制中心	田　侠　单文华　张家棒　马　震　胡　生
	界首市	界首市疾病预防控制中心	项莉红　卢晓东　段玉玺　程允萍　肖　帆
	宿州市埇桥区	埇桥区疾病预防控制中心	张园园　黄　磊
	灵璧县	灵璧县疾病预防控制中心	周永刚　赵　辉
	六安市金安区	金安区疾病预防控制中心	郭　正　王　玲
	寿县	寿县疾病预防控制中心	杨茂敏　蔡传毓　陈多状　黄　奎　唐晶晶
	金寨县	金寨县疾病预防控制中心	俞　亮　廖家胜　张礼兵
	蒙城县	蒙城县疾病预防控制中心	丁　浩　李银梅　刘　翔　刘珊珊
	东至县	东至县疾病预防控制中心	吴泽宁　景燕平　刘芳圆　张　瑶　章辰鹏　陆　鑫

省（自治区、直辖市）Province（autonomous region，municipality）	肿瘤登记处 Cancer Registry	登记处所在单位 Affiliation	主要工作人员 Staff				
	泾县	泾县疾病预防控制中心	刘安阜 程渡西	吴 鹏	马雄梅	李 婷	蒋丹丹
	宁国市	宁国市疾病预防控制中心	胡倩华	付 超	朱韦辰	唐 雯	阚咏琪
福建省	福建省	福建省肿瘤医院	周 衍	马晶昱	相智声		
	罗源县	罗源县疾病预防控制中心	叶奕宁				
	永泰县	永泰县疾病预防控制中心	郭朝峰				
	福清市	福清市疾病预防控制中心	何道逢	钟女娟	翁瑜瑶	王小阳	
	福州市长乐区	福州市长乐区肿瘤防治研究所	陈建顺 张祖霞	陈礼慈	陈 英	陈心聪	陈聪明
	厦门市	厦门市疾病预防控制中心	伍啸青 张卓平 谢丽珊	池家煌 连真忠	林艺兰 张琼花	陈月珍 易艺鹏	陈 沁 谭林华
	厦门市同安区	厦门市同安区疾病预防控制中心	陈上清	洪雅倩			
	厦门市翔安区	厦门市翔安区疾病预防控制中心	柯金练	苏辉耀	林雅秀		
	莆田市涵江区	莆田市涵江区疾病预防控制中心	林玉成	陈 震	吴小芬		
	明溪县	明溪县疾病预防控制中心	黄若瑶				
	大田县	大田县疾病预防控制中心	陈美美				
	建宁县	建宁县疾病预防控制中心	朱 婧				
	永安市	永安市疾病预防控制中心	李杭生	李丽丽	范 光		
	惠安县	惠安县疾病预防控制中心	刘庆烟	张冬雪			
	漳州市长泰区	漳州市长泰区疾病预防控制中心	郑冬柏	许宛意			
	建瓯市	建瓯市疾病预防控制中心	裴振义	官文婷	徐肖健		
	龙岩市新罗区	龙岩市新罗区疾病预防控制中心	廖凌玲	赖庆斌			
	龙岩市永定区	龙岩市永定区疾病预防控制中心	黄远田				
	上杭县	上杭县疾病预防控制中心	张亚平				
	武平县	武平县疾病预防控制中心	方丽娟				
	连城县	连城县疾病预防控制中心	周 叁				
江西省	江西省	江西省疾病预防控制中心	颜 玮	陈小娜	朱 瑶	卢飞豹	
	南昌市东湖区	南昌市东湖区疾病预防控制中心	黄恢淑	王信颖	刘 璐	聂甜甜	陈晶婷
	南昌市青山湖区	南昌市青山湖区疾病预防控制中心	黄 静	陈昔梅	蔡丹桃	杨盈华	周 莹
	南昌市新建区	南昌市新建区疾病预防控制中心	熊 炜	曹丽萍	万 信	孙雪华	万冬明
	萍乡市安源区	萍乡市安源区疾病预防控制中心	吴晓娟	房 泰	杨乐天琪	邬思璇	许兰萍
	萍乡市湘东区	萍乡市湘东区疾病预防控制中心	肖 绮	李玉芳	钟 婷	江 微	袁晓凤

续表

省(自治区、直辖市) Province (autonomous region, municipality)	肿瘤登记处 Cancer Registry	登记处所在单位 Affiliation	主要工作人员 Staff
	芦溪县	芦溪县疾病预防控制中心	张　莉　蔡建新　刘裕坤
	九江市浔阳区	九江市浔阳区疾病预防控制中心	伍　燕　万耀莲　周逸平　田绍进　邓如蕙
	武宁县	武宁县疾病预防控制中心	张赣湘　华　珊
	新余市渝水区	新余市渝水区疾病预防控制中心	杨　竹　周　林　晏琳春　彭娟丽　毛　麒　蔡小猫　胡蓉芳
	鹰潭市余江区	鹰潭市余江区疾病预防控制中心	陈紫云　危安安　上官千皓
	赣州市章贡区	赣州市章贡区疾病预防控制中心	廖　顺　苏德云　任学纳　胡小红
	赣州市赣县区	赣州市赣县区疾病预防控制中心	罗文云　黄文姬
	信丰县	信丰县疾病预防控制中心	王昱云
	大余县	大余县疾病预防控制中心	黄飞平　汪　楠
	上犹县	上犹县疾病预防控制中心	田玉平
	崇义县	崇义县疾病预防控制中心	冯云洪　卢致强
	龙南市	龙南市疾病预防控制中心	袁　菁　彭旻微　龙慧红
	于都县	于都县疾病预防控制中心	刘冬秀　何九凤　邹于生
	峡江县	峡江县疾病预防控制中心	陈志虹　袁怿飞　晏　可　张梅生
	新干县	新干县疾病预防控制中心	陈　冲
	安福县	安福县疾病预防控制中心	王　剑　胡水斌　王玉婷　刘忠明
	万载县	万载县疾病预防控制中心	郭巧红　汤丽珍　卢　萍
	上高县	上高县疾病预防控制中心	左　程　王紫琴
	靖安县	靖安县疾病预防控制中心	赵朝强　舒小裕　刘志英
	樟树市	樟树市疾病预防控制中心	张　思　周文群　谢　丹　葛晗雨　郑国林　万泓妗
	崇仁县	崇仁县疾病预防控制中心	孙　盼　杨　琴　杨　萍
	乐安县	乐安县疾病预防控制中心	郭　敏　刘　玲　黄　菜
	宜黄县	宜黄县疾病预防控制中心	徐媛锋
	抚州市东乡区	抚州市东乡区疾病预防控制中心	陈　霞　习哲浩　聂亚汀
	上饶市信州区	上饶市信州区疾病预防控制中心	李诗钰　叶栩艺　刘　禹
	上饶市广丰区	上饶市广丰区疾病预防控制中心	姚信飞　姚佳丽　黄莉莉
	上饶市广信区	上饶市广信区疾病预防控制中心	汪尚勇　朱光宇　祝君芳
	铅山县	铅山县疾病预防控制中心	暨丽敏　滕　辉
	横峰县	横峰县疾病预防控制中心	毛术霞　杨　帆
	弋阳县	弋阳县疾病预防控制中心	胡素华　林水旺　陈　敏

省（自治区、直辖市）Province (autonomous region, municipality)	肿瘤登记处 Cancer Registry	登记处所在单位 Affiliation	主要工作人员 Staff
	余干县	余干县疾病预防控制中心	董亚平　徐建强　段　叠　洪丽娟
	鄱阳县	鄱阳县疾病预防控制中心	陈晓春　陈　婵
	万年县	万年县疾病预防控制中心	盛根英　陶　婷
	婺源县	婺源县疾病预防控制中心	叶鹏华
	德兴市	德兴市预防疾病控制中心	李彬明　许晓丹
山东省	山东省	山东省疾病预防控制中心	郭晓雷　付振涛　姜　帆
	济南市	济南市疾病预防控制中心	张先慧　亓爱玲　宫舒萍　刘　冰　姜　超　王玉恒　张惠娟　李宗燕　刁燕飞
	济南市章丘区	济南市章丘区疾病预防控制中心	刘庆皆　颛孙宁宁　辛　佳　孙　健
	济南市莱芜区	济南市莱芜区疾病预防控制中心	常　安
	青岛市	青岛市疾病预防控制中心	杨雪纷　孙晓晖　张　婧　辛乐忠　郑晓燕　毛丽燕
	青岛市黄岛区	青岛市黄岛区疾病预防控制中心	廖　倩　张金太　谭　坦　管晓蕾
	淄博市临淄区	淄博市临淄区疾病预防控制中心	卢　斌　韦　洁　张城倩
	沂源县	沂源县疾病预防控制中心	孙　璞　李东芝　陈义菊　张　琪
	滕州市	滕州市疾病预防控制中心	徐玉銮　吴朋利　王　茹　龚　理　韩　瑜　李肖旋
	东营市东营区	东营市东营区疾病预防控制中心	张少强　季林林　刘明涛
	广饶县	广饶县疾病预防控制中心	徐海霞
	烟台市	烟台市疾病预防控制中心	于绍轶　王倩倩
	烟台市芝罘区	烟台市芝罘区疾病预防控制中心	袁金环
	烟台市福山区	烟台市福山区疾病预防控制中心	孙　昕　张　妮　赵菲菲　王美霞
	烟台市牟平区	烟台市牟平区疾病预防控制中心	李东洪
	烟台市莱山区	烟台市莱山区疾病预防控制中心	赵万里
	烟台经济技术开发区	烟台经济技术开发区疾病预防控制中心	孙溪盛
	莱州市	莱州市疾病预防控制中心	孙秋丽
	招远市	招远市疾病预防控制中心	翟玉庭
	潍坊市潍城区	潍坊市潍城区疾病预防控制中心	赵秋萍　刘盼盼　李承霖
	临朐县	临朐县疾病预防控制中心	郭　超
	青州市	青州市疾病预防控制中心	张淑萍　钟　鸣　鲍　菡　张　瑞
	高密市	高密市疾病预防控制中心	黄一峰　冷冠群　谢　珍　马瑞花　宋　娟
	济宁市任城区	济宁市任城区疾病预防控制中心	段世彬　唐　琪　郗帅帅　王仲霞　徐白璐

省（自治区、直辖市）Province（autonomous region, municipality）	肿瘤登记处 Cancer Registry	登记处所在单位 Affiliation	主要工作人员 Staff				
	汶上县	汶上县疾病预防控制中心	曹景军	杨庆杰	李彬彬	张紫怡	
	梁山县	梁山县疾病预防控制中心	张建鲁 孔甜甜	谢书丹 任仲凯	冯昌红	王春秀	张宝帅
	曲阜市	曲阜市疾病预防控制中心	孔　超 乔　乔	侯爱平	颜　俊	王　蕊	孔　晖
	邹城市	邹城市疾病预防控制中心	骆秀美 李　娜	张廷番	杨建宁	刘亚琪	王　薇
	宁阳县	宁阳县疾病预防控制中心	刘婷婷	马学成	董芙蓉	张丽杰	
	肥城市	肥城市人民医院	李琰琰	武亮亮	尹晓燕	姜　敏	
	乳山市	乳山市疾病预防控制中心	邹跃威	李立科	张玉佳	姜雪婧	于梦晨
	日照市东港区	日照市东港区疾病预防控制中心	尚明凤				
	莒　县	莒县疾病预防控制中心	刘　娣				
	沂南县	沂南县疾病预防控制中心	华国梁	魏　强	徐　君		
	沂水县	沂水县疾病预防控制中心	王维霞 王翠翠	杨登强	张江宝	马龑玲	伏祥浩
	莒南县	莒南县疾病预防控制中心	文章军	张斌磊	邓　花	王丽君	闫宝华
	德州市德城区	德州市德城区疾病预防控制中心	马莉莉	屠永梓			
	临邑县	临邑县疾病预防控制中心	苏　莹	邢念坤			
	聊城市东昌府区	聊城市东昌府区疾病预防控制中心	徐　伟	刘　艳			
	高唐县	高唐县疾病预防控制中心	王秀珍	刘淑梅			
	滨州市滨城区	滨州市滨城区疾病预防控制中心	范美霞	王　玲	赵贝贝	付立平	
	菏泽市牡丹区	菏泽市牡丹区疾病预防控制中心	秦　舒 刘洋洋	国　锦	仇翠梅	邱雪梅	周　娜
	菏泽市定陶区	菏泽市定陶区疾病预防控制中心	许忠华	谷洪梅			
	单县	单县疾病预防控制中心	赵海洲	邵光勇	李　锦		
	巨野县	巨野县疾病预防控制中心	高扬波	汪晓丽	孔诗语	张　晋	肖艳玲
河南省	河南省	河南省肿瘤医院	张韶凯	陈　琼	刘曙正		
	郑州市	郑州市疾病预防控制中心	李建彬	宋彩娟	刘建勋	闫瑞平	
	郑州市中原区	郑州市中原区疾病预防控制中心	尚小钰	孙文娟	于成林		
	郑州市二七区	郑州市二七区疾病预防控制中心	杨金秀	齐梦媛	阎　岩		
	郑州市上街区	郑州市上街区疾病预防控制中心	张旭婷	张文芳			
	开封市祥符区	开封市祥符区疾病预防控制中心	马　师	李慎榜	田艳玲	朱方敏	
	洛阳市	洛阳市疾病预防控制中心	闫云燕 马昊翔 齐虹飞	常　颖 魏冰燕 赵晓丽	马　凯 石晓红 邢建乐	吴志豪 陈亚楠	袁瑞姣 平　莉

省(自治区、直辖市) Province (autonomous region, municipality)	肿瘤登记处 Cancer Registry	登记处所在单位 Affiliation	主要工作人员 Staff				
	洛阳市孟津区	洛阳市孟津区疾病预防控制中心	张菲菲	许瑞瑞	张琰琰		
	新安县	新安县疾病预防控制中心	关 勇	龚进国	李 辉	付文莉	翟亚楠
	栾川县	栾川县疾病预防控制中心	刘爱坡	刘杏杏	崔妙丽	郭钊均	唐巾阁
	嵩县	嵩县疾病预防控制中心	马振卫 姜开霞	杨欣欣 万晓琦	乔 幸	石梦瑶	梁秋霞
	汝阳县	汝阳县疾病预防控制中心	耿振强	李白鸟			
	宜阳县	宜阳县疾病预防控制中心	楚玉梅	楚淑英	李若男	苏亚维	
	洛宁县	洛宁县疾病预防控制中心	段乐永	刘龙安			
	伊川县	伊川县疾病预防控制中心	刘 峰	王蜓蜓			
	洛阳市偃师区	洛阳市偃师区疾病预防控制中心	秦延锦	杨惠芳	周 鹏	张 丹	
	平顶山市	平顶山市疾病预防控制中心	王 轶 郭晏强 郑红云	宋 波 马西平 李新鹏	张泽华 李爱军 温红旭	颜欣颖 仲晓伟 郭淑乐	许艺苑 张小亚
	鲁山县	鲁山县疾病预防控制中心	王一博	李保瑞	刘中伟	郭启民	田广恩
	郏县	郏县疾病预防控制中心	张晓芳	王晓艳	昝哲	陈旭姣	王春燕
	舞钢市	舞钢市疾病预防控制中心	刘青兰	尹馨可	李晓杰		
	林州市	林州市肿瘤医院	郭贵周 王 丽	付方现 侯 凯	王振海 刘 畅	李变云	于晓东
	鹤壁市	鹤壁市人民医院	钞利娜 郭雪琴	王冰冰 裴树英	王梦媛	胡凤琴	任红勤
	浚县	浚县疾病预防控制中心	韩晓康	张士民	杨 莹		
	淇县	淇县疾病预防控制中心	李艳辉	王颖超			
	新乡市	新乡市肿瘤医院	朱智玲	曹河璐			
	辉县市	辉县市疾病预防控制中心	孙花荣	赵小聪	李 颖		
	温县	温县疾病预防控制中心	闫 楠	夏小燕	李 岩		
	濮阳市华龙区	濮阳市华龙区疾病预防控制中心	王培贤	王新杰	毛利娟		
	清丰县	清丰县疾病预防控制中心	高铁柱	姚粉霞	刘 欢		
	南乐县	南乐县疾病预防控制中心	王青辉	宋黎霞	徐晓文	王晓静	
	范县	范县疾病预防控制中心	田军艳	邢秀娟	薛 辉	段晓琦	
	濮阳县	濮阳县疾病预防控制中心	郭秋献	穆晓红	刘 军		
	许昌市魏都区	许昌市魏都区疾病预防控制中心	郑云枝 王旭光	崔亚辉 侯灿灿	信保祥 杨彦彦	廖 飞	张 方
	禹州市	禹州市疾病预防控制中心	王全新	郭 影	李 蔚	张亚楠	杨宗慧
	漯河市源汇区	漯河市源汇区疾病预防控制中心	王宏博 王春玲	张 祥	牛艳丽	叶 静	刘一培
	漯河市郾城区	漯河市郾城区疾病预防控制中心	李爱会 何怡聪	袁兵翔 常帅奇	杨莹莹	邓 婕	张 楠

省（自治区、直辖市） Province （autonomous region, municipality）	肿瘤登记处 Cancer Registry	登记处所在单位 Affiliation	主要工作人员 Staff				
	漯河市召陵区	漯河市召陵区疾病预防控制中心	任东洋	崔一齐	鞠晨云	樊永立	
	舞阳县	舞阳县疾病预防控制中心	周小佳 杨艳芳	马永晓 张艳丽	何 洁	徐慧杰	谷来君
	临颍县	临颍县疾病预防控制中心	米富德 张彩铃	罗 婷	吴 真	马玉智	秦苏丹
	三门峡市湖滨区	三门峡市湖滨区疾病预防控制中心	李粉妮	孟素萍	刘润娣	罗 丹	
	义马市	义马市疾病预防控制中心	江 红	管志毅	方新萍	彭丽英	张怡宁
	南阳市卧龙区	南阳市卧龙区疾病预防控制中心	武 霞	刘 凯	周 静	张 爽	黄佳佳
	南召县	南召县疾病预防控制中心	靳万春 樊 璞	王 珂	陈立明	朱广博	张 营
	方城县	方城县疾病预防控制中心	任礼飞 张禄军	王荣记 张 娟	马璟颖	李 谱	倪林静
	内乡县	内乡县疾病预防控制中心	李亚波	金 花	黄 健	代 阳	
	虞城县	虞城县疾病预防控制中心	高为民 江 培	冯金洪	马 宁	刘 威	毕兴华
	夏邑县	夏邑县疾病预防控制中心	班 硕	陈婷婷	李 玲	王丰收	
	信阳市浉河区	信阳市浉河区疾病预防控制中心	兰宏旺	周 娣	楚尚兰	李 刚	耿祎祎
	罗山县	罗山县疾病预防控制中心	徐蔚静	王明阳			
	沈丘县	沈丘县疾病预防控制中心	徐 玲	李庆文	郭丽花	李旭东	孙梦洋
	郸城县	郸城县疾病预防控制中心	张吉志	孙 忠	郭德银	马 慧	李慧珍
	太康县	太康县疾病预防控制中心	董 洪	魏国成	李 昂	刘西彬	
	项城市	项城市疾病预防控制中心	王玉华 马冠军	朱 琳	袁 媛	靳冰洁	杨欣雨
	西平县	西平县疾病预防控制中心	周丽萍	邵天堂	刘彩霞	毛小辉	
	济源市	济源市疾病预防控制中心	刘 磊	郑莹茹	马璐瑶		
	巩义市	巩义市疾病预防控制中心	蒋蔚林	王燕青	张文君		
湖北省	湖北省	湖北省肿瘤医院	姚 霜 夏雅芬	庹吉妤	张 敏	秦 宇	孟繁地
	武汉市	武汉市疾病预防控制中心	金琦曼 张晓霞	严亚琼	杨念念	代 娟	赵原原
	大冶市	大冶市疾病预防控制中心	司媛媛	柯云峰	徐 鹏	杨 薛	
	十堰市郧阳区	十堰市郧阳区疾病预防控制中心	左顺彦 黄 进	柯 华 曹 琳	郭 萍 杨 丽	吴君君 何 锐	杨 伟
	丹江口市	丹江口市疾病预防控制中心	王亚雪 闫 芳 郑 琼 徐 文	王建新 李 坪 徐红雨	杨 俊 朱志娟 李雪飞	王 芳 李学梅 王 珊	贾均江 刘春梅 郑 芳

省（自治区、直辖市） Province （autonomous region，municipality）	肿瘤登记处 Cancer Registry	登记处所在单位 Affiliation	主要工作人员 Staff
	宜昌市	宜昌市疾病预防控制中心	杨佳娟　胡　池　朱　婕　吴　婵　易丽萍 谭江娥　杨玉芝
	秭归县	秭归县疾病预防控制中心	杜万清　颜小芹　陈　蓉
	五峰土家族自治县	五峰土家族自治县疾病预防控制中心	熊　斌　田恩红　汪北阶　杨谢东　覃　涵
	宜都市	宜都市疾病预防控制中心	肖　翔　郑方金　柳登月
	襄阳市	襄阳市疾病预防控制中心	陈小慧　刘　杰　龚文胜　鲲　鹏
	枣阳市	枣阳市疾病预防控制中心	牛永霞　孙晶晶　姜义国　张吉保　段胜仁 张玉玲
	宜城市	宜城市疾病预防控制中心	龚新洪　张家乐　胡院芳　曾卓璇　杨波
	京山市	京山市疾病预防控制中心	李　宏　杨　丹　容艳红
	钟祥市	钟祥市疾病预防控制中心	赵　丽　廖金凤　霍军荣
	云梦县	云梦县疾病预防控制中心	周　浩　李纯波　刘　妍
	荆州市	荆州市疾病预防控制中心	孙　春　刘陈慧　颜　杰　杨　程
	公安县	公安县疾病预防控制中心	申立琼　洪　杰　文良军　张　丹　肖　瑶 胡长贵　王来君
	洪湖市	洪湖市疾病预防控制中心	廖　涛　向代成　徐海涛　刘登洪
	麻城市	麻城市疾病预防控制中心	徐胜平　库守能　项维红　王金荣　丁　成
	嘉鱼县	嘉鱼县疾病预防控制中心	刘晓玲　刘　庆　黄忠文　肖德顺　唐　文 姚志敏　王　愉　杜清华　孟　烨　李文飘 杨　士　易　念　鲁金枝　耿幼兰　张巧敏
	通城县	通城县疾病预防控制中心	熊新征　杨　劲　熊子鹏
	恩施市	恩施市疾病预防控制中心	张玉蓉　王　斌　刘迪军　叶魏莎　陈　飞
	天门市	天门市疾病预防控制中心	刘　积　罗　芬　何明辉　倪亚敏　王佳齐 刘　洋　龚红雨　江　菲　陈志芳　吴艳丽 苏　敏　段格格
湖南省	湖南省	湖南省肿瘤防治研究办公室	肖亚洲　欧阳煜　王　静　颜仕鹏　廖先珍 许可葵　李　灿　邹艳花　肖海帆　曹世钰 石朝晖　王石玉　郭　佳
	长沙市芙蓉区	长沙市芙蓉区疾病预防控制中心	朱　丽　胡辉伍　陈海燕　罗霜艳　张航宇
	长沙市天心区	长沙市天心区疾病预防控制中心	兰泽龙　黄　佳　刘严玲　黄　洁
	长沙市岳麓区	长沙市岳麓区疾病预防控制中心	胡艳红　徐　蕾　陈继怀　谢　婷　易　耀
	长沙市开福区	长沙市开福区疾病预防控制中心	任　敏　陈腊梅　陈　偲　宋香玲　刘　玲
	长沙市雨花区	长沙市雨花区疾病预防控制中心	周建湘　黄　芬　龙花君　廖丽艳　段利霞 赵子瑜

省(自治区、直辖市) Province (autonomous region, municipality)	肿瘤登记处 Cancer Registry	登记处所在单位 Affiliation	主要工作人员 Staff			
	长沙市望城区	长沙市望城区疾病预防控制中心	赵劲良 熊 浩 肖炜琪 邹思伟 王梅芳 张文静			
	长沙县	长沙县疾病预防控制中心 长沙县第一人民医院	李 力 刘宗奇 何 花 罗辉琴 刘 丹 黄雅兰 刘遂怡 钟志军 邹 满 龙志刚 左 丽 王清丽 李 娟			
	宁乡市	宁乡市疾病预防控制中心	徐红斌 文红军 周茂林 喻灵芝 郭 亮 刘 飒			
	浏阳市	浏阳市疾病预防控制中心	许 欣 陈建伟 彭 媛 龙花君 李 跳 陈 诚 邓 立 谭诗花 李光辉 刘 威			
	株洲市芦淞区	株洲市芦淞区疾病预防控制中心	何 礼 唐 晶 卞晓嘉 刘慧颖			
	株洲市石峰区	株洲市石峰区疾病预防控制中心	刘 杰 黄 平 朱 江 刘 宏 彭玉梅 袁 敏 齐佳锐 李 洁			
	攸县	攸县疾病预防控制中心	杨体吾 周 义 刘孳雄 刘志军 杨华艳 夏冬艳			
	湘潭市雨湖区	湘潭市雨湖区癌症防治中心	夏 红 谭建中 刘 政 邓莉芳 袁芳华 杨玉环 马超颖 乔光凤 丁 林 彭旻婧 赵媛兰 韩自力 马超颖 蔡文迪			
	衡东县	衡东县疾病预防控制中心	尹 炜 单健生 罗剑武 刘早红 肖静娴 李俊华 周 玲 胡志兰 刘志艳			
	常宁市	常宁市疾病预防控制中心	曹诗鹏 欧 琦 滕德伟 吴良元 唐 毅 郭 兰			
	邵东市	邵东市疾病预防控制中心	曾 平 尹超平 田 丽 陈文伟 谢 玉 刘冬梅			
	新宁县	新宁县疾病预防控制中心	邓海名 周前富 陈 富 刘倩文			
	岳阳市岳阳楼区	岳阳市岳阳楼区疾病预防控制中心	殷建湘 陈艳芳 宋 婷 陈典典			
	常德市武陵区	常德市武陵区疾病预防控制中心	管元平 涂林立 张志刚 彭学文 朱晓辉 周宏惠			
	安乡县	安乡县疾病预防控制中心	何玉龙 贺福丽 杨 玲 王月玲			
	津市市	津市市疾病预防控制中心	文 杰 韩绍楚 万贤珍 雷 力 杨 敏 钱兰芬			
	张家界市永定区	张家界市永定区疾病预防控制中心	袁继卫 胡 剑 徐 宣 杜 雯			
	慈利县	慈利县疾病预防控制中心	朱从喜 向 英 吴 双 庹先锋 陈华云			
	益阳市资阳区	益阳市资阳区疾病预防控制中心	李 艳 肖宏才 鲁 容 王玲玲			
	桃江县	桃江县人民医院	刘 军 廖亚男 薛媚娟 邹 平 谢 真 黄 德 邹朝霞 郭 纯			

省(自治区、直辖市) Province (autonomous region, municipality)	肿瘤登记处 Cancer Registry	登记处所在单位 Affiliation	主要工作人员 Staff
	临武县	临武县疾病预防控制中心	李伟生　曹玉兰　李慕雪　曹玲芳　何　鑫
	资兴市	资兴市疾病预防控制中心	夏云磊　李雄豹　黎利文　王英籍
	道县	道县疾病预防控制中心	肖拥军　邹四妹　黄兰婷　许洪平　邓　红
	宁远县	宁远县疾病预防控制中心	李万忠　欧阳晓芳　陈颖香　李　玮
	新田县	新田县疾病预防控制中心	欧阳乐　谢众麟　黄　锋　何忠勇　段良祥 刘君红　刘　波
	麻阳苗族自治县	麻阳苗族自治县疾病预防控制中心	张春玉　向　华　陈　琳　谭江勇　陈启佳
	洪江市	洪江市疾病预防控制中心	杨小琴　胡小玲　易思连　寻英姿
	双峰县	双峰县疾病预防控制中心	刘国贤　戴凯亭　刘伏香　李　想
	冷水江市	冷水江市疾病预防控制中心	方吉贤　张彬彬　罗三峰　杨　娟　陈元玲
	涟源市	涟源市疾病预防控制中心	文申根　肖红军　李秀兰　周红大　张小勇 肖艳慎　李　清
	泸溪县	泸溪县疾病预防控制中心	杨秀亮　石湘燕　陈晓华　代小燕
广东省	广东省	广东省疾病预防控制中心	赵德坚　廖　羽　孟瑞琳　王　晔
	广州市	广州市疾病预防控制中心	王穗湘　许　欢　梁伯衡
	韶关市曲江区	韶关市曲江区疾病预防控制中心	刘素谦　曾翠梅
	翁源县	翁源县疾病预防控制中心	李育清　高志锋
	南雄市	南雄市疾病预防控制中心	张艳艳　邬香华　钟建良　陈四娇　王拨雄
	深圳市	深圳市慢性病防治中心	雷　林　刘芳江　林铠浩　蔡伟聪
	珠海市	珠海市疾病预防控制中心	陈国荣　邓韶英　汤小鸥　赵泳瑜
	汕头市澄海区	汕头市澄海区疾病预防控制中心	陈　铿
	佛山市	佛山市疾病预防控制中心	古嘉诚　隋丹丹　孙宝志　祝巧英　张雅智 陆鹏宇
	佛山市禅城区	佛山市禅城区疾病预防控制中心	黄锦航　李彩霞　何锦森
	佛山市南海区	佛山市南海区疾病预防控制中心	谢威龙　谢冬怡　黄杰周
	佛山市顺德区	佛山市顺德区慢性病防治中心	杨俊杰　罗洁莹　王谦可　陈　榕　吴　焜 詹　珏
	佛山市三水区	佛山市三水区疾病预防控制中心	李忠平　梁佳炜　何惠娟　魏文玉
	佛山市高明区	佛山市高明区疾病预防控制中心	黄学敏　李柱宁　林少英
	江门市城区	江门市疾病预防控制中心	于雪芳　李一鹏
	湛江市	湛江市疾病预防控制中心	曾小任　周晓媚　游小倩
	湛江市赤坎区	湛江市疾病预防控制中心	戚佩玲　叶桂梅
	湛江市霞山区	湛江市疾病预防控制中心	赖向昌　陈紫娟　董小洁　王　靖

省(自治区、直辖市) Province (autonomous region, municipality)	肿瘤登记处 Cancer Registry	登记处所在单位 Affiliation	主要工作人员 Staff			
	湛江市坡头区	湛江市疾病预防控制中心	符 咏	吴彩燕		
	湛江市麻章区	湛江市疾病预防控制中心	陈紫娟	吴肖芳	王 靖	何振杰
	遂溪县	遂溪县疾病预防控制中心	李秀梅	梁 乐		
	徐闻县	徐闻县疾病预防控制中心	符悦瑾	吴启花		
	廉江市	廉江市疾病预防控制中心	李小琼	彭东文		
	雷州市	雷州市疾病预防控制中心	周 贤	曾春光		
	吴川市	吴川市疾病预防控制中心	李国平			
	茂名市茂南区	茂名市疾病预防控制中心	莫文康	蔡 娟	林燕珠	苏钰婷
	高州市	高州市疾病预防控制中心	莫文康	蔡 娟	吴小玲	张峰华
	肇庆市端州区	肇庆市疾病预防控制中心	陆素颖	方艺娟	梁大艳	冼国佳
	肇庆市鼎湖区	肇庆市疾病预防控制中心鼎湖区办事处	谢美兰	陈剑雄		
	肇庆市高要区	肇庆市高要区疾病预防控制中心	苏伟华	宋正杰	黄玉红	
	肇庆市高新区	肇庆市疾病预防控制中心高新区办事处	莫淦华	陈润麒	郑肇沂	
	广宁县	广宁县疾病预防控制中心	李秋月	谢欣谊		
	怀集县	怀集县疾病预防控制中心	李志耀	莫润元		
	封开县	封开县疾病预防控制中心	张 弘	蔡小敏	方文坚	
	德庆县	德庆县疾病预防控制中心	李垚俊	苏舒婷	韦健梅	
	四会市	四会市惠民平价门诊部(四会市肿瘤研究所)	卢玉强	李晓翌	谭燕梅	
	惠州市惠阳区	惠州市惠阳区疾病预防控制中心	陈 萍	黄惠玲	李琼燕	
	梅州市梅江区	梅州市梅江区疾病预防控制中心	刘明珍	谢菊桂	古彩红	杨润威
	梅州市梅县区	梅州市梅县区疾病预防控制中心	杨 慧	李加宁	古彩红	杨润威
	大埔县	大埔县疾病预防控制中心	徐伟晓	温 婷	古彩红	杨润威
	汕尾市城区	中山大学孙逸仙纪念医院深汕中心医院	陈依琳			
	河源市源城区	河源市疾病预防控制中心	刘翠娟	刘惠珍		
	阳江市阳东区	阳江市阳东区疾病预防控制中心	谭家伟	关 设	李海凤	雷玉燕 陈 文
	清远市清城区	清远市清城区疾病预防控制中心	汤嘉慧 罗汝良 凌水权 王 馨 陈瑞贞 柳爱兰 欧爱平 杨少玲 蔡文勇 罗伟观 潘龙兴 朱颖珊 陈伟谦 冯志谦 温友银			
	阳山县	阳山县疾病预防控制中心	黄永杰	梁时力	毛智趣	丘银霞

省(自治区、直辖市) Province (autonomous region, municipality)	肿瘤登记处 Cancer Registry	登记处所在单位 Affiliation	主要工作人员 Staff				
	东莞市	东莞市疾病预防控制中心	陈妙嫦	钟洁莹	黄雅卿	魏建坤	殷茵蕾
	中山市	中山市人民医院(中山市肿瘤研究所)	魏矿荣	梁智恒	李柱明	刘 宁	
	潮州市潮安区	潮州市潮安区疾病预防控制中心	郭慧斌	陈秀萍			
	揭西县	揭西县疾病预防控制中心	贝晶利	刘洁霜			
	普宁市	普宁市疾病预防控制中心	杨锦雄				
	罗定市	罗定市疾病预防控制中心	张乔珍 郑建国	梁惠玲 张 冰	蔡大杰 李惠瑜	温海锐 陈红艳	叶炽娟 黎杰文
广西壮族自治区	广西壮族自治区	广西医科大学附属肿瘤医院	李秋林 容敏华	余家华 周子寒	余红平	葛莲英	曹 骥
	南宁市	南宁市疾病预防控制中心	黄秋兰	周 吉	朱荣健	叶 琳	梁 竹
	南宁市兴宁区	南宁市兴宁区疾病预防控制中心	梁翠敏	欧阳丽华			
	南宁市青秀区	南宁市青秀区疾病预防控制中心	卢志玲	黄绍旎	黄中学		
	南宁市江南区	南宁市江南区疾病预防控制中心	戴 姮				
	南宁经济技术开发区	南宁市经开区疾病预防控制中心	覃燕红				
	南宁市西乡塘区	南宁市西乡塘区疾病预防控制中心	苏升灿	唐盛志	何雨澄		
	南宁市良庆区	南宁市良庆区疾病预防控制中心	李晶晶				
	南宁市邕宁区	南宁市邕宁区疾病预防控制中心	廖柳艳				
	南宁东盟经济开发区	广西-东盟经济技术开发区疾病预防控制中心	宁 栈				
	南宁市武鸣区	南宁市武鸣区疾病预防控制中心	潘文川	谢 维	李盛剑	吴世鲜	
	隆安县	隆安县疾病预防控制中心	陈珍莲	黄建云			
	马山县	马山县疾病预防控制中心	陆家龙	黄海洪	黄春梦		
	上林县	上林县疾病预防控制中心	罗莉菲				
	宾阳县	宾阳县疾病预防控制中心	韦柳青 龚冰冰	莫少梅 张 华	李秀霞	孙华娟	陈伟强
	横县	横县疾病预防控制中心	何保华	陆丽群	陈江标		
	柳州市	柳州市疾病预防控制中心	梁佳佳 刘 芸 谭金雪	周丽芳 陈宁钰 周 琳	谢昌平 朱庭萍	蓝 剑 谭晓萍	王晓伟 欧 蕾
	柳城县	柳城县疾病预防控制中心	韦小凤	赵文官	林佳佳	毛青青	
	鹿寨县	鹿寨县疾病预防控制中心	阳 立	银星腾	陈献军	黄仪颖	

省（自治区、直辖市） Province（autonomous region，municipality）	肿瘤登记处 Cancer Registry	登记处所在单位 Affiliation	主要工作人员 Staff
	融安县	融安县疾病预防控制中心	袁彩红　贾合东
	桂林市	桂林市疾病预防控制中心	石朝晖　蒋富生　汤　杰　石　瑀　黄　灵
	阳朔县	阳朔县疾病预防控制中心	秦大武　吴海波　欧俊宏
	灵川县	灵川县疾病预防控制中心	李国春　全文郎
	兴安县	兴安县疾病预防控制中心	李海燕　杨德保　唐晓丽
	灌阳县	灌阳县疾病预防控制中心	陆　润　吴承芳　黄婷云　吴荣荣
	龙胜各族自治县	龙胜各族自治县疾病预防控制中心	代典凤　姚　群　张岚　石昌胜　梁新星
	资源县	资源县疾病预防控制中心	潘希平　刘建华　马　静
	平乐县	平乐县疾病预防控制中心	蒋东原　李春松　黎　彬　黎晓莉　邓日春
	荔浦市	荔浦县疾病预防控制中心	黎志芬　蒋宏文　徐蕴琦　唐秀香
	恭城瑶族自治县	恭城瑶族自治县疾病预防控制中心	周青霞　卢恩辅　邝绍玉
	梧州市	梧州市红十字会医院	郑裕明　汤敏中　汤伟文　苏韶华　苏阳红 黄金菊　陈骐炜
	苍梧县	苍梧县疾病预防控制中心	李汉福　杨敏生　李连荣　谭夏敏　麦新苗 苏石汉　李北金　余思洁
	北海市	北海市疾病预防控制中心	谢　平　梁耀洁
	合浦县	合浦县疾病预防控制中心	苏福康　曹　松　张　强　秦晓丽　罗世琼 邓丽华　陈鑫祖
	防城港市港口区	防城港市港口区疾病预防控制中心	陈志艳
	钦州市钦南区	钦州市钦南区疾病预防控制中心	陆玉培　黄红英
	浦北县	浦北县疾病预防控制中心	洪　波　叶海燕　谢源民　陈　亮　罗　梅 梁海辉
	贵港市	贵港市疾病预防控制中心	宋开玲　陈文静　韦奉泽
	贵港市港北区	贵港市港北区疾病预防控制中心	韦坚峥　李美春　方丽声
	贵港市港南区	贵港市港南区疾病预防控制中心	李雪芳
	贵港市覃塘区	贵港市覃塘区疾病预防控制中心	李悦凤
	平南县	平南县疾病预防控制中心	冯　翠
	桂平市	桂平市疾病预防控制中心	曹良清
	北流市	北流市疾病预防控制中心	陈金武　黎　丹　黄　胜　邹鸿蔚
	百色市右江区	百色市右江区疾病预防控制中心	吴美秀　杨丽敏
	百色市田阳区	百色市田阳区疾病预防控制中心	李洁玲　黄志刚　甘珍妮
	田东县	田东县疾病预防控制中心	李　玲　辛华恒　农凤兰

省(自治区、直辖市) Province (autonomous region, municipality)	肿瘤登记处 Cancer Registry	登记处所在单位 Affiliation	主要工作人员 Staff
	凌云县	凌云县疾病预防控制中心	覃凌峰　倪荣红　王秀兵
	贺州市八步区	贺州市八步区疾病预防控制中心	林海霞　罗亚娣　陈健苗
	钟山县	钟山县疾病预防控制中心	刘奕
	河池市金城江区	河池市金城江区疾病预防控制中心	覃向清　黄富荣
	罗城仫佬族自治县	罗城仫佬族自治县疾病预防控制中心	韦政兴　韦愿　梁玉春　卢永钧　罗黎霞
	来宾市兴宾区	来宾市兴宾区疾病预防控制中心	闫萍　兰舒婷　陈年媛　周静　吴卫　范凯
	合山市	合山市疾病预防控制中心	黄海浪
	崇左市江州区	崇左市江州区疾病预防控制中心	周静静　梁阳杨
	扶绥县	扶绥县人民医院	李云西　李海华　黄志斌　韦忠亮
	龙州县	龙州县疾病预防控制中心	杨慧君
	大新县	大新县疾病预防控制中心	何新桂　马燕英　赵华清
	天等县	天等县疾病预防控制中心	农锋丽　农建宏
海南省	海南省	海南省肿瘤防治中心	张旭　华婧　范康琼　王定彬　苏良苹
	海口市	海口市疾病预防控制中心	朱庆　吴叶青
	三亚市	三亚市疾病预防控制中心	黄炯媚　潘超
	儋州市	儋州市疾病预防控制中心	霍德芳　高冠斌
	五指山市	五指山市疾病预防控制中心	符美艳　卢耿慧
	琼海市	琼海市疾病预防控制中心	符芳敏　颜李丽
	东方市	东方市疾病预防控制中心	孙发睿
	定安县	定安县疾病预防控制中心	黎才刚　郭芳华
	昌江黎族自治县	昌江黎族自治县疾病预防控制中心	梁赛文　黄存
	陵水黎族自治县	陵水黎族自治县疾病预防控制中心	许声文
重庆市	重庆市	重庆市疾病预防控制中心	吕晓燕　丁贤彬
	重庆市万州区	重庆市万州区疾病预防控制中心	屈秋琼
	重庆市涪陵区	重庆市涪陵区疾病预防控制中心	王杨凤　王琪　周义芬　陈晓明
	重庆市渝中区	重庆市渝中区疾病预防控制中心	周琦　凌瑜双　汤洪秀　张雍
	重庆市大渡口区	重庆市大渡口区疾病预防控制中心	陆小峰　刘勇言

省(自治区、直辖市) Province (autonomous region, municipality)	肿瘤登记处 Cancer Registry	登记处所在单位 Affiliation	主要工作人员 Staff
	重庆市江北区	重庆市江北区疾病预防控制中心	郭 梅 雷 勇 刘 静
	重庆市沙坪坝区	重庆市沙坪坝区疾病预防控制中心	蒙 怡 李廷荣 支 倩 黎 瞳
	重庆市九龙坡区	重庆市九龙坡区疾病预防控制中心	贺 明 汤 成
	重庆市南岸区	重庆市南岸区疾病预防控制中心	廖晓澄 黄治兰 张 楠 钟 韵 李高婷
	重庆市北碚区	重庆市北碚区疾病预防控制中心	李大兵 邓小霞 陈 洁
	重庆市綦江区	重庆市綦江区疾病预防控制中心	罗春亮 李华梅 周梦雪
	重庆市大足区	重庆市大足区疾病预防控制中心	任香勇 李万华 王爱民
	重庆市渝北区	重庆市渝北区疾病预防控制中心	张晓慧 王忠菊 郭昌融
	重庆市巴南区	重庆市巴南区疾病预防控制中心	陶小红 余兰英 刘成果
	重庆市黔江区	重庆市黔江区疾病预防控制中心	吴 畅 郭 峰 吴彩霞 王 敏 李 卫
	重庆市长寿区	重庆市长寿区疾病预防控制中心	杨 亮 陈 娜 邓 静 毛晓锋
	重庆市江津区	重庆市江津区疾病预防控制中心	杨 媚 付小燕 赵祖敏 刘乐其
	重庆市合川区	重庆市合川区疾病预防控制中心	贺 玲 王绍梅
	重庆市永川区	重庆市永川区疾病预防控制中心	吴 欢 程莉莎 刘 琳
	重庆市南川区	重庆市南川区疾病预防控制中心	张世勇 钟 静 周 涛
	重庆市万盛经济技术开发区	重庆市万盛经济技术开发区疾病预防控制中心	杨 琴
	重庆市潼南区	重庆市潼南区疾病预防控制中心	陈雪莲 郝真强 龙 凤
	重庆市铜梁区	重庆市铜梁区疾病预防控制中心	田 燕
	重庆市荣昌区	重庆市荣昌区疾病预防控制中心	熊华利 于均梅 舒 强
	重庆市璧山区	重庆市璧山区疾病预防控制中心	徐 玲 张 瑜 陈 静
	重庆市梁平区	重庆市梁平区疾病预防控制中心	张 涛 谢秋虹 肖 佳 邱虹蛟 陈 靓
	城口县	城口县疾病预防控制中心	靳双红
	丰都县	丰都县疾病预防控制中心	刘 琳 熊 薇 付 军 彭庆华 秦雪花
	垫江县	垫江县疾病预防控制中心	谭 格
	重庆市武隆区	重庆市武隆区疾病预防控制中心	冯 静 刘兴建 李婷婷 王登嵘 陈一语
	忠县	忠县疾病预防控制中心	袁 英 朱红云 熊晓世 方 君
	重庆市开州区	重庆市开州区疾病预防控制中心	肖幸平 崔喜闻
	云阳县	云阳县疾病预防控制中心	张 林 张 星 王伟仁
	奉节县	奉节县疾病预防控制中心	张克燕 罗 宇

省（自治区、直辖市）Province（autonomous region, municipality）	肿瘤登记处 Cancer Registry	登记处所在单位 Affiliation	主要工作人员 Staff
	巫山县	巫山县疾病预防控制中心	何成丹　梁　辉　图门阿拉腾　黄　鑫　张　元
	巫溪县	巫溪县疾病预防控制中心	王发辉
	石柱土家族自治县	石柱土家族自治县疾病预防控制中心	杨　帆　冉丽君　汤剑峰
	秀山土家族苗族自治县	秀山土家族苗族自治县疾病预防控制中心	郭　敏　孙志军　曾　琼
	酉阳土家族苗族自治县	酉阳县疾病预防控制中心	王　政
	彭水苗族土家族自治县	彭水苗族土家族自治县疾病预防控制中心	陈　节　郭　超　杨　璇
四川省	四川省	四川省疾病预防控制中心	成姝雯　邓　颖　董　婷　胥馨尹　袁芝佩　张　新　李　尤
	成都市锦江区	成都市锦江区疾病预防控制中心	江　珊　阴红燕　柳建超　罗熙平
	成都市青羊区	成都市青羊区疾病预防控制中心	彭长燕　蔡　鹏　刘　嘉　韩湘意
	成都市金牛区	成都市金牛区疾病预防控制中心	李彦青　雷　方　曾海宁　余　林
	成都市武侯区	成都市武侯区疾病预防控制中心	程　谧　张　静
	成都市成华区	成都市成华区疾病预防控制中心	胡　莹　周　静　赵子君
	成都市高新区	成都市高新区疾病预防控制中心	何　柳
	成都市龙泉驿区	成都市龙泉驿区疾病预防控制中心	阮红海　刘明艳　郑沾福　熊林森
	成都市青白江区	成都市青白江区疾病预防控制中心	徐　仙　郭　敏　周思敏　陈　丹
	成都市新都区	成都市新都区疾病预防控制中心	刘　芳　焦　娇　赵子贺　李　敏　刘　燕　叶　雨
	成都市温江区	成都市温江区疾病预防控制中心	聂　炜　郭毅梅
	金堂县	金堂县疾病预防控制中心	李林容　叶立力
	成都市双流区	成都市双流区疾病预防控制中心	叶永利　潘　飞　胡　容　黄先志　唐　爽
	成都市天府新区	成都市天府新区疾病预防控制中心	袁晓宇　郭　丹
	成都市郫都区	成都市郫都区疾病预防控制中心	林超兰
	大邑县	大邑县疾病预防控制中心	曾　纪　岳　涛　周正蓉
	蒲江县	蒲江县疾病预防控制中心	李朋林　韩艳艳　丁　伟　周凤英　曾　智
	成都市新津区	成都市新津区疾病预防控制中心	刘凤容　杨　杰　苟念秋　童书勤

省(自治区、直辖市) Province (autonomous region, municipality)	肿瘤登记处 Cancer Registry	登记处所在单位 Affiliation	主要工作人员 Staff				
	简阳市	简阳市疾病预防控制中心	敬　琳	谭晓桃	李红燕	张　静	周良莹
			曾　近	谢君娅			
	都江堰市	都江堰市疾病预防控制中心	伍轩民	凌　波	曾红梅	蒋晓宏	马　艳
			冯先礼	王泽芳	罗　丽	罗　炯	
	彭州市	彭州市疾病预防控制中心	蒋　微	陈小芳	王　建	伍　霞	孙　强
			刘佳秋	李　娜			
	邛崃市	邛崃市疾病预防控制中心	王　丹	陈　益	周　翔		
	崇州市	崇州市疾病预防控制中心	广嘉欣	向秀蓉	冯　艳		
	自贡市自流井区	自贡市自流井区疾病预防控制中心	李　刚	高志赟	商　静	魏丽娟	
	自贡市贡井区	自贡市贡井区疾病预防控制中心	邱玉琼	江　超	毛喜艳	陈　丽	向　情
	自贡市大安区	自贡市大安区疾病预防控制中心	倪　嘉	张小林	王　琦		
	自贡市沿滩区	自贡市沿滩区疾病预防控制中心	明晓雪	苟俊伟	王旭萌	易洪安	
	荣县	荣县疾病预防控制中心	赵梦琳	代　飞	杨　玲	陈　莉	范小桃
	富顺县	富顺县疾病预防控制中心	刘兴莉	黄帮雨	关晓旭	徐小丽	刘海燕
			宋　敏				
	攀枝花市东区	攀枝花市东区疾病预防控制中心	周川楠	陈　莹			
	攀枝花市西区	攀枝花市西区疾病预防控制中心	贺绍琼	李　英			
	攀枝花市仁和区	攀枝花市仁和区疾病预防控制中心	毛　鹏	汪　杰	赫永新		
	米易县	米易县疾病预防控制中心	曹　珊	董家君	罗　欢		
	泸州市江阳区	泸州市江阳区疾病预防控制中心	李娅凌	邵　红	晏艺涵		
	泸州市纳溪区	泸州市纳溪区疾病预防控制中心	林　利	李华梅	杨　凤		
	泸州市龙马潭区	泸州市龙马潭区疾病预防控制中心	李春艳	唐　伟	徐梅钦		
	泸县	泸县疾病预防控制中心	熊　君	谢　婧	汪正刚	陈平平	
	合江县	合江县疾病预防控制中心	胡　东	刘明海			
	叙永县	叙永县疾病预防控制中心	谈洪芬	刘　瑶	雷宇鸿		
	德阳市旌阳区	德阳市旌阳区疾病预防控制中心	周小华	郑　伟	陈　思	何盛嘉	苏小波
			李佳滨	瞿志明	张长龙		
	中江县	中江县疾病预防控制中心	邹　红	蒋文斌	邓绍清	谢　伟	邓　庆
	德阳市罗江区	德阳市罗江区疾病预防控制中心	管小琴	肖寿宝	刘怀淑	彭　茹	
	广汉市	广汉市疾病预防控制中心	刘丹丹	肖昌华	王　玲	龙小刚	吴　浩
	什邡市	什邡市疾病预防控制中心	邢婷婷	郑小军	肖家慧	蒋　丽	邓利英
			孙贵茜				

省(自治区、直辖市) Province (autonomous region, municipality)	肿瘤登记处 Cancer Registry	登记处所在单位 Affiliation	主要工作人员 Staff
	绵竹市	绵竹市疾病预防控制中心	张 桃 周道兴 周 萍 魏 佳 赵海川 伍 琦 刘 强
	绵阳市涪城区	绵阳市涪城区疾病预防控制中心	周晓凤 李 洁 王蒙杰
	绵阳市游仙区	绵阳市游仙区疾病预防控制中心	安水玲 王 慧
	绵阳市安州区	绵阳市安州区疾病预防控制中心	吴春陶 刘宝英 王佳雨
	三台县	三台县疾病预防控制中心	李长剑 周 欢 赵 丹
	盐亭县	盐亭县肿瘤医院	李 林 李 军
	梓潼县	梓潼县疾病预防控制中心	帖映伟 谢锦言 杨海蓉 宋灵巧 应宇辉
	北川羌族自治县	北川羌族自治县疾病预防控制中心	蒋素红 刘 飞 韩 丽
	平武县	平武县疾病预防控制中心	严松林 刘严娇 罗 健
	江油市	江油市疾病预防控制中心	夏丽莉 李 宁 王定邦 孙甫飞 曹 婕
	广元市利州区	广元市利州区疾病预防控制中心	张小玲 王 平 王 茜
	广元市昭化区	广元市昭化区疾病预防控制中心	李小建 薛春香 曹 智
	广元市朝天区	广元市朝天区疾病预防控制中心	何 磊 马凤奎 刘艳平 徐 燕 李清泉
	旺苍县	旺苍县疾病预防控制中心	杨显路 杨红梅 周军勇
	青川县	青川县疾病预防控制中心	胥璟宸 宋友科 袁伟贤 柳青蓉 王桂花 袁 双
	剑阁县	剑阁县疾病预防控制中心	田 辉 赵志刚
	苍溪县	苍溪县疾病预防控制中心	史 千 吴德明 何 楠
	遂宁市船山区	遂宁市船山区疾病预防控制中心	刘 淼 杨 翀 谭 凯
	遂宁市安居区	遂宁市安居区疾病预防控制中心	李 谦 陈胜春 冯裕如
	蓬溪县	蓬溪县疾病预防控制中心	邱 林
	射洪市	射洪市疾病预防控制中心	刘 扬 董 胜
	大英县	大英县疾病预防控制中心	夏 冰
	内江市市中区	内江市市中区疾病预防控制中心	董永年 唐纯丽 尤 霄
	内江市东兴区	内江市东兴区疾病预防控制中心	冷江涛 黄 艳 刘念奴 甘丁羽
	威远县	威远县疾病预防控制中心	陈 娜 杨卉玲
	资中县	资中县疾病预防控制中心	梁英凤 陈 璐 孙于茹
	隆昌市	隆昌市疾病预防控制中心	游大勇 罗 睿 高雪娅
	乐山市市中区	乐山市市中区疾病预防控制中心	张 翼 赵彬茜 钟 钰
	乐山市沙湾区	乐山市沙湾区疾病预防控制中心	朱 攀 苟 伟 张春霞
	乐山市五通桥区	乐山市五通桥区疾病预防控制中心	侯 亮

省(自治区、直辖市)Province (autonomous region, municipality)	肿瘤登记处 Cancer Registry	登记处所在单位 Affiliation	主要工作人员 Staff
	乐山市金口河区	乐山市金口河区疾病预防控制中心	刘廷清　吕伟华　刘海燕　江旭婷　田　玉
	犍为县	犍为县疾病预防控制中心	袁　叶　杨海燕
	井研县	井研县疾病预防控制中心	税智群　何　芳
	夹江县	夹江县疾病预防控制中心	晏　荧　干晓辉
	沐川县	沐川县疾病预防控制中心	郑　玲　周玉萍
	峨眉山市	峨眉山市疾病预防控制中心	吴　洁　费　琳
	南充市高坪区	南充市高坪区人民医院	邢　丽　廖　波
	南充市嘉陵区	南充市嘉陵区疾病预防控制中心	祝　倩　黄　维
	营山县	营山县疾病预防控制中心	苟军平　彭　勇
	蓬安县	蓬安县疾病预防控制中心	蒲泓兵　罗　容　母书豪
	仪陇县	仪陇县疾病预防控制中心	曹秋菊　曹　成　吴相遇
	西充县	西充县疾病预防控制中心	孙青青　赵　辉
	阆中市	阆中市疾病预防控制中心	游宁静　刘　刚
	眉山市东坡区	眉山市东坡区疾病预防控制中心	陈兰芬　李燕华　徐　欢　吴微娜　王晓玉
	眉山市彭山区	眉山市彭山区疾病预防控制中心	周建容　余志祥
	仁寿县	仁寿县疾病预防控制中心	黄佳玲　瞿遥来　宁　芳　陈春俊　杨　红 邓　科
	洪雅县	洪雅县疾病预防控制中心	吴　莹　罗大春　赖　兵　杨利琴
	丹棱县	丹棱县疾病预防控制中心	罗　源　梁学祥
	青神县	青神县疾病预防控制中心	张　邻　徐　琴　黄彬鑫
	宜宾市翠屏区	宜宾市翠屏区疾病预防控制中心	马坤容　刘如葵　戴自强　陈志富　应元玲 黄昌学　朱德琴
	宜宾市南溪区	宜宾市南溪区疾病预防控制中心	李　凤
	宜宾市叙州区	宜宾市叙州区疾病预防控制中心	陈小芳　胡友平　周　刘
	江安县	江安县疾病预防控制中心	王　芳　杨　晴　李必容
	长宁县	长宁县疾病预防控制中心	王　宇
	兴文县	兴文县疾病预防控制中心	唐明月　邵世宗　唐　华
	屏山县	屏山县疾病预防控制中心	程　伟　汪　群
	广安市广安区	广安市广安区疾病预防控制中心	苏中婷　杜承彬　李荣川
	广安市前锋区	广安市前锋区疾病预防控制中心	黄春凤　王　维　谢　婵
	岳池县	岳池县疾病预防控制中心	李晓琴　聂　勇
	武胜县	武胜县疾病预防控制中心	米慧琼　王文婷
	邻水县	邻水县疾病预防控制中心	廖冬娟　彭晓君

省(自治区、直辖市)Province (autonomous region, municipality)	肿瘤登记处 Cancer Registry	登记处所在单位 Affiliation	主要工作人员 Staff				
	华蓥市	华蓥市疾病预防控制中心	彭书灵	韩小月	左 超	杜东森	雷德琼
	达州市达川区	达州市达川区疾病预防控制中心	罗 玲	段凯岚	周 莉	熊舒书	
	宣汉县	宣汉县疾病预防控制中心	张冬梅	桂国尧	张 涛		
	开江县	开江县疾疾病预防控制中心	卢有见	舒进川	陈 红		
	大竹县	大竹县疾病预防控制中心	王大骞	叶明兰	师小林		
	渠县	渠县疾病预防控制中心	李 平	王秀瑛			
	雅安市雨城区	雅安市雨城区疾病预防控制中心	王登琪				
	雅安市名山区	雅安市名山区疾病预防控制中心	王修华				
	荥经县	荥经县疾病预防控制中心	吴玉福				
	汉源县	汉源县疾病预防控制中心	廖卓航				
	石棉县	石棉县疾病预防控制中心	李桂芬				
	天全县	天全县疾病预防控制中心	高鸿敏				
	芦山县	芦山县疾病预防控制中心	王 鸿	李唐芳	熊 欣		
	宝兴县	宝兴县疾病预防控制中心	徐新红				
	巴中市巴州区	巴中市巴州区疾病预防控制中心	李俊杰 王彩云	于冬梅	曾婷婷	叶南宁	朱玉林
	通江县	通江县疾病预防控制中心	赵廷明	徐 畅	王 丽	张 劲	陶小娥
	南江县	南江县疾病预防控制中心	王光秀	杨浩菁	刘 兰	罗 雯	
	平昌县	平昌县疾病预防控制中心	钟 鑫	何 勇			
	资阳市雁江区	资阳市雁江区疾病预防控制中心	李仕海	李成维	王红艳		
	安岳县	安岳县疾病预防控制中心	江 霁	谢益琼			
	乐至县	乐至县疾病预防控制中心	吴志敏	雷方君	李 光	肖 洋	卢心悦
	汶川县	汶川县疾病预防控制中心	余小芳	姚 云	张诗卓		
贵州省	贵州省	贵州省疾病预防控制中心	刘 涛	周 婕	张 骥	吉 维	
	开阳县	开阳县疾病预防控制中心	颜克梅	陈佐俊	李 卫		
	息烽县	息烽县疾病预防控制中心	吴 会				
	修文县	修文县疾病预防控制中心	沈 婧	肖丽梅			
	清镇市	清镇市疾病预防控制中心	付 敏				
	六盘水市钟山区	六盘水市钟山区疾病预防控制中心	张 薇	朱 娟			
	六盘水市六枝特区	六盘水市六枝特区疾病预防控制中心	张徐巾				
	盘州市	盘州市疾病预防控制中心	章有健	王 英			
	遵义市汇川区	遵义市汇川区疾病预防控制中心	杨 琴	冉隆梅			

省(自治区、直辖市) Province (autonomous region, municipality)	肿瘤登记处 Cancer Registry	登记处所在单位 Affiliation	主要工作人员 Staff				
	绥阳县	绥阳县疾病预防控制中心	李秀丽	李顺顺	何应琴	李家成	
	习水县	习水县疾病预防控制中心	张 文	穆洪莲	张倩影		
	赤水市	赤水市疾病预防控制中心	杨国旗	邓金勇	钟方前	姜 霞	王雨笛
	安顺市西秀区	安顺市西秀区疾病预防控制中心	钟鲜鲜				
	镇宁布依族苗族自治县	镇宁布依族苗族自治县疾病预防控制中心	杨 琳				
	金沙县	金沙县疾病预防控制中心	王天赐				
	铜仁市碧江区	铜仁市碧江区疾病预防控制中心	杜婷婷	杨江艳	曾群花	谢妮娜	
	江口县	江口县疾病预防控制中心	刘淑芬				
	玉屏侗族自治县	玉屏侗族自治县疾病预防控制中心	张乙中	陆承凯	吴 蓉	刘甜甜	王 艳
	印江土家族苗族自治县	印江土家族苗族自治县疾病预防控制中心	田 阳	杨红丽	杨 瑞	李 婷	
	册亨县	册亨县疾病预防控制中心	覃明江	韦永琴	潘 可	忙光积	侯先品
	黄平县	黄平县疾病预防控制中心	杨 玲				
	镇远县	镇远县疾病预防控制中心	黄小容 陈 沙 石大为	周稚爽 莫海燕 李泽斌	李慧平 欧阳佳航 汪庆兰	杨雅竹 刘利芬 唐 林	王丽琼 肖 艳 曾萍萍
	天柱县	天柱县疾病预防控制中心	罗世华				
	锦屏县	锦屏县疾病预防控制中心	杨通平	吴玉琼	龙俊贵	王 静	石云昌
	台江县	台江县疾病预防控制中心	欧 玲				
	榕江县	榕江县疾病预防控制中心	吴永莲				
	雷山县	雷山县疾病预防控制中心	毛 海 白坐顺 吴寿美	杨 军 鲍江国	杨洁玉 田应彰	吴晓花 龚玉娟	吴成彪 张英梅
	麻江县	麻江县疾病预防控制中心	吴晓云				
	丹寨县	丹寨县疾病预防控制中心	李 玲	杨秀权	唐海玉		
	都匀市	都匀市疾病预防控制中心	李国叶	陈 珺			
	福泉市	福泉市疾病预防控制中心	孙仕丽	杨 飞			
	荔波县	荔波县疾病预防控制中心	覃荣盼 何凤甜 赵永娟	李银春 韦小强 白明伟	杨本力 韦 彬	沈 睿 覃富春	刘 霞 岑扬慧
	瓮安县	瓮安县疾病预防控制中心	陈永群 陈 虹	马盆静 宋居翔	胥 奎 余 欢	王 均	伍 菲
	龙里县	龙里县疾病预防控制中心	杜月清 杨昌灵 岑德勇	代远应 张 毅 邹宇航	罗 志 王启芬 陶 欢	张胜娟 刘太敏 徐 芸	林品琛 罗 艳 陈道兴

省（自治区、直辖市） Province （autonomous region， municipality）	肿瘤登记处 Cancer Registry	登记处所在单位 Affiliation	主要工作人员 Staff				
云南省	云南省	云南省疾病预防控制中心	文洪梅	伍福仙	陈 杨	石青萍	任思颖
			朱云芳	绍 英			
	昆明市	昆明市疾病预防控制中心	李 吉	杨 昭	李志坤	李云涛	
	昆明市五华区	昆明市五华区疾病预防控制中心	周 丽	王紫玉	许秋婧	曾成琴	刘 畅
			谢 颖				
	昆明市盘龙区	昆明市盘龙区疾病预防控制中心	何丽明	王睿翊	许秋婧	何开浚	雷 娇
	昆明市官渡区	昆明市官渡区疾病预防控制中心	王 丽	张睿凌	孟 雨	陈月月	段培华
	昆明市西山区	昆明市西山区疾病预防控制中心	袁聪玲	李绍叶	李杰	周欣瑕	李赛云
	昆明市东川区	昆明市东川区疾病预防控制中心	韩贵卫	赵亚楠	杨雁萍		
	昆明市呈贡区	昆明市呈贡区疾病预防控制中心	张永丽	肖凯伦			
	昆明市晋宁区	昆明市晋宁区疾病预防控制中心	张美莲	赵浚如			
	富民县	富民县疾病预防控制中心	李俊兴				
	宜良县	宜良县疾病预防控制中心	段陈丽				
	石林彝族自治县	石林彝族自治县疾病预防控制中心	李成艳	虎 洁	李丽菊	袁逸爽	
	嵩明县	嵩明县疾病预防控制中心	郭树岚	保 尚			
	禄劝彝族苗族自治县	禄劝彝族苗族自治县疾病预防控制中心	钟玉美				
	寻甸回族彝族自治县	寻甸回族彝族自治县疾病预防控制中心	李从美	弥鹏飞	朱亚华		
	安宁市	安宁市疾病预防控制中心	赵会联	杨文功			
	曲靖市	曲靖市疾病预防控制中心	李继华	牛文倩	李 云		
	曲靖市麒麟区	曲靖市麒麟区疾病预防控制中心	雷芸华	关秋艳	施红娟	丁鹏俊	徐彩阳
	曲靖市沾益区	曲靖市沾益区疾病预防控制中心	雷宝琼				
	曲靖市马龙区	曲靖市马龙区疾病预防控制中心	王慈蓉				
	师宗县	师宗县疾病预防控制中心	马晓燕				
	罗平县	罗平县疾病预防控制中心	牛文倩	刘曼青			
	富源县	富源县疾病预防控制中心	王 云				
	宣威市	宣威市疾病预防控制中心	宁伯福				
	玉溪市	玉溪市疾病预防控制中心	马真飞	李 吉	王艳波		
	玉溪市红塔区	玉溪市红塔区疾病预防控制中心	瞿 媛	张 莉	刘 蕊	林 蕾	管 颖
			白光宝	陶 然	邹 容	赵明洪	孟源珂
	玉溪市江川区	玉溪市江川区疾病预防控制中心	赵媛丽				
	澄江市	澄江市疾病预防控制中心	董志鹏	周红云	杨 晶	李 颖	侯 瑞
			马重义				

省(自治区、直辖市) Province (autonomous region, municipality)	肿瘤登记处 Cancer Registry	登记处所在单位 Affiliation	主要工作人员 Staff				
	通海县	通海县疾病预防控制中心	高瑞芳	杨春琼	任晶晶		
	华宁县	华宁县疾病预防控制中心	施云丽	王志鹏	杨 蓉	李宇婷	杨 琳
	易门县	易门县疾病预防控制中心	樊学琼	许 葵	赵永琼	王冬梅	段臣康
			阮 伟	吕 宏	周永斌		
	峨山彝族自治县	峨山彝族自治县疾病预防控制中心	李晓燕 温雅淇	何仕友	罗忠玉	金自萍	巴园清
	新平彝族傣族自治县	新平彝族傣族自治县疾病预防控制中心	赵 青	刘晓冬	殷文学	但文娅	
	元江哈尼族彝族傣族自治县	元江哈尼族彝族傣族自治县疾病预防控制中心	张坤平 陆拾妹	卫 芳	杨太专	杨生宝	杨忠强
	保山市	保山市疾病预防控制中心	徐仙会	李明松	邓 丽		
	保山市隆阳区	保山市隆阳区疾病预防控制中心	杨璐竹 赵婧屹	杨善华 杨保国	董全玉 张永新	陈 浩	王 伟
	施甸县	施甸县疾病预防控制中心	吴新会	朱海燕	杨丝丝	杨邱云	杨继虎
	龙陵县	龙陵县疾病预防控制中心	杨福娣 王云春	寸勐震	李顺芹	李菊云	刘 娟
	昌宁县	昌宁县疾病预防控制中心	曾映竹	禹月曦	黄丽琼		
	腾冲市	腾冲市疾病预防控制中心	刘晓丽 封占益	杨艳芳 李自娇	李亚丹	李相妹	段立敏
	昭通市	昭通市疾病预防控制中心	戴堂艳	马东琼			
	绥江县	绥江县疾病预防控制中心	刘晓静	李 飞	刘 洁		
	彝良县	彝良县疾病预防控制中心	刘应菲	吴丽丽			
	水富市	水富市疾病预防控制中心	朱晓蕾	杨 姣			
	丽江市	丽江市疾病预防控制中心	杨丽梅 杨永寿	冉钦玉	段 珏	王恭汉	李光聪
	丽江市古城区	丽江市古城区疾病预防控制中心	和臣慧	杨志晖	高 明	杨雄美	
	玉龙纳西族自治县	玉龙纳西族自治县疾病预防控制中心	杨 俊	和致祥	杨翠香	黄晓蓉	
	永胜县	永胜县疾病预防控制中心	史记萍	杨贤梅	王发薪		
	华坪县	华坪县疾病预防控制中心	王正英	卢国春			
	宁蒗彝族自治县	宁蒗彝族自治县疾病预防控制中心	李文华	杨 英			
	普洱市	普洱市疾病预防控制中心	周锦涛	唐 颖			
	宁洱哈尼族彝族自治县	宁洱哈尼族彝族自治县疾病预防控制中心	刘新玉	赵桂兰	段美鸾		
	景东彝族自治县	景东彝族自治县疾病预防控制中心	祝章美	龚 晨	陶 梅	周晓波	

省（自治区、直辖市）Province (autonomous region, municipality)	肿瘤登记处 Cancer Registry	登记处所在单位 Affiliation	主要工作人员 Staff				
	景谷傣族彝族自治县	景谷傣族彝族自治县疾病预防控制中心	周新玉	王丽娇	李发有		
	镇沅彝族哈尼族拉祜族自治县	镇沅彝族哈尼族拉祜族自治县疾病预防控制中心	吴容容	自家梅	罗开萍	王　毅	
	江城哈尼族彝族自治县	江城哈尼族彝族自治县疾病预防控制中心	鲍月月				
	澜沧拉祜族自治县	澜沧拉祜族自治县疾病预防控制中心	苏　琪	李红梅	刘　河		
	临沧市	临沧市疾病预防控制中心	李秋圆	曹建英	胡　红		
	临沧市临翔区	临沧市临翔区疾病预防控制中心	王　强	廖俊华	王新梅		
	凤庆县	凤庆县疾病预防控制中心	沈嘉航	黄淑娟			
	云县	云县疾病预防控制中心	沈羽翎	潘继超	李德会		
	永德县	永德县疾病预防控制中心	吴锦月	李艳萍			
	镇康县	镇康县疾病预防控制中心	刘志梅	杨　凤			
	双江拉祜族佤族布朗族傣族自治县	双江拉祜族佤族布朗族傣族自治县疾病预防控制中心	俸世元	杞志艳	张　俊	周新民	李光统
	沧源佤族自治县	沧源佤族自治县疾病预防控制中心	李　瑶	赵福芳	杨文军		
	楚雄彝族自治州	楚雄彝族自治州疾病预防控制中心	赵会勇	李洪祥	蒋大启		
	楚雄市	楚雄市疾病预防控制中心	刘家早	仇剑芝	陈　露	肖建萍	
	双柏县	双柏县疾病预防控制中心	胡　萍				
	牟定县	牟定县疾病预防控制中心	何　磊	李燕龄			
	南华县	南华县疾病预防控制中心	吕美英	费建琼			
	姚安县	姚安县疾病预防控制中心	苏菊芬				
	大姚县	大姚县疾病预防控制中心	班琼珍	赵宗和			
	永仁县	永仁县疾病预防控制中心	汪家承				
	元谋县	元谋县疾病预防控制中心	仲丽红	张金平			
	武定县	武定县疾病预防控制中心	罗丽琼	凤海丽	丁启艳	郑曙娇	
	禄丰市	禄丰市疾病预防控制中心	刘雪丽 沈丽琼	毕志梅	刘清秀	李红芝	杞发洪
	红河哈尼族彝族自治州	红河哈尼族彝族自治州第三人民医院	潘龙海	王　娴	苏　倩		
	个旧市	个旧市肿瘤防治工作领导小组办公室	王建宁	高美蓉			

省(自治区、直辖市) Province (autonomous region, municipality)	肿瘤登记处 Cancer Registry	登记处所在单位 Affiliation	主要工作人员 Staff				
	开远市	开远市疾病预防控制中心	杜晓芳	顾春芳	陈亚苏	闫友芸	
	蒙自市	蒙自市疾病预防控制中心	杨 涛				
	屏边苗族自治县	屏边苗族自治县疾病预防控制中心	吴 娅	冯 伟	保功成		
	建水县	建水县疾病预防控制中心	周艳梅	张艳芳	刘 怡	白玉仙	
	石屏县	石屏县疾病预防控制中心	王昌钰	高 霞	朱婷婷	苏 舟	朱梦圆
	弥勒市	弥勒市疾病预防控制中心	杨晓静	徐建华			
	泸西县	泸西县疾病预防控制中心	戴 丽	王秋婷			
	文山市	文山市疾病预防控制中心	马忠水	孙兴悦	罗世梅		
	砚山县	砚山县疾病预防控制中心	祁红芬	杨志方			
	西畴县	西畴县疾病预防控制中心	袁 丽	黄 巧			
	麻栗坡县	麻栗坡县疾病预防控制中心	王 莉	韦跃海	胡美欣		
	马关县	马关县疾病预防控制中心	恩荣琳				
	丘北县	丘北县疾病预防控制中心	杨燕琼				
	富宁县	富宁县疾病预防控制中心	陆 佩	何莉华			
	西双版纳州	西双版纳州疾病预防控制中心	陈 萍	范芸苑	张双权		
	景洪市	景洪市疾病预防控制中心	石保英	依旺叫	杨舒寒	杨 娜	
	大理州	大理州疾病预防控制中心	杨瑞雪	曹占南	左丽娟	施照云	
	大理市	大理市疾病预防控制中心	袁 涵 张 莹	杨 清 章燕玲	赵庆平 魏朝晖	杜雅素	夏春秋
	祥云县	祥云县疾病预防控制中心	杨永翠				
	宾川县	宾川县疾病预防控制中心	陈建梅				
	弥渡县	弥渡县疾病预防控制中心	孙海欧	白仙玉	吴梦绮		
	南涧彝族自治县	南涧彝族自治县疾病预防控制中心	刘一桂	徐思平			
	永平县	永平县疾病预防控制中心	李亚芳	马迎春			
	洱源县	洱源县疾病预防控制中心	赵应吉 杨金玉	杨刘佳	王秀美	冉学军	李 书
	德宏傣族景颇族自治州	德宏傣族景颇族自治州疾病预防控制中心	李家才	高右东			
	梁河县	梁河县疾病预防控制中心	杨 莹	方永兴			
	陇川县	陇川县疾病预防控制中心	刘淑红	王金梅			
	怒江傈僳族自治州	怒江傈僳族自治州疾病预防控制中心	杨卫美	王新琳	李晓霞		

省(自治区、直辖市) Province (autonomous region, municipality)	肿瘤登记处 Cancer Registry	登记处所在单位 Affiliation	主要工作人员 Staff
	泸水市	泸水市疾病预防控制中心	欧国琴　黎庆莲
	贡山独龙族怒族自治县	贡山独龙族怒族自治县疾病预防控制中心	汉琳芸　许荣芳　周坤花　康钰苹
	迪庆藏族自治州	迪庆藏族自治州疾病预防控制中心	曹慧芳　杜晓霞　熊子茹
	香格里拉市	香格里拉市疾病预防控制中心	和桂芬　邓芬　杨丽
西藏自治区	西藏自治区	西藏自治区疾病预防控制中心	扎西宗吉
	拉萨市城关区	拉萨市城关区疾病预防控制中心	魏翠兰
	日喀则市	日喀则市疾病预防控制中心	格吉
	昌都市	昌都市疾病预防控制中心	卓玛
陕西省	陕西省	陕西省疾病预防控制中心	邱琳　王艳平
	西安市新城区	西安市新城区疾病预防控制中心	付艳玲　凌敏珍
	西安市碑林区	西安市碑林区疾病预防控制中心	范颖　李福强　周鼎
	西安市莲湖区	西安市莲湖区疾病预防控制中心	王宁　薛静怡　刘少龙　刘婷
	西安市未央区	西安市未央区疾病预防控制中心	吴爽　杨梦
	西安市雁塔区	西安市雁塔区疾病预防控制中心	高盼盼　于丹丹　高玮
	西安市阎良区	西安市阎良区疾病预防控制中心	李美萍　韩梅
	西安市临潼区	西安市临潼区疾病预防控制中心	岳婷　郑斌　张丽莎　魏巍
	西安市长安区	西安市长安区疾病预防控制中心	刘小霞
	西安市高陵区	西安市高陵区疾病预防控制中心	潘熙
	西安市鄠邑区	西安市鄠邑区疾病预防控制中心	张莹　刘言　石明娟
	蓝田县	蓝田县疾病预防控制中心	闫红梅
	铜川市耀州区	铜川市耀州区疾病预防控制中心	陈雯雯　文静妮
	宝鸡市渭滨区	宝鸡市渭滨区疾病预防控制中心	李晨　田宏兵　赵军艳
	宝鸡市金台区	宝鸡市金台区疾病预防控制中心	张晓林　温晓叶
	宝鸡市陈仓区	宝鸡市陈仓区疾病预防控制中心	王新梅
	宝鸡市凤翔区	宝鸡市凤翔区疾病预防控制中心	周晓梅　杨晓宏　梁向红　刘向
	岐山县	岐山县疾病预防控制中心	上官小博　王晓强　邓玉洁　白小光　武肖玉 巨磊　张格平　袁小红
	扶风县	扶风县疾病预防控制中心	狄苗
	眉县	眉县疾病预防控制中心	刘剑飞　高歌　赵云
	陇县	陇县疾病预防控制中心	闫建军　段亚琴
	千阳县	千阳县疾病预防控制中心	吕瑞娟　茹夏丽　张文博　张玉梅
	麟游县	麟游县疾病预防控制中心	马方伟　何雅梅

省(自治区、直辖市) Province (autonomous region, municipality)	肿瘤登记处 Cancer Registry	登记处所在单位 Affiliation	主要工作人员 Staff
	凤县	凤县疾病预防控制中心	郭宏祥 雷茹
	太白县	太白县疾病预防控制中心	净昭 沈洁 荔群辉 王栋 刘淑芹 李枝员 曾宪颜 戚平康
	泾阳县	泾阳县疾病预防控制中心	闫阿妮 马娟
	武功县	武功县疾病预防控制中心	赵海荣 张鹏
	渭南市临渭区	渭南市临渭区疾病预防控制中心	权巧玲
	渭南市华州区	渭南市华州区疾病预防控制中心	张亚莹
	潼关县	潼关县疾病预防控制中心	陈娜
	大荔县	大荔县疾病预防控制中心	陈艳萍
	合阳县	合阳县疾病预防控制中心	梁忠义
	蒲城县	蒲城县疾病预防控制中心	赵莹
	富平县	富平县疾病预防控制中心	苏木兰
	华阴市	华阴市疾病预防控制中心	郝青青
	延安市宝塔区	延安市宝塔区疾病预防控制中心	贺军宏 尹明萍 孙婧
	志丹县	志丹县疾病预防控制中心	鲁婷婷 白江 张兴伟
	富县	富县疾病预防控制中心	王忠学 吕亚军 杜悠悠
	黄龙县	黄龙县疾病预防控制中心	贾文虎 徐晓红 乔媛
	黄陵县	黄陵县疾病预防控制中心	杨明霞 雷云云 张铁军
	汉中市汉台区	汉中市汉台区疾病预防控制中心	刘轩岐 张淼
	城固县	城固县疾病预防控制中心	张振财 杨俊明 尹勇 高智平
	宁强县	宁强县疾病预防控制中心	王忠宝 彭兆生 向风义
	绥德县	绥德县疾病预防控制中心	刘成
	安康市汉滨区	安康市汉滨区疾病预防控制中心	李世艳 杨锐 陈静 张果 洪刚
	汉阴县	汉阴县疾病预防控制中心	吴丹 刘厚明
	宁陕县	宁陕县疾病预防控制中心	代鹏 徐滟 张洁
	紫阳县	紫阳县疾病预防控制中心	余汉春 许金华
	旬阳县	旬阳市疾病预防控制中心	刘娟 冯佩 杜小菊
	商洛市商州区	商洛市商州区疾病预防控制中心	王天军 张琪
	丹凤县	丹凤县疾病预防控制中心	彭粉茹 杨岚
	镇安县	镇安县疾病预防控制中心	王雯 刘家政
甘肃省	甘肃省	甘肃省肿瘤医院/甘肃省癌症中心	刘玉琴 丁高恒
	兰州市城关区	兰州市城关区疾病预防控制中心	韩霞 杨菁

省(自治区、直辖市) Province (autonomous region, municipality)	肿瘤登记处 Cancer Registry	登记处所在单位 Affiliation	主要工作人员 Staff		
	兰州市七里河区	兰州市七里河区疾病预防控制中心	苗佳丽	唐明华	王志龙
	兰州市西固区	兰州市西固区疾病预防控制中心	徐 梅		
	兰州市安宁区	兰州市安宁区疾病预防控制中心	殷 行	何秀芬	
	兰州市红古区	兰州市红古区疾病预防控制中心	张 青	李巩业	
	白银市白银区	白银市白银区疾病预防控制中心	李顺翠	张小琴	
	白银市平川区	白银市平川区疾病预防控制中心	李 霞	刘祥祖	张小燕
	靖远县	靖远县疾病预防控制中	欧志秀	妙文丽	住国蓉
	会宁县	会宁县疾病预防控制中心	党丽琴	程永莲	李 霞
	景泰县	景泰县疾病预防控制中心	王生芸	周福新	
	天水市秦州区	天水市秦州区疾病预防控制中心	安珊珊		
	天水市麦积区	天水市麦积区疾病预防控制中心	杨 慧		
	武威市凉州区	甘肃省武威肿瘤医院	秦天燕	高彩云	
	民勤县	民勤县疾病预防控制中心	石 芳	姜玉平	薛昌瑞
	古浪县	古浪县疾病预防控制中心	许存洁		
	天祝藏族自治县	天祝藏族自治县疾病预防控制中心	陈 娟		
	张掖市甘州区	张掖市甘州区疾病预防控制中心	王金金	赵文雅	陈国辉
	高台县	高台县疾病预防控制中心	张 军	黄充盈	许丽娟
	静宁县	静宁县疾病预防控制中心	杨 娟	闫润芳	薛娟娟
	敦煌市	敦煌市疾病预防控制中心	淳志明	殷海燕	杜文倩
	庆城县	庆城县疾病预防控制中心	项霞霞		
	临洮县	临洮县疾病预防控制中心	康玉霞		
	临潭县	临潭县疾病预防控制中心	祁少华	冯锦芳	朱彦红
青海省	青海省	青海省疾病预防控制中心	周素霞		
	西宁市	西宁市疾病预防控制中心	汤海霞		
	西宁市城东区	西宁市城东区疾病预防控制中心	马丽娟	王占青	
	西宁市城中区	西宁市城中区疾病预防控制中心	马晓萍		
	西宁市城西区	西宁市城西区疾病预防控制中心	王 舒	陈晓萍	
	西宁市城北区	西宁市城北区疾病预防控制中心	徐晓晴		
	大通回族土族自治县	大通回族土族自治县疾病预防控制中心	朱彩虹		
	西宁市湟中区	西宁市湟中区疾病预防控制中心	汪有库		
	海东市	海东市疾病预防控制中心	魏 青		

省(自治区、直辖市) Province (autonomous region, municipality)	肿瘤登记处 Cancer Registry	登记处所在单位 Affiliation	主要工作人员 Staff
	海东市乐都区	海东市乐都区疾病预防控制中心	谢淑雯
	民和回族土族自治县	民和回族土族自治县疾病预防控制中心	张学强
	互助土族自治县	互助土族自治县疾病预防控制中心	王小庆
	循化撒拉族自治县	循化撒拉族自治县疾病预防控制中心	陕国清
	海南藏族自治州	海南藏族自治州疾病预防控制中心	拉毛才让 马 兰 卓根措 贺永庆 张 琼 代晓倩
宁夏回族 自治区	宁夏回族自治区	宁夏疾病预防控制中心	马 芳 杨 艺 魏 嵘
	银川市兴庆区	银川市兴庆区疾病预防控制中心	吴春燕 王 晶 王洪丽 侯静雅 王雁德 杨文杰 何沿虹 王丽珠 徐天贞 王艳芳 彭旺龙 孙志清 廖 静 程 旺 高晓燕
	银川市西夏区	银川市西夏区疾病预防控制中心	刘纪红 王 娟 王冬梅
	银川市金凤区	银川市金凤区疾病预防控制中心	保红莉 张 梦 魏慧娴 伊玲玲
	贺兰县	贺兰县疾病预防控制中心	陈海荣 姜旭红 陈 娥 董 威
	石嘴山市大武口区	石嘴山市疾病预防控制中心	张平稳 马 洁 刘 英 仇祖训 赵旭辉 张 悦 吴永军
	石嘴山市惠农区	石嘴山市惠农区疾病预防控制中心	郎红霞 李冬梅 冯 羽
	平罗县	平罗县疾病预防控制中心	刘凤香
	青铜峡市	青铜峡市疾病预防控制中心	赵仲刚 马 丽 哈艳茹
	固原市原州区	固原市原州区疾病预防控制中心	南 艳 杨志敏 王耀芳
	中卫市沙坡头区	中卫市疾病预防控制中心	姚永红 田彦军
	中宁县	中宁县疾病预防控制中心	康文慧 赵寿桃 王 静 杨晓静
新疆维吾尔 自治区	新疆维吾尔自治区	新疆维吾尔自治区疾病预防控制中心	张 荣 阿迪拉·苏力旦 董 言
	乌鲁木齐市天山区	乌鲁木齐市天山区疾病预防控制中心	郭颖贞
	乌鲁木齐市新市区	乌鲁木齐市新市区疾病预防控制中心	刘江荣
	乌鲁木齐市水磨沟区	乌鲁木齐市水磨沟区疾病预防控制中心	程新雷 玛尔哈巴
	乌鲁木齐市达坂城区	乌鲁木齐市达坂城区疾病预防控制中心	孔海滨

省(自治区、直辖市) Province (autonomous region, municipality)	肿瘤登记处 Cancer Registry	登记处所在单位 Affiliation	主要工作人员 Staff
	乌鲁木齐市米东区	乌鲁木齐市米东区疾病预防控制中心	赵生明　刘馨
	乌鲁木齐县	乌鲁木齐县疾病预防控制中心	海燕
	克拉玛依市	克拉玛依市疾病预防控制中心	陈文俊　朱伟敏　黄芸　许德民　聂银燕 陈雪滢　李学智　古力米拉·艾力　马贞 杨泽浩　邓青文
	克拉玛依市乌尔禾区	克拉玛依市乌尔禾区疾病预防控制中心	苏蕾　贾琛
	吐鲁番市高昌区	吐鲁番市高昌区疾病预防控制中心	王英
	鄯善县	鄯善县疾病预防控制中心	墨祥敏　刘维芹　木旦力甫　帕提古丽
	巴里坤哈萨克自治县	巴里坤哈萨克自治县疾病预防控制中心	冉燕　范小荣
	伊吾县	伊吾县疾病预防控制中心	王菊红
	昌吉市	昌吉市疾病预防控制中心	冶雪婷　杨锦
	阜康市	阜康市疾病预防控制中心	姜海娟　张静
	呼图壁县	呼图壁县疾病预防控制中心	成月华　王杨　李杰
	玛纳斯县	玛纳斯县预防控制中心	努尔吉别克
	奇台县	奇台县疾病预防控制中心	库拉西　马爱国　徐春风
	吉木萨尔县	吉木萨尔县疾病预防控制中心	古丽巴努·热伊木江　樊艳军　徐建勤
	木垒哈萨克自治县	木垒哈萨克自治县疾病预防控制中心	杨琳
	博乐市	博乐市疾病预防控制中心	新才　吐尔买买提
	阿拉山口市	阿拉山口市疾病预防控制中心	阿布都买吾兰·买合玛洪　阿迪莱·艾克拜尔
	精河县	精河县疾病预防控制中心	杨林芳
	温泉县	温泉县疾病预防控制中心	景世忠
	库尔勒市	库尔勒市疾病预防控制中心	木克热木·于努斯
	尉犁县	尉犁县疾病预防控制中心	刘建西
	焉耆回族自治县	焉耆回族自治县疾病预防控制中心	相玉华
	和静县	和静县疾病预防控制中心	吾买尔·艾合买提　金花　那仁才次克
	博湖县	博湖县疾病预防控制中心	阿尔祖古丽·热西提
	阿克苏市	阿克苏市疾病预防控制中心	阿孜古丽·丘尕尼亚孜
	温宿县	温宿县疾病预防控制中心	阿塔吾拉·尼扎麦提
	库车市	库车市疾病预防控制中心	吴秀花

省(自治区、直辖市) Province (autonomous region, municipality)	肿瘤登记处 Cancer Registry	登记处所在单位 Affiliation	主要工作人员 Staff
	沙雅县	沙雅县疾病预防控制中心	阿依努尔·艾则孜
	拜城县	拜城县疾病预防控制中心	宏千木·库尔班
	阿瓦提县	阿瓦提县疾病预防控制中心	阿依吐热木·如孜
	柯坪县	柯坪县疾病预防控制中心	热娜古丽·提来木
	阿图什市	阿图什市疾病预防控制中心	古丽先·沙比尔　阿吉·努尔买买提
	阿克陶县	阿克陶县疾病预防控制中心	古丽米热·艾海提
	阿合奇县	阿合奇县疾病预防控制中心	阿曼古丽·加帕尔　阿依吐尼克·托合提巴依
	疏附县	疏附县疾病预防控制中心	努尔麦麦提·依明　罗晓峰
	疏勒县	疏勒县疾病预防控制中心	如斯太木·热合曼　穆再排
	英吉沙县	英吉沙县疾病预防控制中心	比丽柯孜·玉斯尹　艾买提江·吾吉 白合提古丽·阿布都瓦伊提
	泽普县	泽普县疾病预防控制中心	肉孜·吐地　段宁莉
	莎车县	莎车县疾病预防控制中心	米开热木·吐尔孙　罗盖琴
	叶城县	叶城县疾病预防控制中心	孙慧欣　雷升萍
	麦盖提县	麦盖提县疾病预防控制中心	艾西丁·吐洪　楚东燕
	岳普湖县	岳普湖县疾病预防控制中心	图罕克孜·图尔迪　努热曼古丽·艾海提 努尔比耶·阿布力米提　冯海箐 吐尔逊姑丽·吾斯曼　姑丽那尔·牙生
	伽师县	伽师县疾病预防控制中心	组力皮牙·艾买提　高玉明
	巴楚县	巴楚县疾病预防控制中心	艾斯艾提·艾买提　阿丽亚·阿布都米吉提
	塔什库尔干塔吉克自治县	塔什库尔干塔吉克自治县疾病预防控制中心	艾尔肯·艾尔西丁　艾斯马尔江·艾尔肯
	和田市	和田市疾病预防控制中心	买哈巴·艾尼玩江　吾尔尼沙·吐尔孙
	和田县	和田县疾病预防控制中心	艾力
	伊宁市	伊宁市疾病预防控制中心	吐尔洪娜依·阿不都哈德　马静　李亚星
	伊宁县	伊宁县疾病预防控制中心	米也赛热·亚力买买提 古丽拜克热木·木力克
	察布查尔锡伯自治县	察布查尔锡伯自治县疾病预防控制中心	邱梅　柏珂
	霍城县	霍城县疾病预防控制中心	祖丽胡玛尔·阿力木江　火照云
	新源县	新源县疾病预防控制中心	田鹏昊　丁得勇　张春英　刘书起 阿勒帕拉比　杨贺霞　陈光照
	特克斯县	特克斯县疾病预防控制中心	李淑恒　阿孜古丽
	尼勒克县	尼勒克县疾病预防控制中心	丁慧云　萨合尼西　王婉霖
	塔城市	塔城市疾病预防控制中心	陈玲　沙比拉　赵永强

省(自治区、直辖市) Province (autonomous region, municipality)	肿瘤登记处 Cancer Registry	登记处所在单位 Affiliation	主要工作人员 Staff
	乌苏市	乌苏市疾病预防控制中心	蔡忠梅　黄国平
	沙湾县	沙湾县疾病预防控制中心	魏　强　潘　萍　杨新涛
	托里县	托里县疾病预防控制中心	塔苏·图斯普汗　阿依努尔·奴尔木哈什 达娜·玛依旦哈里
	裕民县	裕民县疾病预防控制中心	努尔兰　莎　娜
	和布克赛尔蒙古自治县	和布克赛尔蒙古自治县疾病预防控制中心	杨志华　兰学文　孟　克
	阿勒泰市	阿勒泰市疾病预防控制中心	朱建红
	布尔津县	布尔津县疾病预防控制中心	库力孜拉·加那泰　拉扎提·马切
	富蕴县	富蕴县疾病预防控制中心	阿依古丽·恰布达尔汗　森巴提·热合买提
	福海县	福海县疾病预防控制中心	臧其鸾
	哈巴河县	哈巴河县疾病预防控制中心	米来依·阿合提　赛尼亚·木合提汗
	青河县	青河县疾病预防控制中心	齐丽丽　彩彩·吉格尔
	吉木乃县	吉木乃县疾病预防控制中心	阿热依古丽·俄特玛克　徐美英
新疆生产建设兵团	新疆生产建设兵团	兵团疾病预防控制中心	李凡卡　罗建忠　余　敏　申嘉丛　王宇婷
	第二师	第二师疾病预防控制中心	闫　澈　文　静　阿孜古力·阿布都热西提
	第七师	第七师疾病预防控制中心	周　倩　龚　耀
	第八师	石河子大学医学院	李　锋　胡建明　胡云华　李述刚　王　悦 何雄伟　陈　瑜　孙　芳　梁伟华　李　曼 杨　兰　费　晶　闫贻忠　陈文娟